Psychiatry

FOR   MEDICAL STUDENTS

SECOND EDITION

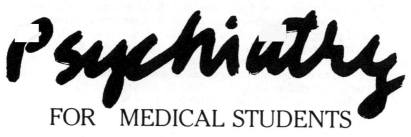

Psychiatry

FOR MEDICAL STUDENTS

SECOND EDITION

BY ROBERT J. WALDINGER, M.D.

Instructor in Psychiatry
Harvard Medical School;
Director of Training
Massachusetts Mental Health Center
Boston, Massachusetts

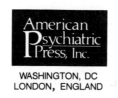

American
Psychiatric
Press, Inc.

WASHINGTON, DC
LONDON, ENGLAND

Diagnostic criteria included in this book are reprinted, with permission, from the *Diagnostic and Statistical Manual of Mental Disorders, Third Edition, Revised*. Copyright © 1987, American Psychiatric Association.

Books published by the American Psychiatric Press, Inc., represent the views and opinions of the individual authors and do not necessarily represent the policies and opinions of the Press or the American Psychiatric Association.

American Psychiatric Press, Inc.
1400 K Street, N.W., Washington, DC 20005

The paper used in this publication meets the minimum requirements of the American National Standard for Information Sciences—Permanence of Paper for Printed Library Materials ANSI Z39.48-1984.   ∞

Library of Congress Cataloging-in-Publication Data

Waldinger, Robert J.

    Psychiatry for Medical Students / Robert J. Waldinger—2nd ed.
      p.   cm.
    Includes bibliographical references.
    Includes index.
    ISBN 0-88048-276-1 (alk. paper).—ISBN 0-88048-373-3 (pbk. : alk. paper)
    1. Psychiatry. I. Waldinger, Robert J., 1951– . II. Title.
    [DNLM: 1. Mental Disorders.]
RC454.W28   1990
616.89
DNLM/DLC
for Library of Congress   90-1151
                                                    CIP

British Library Cataloguing in Publication Data

A CIP record is available from the British Library.

To the memory of my parents,
David and Miriam Waldinger

Additional Contributors

Don R. Lipsitt, M.D., coauthor of Chapter 11, is Clinical Professor of Psychiatry at Harvard Medical School and Chairman of the Department of Psychiatry at Mt. Auburn Hospital in Cambridge, Massachusetts.

Sheldon Benjamin, M.D., author of Chapter 12, is Assistant Professor of Psychiatry and Neurology in the Department of Psychiatry at the University of Massachusetts Medical Center in Worcester, Massachusetts, and Director of Neuropsychiatry at the Westborough State Hospital in Westborough, Massachusetts.

Contents

Introduction   ix
Acknowledgments   xi

Part I Assessment Skills   **1**

1 The Clinical Interview: Fundamentals of
   Technique   3
2 Psychodynamics: Some Basic Concepts   19
3 Taking a Psychiatric History   37
4 The Mental Status Examination   55

Part II Basic Psychopathology   **77**

5 Schizophrenia   79
6 Mood Disorders   103
      Unipolar Disorders (Depressive Disorders)   105
      Bipolar Disorders (Manic-Depressive Illness)   127
7 Personality Disorders   145
8 Anxiety, Phobias, Dissociative Disorders,
   and Somatoform Disorders   199

Part III Special Populations **231**

9 Geriatric Psychiatry 233
10 Children and Adolescents 271
11 Consultation-Liaison Psychiatry 325
12 Neuropsychiatry 345

Part IV Special Problems **381**

13 Human Sexuality: Function and Dysfunction 383
14 Substance Abuse and Eating Disorders 413
15 Suicide 443
16 Violence 459

Part V Treatment **481**

17 Psychotherapies 483
18 Somatic Therapies 515
   Psychotropic Medications 515
      Antipsychotic Medications 527
      Antidepressants 541
      Lithium 556
      Anticonvulsants 561
      Antianxiety Agents 563
   Electroconvulsive Therapy 569

   Appendix A Sample Psychiatric Evaluation 575
   Appendix B Table of Commonly Abused
             Drugs 581
   Appendix C Global Assessment of Functioning
             (GAF) Scale 585
   Appendix D Some Common Psychotropic
             Medications (classified by type) 587
   Appendix E Trade Names of Psychotropic
             Medications 589

   Index 591

Introduction

THIS IS A BOOK FOR BEGINNERS. It was written for medical students who are taking a first course in psychiatry or doing a first clinical clerkship. It is also meant for nurses, social workers, psychologists, and others who are trying to make sense of their first encounters with people who are emotionally disturbed. The book assumes no prior knowledge of psychiatry.

I wrote this book because I wished it had been written for me. When I was a medical student, I was skeptical of psychiatry with all of its jargon, and I was bewildered by the complicated illnesses and profound emotional distress that I encountered among psychiatric patients during my first experience in mental health care. At the local bookstore, I found quite a few massive comprehensive textbooks, and many excellent books devoted to particular areas of psychopathology. But what I wanted was one book that would give me the basics—that would provide me with an introduction to topics like schizophrenia, electroconvulsive therapy, transference, and tranquilizers—and would do so in plain English.

That is what this book is meant to do. My aim has been to write chapters that can be read and referred to quickly while you are in the midst of a busy student rotation. Then, when you have time, you can do further reading to pursue in more detail those areas that particularly interest you.

A second goal of this book is to help you make sense of your own reactions to what you see clinically—because your feelings about patients and their problems often provide you with crucial diagnostic information. And the experience of working with people who are in severe emotional distress can be grueling, particularly when you are new at it. In order to take care of other people, you have to take care of yourself—and that means paying attention to your own reactions to clinical work and knowing when to get support from friends, colleagues, and teachers. Throughout these chapters, I have tried to help you focus on yourself as well as on your patients.

The second edition incorporates the changes in the *Diagnostic and Statistical Manual of Mental Disorders, 3rd Edition, Revised* (DSM-III-R). In addition, I have expanded the book to cover topics not included in the first edition, including four new chapters on child psychiatry, geriatrics, neuropsychiatry, and consultation-liaison psychiatry. I have also added discussions of recent developments in numerous areas of the field to bring the text into the 1990s.

The text is laid out in five sections. Chapters 1 through 4 are designed to give you the basic skills with which to carry out a diagnostic evaluation. Chapters 5 through 8 cover some of the most common psychiatric disorders, while Chapters 9 through 12 cover particular groups of patients and specialized fields of psychiatry. Chapters 13 through 16 deal with special problems encountered among patients who have a broad range of psychiatric diagnoses—problems that are of clinical concern to everyone who works in mental health care. Chapters 17 and 18 describe psychotherapies and somatic therapies, respectively.

Despite its expanded form, this text is deliberately *not* encyclopedic. Much is left out. But it will provide you with a place to start. And if these chapters make psychiatry more accessible to you and prompt you to delve further into the field, then the book will have accomplished its purpose.

Acknowledgments

Many generous and capable people contributed to the writing of this book. I am indebted to my colleagues at McLean Hospital, who commented on the early drafts of the first and second editions:

Ross J. Baldessarini, M.D.
Jonathan O. Cole, M.D.
Robert Fein, Ph.D.
Arlene Frank, Ph.D.
John G. Gunderson, M.D.
Douglas Jacobs, M.D.
Cynthia N. Kettyle, M.D.
Benjamin Liptzin, M.D.
Margaret McKenna, M.D.
Arthur Rosenberg, Esq.
Anthony J. Rothschild, M.D.
Alan F. Schatzberg, M.D.
Chester Swett, M.D.
Mauricio Tohen, M.D.
Sharon R. Weinstein, M.D.
Roger Weiss, M.D.
Kerrin White, M.D.

Carolyn B. Robinowitz, M.D., Deputy Medical Director of the American Psychiatric Association, offered valuable perspectives on medical student education. I owe special thanks to Diane Mosbacher, M.D., Ph.D., who somehow found the time and energy during her fourth year of medical school to examine the entire text of the first edition from a student's vantage point. She heightened my awareness of many social and political issues, and helped me to free the text of some of its cumbersome jargon.

Philip L. Isenberg, M.D., Director of Residency Education at McLean Hospital, helped me to conceptualize the textbook and to maintain its focus on the needs of beginning students. His support continues to this day. Evelyn Stone shepherded the original text through each stage of production. Without her knowledge of psychiatric publications and her constant willingness to listen and advise, the first edition would not have been realized.

Don R. Lipsitt, M.D., and Sheldon Benjamin, M.D., have made major contributions to the second edition. Their chapters on consultation-liaison psychiatry and on neuropsychiatry, respectively, broaden the scope of the text in two essential areas. Their interest in and enthusiasm for the goals of this book have been of great support in the long process of preparing a new edition. Timothy F. Dugan, M.D., brought his considerable expertise in child psychiatry to bear on the chapter on children and adolescents.

Ron McMillen, Tim Clancy, and Richard Farkas of the American Psychiatric Press have supported my work for close to a decade, and their editorial skills have made my task infinitely easier. Carol C. Nadelson, M.D., added her support to theirs when she became Editor-in-Chief at APPI.

Finally, Jennifer Stone, Ph.D., provided important perspectives on psychotherapy and on work with children. And—more to the point— her optimism, patience, and unflagging moral support were essential in enabling me to finish this project.

For all of their assistance and encouragement, I am very grateful.

Part I   Assessment Skills

1 The Clinical Interview:
  Fundamentals of Technique   3
2 Psychodynamics: Some Basic Concepts   19
3 Taking a Psychiatric History   37
4 The Mental Status Examination   55

INTRODUCTION

The problems that people bring to the psychiatrist run the gamut from memory loss to marital difficulties, from palpitations to hallucinations. The first section of this book is designed to offer you basic tools with which to approach this vast array of problems.

The primary diagnostic tool available to the psychiatrist is the clinical interview. Chapter 1 presents the fundamentals of interviewing technique, discusses how good interviewing differs from everyday conversation, and reviews some of the more common problems encountered by interviewers, particularly those with limited experience.

Chapter 2 is a brief summary of the fundamentals of psychodynamic psychology, presented in an attempt to demystify such basic psychodynamic concepts as the id, ego, and superego, and the unconscious mind. This chapter will also introduce you to the stages of human development and ideas about psychological conflict and mechanisms of defense—concepts that can be invaluable to you in understanding what people tell you about themselves and their past.

In Chapter 3, the focus is specifically on how to do a psychiatric evaluation, because that is usually the first task confronting the student in any health care setting. This chapter outlines the aspects of a person's life you will need to explore as part of an initial evaluation, and it provides examples of interview questions that will help you to gather this information.

Chapter 4 complements Chapter 3 in that it describes the mental status examination, which is a fundamental part of every psychiatric evaluation. In addition to describing the exam and offering suggestions

1

for the best way to conduct it, Chapter 4 is designed to serve as a glossary, defining many of the terms used to label the symptoms of mental disorders. It is important that you become familiar with these terms so that you use them correctly in your work.

These first four chapters serve as a prelude to the rest of the book. Once you have grasped the essentials of interviewing, some basic psychological concepts, and the process of doing an evaluation, you will be prepared to take a closer look at specific mental disorders and the methods we have for understanding and treating them.

1

The Clinical Interview:

Fundamentals of Technique

AN INTERVIEW IS, in essence, a conversation. So a chapter on interviewing technique may seem a waste of time. After all, most of us are well practiced in everyday conversation.

However, the clinical interview is a very particular kind of conversation and differs from daily discourse in many important respects. These differences are subtle, and interviewing is a skill that takes time and practice to master. The concepts discussed below are important tools in all branches of medicine. The basic principles of clinical interviewing apply equally to evaluating congestive heart failure, conducting an emergency-room psychiatric consultation, or embarking on long-term psychotherapy. This chapter places particular emphasis on how to interview a new patient as part of a diagnostic evaluation, because that is usually one of your first tasks as a student in a mental health care setting.

The aim of interviewing is not simply to gather information about someone's past, but to arrive at an empathic understanding of how that person feels. Such understanding is essential to accurate diagnosis and effective treatment, and the success of the interview hinges on its development. The more sensitive you are as an interviewer, the greater will be your grasp of your patient's problems, and the easier it will be for patients to elaborate on the nature of their pain. Emotional distress is often quite isolating, and the experience of sharing one's problems with a concerned listener can be enormously relieving. In a sense, the initial interview is actually the start of treatment.

To evaluate effectively, you must discover as much as you can about how your patient's mind works. During the interview, people will offer many clues, both in what they tell you (the *content* of the interview) and in how they tell it (the *process* of the interview).

3

Being aware of the process of the interview is essential to understanding someone's problems. But process is much more difficult to focus on than content, because most of us are not accustomed to doing so. Attending to process means listening with a "third ear," mentally stepping back from a conversation and watching it even while you participate. It means taking note of how people speak, what topics they bring up and in what order, which subjects they emphasize and which they avoid, how they sit or gesture, what responses they elicit from you, and how they make you feel. This style of listening does not come naturally to most of us, because in everyday conversation we focus on the content of what is said, and think about process only when there is some obvious discrepancy between the two (such as when a friend screams at you, "I am *not* angry!"). Paying attention to process is hard work, but it is a skill worth developing. Through process, people will give you a glimpse of how they cope with their world and how they approach new relationships. Consider the following case example:

> A young man has just been fired from his most recent job and complains to you that he is "depressed" because he cannot get along with a series of "difficult" employers. He also notes that his romantic relationships have never worked out "because women just don't understand me." In your interview, you find that he drones on and on about minute details of his work as an actuary. He becomes frustrated and momentarily angry whenever you attempt to introduce a new topic, saying, "I'll get to that—but first let me finish my story." When you ask about his feelings of depression, he invariably changes the subject back to his work. At the end of the interview, you find that you have gathered little information about his life or about the specific problems that brought him to see you. You also find yourself feeling angry and impatient with him. The content of the interview is of little help to you. However, your attention to the process of the interview provides you with a glimpse of this man's difficulties. He has rigidly insisted on imposing his own order on your meeting, and he has avoided any subject that might arouse unpleasant feelings. You might infer that his inflexibility and need to flee from emotion hamper both his relationships with women and his ability to work with employers. You might also infer that he makes other people feel angry and impatient with him, just as he has done with you.

Clearly, patients must be given the opportunity to show you the processes by which they form a relationship. They will do this in even a single interview, provided that you give them the freedom to do so. The interviewer who subjects the patient to an endless stream of specific questions will never gather this kind of information. This interviewer will not learn, for example, how the person handles silences or sadness. What's more, the interviewer who tends to talk a lot leaves less time to listen and will likely lose touch with his or her own feelings about the patient. Therefore, you should try to be as nondirective as possible. Guide people only when they seem to stray from the themes that are relevant to the interview. Obviously, this is not always an easy task, especially for the neophyte interviewer.

Your first goal is to stay out of the way, so that the patient can talk and you can listen. You must begin by taking steps to create an atmosphere that is conducive to free-flowing conversation.

SETTING THE TONE

Place

In order to devote your full attention to the work at hand, you and your patient must be physically at ease. Choose a quiet place for the interview where you are likely to have as few interruptions as possible. Ideally, this will be a place where you cannot be overheard, so that the patient will feel free to discuss confidential matters, and so that noises will not distract either of you.

Meeting the Patient

You may be the first person to whom your patient has come for help. New patients almost certainly will be anxious about talking to a stranger. They are likely to be worried by their symptoms and apprehensive about what your assessment will be. They may feel embarrassed about personal matters that must be discussed in the interview. Thus, patients are made vulnerable not only by the problems for which they seek help but also by the very nature of the encounter with you. To minimize these natural feelings on the part of new patients, you must make a special effort to put them at ease and treat them with particular courtesy.

Upon meeting each new patient, shake hands and introduce yourself. It is always appropriate to use formal address (i.e., Mr., Ms., Mrs.), both as a courtesy to the patient and as part of professional decorum. Initially, you may be tempted to put yourself and your patients on a first-name basis, but this usually hinders, rather than helps, a professional therapeutic relationship. After all, since this is your first encounter, the patient has not previously granted you the privilege of using his or her first name, and your doing so will seem presumptuous. Moreover, in using familiar forms of address, you convey the impression that the interview is something other than a professional encounter. Since patients are about to reveal intimate information about themselves, your professional attitude will be reassuring to them. You can convey warmth and concern without using terms that imply that you are close friends. Of course, children and adolescents are exceptions to this rule, as it is customary to call them by their first names in business as well as in social settings.

Invite your patient to sit down. If the patient is offered a choice of seats, note whether he or she sits near or far from you. Chairs should be arranged comfortably for conversation. You should sit so as to feel physically relaxed. If you are comfortable, you will be better able to listen, and your relaxed appearance will help put the patient more at ease. Initiate and maintain eye contact, but do not overdo it. A fixed stare is bound to disquiet your patient. You will find that varied eye contact will be most effective in establishing rapport.

Recording the Interview

Take notes if you feel comfortable doing so. If the patient asks about your note taking, you should explore his or her concerns about the confidentiality of your meetings, and you can use this opportunity to reassure the patient that his or her privacy will be respected. In some settings, students are encouraged to tape-record or videotape the interview. This can be a valuable learning experience, in that you and your supervisor can review a recording to study aspects of your interviewing style, your patient's style, and the doctor-patient interaction that may not be apparent to you as you perform the interview. Obviously, you must obtain the patient's permission to tape an interview *before* you begin recording. This may involve verbal or written consent, depending on the policies of the institution in which you work. Many patients will want to know the purpose of taping the interview and who will have access to it. Pay careful attention to any concerns your patient raises, answer the patient's questions, and do not proceed with recording until you are convinced that the patient is comfortable with the arrangement. Remember: Your alliance with the patient is your primary concern, and maintaining an atmosphere of trust and confidentiality takes precedence over any note-taking or recording assignments you may be given.

Time

Let the patient know at the outset how much time there is to talk. Traditionally, psychotherapy interviews last 45 to 50 minutes. Of course, some evaluation interviews (such as an emergency-room consultation) require more time than this, while very agitated patients may not tolerate a meeting lasting longer than a few minutes.

Be prompt for any arranged meeting with a patient. If you must be late for a first meeting, an apology is in order. If you are late for subsequent meetings, you should listen for the patient's reaction (anger, hurt, relief). You should also examine your own feelings if you are repeatedly late for meetings with a particular patient; uncharacteristic lateness on your part may be a reflection of unresolved problems between yourself and the patient (such as when a patient makes you feel helpless or incompetent).

Note how the patient uses time. For example, some patients will arrive far in advance of their appointments; others will arrive late. You will want to pay close attention to lateness as a possible indication that your patient has some feeling about meeting with you that he or she is not directly expressing (e.g., anger at you, or fear of discussing a painful subject in the interview). When patients arrive late and apologize, do not reassure them that lateness is "OK." Instead, inquire about the circumstances. Obviously, lateness is sometimes unavoidable, especially for someone trying to find the way to an unfamiliar location. But often excuses will be vague ("I forgot to set my alarm clock," "I was engrossed in work and forgot the time") and indicate a lack of attention on the patient's part or ambivalence about seeing you. So you may want to ask, "How did you feel about coming today?" to elicit the patient's feelings about the interview. Remember: If people truly want to be on time, they can almost always manage to be. When patients arrive late, be sure to end the session on time regardless of when it began, so that your patients will see that it is not in their interest to arrive late.

Defining the Goals of the Interview

A simple statement at the beginning about the length and purpose of the interview will set the stage for your evaluation. Be sure your patient understands from the outset the reason for your meeting (e.g., to evaluate the problems brought to you by the patient and to determine what interventions, if any, would be of help). Discuss how many meetings the patient will have with you, and whether you are likely to continue seeing the patient when the evaluation is finished or refer the patient to someone else for treatment. This is especially important if you are spending a short period of time in a hospital or an outpatient clinic as part of your training. Your patients will develop feelings for you (often, feelings of attachment and trust) as they tell you about their lives and problems. They must be prepared to lose their relationship with you when your work together is finished or when you leave this particular assignment.

YOUR INTERVIEWING STYLE: HELPING YOUR PATIENT TELL YOU WHAT IS WRONG

We all have preconceived notions about psychiatry. Stereotypically, the psychiatrist is a cold and distant person who never speaks except to ask a question and who remains unmoved by patients' distress. Yet, working with people who are in pain can be a very moving experience. In your first few interviews, you may feel as if you were having an intimate discussion with a close friend.

A good clinical interview is not a cold interrogation, nor is it a friendly chat, for neither style offers the patient the security and the freedom to speak openly about intimate problems. Effective interviewing is not stilted or artificial; in fact, it may even sound like everyday conversation. But interviewing differs from daily discourse in that it is specifically designed to give the patient as many opportunities as possible to tell the interviewer what is wrong. The specific techniques discussed below (and summarized in Table 1-1) can help you to do just that.

Interviewing Techniques

Opening the interview. Once you have introduced yourself and agreed upon the purpose of the meeting, ask a general question that allows your patient to begin wherever he or she chooses. You might begin with, "What brings you to see me today?" or "Can you tell me what has been troubling you?"

If a patient seems very anxious at the start of your interview and has difficulty responding to an open-ended question, you might ask some specific neutral questions concerning age, marital status, and living situation, to allow the patient some time to get more comfortable.

Allow the interview to flow freely. Let patients describe the events

Table 1-1. Some interviewing principles

Allow the interview to flow freely rather than jumping from one topic to another.
Provide structure for patients who have trouble ordering their thoughts.
Phrase your questions to invite the patient to talk.
Avoid leading questions.
Help patients to elaborate on thoughts and feelings.
Avoid jargon.
Use the patient's words whenever possible.
Avoid asking questions that begin with "why?"
Take note of the patient's strengths.

---

of their lives in any order they choose. Your comments and questions should flow naturally from what the patient says. Rather than jump from one topic to another, stay with the patient; encourage him or her to elaborate on thoughts and feelings. Later in the interview, you can guide the patient to fill in any gaps in the story without abruptly changing the subject. For example, if a patient has spent the first half of the interview reviewing recent events, you might turn the conversation to the patient's past with, "You mentioned your family; could you tell me more about your background?" If you keep in mind an outline of what needs to be covered, you can later rearrange what the patient has said in an orderly form for your written report.

The inexperienced interviewer is often tempted to ask a prepared list of questions and follow a prescribed order in gathering information. However, this will simply restrict the patient's options to tell you what is wrong, and this approach will give the impression that you are not really listening.

Provide structure for patients who have trouble ordering their thoughts. Some people—such as those suffering from severe anxiety or psychosis—may be confused by open-ended questions and may respond to them by rambling incoherently. In such cases, you must more actively structure the interview, both so that you can gather information about the patient and so that the patient does not become increasingly anxious and disorganized. A general question like "Tell me about your background" is not likely to evoke a cogent response from such a patient. Instead, you must show the patient precisely where you want the interview to go, with specific questions such as "What was your father's occupation?" and "How old were you when he died?" You may shift back and forth from a more-structured to a less-structured interviewing style as the interview proceeds; your goal is to tailor the specificity of your questions to your patient's needs.

Phrase your questions to invite the patient to talk. How you phrase questions will have an enormous impact on the information you gather. *Open questions* allow the patient to elaborate; *closed questions*, which require short answers (often "yes" or "no"), leave little room for detail. The following are some examples:

Closed: Have you felt depressed for a long time?
Open: Can you tell me how you feel when you are depressed?

Closed: Are you from a large family?
Open: Tell me about your family.

Open questions help people reveal relationships between their symptoms and events in their lives. Closed questions keep patients quiet and make *you* do all the work. Using closed questions leaves you with the impossible task of knowing which out of possibly hundreds of closed questions will get to the root of the patient's problems. And unless you prepare these questions ahead of the interview, you will be compelled to concentrate so hard on thinking them up as you go that you will lose touch with what the patient is saying.

Avoid leading questions. Like closed questions, leading questions are conversation-stoppers. They imply that you already know how the patient feels. In the case of a man whose brother had just died, a typical leading question would be, "Did you feel sad when your brother died?" This question sends a clear message that you expect the patient to feel sad. In fact, the patient may have hated his brother and must then confront the choice of challenging your expectation or concealing his real feelings. The obvious nonleading question in this instance would be, "How did you feel when your brother died?"

In short, do not assume that patients will react to events as you do. Leave them ample opportunity to explain how they really feel.

Help patients to elaborate. When patients seem to run out of steam or come to a stopping point, a nod may suffice to show them that you are eager to hear more. Or you may offer an encouraging comment like, "Tell me more about that," "Please go on," "Oh?" or "And?" You may also echo a key word or phrase from the patient's statement. For example, if the patient said, "My wife thinks I'm impossible to live with," you could say, "Impossible to live with?"

You may want to help the patient focus on feelings. For example, you could ask, "How did you feel about that?" or "How did you feel when that happened?" And to get the patient to be more specific when he or she is speaking in generalities, you could ask, "Can you give me a specific example?" or "What do you mean when you say 'crazy'?"

Reflect your patients' feelings back to them. This technique involves echoing the *tone* the patient has conveyed. This helps in two ways. First, when you show patients that you are trying to understand how they feel, you communicate your concern and thereby encourage them to open up. Second, reflecting patients' feelings in this way serves to test your own perceptions—that is, to confirm or deny that you have understood. Here are some examples:

> *Patient:* I can't seem to accomplish anything. Nothing has worked out for me in my life. Why should I expect the future to be different?
> *Interviewer:* You seem pretty discouraged.

*   *   *

Patient: It just isn't fair. My husband walked out and left me flat. He had no right.
Interviewer: You sound pretty angry with him.

When you do correctly verbalize patients' feelings, they will confirm it by elaborating further. You may help them in this way to see their feelings more clearly. But if you have not understood your patients, they will then have a chance to correct you.

Remember: Reflecting the patient's tone does not involve *sympathy.* Avoid making statements like, "Your story makes me feel terrible," or "That's absolutely awful!" Your goal is *empathy,* which means understanding how the other person feels, and not necessarily sharing those feelings.

Paraphrase the patient's thoughts. This technique is similar to reflecting the patient's feelings, but focuses on ideas more than emotions. Like reflecting feelings, paraphrasing the patient's thoughts lets the patient know that you are listening and trying to understand. It provides a check on your perceptions and helps the patient clarify his or her comments. Examples of paraphrasing include the following:

Patient: That medicine I'm taking is no good.
Interviewer: You mean, when you took it you did not feel better?

Patient: I come in here and talk to you, but what good is it doing me?
Interviewer: You're wondering whether our talks have helped you.

Another useful technique is *summarization*—recapitulating and condensing what the patient has said. Summarization encompasses both thoughts and feelings. It is similar to reflecting feelings and paraphrasing, but summarizing allows you to cover more material or a longer time span. The following are a few instances in which summarizing may help clarify what the patient has said:

- When the patient's discussion has been long-winded, rambling, or confusing
- When the patient appears to have talked about everything important on a specific subject
- When you want to ensure that you and the patient have a mutual understanding of what has been discussed so far, so that you may move on to other matters
- When you want to highlight certain ideas or events that you believe to be particularly important

Here are some examples of summarization:

> *Interviewer:* So for the past three months you have been hearing your dead mother's voice tell you that you should kill yourself. Since this began, you have been unable to go to work and have refused to leave your bedroom.

> *Interviewer:* So you have felt depressed ever since your brother became ill, and for the past several days you have had trouble falling asleep and have not felt like eating.

Additional Tips on Interviewing

Avoid jargon. Our daily language has become increasingly "psychologized" in recent years, but psychological jargon usually confuses rather than clarifies. Also, your use of jargon may make the patient feel dehumanized. Patients themselves sometimes use jargon to avoid genuine feelings. For example, the patient who "explains" his recent suicide attempt as "a temporary decompensation due to a reactive depression" has told you absolutely nothing about what prompted him to try to kill himself, or how he feels about it. Therefore, take care not to use jargon, and when patients (or colleagues) use it, be sure to ask them what they mean. Inexperienced interviewers are often reluctant to ask patients to explain such terms as "depression" or "psychosis." However, if you ask for such explanations, you will be surprised at the many meanings offered. In addition, you will begin to understand more about your patient's particular language.

Be careful, too, about assigning a diagnostic label to the patient's problem during the interview. Such labels are rarely of any use to the patient at this point and may be frightening or confusing.

Use the patient's words as frequently as possible, rather than your own. This is particularly important, for example, in dealing with sexual matters. People describe their sexual experiences in language that is infinitely varied. If a patient says that he or she is "gay," use the patient's term during the interview rather than a word like "homosexual," which may have different connotations for the patient. Of course, if a patient should use a self-denigrating term, like "queer," you might want to note the patient's word choice and substitute a more neutral choice of words in your own speech. The principle of using the patient's terminology applies to virtually all subjects, but particularly to matters about which the patient is likely to be sensitive.

Avoid asking questions that begin with "why." Patients do not usually know "why," and asking implies that you expect them to produce facile explanations. With your help, patients will discover more about the roots of their problems as they reflect upon their lives during the interview and in subsequent sessions. When you are tempted to ask "why," rephrase your question so that it elicits a detailed response, such as, "What happened?" "How did that come about?" or "What thoughts do you have about that?"

Thoughts versus feelings. In the interview, most people will use a mixture of ideas and emotions to paint a picture of their lives. However, some people keep a tight rein on their emotions and will dwell exclusively on ideas and explanations—that is, they will intellectualize to protect themselves from uncomfortable feelings. With such people, it is very helpful to emphasize emotion in your interview by asking how they *feel*. Conversely, other people deal with problems and anxiety almost exclusively in emotional terms, such as, "Oh, I get so upset I just can't think straight." For them, it helps to emphasize their capacity to think by asking questions like, "What do you think about that?"

Often, the patient's immediate response to a difficult or anxiety-provoking question is, "I don't know." Rather than immediately asking another question, you may get more information if you just sit quietly after an "I don't know" response, or ask the patient, "What comes to mind?" and see what happens.

Sensitive subjects should be approached tactfully but not avoided. After initially refusing, the patient may discuss difficult or embarrassing material if you rephrase your question or return to the topic at a later time.

Take note of the patient's strengths. People seek psychiatric help because they have problems, and these often obscure positive personality traits and accomplishments. If you listen for strengths and show interest in them, you will convey to your patients a sense that you want to get a balanced view of their situation. If patients do not offer any examples of how they feel good about themselves, you might ask, "What are you proud of?" or "What do you like about yourself?" The reply will give you important information about self-esteem.

Humor. Humor can be a wonderful tool in building an alliance with your patient. Be careful, though, for it can backfire. Patients may use humor defensively to avoid unpleasant feelings or to keep you amused. Your own use of humor may be misunderstood as ridicule. The key is to stay in tune with how your patient is feeling—and when you are not sure of those feelings, ask.

Keep track of where the interview is going. While it is important to allow patients to tell their stories as they choose, the time in which you must complete the evaluation is usually limited. Thus, you should not hesitate to guide patients to more relevant matters if they ramble or repeat themselves. Keep track of time, so that you have a chance at the end of the interview to ask about topics that may have been ignored or that need to be explored further.

Avoid premature reassurance. You may be tempted to allay the patient's fears with such assurances as,"Everything will be fine," or "There is nothing seriously wrong with you." However, reassurance is only genuine when 1) you have explored the precise nature and extent of the patient's fears, and 2) you are certain of what you are telling the patient. Premature reassurance can heighten the patient's anxiety, by giving the impression that you have jumped to a conclusion without doing a thorough evaluation, or that you are just saying what you think the patient wants to hear. It also leaves the patient alone with his or her fears about what is "really" wrong. Instead of minimizing these fears, try to find out more about them. When, for example, the patient expresses fears of being incurable, you might explore this area with an open-ended question: "What do you mean by incurable?" Or you might say, "You seem quite worried about this. Tell me more about it."

Address what is going on in the room. If the patient speaks incoherently, for example, or is actively hallucinating in your office, it will most likely be a relief to both of you if you acknowledge the patient's distress and try to clarify what you do not understand. Even the most disorganized patients often know when they are not making sense. If you are confused, say so. You might begin with a comment such as, "I am having trouble understanding what you are saying. Perhaps if I ask some specific questions we can more clearly focus on what is concerning you," or "It seems that you are reacting to something in the room that I cannot see or hear. Could you tell me about it?"

Set limits on inappropriate behavior. Although understanding is your goal in the interview, there are times when you must simply put a stop to what the patient is doing. This includes threats and menacing behavior, refusal to leave the office, and disruptive behavior in the office or waiting area. When, for example, a manic individual wants to remove his clothing, or an angry patient threatens to throw an ashtray through your office window, you must put a stop to such behavior before you can go on with the interview. You might acknowledge the patient's distress with a comment like, "You seem to be having difficulty controlling yourself. We'll have to stop our meeting until you are able to sit quietly again." As discussed in more detail in Chapter 16, you should never continue an interview when you feel that you or the patient may be physically harmed. If a patient's behavior becomes unmanageable, do not hesitate to stop what you are doing and summon help.

YOUR REACTIONS TO THE PATIENT

In the psychiatric interview, you are your own best and most important diagnostic instrument. Thus, your emotional reactions to the patient constitute invaluable data. Your reactions not only tell you how the patient makes others feel, but they may tell you how the patient feels behind all of his or her defenses. (For example, the helplessness you feel in talking with a woman who intends to commit suicide may reflect her sense of helplessness in the face of intolerable emotional pain.) If the patient awakens in you strong feelings of anger, depression, sexual arousal, or anxiety that you do not acknowledge, you may be rendered incapable of effective listening and may miss key aspects of the patient's problem.

Anxiety is probably the most common obstacle to effective listening. It is only natural to be somewhat anxious as a beginning interviewer. But sometimes particular patients (such as threatening ones) or particular topics (such as suicide) arouse so much anxiety that the interviewer screens out anxiety-provoking information. For example, when a depressed patient speaks casually of having a loaded gun in the house, the interviewer may become so frightened that he or she does not hear what has been said or minimizes the seriousness of the situation. The anxious interviewer may even unwittingly change the subject and leave the patient's suicidal thoughts unexplored. If you allow yourself to be aware of your anxiety and examine its source, you will be much less likely to retreat from difficult subjects during the interview. (For more detailed discussion of anxiety in dealing with violent patients, see Chapter 16.)

Identifying with the patient is another common occurrence among inexperienced interviewers, and this can hinder an accurate assessment of the patient's problems. You may mistakenly assume that you share certain feelings or experiences with your patient. This assumption could distort the facts and hamper your work, as in the following case example:

> A young man seeks a psychiatric evaluation at his college health service, complaining that he can never complete his term papers on time and that he is in jeopardy of flunking out of college. The psychiatrist, a second-year resident, comments to the patient that she, too, had difficulty completing assignments on time during college and medical school. She assumes that she and her patient are alike in this respect, that his symptom, like hers, is confined to his schoolwork, that he will "grow out of it," and that his fears of academic failure are exaggerated. The resident reassures him that the problem is not serious and sends him home.

In this case, the resident has failed to learn that her patient procrastinates in every area of his life: He is routinely late for appointments, never pays bills on time, and always keeps his dates waiting (apologizing profusely for his lateness when he finally arrives). His problem is much more pervasive than hers, and it causes him to be much more dysfunctional.

In addition, the resident does not recognize that their respective symptoms have very different roots. The resident struggles with her concerns about surpassing her mother in terms of professional education and advancement, and her trouble meeting deadlines in her work reflects a conflict between her wish to excel and her fear of losing her mother's love if she does. The undergraduate, by contrast, is caught in a more global struggle to exert control over all aspects of his life, and he stubbornly refuses to submit to what he sees as other people's demands. Because she has mistakenly equated her patient's situation with her own, the resident does not get an accurate picture of this man's problem, and she intervenes in a way that is not likely to be helpful.

When you start to feel that you and your patient are in some way alike, tread carefully. Make sure you differentiate what you know about yourself from what you know about your patient. As a general rule, avoid talking about your own life. Doing so usually diverts the focus from the patient's problems.

CLOSING THE INTERVIEW

As the interview comes to a close, leave a few minutes for any comments or questions that the patient has yet to voice. Often, patients will save critical information or profound concerns for the end of the session.

You might signal the close of the interview with a question such as, "In the minutes remaining, is there anything you'd like to add?" or "Is there anything else you think I should know?"

Also, ask your patient if he or she has any questions for you. People are understandably anxious about their problems and may ask you such questions as "What do you think is wrong?" or "So tell me, can you help me?"

Obviously, there are no pat answers to such questions, in part because the feelings and fears that prompt them are unique to each patient. Your job is to provide as straightforward a reply as possible. Do not be afraid to admit that you do not yet know the answer and that it may take more time to fully understand your patient's problems. You may, for example, want to obtain laboratory tests or psychological testing, and toward the close of the interview you can let the patient know that you think these measures are indicated. Or you may be unclear about what to do next, and it is perfectly legitimate to explain to the patient that you want to consult with a colleague or supervisor before determining how to proceed. Most patients will tolerate uncertainty better than false reassurance.

This chapter has focused on the fundamentals of conducting a clinical interview. Chapter 2 will give you a brief introduction to psychodynamic concepts and terminology. You can then use these concepts to help you make sense of what your patients tell you about their lives.

BIBLIOGRAPHY

MacKinnon RA, Michaels R: The Psychiatric Interview in Clinical Practice. Philadelphia, PA, WB Saunders, 1971

Nicholi AM Jr (ed): The New Harvard Guide to Psychiatry. Cambridge, MA, Harvard University Press, 1988, pp 7-28. (Chapter 1 contains a general discussion of interviewing technique and the therapist-patient relationship.)

Sullivan HS: The Psychiatric Interview. New York, WW Norton, 1954

2

Psychodynamics: Some Basic Concepts

PSYCHODYNAMICS REFERS TO the study of mental forces and how they motivate behavior. For thousands of years, human beings have struggled to elucidate and schematize the nature of mental life, and a great many models of the mind have been put forward.

Modern psychodynamic theory is founded on the work of Sigmund Freud (1856–1939). His ideas about mental structure and functioning have been widely applied clinically to help understand and relieve many of the symptoms of the mentally ill.

Freud has been a controversial figure in Western culture for nearly a century, and his ideas continue to be closely scrutinized and hotly debated among thinkers in virtually all areas of the social and biological sciences. Freud's work did not arise out of a vacuum and was in many respects evolutionary rather than revolutionary. Specifically, Freud incorporated the concepts of many important eighteenth- and nineteenth-century theorists into his schemata of mental life. There is much that remains controversial in Freud's work, and, as he himself was quick to point out, there is much that is in need of revision. Nevertheless, Freud's ideas have profoundly influenced our way of thinking about the human mind and human behavior. His concepts have permeated virtually every aspect of our culture, including the arts, politics, philosophy, and even education.

This chapter does not attempt to teach Freudian psychology. Much of Freud's initial work has been modified by later theorists, so a description of Freud's theories would not be an adequate representation of psychodynamic psychiatry as it exists today. Instead, this discussion aims to define some of the "household words" in the language of psychodynamics that were initially coined by Freud and that you are bound to encounter in your clinical work. To the student who has had no prior clinical experience in mental health, psychodynamic theories will likely seem confusing and even nonsensical. Phrases like "the unconscious mind" and "oedipal rivalries" may seem, to the uninitiated, abstract and removed from real experience. Psychodynamic concepts are best learned not from books, but by talking with patients, watching others perform interviews, and discussing your clinical experiences with colleagues and supervisors. Once you have developed a curiosity about the forces that cause your patients emotional distress, you will be much more likely to find psychodynamic theories intelligible, helpful, and even exciting.

MAPS OF THE MIND

Freud put forth two major models for understanding mental life: the topographic model and the tripartite model. Modern psychodynamic theory rests on both of these.

The Topographic Model: Conscious, Preconscious, and Unconscious

The discovery of the unconscious may well be Freud's most important contribution to modern thought. The idea that each of us has an ongoing mental life that operates *without our awareness* is an astounding concept. Freud first presented this idea in 1900, in *The Interpretation of Dreams*, in order to explain such phenomena as the forgetting of dreams and our ability in dreams to recall hitherto forgotten events from early life.

His topographic model divides the mind into three "agencies," based on the extent to which the thoughts, feelings, and perceptions in each agency are accessible to our awareness. These agencies of the mind are not tangible—they do not occupy physical space in the brain—but are simply metaphors; that is, they are theoretical constructs that help us organize our clinical observations.

The **conscious** includes all thoughts and feelings we are aware of, including sensory input from the environment as well as input from within (i.e., from the preconscious).

The **preconscious** contains all those ideas, feelings, and memories available to us when we choose to focus attention on them. For example, most of us do not maintain the threat of nuclear war in the forefront of consciousness, but the thought is available when we choose to focus on it. A primary function of the preconscious is to censor—to police our psyche and to prevent unconscious thoughts that might generate anxiety from reaching consciousness. The censor operates either by completely blocking access of unconscious material to consciousness, or by disguising unconscious material so that the conscious mind cannot recognize it.

For example, a young girl's unconscious sexual longing for her father would arouse considerable anxiety if she became aware of it, so her censor represses her incestuous impulses. The censor may block these sexual feelings entirely, or disguise them as their opposite (i.e., hatred). In the latter case, the girl would be using the defense of *reaction formation* (see below) and would be aware only of an aversion for her father. Her sexual yearnings would remain buried in the unconscious. (Of course, this is only one possible explanation for a girl's aversion to her father. Another might be that she has suffered some real trauma at his hands in the past.)

The **unconscious** contains ideas, impulses, feelings, and fantasies that lie out of reach of the conscious mind and cannot be made conscious by focusing one's attention. This material has been banished from awareness—that is, it has been repressed because it is in some way unacceptable, as in the example noted above. Unconscious material may reach consciousness when the censor is relaxed, as in dreams, or when it is overpowered and neurotic symptoms result. (For example, if the young girl's repressed incestuous impulses toward her father intensify, she may develop a conscious reaction against these impulses that takes the form of a snake phobia.) Along with these three aspects of the mind, Freud's topographic model includes two types of thought processes: primary process and secondary process.

Secondary process is the mode of thinking with which we are most familiar. Our conscious and preconscious mental activities are carried out in secondary-process thought, which makes sense to us and to the people with whom we communicate. It is logical, it is not filled with gross inconsistencies, and it is relatively well organized. Secondary-process thought is governed by the *reality principle*—that is, it respects the constraints of the real world. Thus, for example, the rules of secondary process dictate that today cannot be yesterday or tomorrow, and one cannot be in two places at once. These are, of course, statements of the obvious, and secondary process seems obvious because it appears to most of us that this is the only type of thinking we do. But there is another type—primary process—that is strikingly different.

Primary process is unorganized mental activity that seems foreign to us because it operates primarily in the unconscious. Primary-process thinking does not respect logic, contains no sense of time, allows for blatant contradictions and inconsistencies, and aims at immediate gratification without regard for the demands of the real world. Dreams are the best examples of primary-process thinking. (For example, in a dream you may be 5 years old but also a college student, the year may be 2005, and your professor may look exactly like your mother.) The rules of logic do not apply in primary-process thinking, but certain other mechanisms operate to make primary process seem bizarre to our conscious minds. The most important of these mechanisms are as follows:

1. *Symbolism.* An object or idea comes to signify something else, based on a resemblance between the original and its substitute (e.g., a banana may symbolize a penis).
2. *Condensation.* Several concepts or objects become fused in a single symbol (e.g., one's father, boss, and minister may become the same person in a dream).
3. *Displacement.* Emotions, ideas, or wishes are transferred from their original substitute (e.g., anger might be displaced from a parent to a teacher).

Dreams exhibit all of these characteristics, and this is why a dream often seems like nonsense after you wake up. Also, in your clinical work you will likely be able to detect primary process in the speech of severely psychotic people, whose ability to censor unconscious material is noticeably impaired.

Primary process is a normal part of conscious mental activity in children below the age of 5. For example, young children commonly use *magical thinking*—that is, they equate thinking with doing, and believe that their wishes actually define what is real. Hence, a child may believe that wishing someone dead will make it happen. As children grow, they become increasingly aware of the proper relationship between fantasy and reality, and cease to use magical thinking. Other primary-process modes of thought (e.g., denial) also gradually disappear under the pressures of the child's expanding knowledge of the real world.

The Tripartite Model: Id, Ego, and Superego

Freud's topographic model categorized mental *content* according to whether or not it was available to consciousness; but this scheme did not account for the different types of mental *functions* that he encountered in his work with patients. Dividing the mind according to functions and forces, he devised the tripartite model of id, ego, and superego. Like the divisions of the topographic model, the id, ego, and superego are not concrete entities but metaphors that clinicians have found useful in differentiating one type of mental function from another.

Id. The *id* is the name given to our most basic biological drives and our most primitive impulses. The guiding force of the id is the *pleasure principle*—the tendency to demand immediate satisfaction of desires, seek immediate pleasure, and avoid pain. The id encompasses states of pain and rage; cravings of sexual longing, hunger, and thirst; and the drive for self-preservation.

Id impulses and instincts are unconscious. The aspects of instinctual drives that do reach our awareness have usually been censored—that is, "laundered" to look more sensible and respectable to our conscious adult selves.

Ego. In everyday language, the word *ego* has come to refer to self-love or self-esteem. The psychological usage of the term, however, is quite different from this. The ego is the part of the personality that mediates between inner strivings and the realities of the world. It comprises all of those faculties of thought, feeling, perception, and action we use to harmonize the urges of the id with the requirements of the external environment and the inhibitions and aspirations of the superego (see below).

The ego strives to maintain mastery over the drives of the id, and it is the ego that delays gratification and substitutes more acceptable pleasures for less acceptable ones. The ego contains the compromising, evaluating, puzzle-solving, and defense-creating aspects of the personality. Ego functions are largely, but not entirely, conscious.

The ego develops as the growing infant interacts with the environment—especially with parents and other caregivers. Ego development includes the acquisition of defensive maneuvers for self-protection, as well as intellectual functions like comprehension, judgment, and language. The mature individual with a healthy ego is someone who is flexible in handling various life stresses, rather than one who must repeatedly resort to inflexible, maladaptive behaviors under pressure.

Superego. The *superego*, like the ego and the id, is a metaphor. The fictional character who most closely personifies the superego is Jiminy Cricket, who sat on Pinocchio's shoulder and acted as his guardian of moral standards and promoter of personal ideals. Freud conceived of the self-critical faculties of the mind as constituting a separate psychic agency that observes and evaluates our thoughts, feelings, and actions, comparing actual ego functioning with ideal standards. The superego consists of what we commonly call the "conscience," as well as the standards known collectively as the *ego ideal*.

Each of us develops an image of the person he or she would like to become. This "ideal image" is derived from the standards of behavior that we perceive in parents, teachers, and other important people in our childhood. The ego ideal is highly individual. It provides our inspiration to achieve and directs our strivings for gratification.

Children also adopt many of the prohibitions and obligations of parents and other important figures, by accepting parental dictates as demands of absolute obedience. This process by which parental standards and morality are incorporated into one's personality is a central part of superego formation and is thought to begin around the age of 4 to 6 years, and continue throughout life. As the child's social sphere expands, parental morality no longer seems absolute, while the standards of peer groups, teachers, and other admired figures take on new importance. Many, though not all, aspects of the superego are conscious.

People who develop harsh and strict superegos are their own cruelest taskmasters. They are often rigid, inhibited, anxious, and very unhappy. Those with more tolerant superegos can be flexible and accept their limitations without giving in to impulses that violate their own or society's fundamental moral ideals.

The id, ego, and superego exist in a constantly changing relationship. A disturbance in the checks and balances of these three agencies often results in mental discomfort, unacceptable behavior, or both. The id and superego largely remain out of our awareness until they cause trouble—for example, when an unacceptable instinctual impulse becomes conscious and arouses anxiety, or when criticism by the superego prompts feelings of guilt. The well-adjusted individual makes compromises intuitively that resolve conflicts among id, ego, and superego.

PSYCHOSEXUAL DEVELOPMENT

Freud postulated the existence of two basic human drives: libidinal instincts and aggressive instincts. *Libido* refers to sexual energy, though the term is also used more broadly to refer to all strivings for pleasurable experience. He put forth the idea that the child's strivings for pleasure are organized and modified in a series of developmental stages. In each stage, the child has particular needs to be met and problems to be solved.

According to Freud, the way we negotiate each of these stages is crucial, for "unfinished business" from any one stage is carried with us as development proceeds, and can become a source of psychopathology in adult life. The stages of psychosexual development are briefly outlined in Table 2-1 and described below. The timetable for these stages is only a crude approximation, since each child develops at his or her unique pace. Moreover, keep in mind that Freud's *instinct theory* remains highly controversial even today. Many argue that it ignores other essential forces that drive the process of human development. Nevertheless, you are likely to hear these psychosexual stages referred to in many case discussions.

Oral Stage (Birth to 18 Months)

The newborn infant needs total care and so must immediately begin to form relationships with other human beings. The mouth is the part of the body through which pleasure is secured and hunger satisfied. The mouth thus becomes the focus for a variety of the infant's sensations, interests, and activities. Because of its pleasure-giving potential at this stage, the mouth is spoken of as an *erogenous zone*. The infant's pri-

Table 2-1. The stages of psychosexual development

Stage	Age	Description
Oral	0 to 18 months	The mouth is the focus for sensations and activities. "Good mothering" now lays the foundation for a sense of security and basic trust in others.
Anal	1½ to 2½ years	The child finds pleasure in experiencing control over bodily needs. This period ideally fosters self-control, independence, the ability to give, and personal pride.
Phallic	2½ to 4 years	The focus of attention shifts to the genitals. The child begins to explore the world more autonomously and learns to take pride in his or her abilities. This stage is crucial in developing a stable sense of self-worth.
Oedipal	4 to 6 years	The child longs for a special relationship with the parent of the opposite sex and has feelings of jealousy and hostility for the parent of the same sex. Resolution requires development of a special relationship with the same-sex parent.
Latency	6 to 12 years	The child masters physical, intellectual, and social skills; identifies with those of the same sex; and learns mastery of impulses.
Adolescence	Teen years	Physical maturation heightens interest in sexual activities. The adolescent is preoccupied with personal identity and how others perceive him or her. The adolescent ideally assumes more responsibilities for self-control and self-direction.

mary relationship is, in most cases, with the mother, although "good mothering" at this stage may actually come from any caregiver(s), male or female, whose attention to the infant is warm and consistent. Such caring lays the foundation for a sense of security and basic trust in others that the infant will carry into later life, whereas a lack of caring may establish a deeply rooted sense of mistrust and insecurity.

The infant must learn to tolerate frustration when his or her urgent demands are not instantly met. Contact with the mother cannot ever be as immediately or constantly gratifying as the infant would wish, and the child must cry in order to make certain needs known. This frustration, if not unduly prolonged, prompts the infant to develop healthy self-soothing techniques and defense mechanisms that protect against overwhelming excitement and rage. It also helps the infant differentiate between self and others, as it becomes clear that mother is a separate being who is not always present when the infant wants her.

We often label adult emotional states *infantile* if they are reminiscent of behavior at the oral stage of development—that is, states characterized by urgent demands, extreme dependence, lack of responsibility for or consideration of others, and a very low tolerance for frustration. People with such characteristics are said to have *oral personalities*, and they are commonly preoccupied with fantasies and needs that focus on the mouth.

Anal Stage (1½ to 2½ Years Old)

As the infant's nervous system matures, it becomes possible to recognize and control the need to eliminate. This is a pleasurable experience for the child, both because of a growing awareness of the sensations involved in the excretory functions and because of the new experience of control over bodily needs. During toilet training, the child and the parent interact around the child's control of bowel and bladder function, and this interaction is thought to influence later personality traits.

The child must make compromises between primitive wishes to do whatever he or she pleases, and the rewards obtained by conforming to the demands of important caregivers. Ideally, this period fosters the beginnings of self-control, independence, the ability to give, and a sense of personal pride. However, if toilet training is harsh and the parents are punitive, the child may develop strong attitudes of shame and disgust, and be both fearful of and enraged at controlling caregivers. In later life, these unresolved problems of self-control may manifest themselves as rigid behavior patterns. The four classic traits of the *anal character* are aptly described by the following mnemonic:

Parsimony
Orderliness
Obstinacy
Punctuality

Obviously, toilet training is only one of the areas of childhood experience in which issues of self-control and societal expectation emerge. It has become a symbol in our culture for a developmental step that all children must take in the process of becoming social beings.

Phallic Stage (2½ to 4 Years Old)

The focus of the child's attention gradually shifts from the mouth to the anus to the genitals. At this stage, the penis or clitoris is a new discovery and a source of pleasure. The differences between the sexes become more discernible to children at this age, promoting the beginnings of identification as male or female. In addition, the child's increasing motor and intellectual capacities make it possible to explore, to be curious, and to take initiative and pride in solving simple problems. Ideally, parents greet such initiatives with pleasure—which mirrors the child's own sense of accomplishment—while setting realistic limits on the child's sense of his or her unlimited power (e.g., not letting the toddler run into the street). This stage is thought to be crucial in developing a stable sense of self-worth—that is, the sense that one is an attractive and lovable human being.

Psychoanalytic theorists trace many of the origins of narcissistic personality disturbance to problems in the phallic stage of development. They posit that children whose self-esteem does not consolidate during this stage develop into adults who are plagued by persistent feelings of inferiority, extreme sensitivity to perceived slights or insults, and constant excessive reliance on the responses of others as measures of their worth.

Oedipal Stage (4 to 6 Years Old)

Oedipus, you will recall, was the tragic hero of Sophocles' drama about a man who unwittingly murdered his father and married his mother. According to Freud, this Greek classic has remained compelling to audiences for centuries because it recaptures a fantasy that children experience and subsequently repress.

The *Oedipus complex* refers to the child's increasing longings for a special relationship with the parent of the opposite sex. Along with these longings go feelings of jealousy and rivalrous hostility toward the competition (i.e., the parent of the same sex). Thus, little boys feel as if they are competing with father for mother's love, and little girls see mother as a rival for father's affections.

Children at this stage both hope and fear that their murderous and incestuous wishes will come true. Because they cannot yet differentiate clearly between fact and fantasy, children develop the concern that their wishes will hurt their rival and that the rival will retaliate. This is the fear that psychoanalytic theorists refer to as *castration anxiety*.

How does the child resolve this romantic dilemma? The normal resolution to the Oedipus complex involves recognizing that this incestuous pursuit is futile, and giving it up in favor of a special relationship with the parent of the same sex. The child identifies with the rival and adopts many of the same-sex parent's goals, standards, and behaviors. Instead of wanting to marry mother, the little boy settles for growing up to be like father and marrying a woman who is like mother. For little girls, the process is similar, but at present there is great controversy among psychological theorists about how little girls deal with the Oedipus complex.

Resolving the Oedipus complex also requires that the child, to some extent, begin to identify with the parent of the *opposite* sex. Thus, the little girl who cannot "have" Daddy can be partly satisfied by becoming like Daddy in some respects, for example, by adopting certain of her father's interests or attitudes. Children normally emerge from the oedipal stage having identifications with both parents.

People who develop neurotic symptoms are thought to have been unable to successfully resolve the Oedipus complex. Thus, you will often hear the term *oedipal* used synonymously with *neurotic.* By contrast, the term *pre-oedipal* (or *pregenital*) is reserved for more severe illnesses like personality disorders and psychoses, implying that these more severe disturbances originate in the oral, anal, or phallic stages of development.

Latency Stage (6 to 12 Years Old)

The term *latency* refers to Freud's observation that sexual curiosity seemed to become dormant or latent during this period, to reemerge in adolescence with renewed force. However, the term is something of a misnomer in that sexual interests do not disappear during this phase, but remain present throughout childhood.

Latency is a time for mastering a host of physical, intellectual, and social skills. The child's world enlarges beyond the nuclear family to include school and other activities outside the home. This affords the opportunity to identify with new role models (e.g., teachers, peers) and to modify or solidify behavior patterns learned in the family. In this period, the child normally identifies strongly with those of the same sex. The emphasis is on learning social skills and mastering one's own impulses—hence the latency-age child's fascination with games that have elaborate rules and rituals (e.g., hopscotch, "tag"). The child learns about the pleasures and pains inherent in dealing with peers. Failure to conform to peer-group standards can result in ostracism and a sense of inferiority, but successful mastery of age-appropriate skills can foster a sense of pride and social acceptance.

Adolescence

The onset of puberty, with the rapid maturation of the genitals, stimulates a heightened interest in sexual activities. However, the adolescent's drive toward maturation is not confined to sexuality. Adolescents become preoccupied with personal identity and how they are perceived by others—hence the adolescent's concern that he or she dress, speak, and act "cool."

Standing on the threshold of independence from parents, adolescents identify strongly with groups of peers as a means of separating themselves from their families. They try out emancipatory behaviors (e.g., smoking, drinking, staying out late with friends), often rejecting many of the values and demands of their parents in favor of peer-group mores. Courtship and first sexual activities normally occur during this phase. Ideally, the adolescent becomes freed from parental controls, while assuming more responsibility for self-control and self-direction. Adolescence lays the groundwork for mature sexual relationships based on mutual respect.

Psychosexual Development in Perspective

Development does not end with adolescence, of course, but continues throughout life. The preceding discussion is a very crude sketch of Freudian developmental theory. The process by which human beings mature is infinitely complex, and our understanding of it is far from complete.

Freud gave us one particular map of how human beings develop psychologically. Many important psychodynamic models have been developed subsequently. Ego psychologists such as Heinz Hartmann explored aspects of behavior and psychic functioning (e.g., speech) that are relatively independent of the id and not entirely under the sway of the sexual and aggressive drives. Object-relations theorists (Klein, Fairbairn,

Guntrip) departed from Freud's belief that gratifying sexual and aggressive urges was the infant's primary motive for relating to other people. Instead, they posited that human beings have an inborn drive to relate to others and will strive toward relating even when they are well fed and all their other biological needs are met. More recently, Heinz Kohut argued that Freud's psychosexual line of development is not sufficient to explain emotional growth, but that human beings follow a path of narcissistic development as well. He postulated that healthy narcissistic development leads to the establishment of a coherent sense of one's self and stable, realistic self-esteem. These and other theories make up a vast body of literature on psychodynamic understanding of normal and abnormal development. (Further discussion of childhood and adolescent development can be found in Chapter 10.)

MECHANISMS OF DEFENSE

Each of us uses a variety of techniques to relieve tension and shield ourselves from painful experiences. However, not all of our self-protective maneuvers are carried out consciously. Those techniques that we employ unconsciously to alleviate anxiety and eliminate conflict are termed *defense mechanisms*. The defenses listed in Table 2-2 and described below are among those most commonly encountered in clinical practice. The first 12 defense mechanisms are "immature" in that they may work to protect the person who uses them from distress but they do so at a significant cost (e.g., by grossly distorting reality). The "mature" defenses do not require such distortions.

Table 2-2. Some common defense mechanisms

Immature	Mature
Repression	Altruism
Denial	Humor
Retroflexion	Suppression
Acting out	Anticipation
Projection	Sublimation
Splitting	
Reaction formation	
Conversion	
Dissociation	
Displacement	
Intellectualization	
Isolation of affect	

Immature Defense Mechanisms

Repression, the fundamental mechanism of defense that underlies all others, is akin to forgetting. It involves forcing thoughts, memories, and feelings into the unconscious and actively keeping them out of awareness. Repression is responsible for lapses of memory (e.g., forgetting the hour of a dreaded examination) or seemingly inexplicable naivete. The apparent ignorance which results from repression is often accompanied by symbolic behavior that suggests that the repressed material is not really forgotten (e.g., the woman who is unaware of her sexual attraction to her therapist, but who dresses seductively for her appointments). Repression prevents us from recognizing our own thoughts and feelings, whereas *denial* prevents the recognition of external reality.

Denial involves disbelieving a fact of external reality in order to avoid pain or anxiety. Denial often results in grossly distorted thinking and behavior, as in the case of the man who refuses to accept the death of his wife and goes on "communicating" with her as though she were still alive. People commonly use denial to avoid recognizing the presence of serious physical illness, and may delay consulting a physician about ominous symptoms until it is too late (e.g., the woman who denies the growing lump in her breast for many months). Denial is not conscious— that is, it involves more than simply pretending that something is not so. Unacceptable facts are banished from awareness entirely, and the individual has no access to them.

Retroflexion (turning against the self) is the process of making an unacceptable impulse or feeling (usually hostile) acceptable by deflecting it from its original object back upon the self. This is most commonly seen among people who are labeled "depressive" or "masochistic" (e.g., the woman who berates herself for being a bad wife after she is abandoned by a physically abusive husband).

Hypochondriasis is related to retroflexion and involves transforming a reproach toward others into somatic complaints. It allows the individual to bemoan his or her condition in lieu of complaining about others.

Acting out is a term used too often and too loosely to describe any patient's behavior that mental health professionals do not approve of. When used correctly, the term *acting out* refers specifically to the process of acting on an unconscious wish or impulse in order to avoid being aware of the emotion that accompanies it. In other words, action is used in the service of remaining unaware of intolerable feelings (e.g., a man who behaves with uncharacteristic promiscuity and who has no awareness of sexual longings for his therapist).

Projection is a process by which motives and feelings unacceptable to the self are unconsciously attributed to others instead. For example, a man who struggles to fend off his own unconscious homosexual impulses may complain, "Every man on the street makes homosexual advances toward me." Projection is used both by people whose thinking is grossly out of touch with reality (as in the example above) and by healthier individuals as well. Racial and other forms of prejudice are based on the use of projection.

Splitting involves dissociating positive and negative aspects of oneself and others, and compartmentalizing them into "all good" or "all bad" images. People who use splitting see themselves and others in black-and-white terms, dividing the world into "good guys" and "bad guys." This relieves the anxiety that comes with recognizing ambivalence (e.g., that one can be mad at someone one loves).

Reaction formation occurs when unacceptable unconscious impulses are disavowed and *opposite* conscious attitudes and behaviors are adopted. For example, a man whose strong sexual urges are severely repressed may lead a campaign for censorship of "salacious" literature in school libraries, or a woman who unconsciously despises her children may smother them with undue affection.

Conversion takes the unconscious conflicts that would otherwise give rise to anxiety and instead gives them symbolic external expression through some bodily symptom—such as hysterical blindness or paralysis (e.g., a woman whose arm suddenly becomes paralyzed due to her unacceptable impulse to stab her unfaithful husband). Conversion is a major defense used in somatoform disorders.

Dissociation involves a temporary but drastic modification of one's character or of one's sense of personal identity to avoid emotional distress. Examples of dissociation include such states as sleepwalking, amnesia, and multiple personality. Even acting in the theater may involve dissociation, as when it allows the actor a "safe" way to express instinctual wishes that would be unacceptable in real life.

Displacement redirects feelings from an original object to a more acceptable or less dangerous substitute. This defense is commonly found in everyday life (e.g., as when a man who is angry at his boss takes it out on his family).

Intellectualization involves thinking about instinctual wishes in affectively bland terms in order to avoid experiencing strong emotions.

Isolation of affect involves separating an idea from the feelings associated with it and generally banishing these feelings from consciousness. This defense is closely related to intellectualization. It is characteristic of people with obsessive-compulsive personality styles. People use isolation to protect themselves from emotions they find threatening or unacceptable (e.g., sexual or angry feelings). Thus, a man who is enraged at his wife may be totally unable to feel his anger, but finds himself preoccupied with emotionless, matter-of-fact thoughts about hurting her. While extensive reliance on isolation can hamper one's ability to form satisfying relationships and to experience life fully, isolation can be useful in certain situations. For example, health care professionals who routinely deal with people who are in pain usually need to isolate thoughts from feelings to prevent being overwhelmed and rendered incapable of performing their jobs.

Mature Defense Mechanisms

All of us, when under stress, occasionally fall back on some of the defenses listed above. However, healthier individuals do not rely heavily on any of these, but instead allay anxiety and diminish intrapsychic conflict by using the following, more adaptive defenses.

Altruism involves constructive and instinctually gratifying service to others, including philanthropy and other activities from which one derives vicarious or more direct pleasure. Unlike reaction formation, altruism is gratifying to the person who uses the defense.

Humor facilitates our ability to express feelings and focus on anxiety-provoking thoughts without causing distress to ourselves or others. Forbidden wishes can be expressed in comic fashion and not acted upon.

Suppression involves a conscious decision to postpone paying attention to an unpleasant subject. This is in contrast to repression, which operates unconsciously and is therefore beyond conscious control. Suppression includes minimizing misfortunes, "keeping a stiff upper lip," and postponing, but not avoiding, difficult experiences. Consider Scarlett O'Hara's famous line in Gone With the Wind: "I'll think about that tomorrow."

Anticipation involves planning for future discomfort in a realistic fashion to effectively decrease anxiety, for example, by carefully planning for an impending separation from a loved one.

Sublimation supports much of civilization. It consists in diverting unacceptable instinctual drives (e.g., sexual and aggressive impulses) into personally and socially acceptable channels. One common example is competitive sports, in which aggression is "tamed" and channeled, but not inhibited. Many artistic endeavors are thought to result from sublimated libidinal energies.

PSYCHODYNAMICS IN CLINICAL PRACTICE

What relevance do these maps of the mind, developmental stages, and mechanisms of defense have to your clinical work? After all, no one has ever seen an ego or measured the size of an Oedipus complex. Yet despite their intangibility, psychodynamic concepts can be invaluable tools in helping you make sense out of symptoms and behaviors that might otherwise seem nonsensical. Indeed, Freud was among the first to advocate the idea that psychological symptoms (such as obsessions and phobias) have meaning and that they represent the human mind's complex and often ingenious efforts at easing intrapsychic distress.

You will not often hear your patients talk directly about these concepts—about their defenses or their developmental problems—but you will hear "derivatives" of them. For example, a patient is not likely to tell you about (or even to recall) his difficulties with a rigid and punitive parent around the issue of toilet training at age 2. But you may see him replay this traumatic situation by struggling with a series of "unreasonable" bosses over his working conditions or by struggling with you over whether or not he will pay his bill.

As you hear more about a patient's life, you will discover recurring themes—like strains of music that thread through a symphony—and you can usually relate these themes to problems the patient experienced at particular stages of development. In attempting to master issues not resolved in childhood, people continually recreate infantile problems in many areas of their adult lives. Much of psychotherapy consists of helping people to discover these leftover problems, along with the defenses used to keep from recognizing them.

Psychodynamic concepts can be of great help to you in organizing the many details of a patient's life story. Even in a single interview, you can learn enough to relate many of the recurrent problems in patients' adult lives to their childhood experiences, and begin to outline some of the defenses and psychological conflicts that cause or exacerbate their current distress. The next chapter discusses the process of taking a history, a process that will be greatly enhanced by your familiarity with the basic ideas about mental functioning discussed above.

BIBLIOGRAPHY

Freud A: The Ego and the Mechanisms of Defense, Revised Edition. New York, International Universities Press, 1966

Gedo JE, Goldberg A: Models of the Mind: A Psychoanalytic Theory. Chicago, IL, University of Chicago Press, 1973. (An excellent review of psychoanalytic theories of mental structure and function, beginning with Freud.)

Greenberg JR, Mitchell SA: Object Relations in Psychoanalytic Theory. Cambridge, MA, Harvard University Press, 1983. (A clear and readable book that compares and contrasts different psychodynamic theories of human development.)

Horowitz MJ: Introduction to Psychodynamics: A New Synthesis. New York, Basic Books, 1988. (An interesting synthesis of psychodynamic and cognitive theories of mental functioning.)

Kolb LC: Personality development, in Modern Clinical Psychiatry, 10th Edition. Philadelphia, PA, WB Saunders, 1983, pp 58–79. (An overview of human development, written from a psychoanalytic perspective.)

Nemiah JC: Foundations of Psychopathology. New York, Oxford University Press, 1961. (A general introduction to psychodynamic concepts, with lively case examples.)

Stone EM (ed): American Psychiatric Glossary, 6th Edition. Washington, DC, American Psychiatric Press, 1988

Vaillant GE: Theoretical hierarchy of adaptive ego mechanisms. Arch Gen Psychiatry 24:107–118, 1971

3

Taking a Psychiatric History

THIS CHAPTER DEALS with two separate but related tasks: taking a psychiatric history and reporting it to someone else. They are related in that the information you gather in your interviews with the patient provides the material for the case report. But that is the extent of their resemblance.

You can almost never adhere strictly to an outline in taking a history. People do not talk about themselves in outline form, nor would you be an effective interviewer if you tried to force them to do so. You must keep an outline in your own mind so that you will know which topics you want to cover in the course of your evaluation. But never use it as a checklist—this will only alienate your patients and limit the amount of information you can gather.

The outline of the case history presented in this chapter includes both a list of subjects to be covered in a psychiatric evaluation and some examples of interview questions that may help you explore these topics.

When reporting a case history, the history must be organized and presented in a way that gives readers (or listeners) a coherent picture of your patient's current condition. Given that virtually any detail of the patient's life may be relevant to his or her emotional state, you are likely to feel overwhelmed by the task of fitting all the information you have collected into a single presentation. It is therefore essential that you 1) pare down the history to include only those details you believe will help others understand your patient's problems, and 2) adhere to an outline when you present a case verbally or in writing.

The psychiatric history is organized much like a standard medical history, as the outline in this chapter shows (see Table 3-1). In addition to familiarizing yourself with this outline, look at Appendix A, which contains a sample case report. This will give you a general idea of how a written evaluation is prepared. However, many mental health care facilities have their own specific formats for these reports, and you should be sure that your evaluation summaries are consistent with the record-keeping system of the particular institution in which you work.

The initial evaluation summary is often the portion of the patient's record that is most widely read—for example, by new staff members coming to a ward or an outpatient clinic. The write-up therefore will be essential in communicating your patient's situation to others. It should be clear, concise, and accurate. Beware of too much detail—after all, no one reads a 50-page treatise.

The outline included here is too detailed for most evaluations. You should take care to elaborate on aspects of the history that are germane to your patient's current problems, but do not hesitate to cover less relevant categories in a cursory fashion. For example, if your patient has a "negative" family history for mental illness, you need only write, "The patient denies any history of mental illness or substance abuse in family members."

At a minimum, every area of the psychiatric history must be mentioned in every summary that you prepare. When in doubt about what to include in a case report, discuss your write-up with a supervisor—for both your own and the patient's benefit.

OUTLINE FOR THE PSYCHIATRIC HISTORY

The evaluation begins with a rough sketch of the patient's situation. Identifying data such as age, sex, and occupation, the source of the patient's referral to you, and the patient's chief complaint orient your

Table 3-1. Organization of the psychiatric history

Identifying data	Medical history
Referral source	Drug and alcohol history
Chief complaint	Mental status examination
History of the present problem	Formulation
Past history	Diagnostic impression
Family psychiatric history	Treatment plan

audience quickly to who the patient is and why he or she has come to see you. Because these statements set the stage for the rest of the case report, they come first.

With this brief introduction, you have prepared your audience to learn about the patient in depth. You begin with a description of the present problem, starting with its onset and proceeding chronologically to the date of your interview. You then place the patient's current difficulties in the context of his or her childhood development and important formative experiences. (The description of the present problem and the past history are usually the most detailed sections of the case report.) Information about the patient's physical health, drug and alcohol use, and mental illness in family members completes the history.

The mental status examination (discussed in Chapter 4) is not actually part of the history. Rather, it is your description of the patient as he or she appears and behaves in the interview. It is the psychiatric counterpart of a physical examination.

With all of this information in mind, your audience is then prepared to understand your assessment of the patient's problems (the formulation of the case), your diagnostic impression, and your plan of treatment. By presenting the report in this order, you permit others to follow the thought processes that brought you to your conclusions about the case. Without such an outline, your report can easily become a barrage of disorganized detail in which you and your audience get lost.

OBTAINING IDENTIFYING DATA

Identifying data include the following:

- Name
- Age
- Marital status
- Sex
- Occupation
- Number of children
- Place of residence
- Number of previous admissions to psychiatric hospitals (if an inpatient)

This information alone can tell you much about the patient's situation. For example, "This is the sixth psychiatric hospitalization for Mrs. Petrocelli, a 38-year-old divorced homemaker and mother of six who lives with her children in a Brooklyn apartment." Also detail the patient's ethnic and religious background if this is particularly relevant to his or her current situation.

REFERRAL SOURCE

Find out how your patient came to you, and you may learn something of his or her expectations. For example, the patient may tell you: "My brother says this is the best clinic in the state."

CHIEF COMPLAINT

Ask the question "What brings you to see me?" to elicit the patient's chief complaint. *In the patient's own words*, record a one-sentence description of what is wrong.

HISTORY OF THE PRESENT PROBLEM

When did the present problem begin? In many cases, the patient will tell you, for example, "My wife died six months ago and I've been depressed ever since."

Determining when the patient's current difficulties truly began is often difficult and requires some judgment about what may have precipitated his or her emotional distress. You may, for example, choose to date the onset of the present problem from the time a prominent symptom appeared (e.g., a first suicide attempt), from the date of a first psychiatric hospitalization, or from the time of a major personal loss (e.g., abandonment by a spouse). Whatever you decide, make sure to arrange the events of the history of the present problem in *chronological* order—that is, bring the reader (or listener) from the onset of the problem right up to the time the patient came for help.

Explore in detail the patient's chief complaint and other problems that hamper his or her life at present (Table 3-2). Note when these problems began, as well as how persistent they have been. Describe any prominent psychological symptoms (e.g., hallucinations, memory loss, panic attacks) and any mood changes reported by the patient. Be particularly thorough in documenting previous suicidal or homicidal thoughts or acts. Pay attention to any physical symptoms that have been present during the illness, and determine the degree to which these problems have impaired the patient's relationships with others and his or her

Table 3-2. Exploration of current problems in the patient's life

Onset of problems (time, setting)
Duration and course (chronic vs. episodic)
Psychological symptoms
   Symptoms of psychosis
   Cognitive problems
   Mood changes (irritability, depression, elation)
Somatic symptoms
   Medical conditions
   Vegetative signs (anorexia, weight loss, insomnia, anergy, agitation or
      retardation, decreased sexual energy and interest, diurnal mood variation)
   Neurological symptoms
   Somatic complaints without organic basis
Severity of problems—degree of impairment in functioning
Possible precipitants

ability to function at work. Also, note any circumstances in the patient's life that may have precipitated the present crisis.

Mapping the Current Problems in the Patient's Life

Onset of problems. Determine, if possible, the time and setting. The time of onset may not be clear (e.g., "I've been depressed all my life").

Duration of problems. Has the problem been present continuously or has it recurred intermittently?

Psychological symptoms. Describe in detail any disturbances of thought or perception that are central to the patient's present problem. Although such symptoms are reported in the mental status examination when the patient actually exhibits them during the interview, they are also included in the history of the present problem when they are part of the patient's history. (For example, "The patient reports that for the last 6 months he has heard his dead father's voice commanding him to kill himself.") These symptoms may include the following:

- Symptoms of psychosis, such as hallucinations, delusions, dissociative states, or ideas of reference
- Cognitive problems, such as impaired memory or concentration
- Mood changes, such as

   Irritability—rage and violent thoughts or acts. Techniques for exploring homicidal thoughts and fantasies are outlined in Chapter 16.

Depression—guilt and hopelessness. Recent suicidal thoughts and acts should be reported in the history of the present problem. Techniques for exploring suicidal feelings are outlined in Chapter 15.

Elation—outline the extent of hyperactivity. (For more discussion of mania and hypomania, see Chapter 6.)

Somatic symptoms. Note medical conditions that seem to be an integral part of the present problem. Describe course of illness and treatment (past and present). Somatic symptoms may include the following:

- Vegetative signs, such as anorexia, weight loss, insomnia, loss of energy, agitation or retardation, decreased sexual energy and interest (see section on unipolar disorders in Chapter 6).
- Neurological symptoms, such as seizures or recent head trauma
- Somatic complaints with no known physical basis

Severity of problems. To what extent have current problems interfered with the patient's ability to work and to participate in relationships? Some patients are totally incapacitated by mental illness, whereas others function very well at daily tasks despite emotional distress.

Possible precipitants. Pay close attention to what was going on in the patient's life at the time symptoms developed, and also pay close attention to changes in important relationships (friends, lovers, family), job or financial situation, school performance, or physical health.

Always Try to Answer the Question "Why Now?"

What prompted the patient to seek help this week rather than last week? this month rather than next month? Many times, the problem has been present for quite a while, but some key event in the patient's life has upset an equilibrium and made life less tolerable.

For example, a woman comes to you seeking help for agoraphobia (a fear of being alone or on her own in public places), from which she has suffered for the past 12 years. During this time, she has been afraid to go out of the house unless accompanied by her husband, and cannot stay alone in the house unless she can speak to him by telephone at regular intervals while he is at work. Why does she seek help now, after 12 years? On close scrutiny, you discover that her husband is about to be promoted to a job that will require him to travel for several days each month, and the patient is enraged that he is "abandoning" her.

Determine Whether the Patient Knows Anyone Who Has Had Similar Problems

For example, you may discover that your 30-year-old depressed patient has a mother who also became depressed at age 30. Identification of this kind often exists just outside the patient's awareness. Yet, it may be very important in determining the types of symptoms the patient develops as well as when during the patient's life these symptoms first took hold.

Determine How the Patient Has Dealt With These Problems to Date

First, detail any efforts patients have made to cope on their own or get help from others. Then, mention the patient's previous history of mental health care and treatments, if any—including psychotherapy, medications, hospitalization—noting the patient's responses in the past to these treatments. How the patient felt about previous therapists may give you clues to the kind of relationship he or she is likely to form with a therapist in the future.

PAST HISTORY

The past history summarizes the patient's life, in chronological order, from infancy until the time when the present problem began. Deciding which details of a patient's past are pertinent to his or her current distress is not always easy. But two aspects of your patient's early life are almost always relevant and deserve particular attention:

Relationships with parents, siblings, and other important people during childhood. As is discussed in Chapter 17, our childhood relationships exert a powerful influence on how we deal with people as adults. In the case of the agoraphobic woman described above, you might discover that she had an intense attachment to her mother, that she felt herself to be like her mother in every way, and that she and mother were "inseparable pals" throughout her childhood.

Major milestones in growing up. How we reacted as children during times of stress or separation from parents—starting school, the onset of puberty, leaving home—often carries over into our behavior under similar circumstances as adults. For example, it would not be surprising to discover that the agoraphobic woman was terrified of going to kindergarten and missed many days of school during the months it took her to overcome her fear. Nor would it be surprising to learn that at age 18 she turned down a scholarship to a college in another city and did not leave her parents' home until she married at age 26.

Past history places the patient's current problems in a broader context, helping you to see patterns of behavior that have persisted throughout the patient's life. Thus, although most people seek mental health care because they are concerned about the present, it is important to spend some time learning about the past in the course of your evaluation.

The points to be explored in a patient's history are outlined in Table 3-3 and described more fully below. Bear in mind that there is more detail here than will be applicable to any one patient's situation.

Family Constellation

List age and occupation of the patient's father, mother, siblings, and others living at home, including relatives, babysitters, and other

Table 3-3. Outline of the past history

Family constellation (father, mother, siblings, others living at home)—
   important family relationships, major separations or losses
Infancy
   Birth order
   Birth history
   Developmental milestones
Childhood
   Preschool years
   Health—hospitalizations
   Starting school—academic performance
   Friendships
Adolescence
   Onset of puberty
   Early sexual experiences
   Peer relationships
   Experimentation with drugs, alcohol
Adulthood
   Education
   Military experience
   Employment
   Social life/friendship
   Romantic relationships
   Sexual history
   Marriage
   Children

caregivers. Describe their personalities and relationship with the patient. Include disruptions in this relationship due to illness, death, or separation. Questions that may be helpful in eliciting this information include the following:

- Tell me about your family.
- Who took care of you when you were small?
- Who were you closest to in your family?
- Who do you feel you are most like among those in your family?

Infancy

The patient's place in the family. A patient's birth order can provide valuable clues about his or her family role (e.g., the "baby" or the "little mother"). Also inquire about how much attention patients received from parents and others. (For example, a mother with four children all under age 6 will obviously have less time and energy to devote to individual children than a mother of two.) The birth of younger siblings is usually a major event in a child's life.

The patient's birth history. Was the pregnancy planned or unplanned? Note any complications of pregnancy or delivery.

Developmental milestones. Did the patient have difficulty in learning to walk or talk? Was the patient considered by parents to be a "bright" or a "slow" child? The patient will not remember the early months of life, but what one has been told about birth and infancy becomes an important part of one's self-concept (e.g., "You were always a fussy, unhappy baby," or "You were smarter than every other kid in the neighborhood").

Childhood

Note any major family events (e.g., illness, death, divorce, separations, moves).

Preschool years. Activities, caregivers, playmates. Helpful questions include, "How far back can you remember?" and "What do you recall about your life before you started school?"

Health. Were there any hospitalizations? Note prolonged separation from family as a result of these.

Starting school. Inquire about the patient's relationships to teachers and peers, school performance, extracurricular activities, what the patient hoped to be when he or she grew up, whether the patient had to change schools because of moves or disciplinary problems. Typical questions include the following:

- What do you remember about starting school?
- What were you like in elementary school?

Adolescence

Ask about the onset of puberty in the patient's life and the accompanying emotional reactions to physical changes. Note where the patient acquired initial information about sex. Detail information about early sexual experiences (heterosexual and homosexual), peer relationships, quality of friendships, and experimentation with drugs and alcohol. Questions might include the following:

- Tell me about junior high school/high school.
- From whom did you learn about sex?
- Did you have any romantic relationships as a teenager?
- Did you have any close friendships?

Adulthood

Information relevant to the present problem should be included in the history of this problem.

Education. Note the level achieved and aspirations for further education, in the past or the present.

Military experience. Every patient of appropriate age should be asked about military experience. Veterans of the Vietnam War may be prone to special problems such as posttraumatic stress disorder stemming from their combat experience.

Employment. Stability, satisfaction, relationships with peers and authorities, and job performance are all factors that should be included.

Social life/friendship. Include leisure activities and religious/moral values.

Romantic relationships. Characterize lovers and stability of the relationships. People commonly choose lovers based on their earliest important relationships—that is, they seek lovers who remind them in some ways of parents and other caregivers.

Sexual history. Note degree of intimacy and satisfaction, sexual orientation, and sexual dysfunction. Many people with mental disorders are troubled by sexual dysfunction, and a simple question may open up an entire area of emotional distress—for example, "Is there anything about your sex life or sexual feelings that is troubling you now?" (For a more detailed discussion of how to take a sexual history, see Chapter 13.)

   Marriage. Describe the patient's relationship with his or her spouse, satisfaction in marriage, separations, and/or divorce.

   Children. List the ages of the patient's children and describe his or her relationship with each. Also describe disruptions in these relationships due to illness, death, or separation. Note any miscarriages or abortions, since these often have a major impact on family life.

FAMILY HISTORY OF MENTAL ILLNESS

This is a critical part of every evaluation. Ask about any relatives of the patient (including grandparents, aunts, uncles, cousins) who have had emotional problems, who have seen a mental health professional, who have been hospitalized for mental illness, or who have had problems with drug or alcohol abuse. Pursue any "yes" responses to these questions by inquiring about the following:

- Symptoms of the illness
- Course of the illness (chronic versus episodic)
- Types of treatment (medication, psychotherapy, "shock treatment," hospitalizations)
- Responses to various treatments

   Relatives are either biological (i.e., "blood relatives") or nonbiological (related to the patient by marriage). Biological relatives may suffer from disorders that are thought to be genetically transmitted (e.g., major affective disorders), which would increase the chances that your patient might suffer from the illness as well. The occurrence of emotional disorders in nonbiological relatives is also important, because what has happened to family members is likely to influence your patient's ideas regarding mental illness (e.g., "I'm afraid I'll be locked up in an asylum like my stepfather was"), as well as your patient's experiences in the family during formative years.

MEDICAL HISTORY

Medical problems should be explored in detail. Note major medical conditions, current treatment for them, disabilities, and any other medical facts that might be pertinent to the patient's psychological state. Pay particular attention to a history of neurological disorders, especially seizures or head trauma. Be sure to list all current medications—including over-the-counter drugs—because these can profoundly affect your patient's emotional state. Obtain relevant medical records from doctors and health care facilities, and be sure that these become a part of the patient's chart in the facility at which you are doing the evaluation. Patients who have physical complaints but who have not obtained a recent physical examination should be advised to do so. When indicated, you should examine the patient yourself and order relevant laboratory studies. Inpatients should be examined upon admission.

DRUG AND ALCOHOL HISTORY

Note types of drugs and alcohol used. Also detail how frequently and in what amounts these are taken as well as symptoms of withdrawal and other complications (e.g., hepatitis or AIDS resulting from the use of contaminated needles). If drug use is a major problem, include it in the history of the present problem. When inquiring about drugs, use terms the patient is familiar with (e.g., "angel dust" instead of PCP or phencyclidine). (See Appendix B for a table of commonly abused drugs.) Also, inquire about so-called "social use" of drugs like alcohol, marijuana, and cocaine. Patients who heavily abuse these substances may rationalize their behavior as "just being sociable" (see Chapter 14).

MENTAL STATUS EXAMINATION

The results of the mental status examination (MSE) can usually be summarized in a short paragraph. (For a detailed discussion of the MSE, see Chapter 4.) Each aspect of the MSE (appearance and behavior, speech, emotions, thought, etc.) must be mentioned. Where no abnormalities are present, you may simply say so without elaborating.

CASE FORMULATION

The case formulation is the clinician's attempt to integrate all the data collected during the evaluation and to arrive at a tentative understanding of the factors contributing to the patient's problems. Your formulation assesses the biological and social forces that have fostered the development of the patient's personality style and current illness. This assessment is based on what you have learned from the patient's history and MSE. In short, your formulation summarizes the case for the reader. It does not include a diagnosis, but musters evidence in support of your diagnostic impression.

Composing a case formulation need not be an intimidating task; two or three well-organized paragraphs will usually suffice. The outline below may help you organize your formulation.

Introduction

In one or two sentences, describe your patient, the presenting problem, and your understanding of why the patient seeks help at this particular time. Summarize the patient's symptoms and the extent to which they cause distress to the patient and/or others. Also note how the symptoms impair the patient's ability to function in his or her usual daily tasks and in ongoing relationships.

Biological Factors

Discuss any organic problems present (e.g., seizure disorder, endocrine abnormality) and how these might contribute to the patient's problem. Include drug or alcohol abuse, if any. Also note any predisposition to illness caused by organic factors (e.g., a history of minimal brain dysfunction in childhood) or family history that might suggest a genetic contribution to the problem. If no biological factors have been noted, state this explicitly.

Psychological Factors

Psychodynamics. Note the patient's major conflicts, defense mechanisms, and personality strengths and weaknesses. Also, describe the type and quality of relationships your patient is capable of forming with men *and* women (see Chapter 2).

Social situation. Comment on your patient's current life situation, including his or her important relationships and occupational status, as well as changes in these.

Mental status. Note any important findings from your mental status examination of the patient (e.g., delusional thinking, paucity of expressed emotion).

Hypotheses About Causes

Try to link the biological and social factors in a coherent statement about how the patient's illness came about. Obviously, this statement will be somewhat speculative, but it may provide you with hypotheses that you can test as treatment proceeds. Note any patterns you see in the course of the illness—recurrent decompensations, a slow but constant deterioration, or specific somatic or environmental precipitants (e.g., a patient who becomes psychotic every time his wife gives birth to another child).

DIAGNOSTIC IMPRESSION

You will be called upon to make a tentative diagnosis based on your formulations. Keep in mind that accurate diagnosis is difficult and often requires observation of the patient over time. Thus, your initial impression may change as you get to know your patient better and watch how he or she responds to your treatment.

The *Diagnostic and Statistical Manual of Mental Disorders*, Third Edition–Revised (DSM-III-R) should be available in the health care facility where you are working. You can compare your patient's signs and symptoms with the various sets of diagnostic criteria in DSM-III-R to see which syndromes most closely fit your patient's condition. Once you have done this, you will probably want to discuss your diagnostic impression with a supervisor.

DSM-III-R organizes diagnosis along a series of five axes (the use of this multiaxial system is explained in detail on pp. 15–24 of DSM-III-R):

Axis I: Clinical syndromes. This axis includes all mental disorders except personality disorders and developmental disorders. It also includes V Codes, which are conditions not attributable to a mental disorder that are a focus of attention or treatment.

Axis II: Personality disorders and developmental disorders. The separation of personality disorders from other disorders is clinically useful, because many patients will have a personality disorder underlying another clinical syndrome. In such cases, patients will be assigned both Axis I and Axis II diagnoses (e.g., bipolar disorder on Axis I and obsessive-compulsive personality disorder on Axis II).

Axis III: Physical disorders or conditions. This category is self-explanatory. Your primary concern in arriving at a diagnostic impression should be with Axis I and Axis II, for all patients with mental disorders will have diagnoses in either Axis I or Axis II, or in both. Patients may have more than one diagnosis in any of the first three axes, but where no diagnosis is made (e.g., when no physical or personality disorder is present), it is sufficient to write "no diagnosis" beside the appropriate axis number.

Axis IV: Severity of psychosocial stressors. This axis allows for the identification of specific psychosocial stresses that have occurred in the preceding year and seem to have precipitated, revived, or exacerbated the patient's current condition. Considered here are interpersonal, family, occupational, financial, legal, developmental, and physical factors.

Axis V: Global Assessment of Functioning. This category allows you to judge how well your patient has been able to function at work, in social relations, and during leisure time. This is done by using the Global Assessment of Functioning (GAF) Scale (see Appendix C) to make two ratings: 1) your patient's level of functioning at the time of the evaluation, and 2) his or her highest level of functioning for at least a few months during the previous year. The patient's current level of functioning will generally reflect his or her need for treatment, and the highest level of functioning in the past year is likely to have some prognostic significance, because patients usually return to their previous levels of functioning after an episode of illness. (For example, a man who is now floridly manic but worked effectively as a corporate executive between manic episodes in the past year is likely to return to this high level of job performance when the current crisis passes.)

You will want to consult DSM-III-R to see how to evaluate your patients' situations with respect to psychosocial stressors (Axis IV) and global assessment of functioning (Axis V). In many health care facilities, the use of Axis IV and Axis V is optional.

An example showing how to use the multiaxial system for diagnosis is included in Appendix A. Further examples can be found in DSM-III-R (p. 21).

Along with your diagnosis, you may want to include one or more diagnoses that have not been ruled out, that is, diagnoses you feel have not been excluded and that still warrant serious consideration. However, avoid entering unsubstantiated diagnoses into a patient's permanent record, because government agencies and insurance companies may have access to such documents and could be misled by inappropriate diagnostic labels.

TREATMENT PLAN

The treatment plan is your recommendation regarding how the patient's problems can best be alleviated. It may include any of the many therapies discussed in Chapters 17 and 18. Often, you will recommend more than one treatment. For example, your plan for a depressed patient who is being seen as an outpatient might read as follows: "Trial of tricyclic antidepressants, supportive psychotherapy once weekly, and one or more meetings with the patient and her husband to assess marital difficulties."

The treatment plan is based on many factors, the most important of which is your assessment of what is wrong. In addition to diagnosis, however, you must consider the following:

What is your patient's most pressing problem? Obviously, you must attend to emergencies first. For example, a severely depressed young man may be an excellent candidate for treatment with antidepressant medication, but his clear suicidal intentions make it impossible to begin any pharmacotherapy until he can be prevented from harming himself. Thus, hospitalization would be the most important recommendation at this time.

How receptive is your patient to various forms of treatment? You might, for example, decide that a woman with anorexia nervosa needs a behavior modification program to help alter her eating patterns, and twice-weekly psychotherapy to work on the severe personality disorder that underlies the eating problem. However, the patient denies that she has any emotional difficulties and vehemently rejects the idea of psychotherapy, despite your emphatic recommendation. She does, however, accept a referral to a behavior therapist, and you list insight-oriented psychotherapy as a possible future treatment in your plan.

What services are available to the patient? To some extent, you must gear your treatment plan to the resources available in your area. Suppose, for example, you are working in a busy urban mental health clinic and a young man comes to you in acute distress over a failed romance. Even though it is apparent that he has persistent difficulties with women and could benefit from long-term insight-oriented psychotherapy, you know that there are no staff members available at this time to provide long-term treatment. However, the clinic can offer short-term psychotherapy that provides the patient with support and helps him weather the current crisis. He may return for long-term therapy at some future time.

What are the patient's financial resources? Ideally, money would never need to be considered in deciding on a treatment plan. But, in fact, mental health care is costly, and patients often need treatment over a period of months or years. Thus, it is imperative that you help patients plan for ongoing care that is financially feasible. For example, a family may be willing to exhaust their life's savings to pay for their schizophrenic son's stay in a private hospital rather than send him to a state-run facility. However, this would not be in the patient's best interest, because he will almost certainly need long-term follow-up care as an outpatient and will require financial assistance from his family for a long time to get the treatment he needs.

In devising a treatment strategy, do not hesitate to recommend further evaluative procedures when you feel that important questions about the patient's condition remain unanswered. These procedures include consultations by other professionals (e.g., a consultation by a neurologist for a suspected seizure disorder), laboratory testing, psychological testing (e.g., an intelligence test to rule out mental retardation), and meetings with rehabilitation specialists (e.g., to assess a patient's ability to work).

The next chapter covers a particular part of the mental health evaluation, the mental status examination. The chapter is designed not only to familiarize you with the structure of this examination, but also to define for you many of the most important terms used to describe the symptoms of psychiatric illness.

BIBLIOGRAPHY

American Psychiatric Association: Diagnostic and Statistical Manual of Mental Disorders, 3rd Edition, Revised. Washington, DC, American Psychiatric Association, 1987, pp 15–24

Cameron PM, Kline S, Korenblum M, et al: A method of reporting formulation. Canadian Psychiatric Association Journal 23:43–50, 1978

Friedman RS, Lister P. The current status of psychodynamic formulation. Psychiatry 50:126–141, 1987

MacKinnon RA, Yudofsky SC: The Psychiatric Evaluation in Clinical Practice. Philadelphia, PA, JB Lippincott, 1986

Nicholi AM Jr: History and mental status, in The New Harvard Guide to Psychiatry. Edited by Nicholi AM Jr. Cambridge, MA, Harvard University Press, 1988, pp 29–45

Perry S, Cooper AM, Michels R: The psychodynamic formulation: its purpose, structure, and clinical application. Am J Psychiatry 144:543–550, 1987

4

The Mental Status Examination

THE MENTAL STATUS EXAMINATION (MSE) is an assessment of the patient's current state of mind. Like a physical examination, the MSE evaluates the patient's functioning in the here and now; like physical findings, the patient's mental status may change over time.

The term "mental status examination" is used to refer both to 1) the process of gathering information about the patient's state of mind during an interview, and 2) the section of the case report reserved for this information. The MSE is recorded separately from the history in evaluation summaries and progress notes, as a way of distinguishing what you observe about the patient from what the patient tells you about himself or herself.

The outline of the MSE presented in this chapter is very detailed (see the summary in Table 4-1). This may give you the impression that an MSE takes 4 or 5 hours to complete. Do not be misled. In most cases, you will not need to devote more than a few minutes of an evaluation interview to a formal exam, because most of the necessary information about mental status will come not from asking specific questions, but from your observations of the patient's appearance, behavior, and manner of speaking in the course of routine conversation.

Table 4-1. Summary outline of the mental status examination

Appearance and behavior
  Dress and grooming
  Posture and gait
  Physical characteristics
  Facial expression
  Eye contact
  Motor activity
  Specific mannerisms
Speech
  Rate
  Pitch, volume, clarity
  Abnormalities
Emotions
  Mood
  Affect (variability, intensity, lability, appropriateness)
Thought
  Process (flow of ideas, quality of associations)
  Content
    Distortions (delusions, ideas of reference, depersonalization)
    Preoccupations (obsession, phobias, somatic concerns)
    Suicidal or homicidal ideation
Perception
  Illusions
  Hallucinations
Sensorium and intellectual functions
  Consciousness
  Orientation
  Concentration
  Memory (immediate, recent, and remote)
  Fund of knowledge
  Abstraction
  Judgment
  Insight
Attitude toward the interviewer

WHEN DO YOU CONDUCT A MENTAL STATUS EXAMINATION?

Actually, you assess a patient's mental status every time you meet, but in most cases, you do this informally. A detailed and careful MSE is usually part of an initial evaluation. This serves as a baseline examination with which to compare your impressions of the patient on subsequent meetings. For example, you may notice that a patient who has just been admitted to the hospital has trouble concentrating on your interview with her because she hears her grandmother's voice telling her to jump out of your office window. As part of your MSE, you test her other intellectual functions and discover that she also has difficulty remembering recent events (e.g., what she ate for breakfast). In your follow-up interviews, you need not go through an entire formal MSE again, but can simply test those areas in which you noted abnormalities on admission—perception, concentration, and recent memory. In this case, as treatment alleviates auditory hallucinations, the patient may recover both her ability to concentrate and her ability to remember recent events.

Do you conduct a formal MSE with every new patient? Clinicians disagree on this issue. Some insist that you can gather all the information you need about a patient's mental state from informal conversation alone. They argue that asking structured questions (e.g., asking the patient to interpret proverbs or do simple arithmetic) alienates you from the patient and destroys any rapport that has developed between you in the course of the interview. Other clinicians warn that abnormalities of mental functioning can be masked by the patient and go unnoticed in an unstructured interview and that formal questioning is the only way to elicit them.

There is no clear way to resolve this debate. With each patient you see, you must use your judgment about the extent to which formal testing of mental functions is necessary to answer your questions about the patient's condition. Certainly, it is incumbent upon you to learn how to do a complete MSE as part of your training in psychiatry.

Often, patients will tell you about abnormalities of mental functioning that are symptoms of their presenting problem and that you need to explore in a formal MSE. For example, if an elderly patient tells you that he has trouble remembering to turn off the stove at home, you will want to do a careful evaluation of his memory, along with other intellectual functions. Patients will usually give you clues to important abnormalities, either in what they tell you (e.g., "I keep hearing voices") or in how they tell it to you (e.g., continually losing the train of thought in midsentence). If you pay attention to these clues and explore in depth anything that seems unusual, you are likely to pick up any important abnormalities in the patient's mental state.

DETERMINING THE PRESENCE OF PSYCHOSIS

One of the most important questions you will need to explore in the MSE is whether the patient is currently psychotic. But first you must understand what we mean when we use the term "psychotic."

Surprisingly, there is some debate among psychiatrists on this point. Many textbooks define **psychosis** as a major mental disorder in which thinking, emotions, communication, and behavior are so severely impaired that this impairment significantly interferes with the individual's capacity to meet the ordinary demands of daily life. This definition emphasizes loss of functioning.

However, many people who are severely impaired in their daily lives (e.g., those with severe personality disorders) would not be considered psychotic. Some people who harbor carefully concealed delusions (e.g., that their thoughts are being monitored by foreign spies) may nevertheless function well at jobs and even manage to maintain a family life.

There is no single definition that will satisfy all clinicians. For practical purposes, psychosis may be defined as an inability to distinguish between what is real and what is not, even when evidence of reality is clearly available. We speak of the psychotic individual as having impaired *reality testing*—that is, being unable to test subjective ideas and experiences against objective facts of the external world.

The loss of the ability to test reality is an essential aspect of psychosis. Those individuals whose misperceptions of reality can be corrected by evidence are not said to be psychotic.

A hallmark of psychosis is confusion between what comes from one's own mind and what emanates from the outside world. The psychotic person loses a sense of boundaries between inside and outside. Some common psychotic beliefs are that one can control others' thoughts, that external forces have put thoughts into one's own head, or that other people can read one's thoughts—all of which involve the notion of a "permeable" mind. Hallucinations, which are by definition psychotic, are internal stimuli (e.g., hearing voices) that are falsely believed to be of external origin.

In the narrow definition given above, psychosis involves false ideas or perceptions about oneself and the world that cannot be altered even when evidence of their falsehood is presented. In reality, there is no precise boundary between psychotic and nonpsychotic thinking, for false ideas and perceptions are held by people with varying degrees of tenacity. You must watch and listen carefully for evidence of psychosis, because it can be well masked in an interview. The most common psychotic symptoms you will see involve disorders of thought content (e.g., delusions) and disorders of perception (e.g., hallucinations); these are described in some detail below. Bizarre forms of speaking and behaving are also commonly associated with psychosis.

Psychosis is not, in and of itself, an illness. It is a symptom of a wide variety of illnesses, ranging from drug overdoses to manic-depressive illness. Some disorders involve psychotic symptoms by definition (e.g., schizophrenia), while others may or may not include psychotic symptoms (e.g., depression). An individual may be psychotic for a period of minutes, or for many years. Psychotic symptoms often wax and wane in their severity, but they may remain unchanged over long periods of time. Thus, each time you interview a patient you must reassess whether psychosis is present.

USING THE MENTAL STATUS EXAMINATION

Although specific mental illnesses are associated with particular abnormal findings in the MSE, beware of jumping to diagnostic conclusions based on the MSE alone. Each symptom in this outline can occur in any of several disorders. A given symptom provides only a small portion of the evidence required to make a diagnosis. The patient's history and course over time will provide critical data. If you rely only on the MSE, you will often be fooled.

Avoid using this outline for the MSE as a checklist; the exam should vary according to each patient's needs. Let the patient's history and your clinical judgment guide you to explore in detail only those areas of mental functioning about which you have specific questions.

In many cases, you will have more than one meeting with the patient you are evaluating, so you need not gather all the necessary information at one sitting. After a first meeting with a new patient, you may find it helpful to seek the advice of a supervisor in deciding which aspects of the MSE to explore in follow-up interviews. Do not, however, neglect to ask about suicidal and homicidal ideation in the first interview with *every* new patient you see. Dangerousness to self or others is a mental health emergency, and its assessment must not be postponed or overlooked.

AN OUTLINE OF THE MENTAL STATUS EXAMINATION

Appearance and Behavior

The patient provides a wealth of information without saying a word. Take care not to overlook the many things you can learn through nonverbal communication.

Dress and grooming. Grooming is an important indicator of a patient's ability to care for himself or herself; manner of dress often provides valuable clues to a patient's self-image. Dress may be seductive or slovenly or overly fastidious. Depression or psychosis may prevent normally well-groomed individuals from attending to personal hygiene, and these individuals may become disheveled and disorganized. Any change in appearance should be explored with the patient and family, documenting when the change occurred and under what circumstances.

Posture and gait. Rigid posture and gait may indicate a patient's anxiety or vigilance. Seriously depressed patients often demonstrate slumped posture and slow gait. Physical handicaps are almost always of great emotional significance to the patient and should be noted.

Physical characteristics. Note the patient's apparent versus chronological age (young-looking, old-looking), physical health (vigorous, frail), and weight (obese, emaciated).

Facial expression. The patient's facial expression often mirrors his or her mental state (e.g., sad, suspicious, angry, silly, bland, immobile).

Eye contact. Note whether the patient makes frequent eye contact with you, avoids a direct gaze, stares into space, or glances furtively about the room. Eye contact often decreases with increasing anxiety or paranoia. Patients with psychosis or dementia who cannot concentrate on the interview may not focus on you visually.

Motor activity. Observe the patient's physical activity during the interview. Constant restlessness and pacing may signal anxiety, agitated depression, or mania. Slow movements and little reactivity are signs of the psychomotor retardation common in depression, drug reactions (e.g., extrapyramidal side effects), and *catatonia*, a state in which the patient becomes immobile, with muscular rigidity or inflexibility. Catatonia may be accompanied by stupor or excitement, or by a refusal to cooperate with others (negativism).

Specific mannerisms. Repetitive gestures such as tics or grimacing should be noted. Also, pay attention to agitated behaviors (e.g., hand-wringing, hair-pulling) that may accompany anxiety or depression. People who are taking antipsychotic medications should be observed for involuntary movements of the tongue and mouth or the extremities (these are suggestive of tardive dyskinesia) and for the general motor restlessness that is characteristic of akathisia. (For an explanation of these side effects, see Chapter 18.)

Speech

This category of the MSE is reserved for observations about the way the patient speaks. By contrast, your observations about what the patient says are included under the category "Thought" (see below).

Rate. *Pressured speech* is very rapid, frenzied speech that may exceed the speaker's physical powers of articulation and/or the listener's ability to comprehend. It is often present in the manic phase of bipolar disorder (manic-depressive illness).

Rapid speech is found in a variety of other conditions, most commonly in acute anxiety states.

Slowed speech is common among depressed people who have generalized psychomotor retardation.

Mutism (i.e., absence of speech) occurs in some severely psychotic people, including catatonic patients.

Pitch, volume, and clarity. Speech may, for example, be described as high-pitched, infantile, loud, whispered, mumbled, or garbled. Some psychotic patients can be inappropriately loud. Shy, withdrawn people may speak in a whisper. Patients with organic brain syndromes or alcohol intoxication may have garbled speech. Some patients who see themselves as "not grown up" may adopt a high-pitched, almost childlike manner of speaking.

Specific abnormalities. *Stuttering* may interfere with conversation; note any circumstances that alleviate or exacerbate stuttering (e.g., anxiety-provoking subjects).

Speech impediments may be subtle or very marked, and can interfere with communication to varying degrees.

Aphasia is the loss of facility in language comprehension or production at the level previously possessed. It is commonly found in people who have brain damage (e.g., secondary to strokes). *Amnesic* (or *anomic*) *aphasia* is the loss of the ability to name objects. *Broca's aphasia* is a syndrome characterized by the loss of the ability to produce spoken and (usually) written language, even though the individual retains the ability to understand language. *Wernicke's aphasia* is a syndrome that involves the loss of the ability to comprehend language, coupled with the production of inappropriate language (e.g., nonsensical speech).

Emotions

The patient's emotional state consists of both mood and affect. *Mood* is a pervasive and sustained emotion experienced by the patient. *Affect* refers to the outward manifestation of mood (i.e., the way the patient shows feelings). Mood and affect are not always the same. The range of emotions patients report and display is vast and includes depression, despair, hopelessness, anger, irritability, tenseness, anxiety, panic, terror, elation, emptiness, guilt, and self-loathing.

Mood

Patients often volunteer information about how they feel during an interview, but it may be helpful to ask about mood (e.g., "How would you describe your general mood recently?"). If it is possible, use the patient's own words to report the quality and intensity of mood, and note whether the patient reports a change in mood in the course of the interview.

Affect

Predominant affect. During the course of the interview, carefully note the patient's predominant expression of emotion (e.g., depression, elation).

Variability. Normally, emotional tone varies in the course of conversation, from animated to subdued, from sad to happy, etc. Disturbances of affect often destroy this variability, so a depressed patient may not brighten up even when discussing pleasant subjects, and a manic patient may be incapable of maintaining a calm and sober attitude in the interview.

Intensity. Emotional reactivity may be increased or decreased. Increased reactivity is common among histrionic individuals, who show intense disproportionate emotional responses (e.g., rage if you arrive 2 minutes late). Decreased reactivity is also common: *blunted affect* refers to a generalized decrease in affective intensity, while *flat affect* describes a more extreme situation—the virtual absence of any evidence of emotion. Blunted and flat affect are classically seen in schizophrenia. Blunted affect is also a symptom of Parkinson's disease. Antipsychotic (neuroleptic) medications commonly cause parkinsonian side effects, and blunted affect is often seen among those patients taking these medications (see Chapter 18).

Lability. Watch for rapidly shifting and unstable emotional reactions, particularly among patients who suffer from affective disorders. Depressed people are often unable to control sudden tearful outbursts, while manic individuals experience uncontrollable bouts of rage or laughter. People with borderline personality disorder often display labile affect.

Appropriateness. You must judge whether the patient's affective responses are appropriate to his or her thought content and to the interview situation. For example, the patient who speaks with apparent indifference about a recent death in the family or abandonment by a spouse may unconsciously be trying to avoid experiencing the consequent emotional pain.

Thought

You evaluate thought processes and thought content based on what the patient says. *Thought process* refers to the way the patient puts ideas together—to the associations between ideas and to the form and flow of thoughts in conversation. *Thought content* refers to ideas the patient communicates. A *thought disorder* is a disturbance of content or process, or of both. A *formal thought disorder* specifically denotes abnormal thought process.

Thought process

Rate and flow of ideas. Patients frequently use the term *racing thoughts* to describe being flooded with ideas and unable to keep up with them. This condition is often seen in anxiety states, as well as in psychosis (e.g., mania, schizophrenia). If you suspect this condition, you might ask, "Do your thoughts ever go so fast you cannot keep up with them?"

In the case of *retarded or slowed thoughts*, people experience their thinking as slowed down, and may consider their minds empty of thoughts. This condition is seen in depressed people.

Circumstantiality involves thinking that is indirect in reaching a goal or getting to the point. This style is common in obsessional people and in schizophrenic patients.

Blocking is a sudden obstruction or interruption in the spontaneous flow of thought, perceived by the patient as an absence or deprivation of thought. It is seen in schizophrenia and in severe anxiety states.

Perseveration is the tendency to emit the same verbal response again and again to varied stimuli. This may range from constant repetition of one word or phrase (e.g., "night and day, night and day, night and day . . . "), to an inability to shift the focus of conversation away from one particular topic.

Associations. Associations are the relationships between ideas. Normally, these relationships are intelligible to the listener (i.e., one idea seems to follow from another). Disturbances in the associative process may be quite subtle, and when one idea does not appear to follow from another, you may erroneously assume that your attention lapsed from what the patient was saying. When something does not appear to make sense, *always* ask for clarification.

Loose associations involve the shifting of ideas from one subject to another in an oblique or unrelated manner; the speaker is generally unaware of the disturbance. An example of a loose association is, "I'm tired; all people have toes." Loose associations are commonly seen in psychotic states.

Flight of ideas is skipping verbally from one idea to another. Speech is fragmented, and associations are determined by chance or by temporal factors. This is commonly seen in patients who are manic.

Tangentiality is a style of speech in which the individual replies to questions in an oblique or irrelevant way. (For example, when asked about his mother's illness, a patient embarks on a lengthy discussion of the various "get well" cards his mother has received.)

Clanging involves using the sound of a word, rather than its meaning, to give direction to the flow of ideas (e.g., "I'm sad, mad, bad.") It is sometimes present in mania.

Punning is used in a similar way, substituting for logic as a means of associating one idea with another; it is seen in mania (e.g., "What's the weather like? Is the sun out? He is out in the yard playing with his new football.").

Other abnormalities of thought process. These may include the following:

Neologisms are new words or condensations of several words that are not readily understood by others. This disturbance is seen in schizophrenia and organic brain syndromes (e.g., a paranoid man used "plickening" to mean "the plot thickens").

Word salad is a jumble of words and phrases lacking comprehensive meaning or logical coherence. It is characteristic of schizophrenia.

Echolalia is a parrot-like repetition of another's speech. It is observed in mania and in organic brain syndromes.

Thought content

Patients' ideas about themselves and the world are frequently at the core of their presenting problems. Careful exploration of unusual or pervasive thoughts will often assist you in making a diagnosis. Here are two helpful rules to keep in mind when assessing thought content:

1. *Always* ask for clarification when you do not understand something the patient has said.
2. Begin with general questions and move on to specific ones.

Some open-ended questions for assessing abnormal thought content are the following: "Have you had any unusual or troublesome experiences?" "Have you had any strange or disturbing thoughts?" "Have you had thoughts you feel other people would not understand?" If you get positive answers to any of these general questions, explore unusual thoughts in more detail, using the categories below.

Delusions. A delusion is a false belief firmly held despite incontrovertible and obvious proof or evidence to the contrary. Further, the belief is not one ordinarily accepted by other members of the person's culture or subculture. Delusions are hallmarks of psychotic illness, although they do not occur in all psychotic individuals. These beliefs may affect all areas of a person's thought and functioning, or they may be "encapsulated" and confined to one particular topic. Examples of delusions are illustrated in Table 4-2.

Delusions of grandeur are exaggerated ideas of one's importance or identity (e.g., "I am the Messiah"). You may discover these with such questions as "Do you feel you have special knowledge or powers?"

Delusions of persecution are ideas that one has been singled out for harassment (e.g., "The FBI is out to get me"). Interview questions might include "Do you think anyone wants to hurt you or has spread lies about you?"

Delusions of control refer to the idea that one's feelings, thoughts, or actions are imposed by some external source (e.g., "A computer puts these angry thoughts in my head") or, conversely, that one can control others' feelings, thoughts, or actions. To elicit such thoughts, you might ask, "Have you felt that your thoughts were influenced or controlled by some outside force?" or "Do you feel that you can control the thoughts of others?"

Somatic delusions are false beliefs about body image or body function (e.g., "I don't care what the doctors say; I know that I have cancer"). You might explore somatic delusions with a general question: "Has anything unusual happened to your body?" or "Do you have any particular worries about your body?"

Table 4-2. Types of delusions

Delusions of grandeur
  "I am the Messiah."
Delusions of persecution
  "The FBI is out to get me."
Delusions of control
  "A computer puts these angry thoughts in my head."
Somatic delusions
  "I don't care what the doctors say; I know that I have cancer."
Thought broadcasting
  "People always know what I'm thinking."
Ideas of reference
  "The President sends me special messages during his television press
  conferences."

Thought broadcasting is the notion that other people can read one's thoughts. Your question could be, "Do you feel that others can hear your thoughts or read your mind?"

Ideas of reference involve incorrectly interpreting casual incidents and external events as having direct personal reference. These ideas often reach delusional proportions; that is, the person believes them despite evidence that they are false (e.g., "That newspaper headline was a secret signal to me from the President that he needs my help in Washington"). You may elicit such ideas with a question like "Do you feel you receive special messages that others do not (on television, over the radio, etc.)?"

Depersonalization and derealization. Depersonalization is a sense of unreality or strangeness concerning the self, manifested by feeling detached from and being an outside observer of one's mental processes or body, or by feeling like an automaton or as if in a dream. A patient who experiences depersonalization may describe feeling like "I have stepped outside of myself and am watching myself do things." Derealization refers to feeling detached from one's environment so that a sense of the reality of the external world is lost (e.g., "I feel as if everything is unreal and those around me are actors in a play"). Depersonalization and derealization are common in anxiety states as well as in borderline personality disorder. Occasional mild *dissociative episodes* (as they are called) are common among people of all ages, particularly adolescents and young adults.

Preoccupations. An *obsession* is a persistent, unwanted idea that cannot be eliminated by logic or reasoning. The obsessive thought is usually consciously distasteful to the person but is often unconsciously desired (e.g., "I'm afraid my father will be hit by a truck"). Obsessive thoughts often occur along with *compulsions*, which are persistent unwanted urges to perform acts that are contrary to one's ordinary wishes (e.g., compulsive hand-washing).

A *phobia* is an obsessive, persistent, unrealistic fear of an object or situation. Some common phobias are *acrophobia* (fear of heights), *agoraphobia* (fear of leaving a familiar home setting, fear of open spaces), *claustrophobia* (fear of closed spaces), *mysophobia* (fear of dirt and germs), and *xenophobia* (fear of strangers). (For a detailed discussion of phobias, see Chapter 8.)

Morbid preoccupations (e.g., with guilt or death) are often found in depressed people. When these concerns with personal guilt and worthlessness are frankly out of touch with reality, they are said to be of delusional proportions.

Suicidal and homicidal ideation. Assessment of suicidal and homicidal thoughts are part of *every* MSE. Actively raise these issues in the first interview with *every new patient*. This includes assessing thoughts, plans, potential for action, deterrents to action, and the patient's feelings about these suicidal and/or homicidal ideas. If you have reason to suspect that a patient may become suicidal or homicidal, you must constantly reassess and monitor these aspects of the patient's mental status. (For a discussion of suicidal and homicidal patients, see Chapters 15 and 16, respectively.)

Perception

Human beings are continually barraged by a wide range of stimuli from the five senses. Perceptual disorders involve misinterpreting sensory input (an *illusion*) or perceiving sensory input in the absence of any actual external stimulus (a *hallucination*). Thus, hearing one's name in a train whistle is an illusion, while hearing one's name called in a silent room is a hallucination.

Illusions

Illusions may be of pathological or nonpathological origin. Seeing a face in a cloud and hearing voices in the rustle of leaves are common experiences, but, in the face of reasonable evidence, the normal person recognizes these as misinterpretations. However, illusions also occur in toxic states (e.g., drug intoxication), in acute anxiety states, and in schizophrenia.

Hallucinations

Hallucinations are perceptions the patient believes to be real despite evidence to the contrary (i.e., the patient perceives something that does not exist). Hallucinations are invariably symptoms of psychosis and may be seen in all types of psychotic illness. They may also be induced by such factors as drugs, alcohol, and stress. They may involve any of the five senses.

Helpful general questions for eliciting reports of hallucinations include the following: "Do you ever hear voices or see things other people do not hear or see?" "Does your mind ever play tricks on you?"

Auditory hallucinations are the most common in psychiatric illness, particularly in schizophrenia. It is useful to document what the patient hears and to ask the identity of the speakers (e.g., "I hear my mother's voice telling me to kill myself").

Visual hallucinations are less common than auditory ones but are often found in toxic psychoses and, less often, in schizophrenia and mania (e.g., "I see a devil with red eyes staring at me").

Olfactory hallucinations (smell) are encountered in schizophrenia and with lesions of the temporal lobe of the brain.

Gustatory hallucinations (taste) are rare and are usually associated with olfactory hallucinations.

Tactile hallucinations (touch) occur mainly in toxic states (e.g., in the toxic state resulting from liver failure) and drug withdrawal syndromes. For example, the sensation that insects are crawling under the skin occurs in delirium tremens ("d.t.'s") and in cocaine toxicity.

In evaluating hallucinatory experiences, it is important to note the *circumstances* in which hallucinations occur, with an eye to possible precipitating factors (e.g., "What was going on when you heard these voices?"). Also note the *content* of the hallucinations (e.g., threatening, benign, grandiose, accusatory, religious, sexual). Content often provides important clues to the patient's fears and wishes, and may identify general areas of intrapsychic conflict. Your questions might include "Whose face did you see in the dark?" or "Whose voice was it, and what did they say?"

Always try to ascertain whether the patient's consciousness is clear or clouded at the time the hallucinations occur. If consciousness is clouded, look to drugs and organic processes (physical illnesses) as likely causes. A careful history of drug and alcohol use is critical to understanding hallucinations diagnostically.

Be sure to differentiate pathological hallucinations from *hypnagogic* hallucinations, which are false sensory perceptions healthy people experience midway between being awake and falling asleep.

Finally, be alert to unreported hallucinatory experiences during the interview—for example, when the patient does not attend well to you and instead appears to be paying attention and even responding to internal stimuli.

Sensorium and Intellectual Functions

Mental illness commonly involves disturbances in cognitive functioning. A person who is overwhelmed with emotional difficulties (as in depression) or flooded with internal stimuli (as in psychosis) is often unable to focus energy and attention on ordinary intellectual tasks. Dementia is a mental disorder in which the primary symptom is a loss of intellectual function.

This area of the MSE is the main one in which specific tests can be of use in the clinical interview (see Table 4-3). However, only test particular intellectual functions if the patient's history or behavior in the interview gives you reason to suspect derangement. Further evaluation can be

Table 4-3. Tests of cognitive functioning

Function	Test
Orientation	
Time	"What is today's date?"
Place	"What is the name of this place?"
Person	"What is your full name?"
Concentration	Serial 7's (or 3's)—ask the patient to subtract 7's (or 3's) in succession, starting from 100.
	Counting backward from 20.
Memory	
Immediate	Digit span—ask the patient to repeat a series of random numbers, first forward and then backward.
Recent	Ask the patient to remember three unrelated objects and recall them after 15 minutes.
Remote	Ask about names and dates from the patient's earlier life; ask the patient to name the U.S. presidents beginning with the current one and going backwards.
Fund of knowledge	"Who is the vice-president of the United States?"
	"What are the colors of the American flag?"
	"How far is it from New York to Los Angeles?"
	"What is a thermometer?"
Abstraction	Proverbs—ask the patient to interpret a proverb (e.g., "A stitch in time saves nine").
	Similarities—ask the patient what two things have in common (e.g., table and chair).
Judgment	Ask what the patient would do in a social situation that requires judgment (e.g., on smelling smoke in a crowded theater).

accomplished by observing the patient over time or by obtaining psychological and neuropsychological testing.

Consciousness

The presence or absence of a clear state of consciousness is a crucial factor in diagnosis. Clouded or fluctuating levels of consciousness suggest an organic etiology (drug or metabolic toxicity, organic brain syndromes). Record whether the patient is *hyperalert, alert, drowsy, confused, stuporous,* or *unconscious*. Note whether alertness is steady or varies during the interview. Patients with altered states of consciousness commonly show some impairment in orientation, although the reverse is not necessarily true.

Orientation

Awareness of *time,* of *place,* and of *person* are basic cognitive capacities that remain intact even in many severely disturbed mental states. Disturbances in orientation are common in delirium, dementia, and drug-induced psychosis, but they are less commonly found in people with acute affective illnesses and schizophrenic disorders. When you have no reason to suspect disorientation from the patient's behavior or your clinical interview, you need not ask about it specifically. You can test for orientation with a few simple questions:

1. *Time.* Ask the time of day (approximate), day of the week, season, and year (for example, "What is today's date?"). People who have been hospitalized for long periods, or even people on long vacations, commonly miss the date by a day or two and miss the day of the week by one. This does not, in and of itself, signify any abnormality.
2. *Place.* To assess orientation to place, ask if the patient knows the building you are in (hospital, office), as well as the street and town (for example, "What is the name of this place?"). If the patient is hospitalized, how long has he or she been there? If the patient knows the name of the hospital but you suspect more subtle disorientation, you might test further by asking the routes by which one would travel to the place of the interview.
3. *Person.* To assess orientation to person, ask whether the patient knows the names of the people who are in the room or involved in the patient's care, and what their relationship to the patient is. Only patients who are severely disoriented cease to know their own names. Among psychiatric patients, it is important to distinguish between disorientation to person and a delusional belief that one is someone else (e.g., Napoleon).

Concentration

Concentration is the ability to focus and maintain one's attention on a desired set of stimuli. A number of disorders can disturb this capacity, but it is most common in depression, anxiety, and psychosis. Severely demented patients also have difficulty with concentration, leaving off tasks in the middle. Gross disturbances in concentration will affect the patient's ability to pay attention and answer your questions during the interview. If you suspect abnormalities, the following tests are useful:

1. *Serial 7's (or 3's).* Ask the patient to subtract 7's (or 3's) in

succession, starting from 100. Most people will be able to perform five or more operations without difficulty, but those who have difficulty concentrating will rapidly lose track of their calculations.

2. *Counting backward.* Particularly if the patient's mathematical ability may be insufficient to perform the task of serial 7's, ask the patient to count backward from 20. Again, those with concentration difficulties are likely to drift away from the task before completing it.

Memory

Memory function is generally divided into three categories: immediate, recent, and remote. Much can be learned about memory as the patient tells his or her story during the interview. Test specific memory functions only when you have reason to suspect memory deficits on the basis of the patient's history and clinical condition.

Immediate memory. Use *digit span* to test immediate recall; that is, ask the patient to repeat a series of random numbers (e.g., 2–6–8–9–3–1–5) immediately after you, first forward, and then backward. Normal people can repeat an average of seven digits forward and five digits backward. However, when concentration is impaired (e.g., in depression), the patient may be unable to attend to the task and will *appear* to have a memory deficit when none exists. Similarly, this test may be difficult for people with minimal brain dysfunction and for those who are extremely anxious, even when no memory deficit is present.

Recent memory. Ask patients how they spent the last 24 hours and what they ate for breakfast, lunch, and dinner. Or ask them to remember three unrelated objects (e.g., lamp, umbrella, telephone) and then to recall these objects in 15 minutes.

Remote memory. Ask the patient important names and dates from his or her earlier life (e.g., birth, marriage, school, jobs), or ask about less personal past events (e.g., "Name as many presidents as you can, starting with the current one and going backward").

If memory impairment is observed, note the patient's reaction to the deficit and any efforts to cope with it. These efforts may include *denial* (acting as if the deficit did not exist), *confabulation* (inventing stories about situations or events that are not remembered), and *circumstantiality* ("beating around the bush" in an effort to mask the memory deficit). Patients who recognize their memory impairment may react to your questions with anxiety, depression, or hostility.

Memory deficits may be confined to particular time spans. In **amne-**

sia, a specific area of experience becomes inaccessible to conscious recall. *Anterograde amnesia* is memory loss for events that occurred after a significant point in time, while *retrograde amnesia* is memory loss for events that occurred before a significant point in time.

The number of disorders that can impair memory is great, but common causes include the following:

1. *Organic lesions as a result of tumors, strokes, or abuse of alcohol.* (Korsakoff's syndrome frequently involves short-term memory loss.) Both presenile and senile dementia also involve recent memory loss, initially without impairment of remote memory.
2. *Trauma.* Posttraumatic amnesia (e.g., after a concussion) is common and is usually predominantly anterograde with a mild retrograde component.
3. *Psychological disorders.* Depression, anxiety, and psychosis impair immediate and recent memory, along with concentration, by distracting the patient and making it difficult for him or her to focus on the environment. Whenever your interview indicates the presence of memory deficits, you should obtain psychological testing to characterize the problem in greater detail.

Fund of knowledge

A person's accumulation of knowledge is lifelong and varies with educational and cultural background. However, a person with chronic psychological disturbances may have difficulty in obtaining and processing information for long periods and will therefore have a poor fund of knowledge. This can usually be judged during the interview as the patient tells you about his or her life. If you need them, specific test questions or requests include the following:

- Who is the president of the United States?
- Who is the vice president?
- What arc the colors of the American flag?
- How far is it from New York to Los Angeles?
- Name three countries in the Middle East.
- What is a thermometer?

Abstraction

For adults, normal thought process involves the ability to shift from the specific to the general and to grasp the whole, as well as the particulars, of a given situation. The mind continually categorizes, relying on symbolic thinking to organize details. *Concrete thinking* involves difficulty in shifting from the specific to the abstract. This disorder is prevalent in the various forms of psychosis, particularly in schizophrenia. Concrete thinking can be masked in conversation, so if you suspect psychosis, use the following specific tests to assess the patient's powers of abstraction:

1. *Proverbs.* Ask the patient to interpret a proverb, couching it in terms of "How would you explain to someone the meaning of (the proverb)?" Use such proverbs as "A stitch in time saves nine," "A rolling stone gathers no moss," and "People who live in glass houses shouldn't throw stones." Obviously, there are no "right answers" in interpreting proverbs. However, people whose thinking is overly concrete will be unable to infer general meaning from the particulars. For example, a concrete interpretation of the "glass houses" proverb might be, "If you throw rocks at others, they'll throw rocks back and break your glass house."

2. *Similarities.* Our ability to see relationships among seemingly different things is based on a capacity for abstract thinking. You can test this capacity by asking about similarities—"What do these things (e.g., apple and orange; table and chair; baseball and tomato) have in common?" A person whose thinking is very concrete will have difficulty seeing any relationships between these objects.

Judgment

As you listen to the patient's history, you should learn a great deal about his or her ability to make and carry out plans and to discriminate accurately and behave appropriately in social situations. People who have poor impulse control or who have been inadequately socialized will often demonstrate faulty judgment. Drug abuse, brain damage, psychosis, depression, and anxiety are among the many causes of impaired judgment.

Formal questions to assess judgment include the following: "What would you do if you smelled smoke in a crowded theater?" (e.g., run, scream "Fire!," get up and leave, tell the usher). "What would you do if you found a stamped, addressed letter on the ground?" (e.g., mail it, or read it).

Insight

Insight refers to patients' awareness and understanding of their illness. People vary enormously in how accurately they perceive themselves and their problems.

Some helpful questions in evaluating insight are the following: "What are your reasons for seeking help?" "Do you feel that you have emotional problems right now?" "Do you feel that you need help in understanding and learning to cope with these problems?"

Attitude Toward the Interviewer

Attitude is the patient's response to you, the interviewer. Mental disorders commonly involve disturbed interpersonal relationships. During a clinical interview, the patient may display such problems by acting them out with you—for example, by adopting an attitude of hostility or seductiveness that is inappropriate to the interview situation. Patients often adopt surface attitudes in an effort to compensate for deeper problems—for example, a frightened man may adopt a hostile and aggressive manner in an effort to hide his fear. Attitudes provide valuable clues to how people defend themselves against unpleasant feelings.

Although it is not sufficient for diagnosis, the patient's attitude can lend support to tentative diagnostic formulations. Paranoid individuals are characteristically suspicious, evasive, and arrogant, while manic people are frequently impatient and uncooperative. Schizophrenic individuals manifest reserved, remote, and seemingly unfeeling attitudes; depressed people are often apathetic, hopeless, and helpless. People with organic brain syndromes (e.g., dementia) classically demonstrate distractibility and apparent indifference to their condition. The following considerations are important in documenting attitude:

- In what ways does the patient engage or distance you?
- Does the patient become more or less comfortable as the interview proceeds?
- Does the patient show an ability to form an alliance and work with you?

REPORTING THE MENTAL STATUS EXAMINATION

When you report a MSE to others orally or in writing, follow the outline in Table 4-1 (see above). Each major category of the MSE (appearance and behavior, speech, emotions, etc.) should be mentioned in its proper order, and when there are no abnormalities you may be brief (e.g., "Speech was clear and normal in rate").

Although you may use many of the terms defined in this chapter, beware of relying heavily on jargon, for it does not convey an adequate picture of a person's mental state. Particularly when you document abnormal findings, use specific examples and quotations from the interview to illustrate your points. For example, it is not enough to report "auditory hallucinations"; instead, note that "the patient reported hearing his mother's voice calling his name during the interview."

Report the MSE with enough detail so that a reader or listener who does not know the patient can get a clear understanding of the patient's state of mind at the time of the interview. The two examples presented below are designed to show you how two very different patients might be described.

Case Examples

The following examples will give you some perspective on what is involved in recording an MSE. It need not be a long and overly detailed endeavor. The MSE report can usually be written in one paragraph, but this will depend on the requirements of the mental health care facility in which you are working. Be sure to report the findings of the MSE in the order given in this chapter.

Example 1. Mr. A is a well-functioning man who presented to an outpatient clinic with mild anxiety and marital difficulties. His MSE is provided below:

> Mr. A presented as a tall, slender, well-dressed, meticulously groomed man who looked his stated age of 35. He sat stiffly during the meeting, with a worried facial expression, and made intermittent eye contact with the interviewer. Speech was clear and normal in rate but at times halting, mood was moderately depressed and anxious, and affect varied appropriately with the content of the interview. No abnormalities of thought or perception were noted, and the patient denied any current suicidal or homicidal ideation. Intellectual functioning was grossly intact with apparent above-average intelligence, good judgment, and moderate insight into the nature of his difficulties. Mr. A related to the interviewer in a formal and deferential manner throughout the meeting.

Example 2. Mrs. B is a chronic schizophrenic woman who was being readmitted to a psychiatric hospital for an acute exacerbation of her psychosis and suicidal impulses. Her MSE is as follows:

> Mrs. B is an obese, disheveled-looking woman who presented with poor

personal hygiene and looked older than her stated age of 46. She sat hunched over in her chair during the interview, with a fixed and bland facial expression, staring at the clock on the wall. She occasionally grimaced and made continuous rapid darting movements with her tongue. Speech was slow and halting, and at times quite loud. She reported "feeling like I'm dead," and her affect was flat and did not vary during the interview. Abnormalities of thought process included occasional episodes of racing thoughts during the interview, loose associations, and tangential replies to questions. The patient also used neologisms infrequently (e.g.,"glidders," "crickly"). She insisted that the CIA was trying to poison her, and she reported believing that CIA agents could hear her thoughts. She denied homicidal ideation but reported urges to harm herself using knives "because I would enjoy seeing the blood run out my veins." She reported seeing men in military uniforms with rifles standing in each corner of the interview room waiting to take her prisoner, but denied any auditory hallucinations. She was oriented to time, place, and person, and her intelligence appeared to be average. There were marked cognitive impairments, notably in concentration (she could only repeat three of seven digits and could not count backwards from 20 beyond 15). Recent memory function was difficult to assess because of her distractibility. Remote memory (date of birth, marital history) was grossly intact. Thinking was markedly concrete on proverb interpretation ("People who have large windows might get them broken with rocks"), judgment was poor, and she had little insight into the nature of her illness. She related to the interviewer in an aloof manner.

BIBLIOGRAPHY

Donnelly J, Rosenberg M, Fleeson WP: The evolution of the mental status—past and future. Am J Psychiatry 126:997–1002, 1970

MacKinnon RA, Yudofsky SC: The Psychiatric Evaluation in Clinical Practice. Philadelphia, PA, JB Lippincott, 1986, pp 58–84

Nicholi AM Jr: History and mental status, in The New Harvard Guide to Psychiatry. Edited by Nicholi AM Jr. Cambridge, MA, Harvard University Press, 1988, pp 29–45

Stone EM: American Psychiatric Glossary, 6th Edition. Washington, DC, American Psychiatric Press, 1988

Part II   Basic Psychopathology

5 Schizophrenia   79
6 Mood Disorders   103
   Unipolar Disorders (Depressive Disorders)   105
   Bipolar Disorders (Manic-Depressive Illness)   127
7 Personality Disorders   145
8 Anxiety, Phobias, Dissociative Disorders, and Somatoform
   Disorders   199

INTRODUCTION

The revised third edition of the *Diagnostic and Statistical Manual of Mental Disorders* (DSM-III-R) lists more than 100 mental disorders. Obviously, you cannot be introduced to all of them at once, nor would such an introduction be of much use to you as a beginning student. You will get a better understanding of mental illness if you familiarize yourself with the more common disorders first and then expand your knowledge to more esoteric subjects as your clinical experience deepens.

This section includes the syndromes you are most likely to encounter as you work in outpatient and inpatient mental health facilities. Chapter 5 focuses on schizophrenia, an illness that accounts for a substantial proportion of those who are chronically mentally ill. Chapter 6 deals with mood disturbances (depression and mania), and Chapter 7, with personality disorders, two categories that encompass much of the psychopathology you will see in your clinical work.

The discussion of personality disorders in Chapter 7 is designed to introduce you to various character styles, as well as to the personality disorders themselves. Because features of human personality such as obsessive-compulsive traits are common both to normal and to neurotic people, as well as to those with personality disorders, an understanding of personality types is relevant to every patient you see, not just those who fit the DSM-III-R criteria for personality disorders.

Chapter 8 deals with anxiety disorders, which are the most prevalent psychiatric disorders in our society, and somatoform disorders, which are commonly seen by general practitioners of medicine. Both agoraphobia and panic attacks have been the focus of much research and public attention in recent years. Dissociative disorders have also been of increasing interest, both to psychiatrists and to the general public.

The literature on each of the disorders in this section is vast. The following chapters are meant to serve as starting points from which you can go on to do further reading.

5

Schizophrenia

MORE THAN A CENTURY ago the French psychiatrist Benedict-Augustin Morel watched a 14-year-old boy deteriorate rapidly because of a severe mental illness. The boy had been a good student, but in a matter of months he seemed to have become "demented"—his thoughts were confused and his behavior disorganized. Morel called this devastating illness *demence précoce* (precocious dementia). The term came to be widely used to describe a syndrome we now know as *schizophrenia*.

Schizophrenia has been described as the "cancer" of mental illness; in fact, the two conditions are similar in many ways. We do not know what causes schizophrenia, nor do we know how to prevent it; our efforts at managing the illness once it occurs have met with limited success. The emotional and financial costs of schizophrenia to those who suffer from the illness and to their families are often astronomical. The pessimism with which many lay people and mental health professionals approach the schizophrenic individual resembles the aversion often shown to cancer victims.

What is schizophrenia? It is a syndrome that involves a highly altered sense of inner and outer reality to which the afflicted person responds in ways that impair his or her life. This altered sense of reality—the psychotic core of the illness—shows itself in disturbances of perception, thinking, emotion, speech, and physical activity. The term literally means "splitting of the mind," and lay people often misuse the word to describe someone with a "split" or multiple personality. But schizophrenia refers instead to incongruity between different mental functions (e.g., between thought content and feeling, or between feeling and motor activity). The schizophrenic may, for example, talk of sad or terrifying events while laughing or showing no emotion whatsoever.

Schizophrenia is a syndrome that probably consists of multiple disorders with varying causes, courses, and treatment outcomes. The diagnostic label covers many different clinical pictures, and symptoms vary so greatly from one individual to another that it is impossible to present a classic picture of the disorder. The diagnosis may, for example, apply equally well to the hypervigilant scientist who suspects others of plotting against him, to the homemaker who believes she is controlled by her dead mother's voice, and to the withdrawn and apathetic teenager who broods incessantly on the reality of existence. Symptoms also vary within the same individual over time, so that a schizophrenic person who is psychotic and totally unable to function one week may next week be capable of better reality testing and able to perform simple menial tasks.

DIAGNOSIS

You must diagnose schizophrenia entirely on the basis of the patient's history and your observations, for we have no independent laboratory tests to verify the presence or absence of the disorder. Because the diagnosis has important implications for prognosis and treatment, mental health professionals have struggled for more than a century to arrive at precise criteria for identifying schizophrenic individuals. The latest effort—by the authors of the revised third edition of the *Diagnostic and Statistical Manual of Mental Disorders* (DSM-III-R)—is summarized in Table 5-1.

Because these criteria emphasize chronicity, you must get a history of psychotic symptoms over at least 6 months, or observe the person for some time, before you can make the diagnosis.

CHARACTERISTIC SYMPTOMS

What are the "characteristic" symptoms that must be present for at least 6 months in order to diagnose schizophrenia? The most common ones are described below. Patients may have only one symptom, or they may exhibit many simultaneously. However, *it is very important that the patient give clear signs of chronically disordered thinking.*

Table 5-1. DSM-III-R criteria (summarized) for the diagnosis of schizophrenia

Characteristic psychotic symptoms—most importantly, hallucinations or delusions.

Continuous signs of disturbance for at least 6 months, including an active phase of characteristic psychotic symptoms for at least 1 week.

Prodromal and/or residual phase of illness may make up some of the 6-month period of illness, characterized by at least two of the following:

1. Social isolation or withdrawal
2. Impaired functioning at job, in school, or at household tasks
3. Peculiar behavior (e.g., hoarding garbage)
4. Deterioration in personal hygiene and grooming
5. Blunted or inappropriate affect
6. Vague, circumstantial, or impoverished speech
7. Odd beliefs or magical thinking
8. Unusual perceptual experiences or illusions (e.g., sensing the presence of a force or person not actually there)
9. Lack of initiative, interests, or energy

Chronic course.

Symptoms are not due to an affective illness, an organic cause, or mental retardation.

Hallucinations. *Auditory hallucinations* are most common. They may consist of sounds, identifiable voices, or even continuous dialogues among several voices. These can be particularly dangerous to the patient, or to others, if hallucinated commands are obeyed. Many schizophrenic patients report hearing voices that comment on their behavior. Visual, tactile, and olfactory hallucinations occur less often in schizophrenia—they are more commonly associated with organic causes of psychosis.

Delusions. Falsely held beliefs that cannot be corrected by presenting the person with the facts are particularly common in schizophrenia. Often these involve erroneous notions about the permeability or transparency of the mind—for example, that one's thoughts are being controlled by an outside force, that thoughts are being inserted or withdrawn by an outside force, or that thoughts are being broadcast to others. Also common are ideas of reference and delusions of persecution (for discussion of these terms, see Chapter 4).

Emotional disturbance. Blunted or flattened emotional tone is the classic affective symptom of schizophrenia. People who exhibit flat affect can remain so expressionless that they appear to be wearing masks. Other emotional disturbances may accompany this disease, in particular, affect that is inappropriate to thought content (e.g., laughing about a friend's death).

Volitional disturbance. The person's will and ability to carry out plans may be paralyzed by negativism or by an irrational fear of his or her own destructive powers. (For example, a patient who believes that he has the power to single-handedly destroy the universe may be terrified lest he do so.)

Disturbed speech. Common disturbances of speech include loose associations, incoherence, concreteness, "private" language understood only by the patient, poverty of speech (little or no speech production), making up new words (neologisms), and echoing the speech of others (echolalia).

Disturbed motor activity. Activity may be markedly decreased, as in catatonia, or increased, as in excited states. Schizophrenic individuals may exhibit robot-like behavior, bizarre repetitive mannerisms, or echopraxia (mimicking others).

CLINICAL PICTURE

By themselves, these symptoms and diagnostic criteria cannot give you a feel for what people with schizophrenia are like. Although the clinical picture may vary greatly from one person to another, certain characteristics are common to most people who have the disease.

A person typically develops schizophrenia in adolescence or early adulthood. For example, the person may be a student whose grades begin to decline for no apparent reason and who begins to spend more time lying in bed "daydreaming." Or the person may be a homemaker who stops spending time with friends, instead spending time apparently lost in thought, and stops paying attention to her appearance. Onset of the disorder is usually insidious. The incipient schizophrenic individual often begins to communicate in ways that seem odd or nonsensical—for example, discussing some special personal meaning in a newspaper headline, or using words in eccentric ways. Performance at daily tasks declines as the person withdraws into his or her own world. The schizophrenic individual may initially show considerable anxiety and hypersensitivity to perceptual and interpersonal stimuli, but increasing absorption in an inner world makes it more and more difficult for him or her to pay attention to what is going on in the environment. This **prodromal phase** may last for days or months. However, some people do not develop schizophrenia in this way but suddenly experience a psychotic "break." Thus, the active phase may be the first sign of illness.

Whether or not there is a prodrome to the illness, all schizophrenic people have what is called an **active phase**, in which their psychosis is most evident and they appear most severely disturbed. It is in this phase that someone is likely to be convinced that he is Jesus Christ, or to believe that the KGB has poisoned his drinking water, or to insist that his intestines are riddled with cancer, despite doctors' assurances to the contrary. In this phase, a patient may believe that her thoughts are controlled by an office computer at her husband's office, or that her 5-year-old son is trying to murder her, or that she receives messages from her dead mother over a radio station. A schizophrenic individual may hear voices commanding him to collect garbage in his bedroom or to lead his family in jumping out a fifth-story window. Or he may see snipers shooting at him whenever he attempts to leave his house. Such delusions and hallucinations sound bizarre to us, but they are quite real to schizophrenic people and may prompt them to act in strange and dangerous ways. To complicate matters, schizophrenic individuals may be so withdrawn and guarded that they are unable to describe their psychotic symptoms to you. Or they may describe them without any show of feeling and thus give the false impression that they are not in any real distress.

The active phase of schizophrenia may last indefinitely or only a few weeks. When this phase subsides (with or without treatment), the schizophrenic person does not return to his or her baseline level of functioning but is left with chronic symptoms that constitute the **residual phase**. In many ways this phase is like the prodromal phase, in that the individual is usually not floridly psychotic or agitated, but is still obviously impaired. If hallucinations or delusions persist in this phase, they are usually less emotionally charged than before. Flattened affect is common, as is poor performance at work, at school, and at household tasks. In fact, impairment of functioning varies, so that some chronic schizophrenic people who are in the residual phase of their illness are able to work (albeit with reduced effectiveness), while others are unable to function at all or even to care for themselves.

Some require chronic care in psychiatric hospitals, but most are able to live either on their own or in community-based programs such as halfway houses (see the discussion of treatment below). Speech and thought commonly remain odd or eccentric, and schizophrenic individuals in the residual phase usually continue to behave in peculiar ways (e.g., talking to themselves in public) and remain socially withdrawn.

The most important feature of the residual phase is that the person remains impaired. A return to normal premorbid functioning is the exception rather than the rule. Thus, if you encounter a "schizophrenic" patient who gets back to baseline functioning after a psychotic episode, you should question your diagnosis and consider other possibilities (e.g., an affective disorder or drug-induced psychosis).

Once a first psychotic episode occurs, the schizophrenic person's clinical course is quite variable. A small number of people recover with little or no residual deficit, but the more common course is one of exacerbations and remissions of the illness throughout life. Some schizophrenic people have increasing residual impairment after each acute exacerbation of their psychosis, while others appear to stabilize at one suboptimal level of functioning.

How do you predict which schizophrenic individuals will have a deteriorating course and which will stabilize or get better? To date, we cannot make such predictions with much reliability. Some factors that have been correlated with specific outcomes among schizophrenic individuals are shown in Table 5-2.

Common and Dangerous Complications

Suicide and *suicide attempts* are common among schizophrenic individuals. Suicide is frequently attempted during the onset of a first psychotic episode, when schizophrenic people feel that something terrible is happening that they do not understand and that is beyond their control. Schizophrenic individuals also try to kill themselves during the periods of depression that occur in the course of the illness. Floridly psychotic individuals are at particular risk for suicide, because hallucinations or delusions may dictate self-destructive acts, and the individuals may obey these internal commands quite impulsively. Roughly 20% of schizophrenic people attempt suicide over the course of their illness, and 2% to 3% of schizophrenic individuals actually kill themselves.

Homicide is much rarer, although catatonic and paranoid people

Table 5-2. Factors that help predict the clinical course of schizophrenia

Poor prognosis	Good prognosis
Premorbidly withdrawn and isolative	Good premorbid social functioning
Premorbid personality disorder	No premorbid personality disorder
No identifiable precipitating events	Precipitating events
Insidious onset	Abrupt onset
Early onset (childhood, adolescence)	Mid-life onset
Little confusion in clinical picture	Confusion prominent in clinical picture
No family history of affective illness	Family history of affective illness

are more prone to violence than those in other categories. The incidence of homicides committed by schizophrenic patients is higher than that among the general population.

SUBTYPES OF SCHIZOPHRENIA

It has long been apparent that schizophrenia as a diagnostic umbrella covers a variety of clinical conditions, and many schemes of subcategories have been proposed that attempt to separate schizophrenic individuals according to symptoms, clinical course, and outcome. None of these schemes has been particularly successful. The subtypes of schizophrenia listed in DSM-III-R are of limited value in this respect, and many schizophrenic people do not fit neatly into any one diagnostic subcategory. Nevertheless, because you will hear these subtypes used in clinical work, they are described briefly below.

Disorganized type. The disorganized type includes the primary symptoms of incoherent speech and blunted or inappropriate affect, with extreme social impairment but without well-developed delusional systems. These people often have a history of poor premorbid functioning, experience an early and insidious onset of the illness, and follow a chronic course without significant remission.

Catatonic type. The catatonic type refers to a clinical picture dominated by psychomotor disturbance. This may take the form of catatonic stupor or rigidity, catatonic excitement, catatonic posturing, or negativism (see Chapter 4). For reasons that are unclear, this type is now relatively rare in Europe and North America.

Paranoid type. The paranoid type is quite common and involves the presence of grandiose, jealous, or persecutory delusions or hallucinations with persecutory or grandiose content. Unlike disorganized or catatonic schizophrenic people, paranoid schizophrenic individuals sometimes show very little impairment in functioning (e.g., a paranoid security expert may function adequately on the job). Gross disorganization of behavior is rare among paranoid schizophrenic individuals—they often speak clearly, and some can behave quite appropriately in social situations that do not arouse their paranoid fears. The onset of this type tends to occur later in life than does the onset of other subtypes, and symptoms remain more stable over time.

Undifferentiated type. The undifferentiated type is simply a category for schizophrenic people whose prominent psychotic symptoms do not fall within any of the main categories listed above.

Subtypes are probably most useful as a kind of shorthand for describing a specific clinical picture of schizophrenia. Do not worry much about classifying an individual by subtype; it is not usually of major importance to the patient's care. What *is* important, however, is that you be certain to take utmost care in differentiating schizophrenia from other diagnoses.

DIFFERENTIAL DIAGNOSIS

Accuracy in diagnosing schizophrenia is of critical importance, but it is the ideal rather than the reality in modern practice. Many disorders mimic schizophrenia, and schizophrenia varies so greatly in its clinical presentation that it is often mistaken for other syndromes. Because "schizophrenia" implies chronicity and intractability, the diagnostic label can have devastating effects on patients and families when applied incorrectly. On the other hand, correct diagnosis may provide some measure of relief to people who are struggling to understand the nature of their illness and to families who are attempting to plan for future care and proper treatment.

The process of differential diagnosis is often difficult, because there are several disorders that are commonly confused with schizophrenia and that must be ruled out before the diagnosis can be made with confidence.

Mood Disorders (Affective Illness)

Mania and psychotic depression often present with hallucinations, delusions, and bizarre behavior; they are easily confused with schizophrenia. (For a detailed discussion of mood disorders, see Chapter 6.) You should suspect a mood disorder in the following cases:

- When the patient develops prominent affective symptoms of depression or mania *before or along with* the onset of psychosis. (Schizophrenic individuals often show affective symptoms, but these symptoms occur *after* psychosis has developed, and often in reaction to it.)
- When the patient has a *complete* remission and functions normally between psychotic episodes.
- When the patient has a biological relative who has a history of a remitting psychotic illness, since this is more suggestive of a mood disorder.

Schizoaffective Disorder

This diagnosis is made when both chronic psychosis and mood disturbance are prominent and you are unable to distinguish between schizophrenia and a mood disorder. DSM-III-R uses the diagnosis to denote conditions that have at one time presented with both a schizophrenic and a mood disturbance, and at another time with psychotic symptoms but without mood symptoms (see Table 5-3).

Organic Mental Disorders

Organically based psychosis may look exactly like schizophrenia with respect to delusions, hallucinations, incoherence, and bizarre affect and behavior. The cause may be drugs (particularly amphetamines or phencyclidine), metabolic disease (e.g., liver failure), a neurological condition, or even infection. If disorientation, confusion, and impaired memory are prominent, it is a good rule of thumb to suspect underlying medical illness or drug toxicity. In evaluating acute psychosis, a thorough history, physical examination, and laboratory screening are essential to rule out medical illness (see Chapters 9 and 14).

Personality Disorders

Transient psychotic symptoms may occur in people with personality disorders—particularly in schizotypal, borderline, and schizoid individuals who become psychotic under stress. However, these people will recompensate completely within hours or days. It is the brevity of the

---

Table 5-3. DSM-III-R criteria for the diagnosis of schizoaffective disorder

A disturbance during which, at some time, there is either a major depressive or a manic syndrome concurrent with characteristic psychotic symptoms of schizophrenia.

During an episode of the disturbance, there have been delusions or hallucinations for at least 2 weeks, but no prominent mood symptoms.

Schizophrenia has been ruled out—that is, the duration of all episodes of a mood syndrome has not been brief relative to the total duration of the psychotic disturbance.

It cannot be established that an organic factor initiated and maintained the disturbance.

psychosis and the fact that the psychotic symptoms are felt to be "alien" that distinguish such people from schizophrenic individuals. Paranoid personality disorder involves pervasive suspicion and mistrust that impairs relationships with others, but it does *not* include delusions or other chronic symptoms of psychosis (see Chapter 7).

Paranoid Disorders

Paranoia is the dominant symptom in this condition. Psychosis may take the form of well-systematized delusional beliefs, but disordered thinking is not prominent, as it is in paranoid schizophrenia.

Brief Reactive Psychosis

This condition, which occurs in individuals under severe stress, may look exactly like schizophrenia. It is here that observing the patient over time is crucial, because reactive psychoses clear rapidly (days to weeks) without residual impairment. Reactive psychosis is frequently seen in adolescents.

EPIDEMIOLOGY

Schizophrenia is ubiquitous. It is found in every culture and in every part of the world, although with varying frequency. It affects men and women equally, and most people develop the illness in their late teens or early twenties. It is estimated that between 100,000 and 150,000 new cases of the disease are diagnosed annually in the United States. Between 500,000 and 1 million cases now exist in this country. At any given time, one-half to one percent of the population is suffering from a schizophrenic disorder.

Schizophrenia is more prevalent among lower socioeconomic groups within urban populations. Among the hypotheses put forward to account for this fact are 1) that downward mobility is forced on people by the debilitating effects of the illness, and 2) that the stresses of lower-socioeconomic class life (e.g., poverty, crime) serve as precipitants in those who are susceptible to schizophrenia. However, neither of these theories has been proven.

ETIOLOGY

The cause of schizophrenia has eluded researchers for years, and few people retain much hope that any single etiologic factor underlies this disorder. Research has been plagued by many difficulties, not the least of which has been the lack of an objective and universally accepted definition of the illness itself. Investigators have looked for a clear relationship between schizophrenia and gross pathological changes in the brain, early childhood development, metabolic disorders, neurochemical abnormalities, and endocrine dysfunction—thus far, without success.

Neurotransmitter Systems

To date, the most widely discussed notion of a biological cause of schizophrenia has been the *dopamine hypothesis*. This hypothesis is based on the idea that the mechanism of action of antipsychotic medications can shed light on the pathophysiology of the schizophrenic disorders that these medications treat.

Antipsychotic agents have been shown to block postsynaptic dopamine receptor sites in the brain. This has led investigators to speculate that schizophrenia might involve excessive levels of activity of dopamine as a neurotransmitter. The clinical efficacy of neuroleptic drugs is related more closely to their ability to block type-II (D_2) rather than type-I (D_1) dopamine receptors, and so the type-II receptor has received much recent attention.

The dopamine hypothesis would explain the therapeutic effects of antipsychotic drugs in schizophrenia, but it presents several problems:

1. Evidence of increased dopamine activity in the brains of schizophrenic patients has *not* been found.
2. Although the dopamine-blocking effects of these medications appear to coincide with their antipsychotic effects, it has *not* been shown that dopamine blockade is the mechanism by which psychosis is ameliorated.
3. These drugs are not specifically antischizophrenic, but have antipsychotic effects in other illnesses, such as mania and psychotic depression.
4. While many studies have found increases in D_2 receptors among schizophrenic patients, it is not clear whether this reflects an underlying disorder or whether this is the secondary effect of neuroleptic treatment.

Thus, the hypothesis of increased dopaminergic activity as a pathological process in schizophrenia remains unproven. Among the other neuroendocrine systems implicated in the pathogenesis of schizophrenia are those involving serotonin, norepinephrine, and gamma-aminobutyric acid (GABA)—but none consistently so. The neurobiology of schizophrenia remains an area of considerable research activity.

Brain Dysfunction

The brains of schizophrenic patients have been extensively studied for possible characteristic lesions. None have been found, and it appears that schizophrenic patients vary considerably in the extent to which they show abnormalities of structure and function. Some patients demonstrate marked cerebral atrophy, enlarged ventricles, diffuse neuropsychological deficits, and electroencephalogram (EEG) abnormalities, whereas other patients show little or no brain pathology or malfunction.

Recent advances in neurodiagnostic techniques have facilitated research in this area. Computed tomography (CT) scanning has shown ventricular enlargement and cortical sulcal enlargement in some series of schizophrenic patients, but these abnormalities have also been observed in patients with bipolar disorder and thus may not be specific to schizophrenia. Positron-emission tomography (PET) scanning has shown decreased levels of glucose metabolism in the frontal cortex of some schizophrenic patients, but these findings have not been replicable in all studies. Studies of regional cerebral blood flow (RCBF) using radioactive xenon have been equivocal: some suggest decreased frontal flow, and others show decreased flow throughout the brains of schizophrenic patients. Magnetic resonance imaging (MRI) is another of the new techniques used to search for brain abnormalities in schizophrenic patients. To date, no consistent findings have emerged from any of these avenues of research.

Heredity Versus Environment

To what extent is schizophrenia rooted in human genes? To what extent is it caused by the environment? Recent research has yielded important but inconclusive findings:

Genetics

The case for a genetic basis in schizophrenic disorders has been supported by a variety of studies, including *adoption studies*, which reveal a significant concentration of schizophrenia in the biological relatives of schizophrenic individuals reared in different environments; and *twin studies*, which show higher concordance for schizophrenia among identical twins than among fraternal twins. (In other words, when one twin is schizophrenic, the other is much more likely to be schizophrenic if the twins have identical genetic makeup.) Such studies lend support to the hypothesis that genetic factors play an important causal role in schizophrenia.

However, different studies of the genetic transmission of schizophrenia yield inconsistent results, suggesting that there is genetic heterogeneity among the group of patients we label "schizophrenic." So, for example, schizophrenic patients with gross brain abnormalities appear to have fewer biological relatives with schizophrenia than do those patients without gross brain pathology. This means that the contribution of genetics to the development of schizophrenia probably varies from patient to patient, and that "schizophrenic" patients must be separated into more homogeneous subgroups before any meaningful information about the genetic basis of this group of disorders can be obtained.

Environment

Genetics alone cannot explain why some individuals become schizophrenic while others do not. This is most clearly seen in pairs of monozygotic twins where only one of the twins is schizophrenic.

In looking for environmental causes, researchers have explored the hypothesis that people with one certain personality type (e.g., schizoid personality) are more vulnerable to schizophrenia than others; but in fact many different personality types are found among people who later develop schizophrenia. Investigators looking at family interactions have found evidence that the families of schizophrenic patients show more communication deviance (i.e., illogical, inconsistent, and/or tangential communications) and lower general competence than families that have no schizophrenia. However, this evidence of preexisting family pathology only establishes a casual (rather than causal) relationship between pathology in family functioning and schizophrenia. The idea of the "schizophrenogenic mother" who literally drives her child crazy has long since been abandoned for lack of empirical support.

No particular environmental factors have been convincingly shown to influence the etiology of schizophrenia. However, there appears to be an association between schizophrenia and perinatal trauma, as well as between schizophrenia and birth during the winter months. Contrary to earlier hypotheses that certain types of families *cause* schizophrenia, there is increasing evidence that the environments in which schizophrenic people grow up are quite diverse. This is important to note, because many families bear terrible burdens of guilt for what they believe to be their responsibility for the patient's illness. You can do an enormous amount of good for families simply by helping them to see that such guilt is unfounded, given our current knowledge about the nature of schizophrenia.

The causes of schizophrenia remain a mystery. Many clinicians posit an interactive relationship between genes and the environment, at least in the course of the illness, if not its etiology. It may be that a *vulnerability* to schizophrenia is transmitted genetically but that the development of the illness itself depends on the presence of environmental factors that have yet to be elucidated.

TREATMENT

The treatment of schizophrenia can be an arduous process for patients, families, and clinicians alike. No cure exists for this tenacious disease, so therapeutic efforts are aimed at management of symptoms and at social and psychological rehabilitation. Like cancer, schizophrenia has invited the discovery of "miracle cures," none of which has proved effective. The major treatment modalities we currently use—medications and psychosocial therapies, including hospitalization (see Table 5-4)—are all of limited efficacy and all have the potential to be harmful as well as helpful. Nevertheless, carefully designed treatment programs can help many schizophrenic patients to regain lost functioning and a greater sense of psychological well-being. Long-term support is necessary for most schizophrenic patients, to maximize both their ability to function and their quality of life.

Table 5-4. Major modalities used in treating schizophrenia

Psychosocial treatments
   Hospitalization
   Psychotherapy
   Rehabilitation—social, vocational
   Aftercare—day treatment, halfway houses
   Education about the illness for patients and families

Somatic therapies
   Antipsychotic medications
   Lithium
   ECT
   Antidepressants

Psychosocial Treatments

Hospitalization

Until the middle of this century, the treatment of choice for schizophrenia was long-term custodial care. Many schizophrenic patients remained in psychiatric hospitals most of their lives. Today, long-term inpatient treatment still occurs, but it has been largely eliminated by programs of *deinstitutionalization.* These programs are based on the idea that hospital stays should be short and used for crisis intervention, to stabilize schizophrenic individuals so they can return to life in their communities.

Advocates of this policy also argue that emphasis on returning to the community promotes greater personal autonomy and higher-level functioning than does a lengthy stay, during which people become accustomed to being cared for by others. Advocates of long-term hospitalization argue that lasting psychological change takes time and is more likely to occur in the protective and structured setting of an inpatient unit. At present, deinstitutionalization is the prevailing policy in mental health care; the number of schizophrenic inpatients in the United States has decreased by more than half in the last 20 years.

When should a schizophrenic patient be hospitalized?:

1. *At the onset of a first psychotic episode.* The patient is hospitalized to facilitate a thorough diagnostic workup, to keep the patient safe, and to initiate medication and psychosocial therapy while the patient is under close observation. These treatments can then be continued in an aftercare program when the patient is discharged.
2. *When the patient poses a danger to self or to others.* Suicidal and homicidal threats or gestures are especially serious among psychotic people, who may lack the judgment and impulse control to keep from acting on hallucinated commands or delusional beliefs.
3. *When the patient is unable to care for himself or herself.* People who cease to be able to protect, clothe, and feed themselves need support until their functioning returns. Some schizophrenic patients have been ill for so long that they have *never* learned to care for themselves. These people can benefit from the intensive social skills programs that are offered in many long-term treatment facilities.
4. *When the patient has lost important social supports.* Patients who function well with a network of supportive people and activities (family, friends, therapists, jobs) may decompensate

when this network is disrupted. Changes in home life, work, or treatment may precipitate loss of functioning, and even psychosis, warranting hospital admission and crisis intervention.

Note that the return of psychotic symptoms is not, in and of itself, an indication for hospitalization of schizophrenic patients. When community support exists and patients are not dangerous to themselves or others, crisis intervention with medication and/or intensified psychosocial treatment can be attempted on an outpatient basis.

Management of hospitalized schizophrenic patients. During acute episodes of psychosis, the schizophrenic patient's behavior may be difficult to manage. Many agitated, suicidal, and violent people require locked inpatient units. Verbal limits may be sufficient to control behavior, and threatening individuals often calm down when confronted with the fact that their behavior is frightening to others. Seclusion rooms (quiet, sparsely furnished areas) are helpful in decreasing the noise and activity around an overstimulated psychotic person who may be flooded with hallucinations and racing thoughts. When verbal limits, reassurance, and seclusion do not suffice to calm the person and control dangerous behavior, physical restraint and/or chemical restraint may be necessary (see Chapter 16).

As the acute symptoms subside, the schizophrenic patient can be integrated into the inpatient community. Ideally, the inpatient unit should have structured activities and group meetings in which people can improve their social skills, modify inappropriate behaviors, and support one another in coping with the stresses of their illnesses. This *milieu therapy* provides the backdrop for the action of medications and the individual and family therapies discussed below. A major focus of hospital admission should be careful planning of comprehensive treatment that can continue when the individual leaves the hospital.

The goals of hospitalization usually include resolution of a suicidal or homicidal crisis, improved hygiene and behavior to allow the person to return to life in the community, improved judgment and reality testing, stable remission of symptoms, the ability to care for oneself (with or without support) outside of the hospital, and the ability to comply with an outpatient treatment program. When these goals are achieved, when the patient has arranged a stable living situation, and when adequate outpatient treatment has been provided for, the patient is usually ready for discharge. Outpatient treatment may include medication, individual and/or group therapy, family therapy, day treatment, and job rehabilitation.

Repeated hospital admissions are the norm in schizophrenia. Nearly

70% of all admissions of schizophrenic people are readmissions. Frequently, a life crisis will prompt the patient to become disorganized, to discontinue medication and other treatment, and to decompensate to the point that hospitalization is required.

Psychotherapy

There is widespread disagreement about the type of psychotherapy that is helpful to schizophrenic patients.

Supportive individual psychotherapy is nonintensive "here and now" treatment in which the therapist actively assists the patient in understanding and coping with the reality of his or her illness and life circumstances. The focus is often on getting and keeping a job, getting along with family and friends, and making sense of social interactions. By contrast, **individual exploratory psychotherapy** is more intensive and focuses on the therapist-patient relationship as a "laboratory" in which patients can gain insight into their psychological makeup and achieve lasting intrapsychic change. Because schizophrenic patients are usually severely handicapped in their ability to be close to others, the first goal of most therapies is to establish a stable, trusting relationship between therapist and patient. Insight-oriented work often emphasizes the importance of helping the schizophrenic patient to label feelings and connect them to life experiences, and to explore feelings that may be so stressful for the patient that he or she lapses into disorganized ways of thinking. The efficacy of individual psychotherapy in the treatment of schizophrenia is a matter of controversy. There is general agreement that psychotherapy alone is not an effective treatment for most schizophrenic patients. However, the strong therapeutic alliance formed in individual therapy is often essential to the success of other forms of treatment such as medication and family work.

Group therapy has been used with some success in helping patients understand and change their inappropriate ways of dealing with others. The focus is often educational, and revolves around social skills training. For example, groups may work on such tasks as learning to start a conversation, learning to listen, being assertive, and giving and receiving criticism and praise. Groups can also focus on tasks of daily living, such as finding a job, planning a meal, and personal grooming.

Family therapy of schizophrenia has become the focus of intense interest in the last decade. Researchers have examined what is termed *expressed emotion* in families and its effect on the course of a schizophrenic person's illness. Expressed emotion refers to the degree to which family members are critical of the patient, the amount of hostility they express toward the patient, and their degree of emotional overinvolvement with the patient. Studies have found that schizophrenic patients who lived with families in which expressed emotion was high were much more likely to have relapses of illness than were patients who lived with families in which expressed emotion was low. Moreover, for patients in families with high expressed emotion, the relapse rate was strongly related to the amount of contact the patient had with the family.

While the amount of expressed criticism and hostility of family members toward a schizophrenic relative seems to be a predictor of relapse, it is not clear that such expressed negative emotion *causes* relapse. Thus, it is not possible to say that expressed emotion is an environmental determinant of poor outcome in schizophrenia. But this research has stimulated the development of psychoeducational techniques that are proving very useful in helping the families of schizophrenic patients, as well as the patients themselves. Family therapy uses education about the genetic and biological bases of schizophrenia to help reduce the family's guilt and self-blame for the patient's illness. It also helps families to become aware of stressors within the home that can increase the likelihood of relapse, and helps them improve their communication skills and problem-solving techniques to better cope with family life and the patient's illness.

The range of approaches to psychotherapy with schizophrenic patients is enormous. While family therapy promises to become a mainstay in the psychosocial treatment of schizophrenia, no single approach is indicated for all patients. The diversity of therapies thought to be effective in schizophrenia reflects the tremendous diversity of needs and personalities among schizophrenic individuals themselves.

Rehabilitation

Patients uniformly lose functioning in some areas of their lives as a result of schizophrenia and must overcome intrapsychic and environmental obstacles to resuming a productive life in the community. All too often, the very process of hospitalization prompts patients to allow others to take over their lives for them—one of the unfortunate side effects of chronic institutionalization. Schizophrenic patients therefore need help in learning or relearning skills for life in the community. Successful rehabilitation can be a tremendous boost to patients' self-esteem as they come to feel more competent at taking care of themselves. Such rehabilitation efforts usually include job training and practice in cooking and other household tasks. Ideally, rehabilitation begins when the schizophrenic patient is in the hospital, and continues after discharge.

Aftercare

The extent to which schizophrenic people can care for themselves outside a hospital setting varies enormously. Some are able to live independently, whereas others need total care on a 24-hour basis. People who can live outside a hospital but who require supervision in their daily activities (e.g., handling money, buying food) often do well in *halfway houses* or *cooperative apartments*, in which residents are supported by mental health professionals who either live in these facilities or staff them on a regular basis. However, such living arrangements are costly, and many schizophrenic people are cared for in private homes by family members or friends.

Along with support in a living situation, schizophrenic people who cannot work full-time or cannot work at all need structured daytime activities. For such people, *day treatment programs* are helpful. These programs are set up so that patients may spend all or part of the day in group activities and meetings designed to increase social and other skills, while providing close supervision of medication regimens for those who have difficulty with compliance. Day treatment programs are usually affiliated with hospitals or community mental health centers.

Somatic Therapies

Antipsychotic medications

Antipsychotic medications are the mainstay of somatic treatment in schizophrenia. They have revolutionized the management of this disease, both because of their acute sedative effects and because of their long-term antipsychotic effects. They do not cure the disease, but they have been shown to reduce confusion, anxiety, delusions, hallucinations, social isolation, and other symptoms of schizophrenia. (The principles of treatment are discussed in detail in Chapter 18.)

Antipsychotic medications are sedating; they may help calm agitated and acutely psychotic people within hours after treatment is begun. However, the maximum antipsychotic effect of these medications may not be reached for 6 weeks. The "positive" symptoms of schizophrenia (e.g., hallucinations, agitation) respond much better to antipsychotic medications than do the "negative" ones (e.g., apathy, negativism).

Once the acute psychotic symptoms of schizophrenia have been controlled (usually in 4 to 12 weeks), the dosage can be reduced to a maintenance level of 10% to 50% of the amount needed in the acute crisis. Carefully monitor the tapering of the dosage over several weeks so that it can be increased again at the first sign of a return of symptoms.

Patients who cannot comply with an outpatient regimen of oral medication may be maintained on intramuscular injections of fluphenazine decanoate (Prolixin) or haloperidol decanoate (Haldol) every 10 to 14 days. Schizophrenic patients who are not maintained on antipsychotic medication after an acute psychotic episode have a relapse rate significantly greater than that of those who continue to take their medication once a crisis has passed. Thus, long-term maintenance therapy with antipsychotic medication is indicated for a great many people diagnosed as schizophrenic.

However, people must not be kept on antipsychotics indefinitely without reevaluation of their need for medication. Patients who have a complete remission that lasts 12 months or more, and those who are stabilized on low maintenance doses of antipsychotics, deserve a trial off all medications for three reasons:

1. To determine whether a first psychotic episode was a reactive psychosis rather than the onset of a schizophrenic disorder. (This is particularly important in young people, many of whom recompensate quickly after a first psychotic break.)
2. To reduce the risk of adverse effects of neuroleptic medication, such as neuroleptic malignant syndrome and tardive dyskinesia, in people for whom maintenance medication is no longer essential (see Chapter 18).
3. To ascertain whether the patient is among a subgroup of schizophrenic individuals who do not require neuroleptic medication for adequate functioning.

The risks of long-term neuroleptic use have prompted clinicians to develop strategies for minimizing the total lifetime exposure of schizophrenic patients to these medications. A low-dose strategy involves maintaining patients on small doses of neuroleptics (as little as 10% of the usual clinical dose), reserving higher doses for periods of exacerbated illness. Intermittent strategies involve complete withdrawal of medication during periods of remission, with use of medication only when the patient seems to be in danger of relapse. Each patient's needs are different, so maintenance therapy must be tailored to the individual through a process of experimentation with different regimens.

Lithium

Lithium therapy has been found to be useful in a minority of people diagnosed as schizophrenic. It is not clear whether this is because lithium-responsive "schizophrenic" patients have been misdiagnosed and are really manic-depressive, or because there are some true schizophrenic patients who happen to respond to lithium. Particularly when the differential diagnosis between schizophrenia and mood disorder is difficult to make, a trial of lithium may be both diagnostic and therapeutic. Certainly, lithium therapy should be considered whenever affective symptoms are a prominent part of a psychotic illness (see Chapter 18).

Electroconvulsive therapy

Electroconvulsive therapy has been found useful in alleviating the symptoms of catatonic stupor and catatonic excitement. However, its efficacy in relieving other symptoms of schizophrenia has not been clearly demonstrated (see Chapter 18).

Antidepressants

Despite the "flat, affectless" stereotype, people with schizophrenic disorders do sometimes become depressed. They are particularly vulnerable to depression after an acute psychotic episode has cleared and they must come to terms with what has happened to them. However, if a schizophrenic patient appears apathetic, inactive, and in low spirits, you must rule out the possibility that he or she has been overtranquilized and is suffering parkinsonian side effects, rather than depression. (This can be done by testing the person's response to an antiparkinsonian drug or to lowering the dosage of the antipsychotic drug.) For people who seem genuinely depressed rather than overmedicated, it is often useful to add an antidepressant to the medication regimen (see Chapter 18). Observe such people closely, because tricyclic antidepressants can precipitate psychosis.

Controversy in the Treatment of Schizophrenia

The introduction of antipsychotic medications has had a powerful effect on the management of schizophrenia. Some psychopharmacologists argue that the only mode of treatment proven effective is medication and that human intervention in schizophrenia is of little use.

On the other hand, advocates of psychotherapy in schizophrenia argue that medication alone is not sufficient, that the effectiveness of medication depends on the psychosocial context in which it is given, and that medication only reduces psychotic symptoms but does not affect the patient's social or personality development.

In fact, there can be no single correct treatment, because "schizophrenia" almost certainly consists of multiple disorders. The range of treatments and combinations of treatments used effectively reflects the variability inherent in the disease itself. In other words, what is useful to some schizophrenic individuals may be useless or even harmful to others. *Most effective treatment regimens combine somatic and psychosocial therapies.*

Despite our best therapeutic efforts, schizophrenic people still occupy nearly half the psychiatric hospital beds in this country. And despite the effectiveness of new antipsychotic medications, the disease continues to leave a significant percentage of schizophrenic people with real deficits, while the prevalence of schizophrenia in the United States remains unchanged.

BIBLIOGRAPHY

American Psychiatric Association: Diagnostic and Statistical Manual of Mental Disorders, 3rd Edition, Revised. Washington, DC, American Psychiatric Association, 1987, pp 187–198. (For a full description of the diagnostic criteria for schizophrenia, you may want to consult this manual.)

Baldessarini RJ: Schizophrenia. N Engl J Med 297:988–995, 1977

Cancro R: Advances in the diagnosis and treatment of schizophrenic disorders, in American Handbook of Psychiatry, Vol 7, 2nd Revised Edition. Edited by Arieti S. New York, Basic Books, 1981, pp 285–296

Carpenter WT, Keith SJ: Integrating treatments in schizophrenia. Psychiatr Clin North Am 9:153–164, 1986

Falloon IRH: Family stress and schizophrenia: theory and practice. Psychiatr Clin North Am 9:165–182, 1986

Faraone SV, Tsuang MT: Quantitative models of the genetic transmission of schizophrenia. Psychol Bull 98:41–66, 1985

Green H: I Never Promised You a Rose Garden. New York, New American Library, 1977. (A moving fictionalized account of a young woman's experience of her illness and improvement during intensive psychotherapy.)

Gunderson JG: Major clinical controversies, in Psychotherapy of Schizophrenia. Edited by Gunderson JG, Mosher LR. New York, Jason Aronson, 1975, pp 3–22

Kanter J, Lamb HR, Loeper C: Expressed emotion in families: a critical review. Hosp Community Psychiatry 38:374–380, 1987

MacKinnon RA, Michels R: The Psychiatric Interview in Clinical Practice. Philadelphia, PA, WB Saunders, 1971, pp 230–258. (Contains useful material on the interview of an acutely psychotic patient.)

Matthysse S, Lipinski J: Biochemical aspects of schizophrenia. Ann Rev Med 26:551–565, 1975

Pope G Jr, Lipinski JF Jr: Diagnosis in schizophrenia and manic-depressive illness. Arch Gen Psychiatry 35:811–828, 1978

Schooler NR: The efficacy of antipsychotic drugs and family therapies in the maintenance treatment of schizophrenia. J Clin Psychopharmacol 6:11S–19S, 1986

Snyder SH: Neurotransmitters and CNS disease: schizophrenia. Lancet 2:970–973, 1983

Williamson P: Hypofrontality in schizophrenia: a review of the evidence. Can J Psychiatry 32:399–404, 1987

6

Mood Disorders

THE MOOD DISORDERS (also called "affective disorders") encompass a spectrum of emotions ranging from deep depression to unbounded elation and mania. An elated or depressed mood dominates the clinical picture, but mood is by no means the only problem for the patient with a mood disorder. Physical symptoms, self-destructive behavior, loss of social functioning, and impaired reality testing frequently go hand in hand with depression and mania, posing difficult and sometimes life-threatening problems for patients and their families.

We are all subject to mood changes in our daily lives. Feelings of sadness and disappointment are a normal part of human existence; fortunately, so are feelings of happiness and elation. How, then, do we distinguish normal moods from abnormal ones? On what basis are mood states labeled abnormal? Here are some questions to use in attempting to identify pathological mood changes:

- *How intense is the mood, and how long does it last?* Pathological mood states are unduly prolonged and severe.
- *Do physical symptoms accompany the mood change?* Impaired body functioning is common, including disturbances of sleep, appetite, and sexual activity.
- *Does the mood disrupt normal daily activities?* Impaired perfor-

mance often occurs in the usual social roles (e.g., home life, work, school, hobbies).

- *Is the patient's ability to recognize reality impaired?* For example, is the mood change accompanied by hallucinations, delusions, or confusion?
- *Does the mood put the patient or others in danger?* The danger may be direct (i.e., suicidal or homicidal intent) or indirect (as a result of impaired judgment).

As in so many other illnesses, the causes of mood disorders remain a mystery and are the subject of intense research and heated debate. Diagnosis rests almost entirely on the patient's history, symptoms, and behavior. However, because depression and elation can present themselves in many ways, diagnosis is not always easy. For years, clinicians have debated how best to fit the mood disorders into diagnostic categories, using different hypotheses about causation and various groupings of symptoms. The most basic and least controversial classification of mood disorders is the bipolar-unipolar dichotomy (Table 6-1).

Bipolar mood disorders are conditions in which both depression and elation are present at different times in the course of the illness, or, more rarely, disorders in which there are only episodes of elation. This category includes *bipolar disorder* (manic-depressive illness) and a milder form of bipolar illness, *cyclothymia.*

Unipolar mood disorders involve episodes of depression, but no episodes of elation. Depression may be chronic or episodic: it may recur again and again or occur only once. This category includes *major depressive disorder* and the milder and more chronic *dysthymia.*

The distinction between unipolar and bipolar illness has been made not only on the basis of symptoms but also on the basis of different genetic and familial patterns, different responses to intervention with medication, and different physical and biochemical characteristics.

Table 6-1. Major forms of affective illness

Type	Key to diagnosis

Bipolar
    Bipolar disorder (manic-depressive
        illness)
    Cyclothymia
	History of episodes of elation, with
	    or without a history of depression

Unipolar
    Major depression
    Dysthymia
	History of depression without any
	    history of elation

UNIPOLAR DISORDERS (DEPRESSIVE DISORDERS)

Depression is one of the most common of mental illnesses. All of us have friends, acquaintances, or relatives who have at some time been clinically depressed. In fact, at least 1 out of 10 adults experiences one or more episodes of depression during his or her lifetime. Researchers estimate the lifetime risk to be as high as 30%.

Some depressed people obtain professional help, but many others do not. Probably only 10% to 25% of those with depressive disorders seek treatment. It is essential that all practicing physicians and other health professionals recognize the signs and symptoms of these ubiquitous disorders.

The clinical picture of depression varies tremendously. One patient may present with tearfulness and self-reproaches, another with lower back pain and chronic fatigue, and a third may be terrified that his spouse is trying to kill him. Yet all three of these patients may have depressive disorders and may even respond to the same treatment modalities. No single symptom is present in all depressive syndromes. Feeling sad or "down in the dumps" is the most common experience of depressed people, but even a depressed mood is not universal. There are patients who report no mood disturbances but have the classic physical signs of depression and respond beautifully to treatment with antidepressant medication.

Symptoms

Given the variety of forms depression assumes, the list of symptoms is long. Some of the most common symptoms of the unipolar disorders are listed in Table 6-2 and described below, grouped according to the mental and physical functions they impair. A patient may be troubled by one or by many of these afflictions at any given time.

Affective symptoms

Depressed mood. More than 90% of depressed people experience prolonged moods of sadness or discouragement, or a sense of "not caring anymore." A depressed mood usually colors the patient's entire mental life; it is pervasive and dominant. A small percentage of depressed people do not experience a depressed mood but manifest other symptoms. One clue to the diagnosis in such cases is that the patient's situation often saddens the interviewer, even though the patient does not report sadness. Depressed children often do not complain of dysphoria but constantly wear sad facial expressions.

Table 6-2. The symptoms of depression

Affective	Motivational
Depressed mood	Loss of interest in usual activities
Anhedonia	Feelings of hopelessness and
Anxiety	helplessness
	Suicidal thoughts or acts
Vegetative	
Sleep disturbance	Cognitive
Appetite disturbance	Sense of guilt, worthlessness, and
Loss of energy	low self-esteem
Decreased libido	Difficulty in concentrating
Psychomotor retardation	Psychosis
Psychomotor agitation	
	Somatic
	Bodily complaints

Anhedonia. The inability to derive pleasure from previously pleasurable activities is an almost universal symptom of depression. Activities that may cease to be enjoyable include eating, sex, hobbies, sports, social events, and family functions.

Anxiety. Most depressed patients experience anxiety—that is, inner distress with dread, fear, or anticipation of danger—along with such autonomic nervous system dysfunctions as sweating, palpitations, rapid pulse, or "butterflies in the stomach." Consequently, because anxiety and depression often go hand in hand, it may be difficult to distinguish patients who are depressed from those who have primary anxiety disorders (see Chapter 8).

Vegetative symptoms

Vegetative symptoms refer to specific physical problems that often accompany a depressed mood. The presence or absence of these symptoms is of primary importance in predicting response to somatic therapies for depression. You should therefore inquire about vegetative symptoms whenever the diagnosis of depression is a possibility.

Sleep disturbance. The majority of depressed patients experience some form of insomnia. This may involve difficulty falling asleep (*early insomnia*); patients with this complaint often report "tossing and turning" while they ruminate on life events. Others complain of waking up during sleep—often from nightmares—and returning to sleep with difficulty (*middle insomnia*). Particularly common is early-morning awakening (*terminal insomnia*); patients wake up at 5:00 or 6:00 A.M. and cannot get back to sleep. Hypnotic medications (e.g., barbiturates, benzodiazepines) are often unsuccessful in prolonging sleep in depressed people, and antidepressants are generally more effective.

Although insomnia is the norm, some people—particularly children, young adults, and those with bipolar illness—experience *hypersomnia*, or sleeping too much.

Appetite disturbance. Many depressed people experience a loss of appetite (*anorexia*) with or without weight loss. In taking a patient's history, you should always document the amount of any weight loss and the period over which it occurred. Weight loss may be small or quite large, even life-threatening. A minority of people—particularly young women and people with bipolar illness—will experience overeating (*hyperphagia*) and binge eating (*bulimia*) as a symptom of depression. In such cases, weight gain usually results.

Loss of energy (anergia). Depressed people commonly experience fatigue and loss of energy in the absence of exertion and describe this as feeling "run down" or "like all the energy has been drained out" of their body. They may believe they suffer from a vitamin deficiency, and some severely depressed people believe that their decreased energy is caused by cancer or tuberculosis. Some experience *diurnal variation* in mood and energy level—that is, depression is worse in the morning and improves somewhat during the day.

Decreased libido. A loss of sexual interest and energy commonly plagues depressed people. It may cause an increase in marital tensions and a lowering of the patient's already fragile self-esteem. In men, the most common presenting symptom is impotence. You must inquire specifically about sexual dysfunction when depression is suspected, because many people are too embarrassed to volunteer such information.

Psychomotor retardation. Many depressed people exhibit an actual retardation of thought, speech, and action. Sparse replies to questions, monotonous and slowed speech, fixed gaze, and slowed body movements are all part of this syndrome, which may be severe enough to resemble catatonia.

Psychomotor agitation. Some depressed people—particularly the elderly—experience agitation rather than retardation. This involves an unpleasant restlessness or tension—an inability to relax or to sit still. Such people appear "fidgety." Unlike elated individuals, whose activity is purposeful, agitated people simply make tension-relieving efforts, such as hand-wringing, pacing, nail-biting, and hair-pulling.

Motivational symptoms

Loss of interest in usual activities. Depressed people experience not only a loss of pleasure but also a decrease in motivation, often in all areas of life. Work, home life, and other pursuits come to seem dull and uninteresting. Ability to perform one's usual tasks may decline.

Feelings of hopelessness and helplessness. People who are very depressed feel they cannot cope with even the smallest of tasks, including personal hygiene and grooming. Work, school, and household duties can suddenly appear unmanageable to the depressed person. The individual who sees nothing but misfortune in the future may lose all impetus to carry on. Getting out of bed in the morning may take hours.

Suicidal thoughts or acts. Suicide is the most serious complication of depressive disorders, and, unfortunately, it is all too common. One percent of all depressed patients kill themselves within 12 months after the onset of a depressive episode. Among patients who suffer from recurrent depressions, 15% eventually commit suicide. Depressed patients are at the highest risk for suicide in the 6- to 9-month period after they have achieved some symptomatic improvement. Why this seeming paradox? It may be because the patient has regained enough energy and motivation to carry out a suicide plan, but has not regained enough of a positive outlook on life to be able to choose an alternative to self-destruction.

Cognitive symptoms

Sense of guilt, worthlessness, and low self-esteem. People who are depressed often berate themselves for perceived shortcomings that they exaggerate but feel are obvious to others. Such people are unable to realistically evaluate their own performance at daily tasks. Their low self-esteem may vary from mild feelings of inadequacy to severely critical auditory hallucinations as described under "Psychosis" below.

Difficulty in concentrating. Depressed people may be so completely preoccupied with inner thoughts that they have difficulty paying attention to their environment. They often complain of "poor memory" or of being unable to keep their minds on such pastimes as reading or watching television. Because demented people also have problems with memory and concentration, it is sometimes difficult in the elderly to differentiate depression from dementia (see Chapter 9).

Psychosis. Depression may be severe enough to include psychotic symptoms, most commonly hallucinations and delusions. The content of these hallucinations and delusions is usually consistent with the depression (*mood congruent*). For example, psychotically depressed people may suffer from the deluded belief that they are being persecuted because they are sinful or inadequate ("My husband is trying to kill me because I'm a bad wife"); hallucinations frequently take the form of voices that berate depressed people for their shortcomings. *Mood-incongruent* psychotic symptoms occur less commonly, sometimes in the form of persecutory delusions.

Somatic symptoms

Besides the classic vegetative symptoms of depression, a variety of somatic symptoms are part of the depressive syndrome. In fact, internists and general practitioners of medicine are barraged with such complaints; the most frequent are headaches, backaches, muscle cramps, nausea, vomiting, constipation, heartburn, shortness of breath, hyperventilation, and chest pain. Many depressed people undergo various examinations, X-rays, and laboratory tests; some even undergo surgery. Too frequently, the diagnosis of depression is only considered after numerous diagnostic studies have failed to reveal an organic basis for the illness and the physician concludes that it is "all in the patient's head." Careful inquiry will often uncover other symptoms besides "aches and pains" that point more clearly to the diagnosis of depression.

Classifying Depressive Disorders—DSM-III-R Diagnostic Categories

The long list above makes it clear that there is tremendous variety among the symptoms of depression. The variations in types of depression become almost infinite when you consider precipitating factors, family histories, and clinical courses. Some people become depressed after obvious traumatic events; others seem to sink into depression for no apparent reason. Some patients have family trees laden with depressed relatives; others have no family history of mental illness. Some people experience discrete, limited episodes of depressive symptoms; others complain that they have been depressed all their lives.

How can we make sense out of this vast array of clinical presentations? Many classification systems have been proposed, most of them based on unproven theories about what causes depression. A newer system, based on symptoms and clinical course, is put forward in the *Diagnostic and Statistical Manual of Mental Disorders*, Third Edition–Revised (DSM-III-R).

DSM-III-R defines two basic depressive disorders: *major depression* (consisting of one or more major depressive episodes) and *dysthymia* (Table 6-3). In major depression, symptoms are severe and persistent, and

Table 6-3. Comparison of major depressive episode and dysthymia

Feature	Major depressive episode	Dysthymia
Dysphoric mood	Yes	Yes
Severity of symptoms	Severe	Mild to moderate
Impaired functioning	Common	Less common
Psychosis	May be present	Not present
Persistence of symptoms	Present every day	Usually fluctuating
Duration of symptoms	Every day for 2 weeks	On and off for 2 years

the illness has a discrete, episodic quality. In dysthymia, symptoms fluctuate and are less severe, psychosis is generally not present, and the illness is chronic and long-term.

Major depression

Major depression is characterized by 1) one or more major depressive episodes, depending on whether the depression is a single episode or recurrent, and 2) no evidence of a manic episode or an unequivocal hypomanic episode (see DSM-III-R, pp. 214–218, for diagnostic criteria of the latter episodes). The diagnostic criteria for a **major depressive episode** are as follows:

1. At least five of the following symptoms have been present during the same 2 weeks, representing a change from previous functioning. At least one of these must be *depressed mood* or *loss of interest or pleasure*:

   - Depressed mood most of the day or nearly every day, either reported by the patient or observed by others
   - Loss of interest or pleasure in almost all activities
   - Significant weight loss without dieting, or decreased appetite nearly every day
   - Insomnia or hypersomnia
   - Psychomotor agitation or retardation
   - Loss of energy or fatigue
   - Feelings of worthlessness, self-reproach, or guilt
   - Impaired ability to think clearly, concentrate, or make decisions
   - Suicidal ideation or recurrent thoughts of death

2. Depression is not due to another condition, such as bereavement, an organic factor, or an underlying schizophrenic disorder.
3. No psychotic symptoms during periods of normal mood.

Two subtypes of a major depressive episode are singled out in DSM-III-R for special mention:

Depression with melancholia (melancholic type): Includes at least five of the following nine symptoms:

- Loss of interest or pleasure in usual activities
- Lack of reactivity to usually pleasurable stimuli
- Worsening of depression in the morning
- Early morning awakening
- Psychomotor retardation or agitation
- Significant anorexia or weight loss
- No significant premorbid personality disturbance
- At least one previous major depressive episode followed by complete (or nearly complete) recovery
- A previous good response to somatic antidepressant therapy

The emphasis in this subtype is on vegetative signs and diurnal variation in mood—the classic picture of what has often been called "involutional melancholia."

Seasonal pattern depression: Involves regular onset and remission of affective episodes (depression and/or mania) at particular times of the year (e.g., onset always during October or November, with recovery in March or April). The diagnosis can be made once the patient has exhibited this pattern of illness in three separate years, and when seasonally timed episodes outnumber nonseasonal episodes by three to one.

Dysthymia

Dysthymia, also called *depressive neurosis*, has the following diagnostic criteria:

1. Depressed mood most of the day and on most days.
2. At least two of the following symptoms during periods of depression:

  - Poor appetite or overeating
  - Insomnia or hypersomnia

- Low energy level or fatigue
- Low self-esteem
- Decreased ability to concentrate; indecisiveness
- Feelings of hopelessness

3. During the 2-year period of dysthymia, a period of normal mood lasts no longer than 2 months at a time.
4. No evidence of a major depressive episode, no history of mania, and no known organic cause (e.g., antihypertensive medication).
5. The disorder is not superimposed on a chronic psychotic disorder (e.g., schizophrenia).
6. Another mental disorder may be present (e.g., a personality disorder or anxiety disorder).

Older Systems of Classification

The DSM-III-R diagnostic categories, now widely used, should replace older and less accurate systems. Some more traditional ways of classifying depression will be briefly described here, for they are still used by many clinicians, and you will continue to hear older diagnostic labels used in day-to-day clinical work.

Endogenous versus reactive depression

Endogenous versus reactive depression reflects a long-standing debate about the cause of depression.

Endogenous depression refers to a syndrome thought to come from inside—that is, it results from internal biological factors and seems to have a life of its own, rather than being dependent on environmental influences. The hallmarks of endogenous depression are prominent physiological disturbances (sleep, appetite, energy); absence of environmental precipitants (deaths, personal losses); and stable premorbid personality patterns without self-pity, hypochondriasis, or self-dramatizing attitudes.

Reactive depression, by contrast, refers to a syndrome triggered by factors in the environment rather than biological factors. Such depressions are characterized by obvious precipitating events and life stresses, the absence of significant vegetative disturbances, fluctuation of symptoms according to psychological and environmental factors, and unstable, "neurotic" premorbid personality patterns.

The value of the endogenous-reactive dichotomy lies in calling attention to the importance of the vegetative signs of sleep disturbance, weight loss, decreased energy, and psychomotor retardation or agitation. It also emphasizes the favorable response of these symptoms to medications and electroconvulsive therapy (ECT). However, the problem with this dichotomy is that very few depressed people fall into one category or the other; most lie somewhere on a continuum between the endogenous and reactive extremes. For example, almost all depressed patients, if pressed, can cite some recent adverse events in their lives that might be termed precipitants. And many depressed people have both obvious life stresses and clear vegetative signs. To further complicate matters, the presence of precipitating life stresses does not rule out a favorable response to medication or ECT.

Psychotic versus neurotic depression

Psychotic versus neurotic depression refers both to the ability to test reality and to the severity of the depression.

Psychotic depression is used quite specifically to denote depression in which the person has lost the ability to test reality. This is often manifested by delusions, hallucinations, or profound confusion. Roughly 10% of all depressed patients have psychotic symptoms. But the term has also been used more broadly to denote depression with severe impairment in social and personal functioning, inability to perform daily tasks, and withdrawal from others. Psychotic depressions are thought to be biologically based.

In *neurotic depression*, reality testing remains intact and, more broadly, day-to-day functioning is not significantly impaired. The term implies social and psychological origins rather than a biological cause.

This distinction is another dichotomy of limited usefulness. Applied to depression, the term psychotic is ambiguous, because it can refer either to specific psychotic symptoms or to the severity of the syndrome. Considering the wide spectrum of severity of depressive disorders, it is rather arbitrary to decide that one person's depression is of psychotic severity while another's is simply neurotic.

However, the presence or absence of specific psychotic symptoms is an essential piece of data in the evaluation of every depressed patient. Besides having implications for long-term treatment (to be discussed later), the presence of psychotic symptoms should alert the clinician to an increased risk of suicide and should prompt consideration of a hospital admission.

In the language of DSM-III-R, psychotic depression would be encompassed by the diagnosis of a major depressive episode, and neurotic depression would generally fall into the category of dysthymia.

Agitated versus retarded depression

Agitated versus retarded depression divides depressive disorders according to the motor disturbances that occur as part of the illness.

Agitated depression refers, quite simply, to the clinical picture that includes psychomotor agitation—excessive, unproductive, and tension-relieving activity such as hand-wringing, hair-pulling, nail-biting, and pacing, along with such vocal expressions of psychic pain as sighing or moaning. Agitated depressions are much more common in older people (peaking in the 50s and 60s) and often include psychotic symptoms. ECT and tricyclic antidepressants are helpful in the treatment of agitated depressions.

Retarded depression refers to a clinical picture that includes psychomotor retardation—slowed, unspontaneous thought and action. The presence of psychomotor retardation predicts a good response to tricyclic antidepressants.

The agitated-retarded dichotomy is of particularly limited usefulness, because many depressed people show a mixture of agitated and retarded features. Also, many depressed people have normal rates of psychomotor activity and do not fall into either category.

Differential Diagnosis

In making the diagnosis of major depression or dysthymia, you must rule out conditions that mimic depression, and underlying illnesses that manifest themselves secondarily as depression.

Organic causes. These are too numerous to list in their entirety, but the more common ones are as follows:

1. *Drugs.* Among the many drugs that can cause depression are reserpine, propranolol, steroids, methyldopa, oral contraceptives, ethanol, marijuana, and hallucinogens. Amphetamine withdrawal can also produce a depressive syndrome, as can withdrawal from benzodiazepines and barbiturates.
2. *Infectious diseases.* Pneumonia, hepatitis, mononucleosis.
3. *Tumors.* These often first present as depression, particularly cancer of the head of the pancreas.
4. *Endocrine disorders,* especially of the thyroid, adrenals, or pituitary. Hypothyroidism, even when subclinical, can exacerbate or cause depression, and thyroid replacement may be the only treatment required (see Chapter 18).

5. *Central nervous system (CNS) disorders.* Brain tumors and strokes.
6. *Systemic diseases,* including anemias and nutritional deficiencies.

The routine evaluation of people with depression should include the screening measures shown in Table 6-4, as well as the additional measures that are done if the patient's history or clinical presentation suggests a particular underlying problem.

Dementia. Because demented people experience memory loss and difficulty in concentrating, it can be difficult to distinguish between depression and dementia, particularly in the elderly (see Chapter 9).

Psychological reaction to a physical illness. People who suddenly find themselves bedridden or functionally impaired because of a medical condition often react by becoming depressed.

Schizophrenia. Differentiating between psychotic depression and schizophrenia may be difficult. In schizophrenia, depressive symptoms usually follow the onset of psychosis; in psychotic depression, the mood disturbance precedes or coincides with the onset of psychosis. A history of normal functioning between psychotic episodes suggests affective illness, as does a family history of affective illness. Also, remember that schizophrenic people may have secondary depressive episodes, particularly upon recovering from an acute psychotic break.

Schizoaffective disorder. This is often called a "wastebasket diagnosis," because the label is given to people whose symptoms and clinical

Table 6-4. The medical workup of the depressed patient

Routine screening measures
    Medical history—including drug use
    Physical examination
    Complete blood count (CBC)
    Routine blood chemistries (SMA-12)
    Thyroid function tests
    Urinalysis

Additional screening measures
    Neurology consultation
    Chest X-ray
    Electrocardiogram (EKG)
    Computed tomographic scan

course make it impossible to differentiate between depression and schizophrenia.

Bipolar disorders. Those who present initially with depression may later manifest elation or mania as well, taking them out of the unipolar category. At this time, we are unable to predict which people who present as unipolar depressive individuals will go on to reveal a bipolar illness instead.

Uncomplicated bereavement. A full depressive syndrome is frequently a normal reaction to the death of a loved one. It may include sleep and appetite disturbance. Such a reaction rarely begins more than 2 or 3 months following a loss, and it does not result in marked or prolonged functional impairment. Remember that the duration of normal bereavement varies widely among different ethnic groups. Grief reactions may last 6 months to 1 year. Somatic therapy is generally not indicated unless depressive symptoms endanger the person's health or result in prolonged inability to function.

Personality disorders. Many people with personality disorders—particularly borderline, histrionic, dependent, and obsessive-compulsive personality disorders—have depressive symptoms as well. The depression is often chronic, has fluctuating symptoms, and usually meets the criteria for dysthymia.

Chronic alcohol dependence. Alcohol addiction is often associated with depressive symptoms. It is thought that many alcoholic people are actually depressed and "self-medicate" underlying depression by drinking, but chronic alcohol abuse can also be the sole cause of depressive symptoms.

Anxiety. Because a large percentage of depressed people also experience anxiety, the task of distinguishing between anxiety disorders and depressive disorders is not always easy. As more and more studies point out the efficacy of antidepressant medication in treating panic disorders, the overlap between depression and anxiety becomes even greater. Anxious patients tend to complain more of bodily symptoms than do depressed patients.

Normal mood fluctuations. Obviously, all of us have experienced depressed feelings at some time in our lives. However, normal mood fluctuations are not as prolonged or as severe as those in dysthymia and major depression. Moreover, normal mood changes do not interfere significantly with day-to-day functioning.

Clinical Course

Major depression. Symptoms of a major depressive episode usually develop over a period of days to weeks, but they may develop quite suddenly—particularly after a severe life stress. The depressive episode is sometimes preceded by several months of milder symptoms, by anxiety, or by panic attacks.

Most acute depressive episodes are self-limiting and have a good prognosis even without specific therapy, but somatic therapies (medications, ECT) decrease the intensity of the symptoms and hasten recovery. Without adequate somatic therapy, most acute depressive episodes last 4 to 6 months, and 80% of the patients recover within 2 years. Between 75% and 80% of those who have a first major depressive episode go on to have one or more recurrences in their lifetime; a minority of people recover completely after one episode.

Most people get back to normal—that is, return to their previous levels of functioning—between depressive episodes. However, about 15% to 30% of those with major depressive episodes never return to their premorbid state of mental health; they have residual symptoms and social impairment. Factors that seem to predispose certain depressed people to a chronic "downhill" course are advanced age, a family history of depression, long-standing personality problems, and lack of social supports.

People who have recurrent major depressive episodes are more likely to go on to develop a manic or hypomanic episode (i.e., bipolar illness) than those who only experience a single depressive episode.

Dysthymia. Unlike major depression, dysthymia has no clear onset, but seems to the patient as if it had always been there. A chronic, rather than episodic, course is the rule. Social and occupational impairment may be mild or even moderate, but this is due to the chronicity of the symptoms rather than to their severity. Hospitalization is rarely necessary unless the patient seriously plans or attempts suicide.

Suicide. A majority (60% to 80%) of people who commit suicide carry a diagnosis of depression. Estimates of the risk of suicide in all mood disorders are as high as 15%, with the greatest period of risk within 5 years after the onset of the disorder. The risk of suicide among people with mood disorders is 30 times that of the general population.

Epidemiology

Depressive disorders are ubiquitous. The following figures give a sketch of their distribution in the general population.

Morbid risk. At least 10% of adults in the general population have one or more major depressive episodes at some time in their lives. Some estimates place an individual's lifetime risk of developing a major depression or dysthymia as high as 30%.

Age at onset. Dysthymia usually begins early in adult life. Major depression may begin at any age, and the most common age of onset ranges from the 20s to the 50s. Contrary to popular belief, depression is no more common among the elderly than among younger adults.

Sex. Major depression is roughly twice as common in women as in men, and dysthymia has been estimated to be four to five times more common in women than men. The reasons for this difference are not fully understood.

Socioeconomic status. No strong or constant trend has been demonstrated, but depression appears to be somewhat more common in the higher socioeconomic strata.

Marital status. There is no appreciable difference among single, married, divorced, and widowed people in the incidence of major depression. Some reports have shown increased incidence of dysthymia among separated and divorced people, but this trend is not striking.

Family history. There is a clear tendency for major depression to run in families, and a family history of depressive episodes doubles or triples one's risk of developing the illness. Familial patterns in dysthymia have not been established.

Etiology

No single causal factor has been identified as the basis of depression. Indeed, the depressive syndromes are so varied in their course and symptomatology that discovery of a single cause of all depressive disorders is highly unlikely. Research points to many factors that seem to contribute to the development of depressive illness.

Genetics

Studies of the incidence of depressive illness in twins, in families, and in the general population have clearly established a genetic basis for at least some depressive disorders. Evidence includes the fact that relatives of people with unipolar depressive illness have a higher frequency of depression than the general population. The prevalence of unipolar depression is greatest among first-degree relatives of unipolar depressive individuals. Also, monozygotic twins have a 65% to 75% concordance rate for depression, while dizygotic twins have only a 14% to 19% concordance rate for the illness. (That is, if one twin suffers from depression, it is much more likely that the other twin will also suffer from depression if he or she is identical rather than fraternal.)

Neurochemical abnormalities

In looking for biochemical correlates of depression, much attention has been focused on chemicals that transmit nerve impulses from one neuron to another in the brain, particularly norepinephrine, serotonin, dopamine, and gamma-aminobutyric acid (GABA).

The **catecholamine hypothesis**, developed in the 1960s, was built on the assumption that depression and mania were biochemically opposite states: depression was thought to be associated with deficits of one or more catecholamine neurotransmitters at critical synapses in the CNS, whereas mania was thought to be connected with an excess of these catecholamines:

1. *Norepinephrine* is found in both the central and the peripheral nervous systems. Evidence suggests that in some forms of depression there is a CNS deficiency of norepinephrine. This is based on studies that reveal abnormally low levels of its major metabolite, 3-methoxy-4-hydroxyphenylglycol (MHPG), in the urine. The concept of a norepinephrine deficiency in depression would be consistent with the fact that certain tricyclic antidepressants (e.g., imipramine, desipramine) block the reuptake of norepinephrine in presynaptic neurons, increasing the amount of norepinephrine that remains active as a neurotransmitter.

2. The possibility of a CNS *serotonin* deficiency has also been explored in studies that measure levels of its metabolite, 5-hydroxyindoleacetic acid (5-HIAA), in the cerebrospinal fluid (CSF). Investigators had hoped to identify a subgroup of depressed patients who had low levels of 5-HIAA in the CSF and who would respond clinically to tricyclic antidepressants that block serotonin reuptake by presynaptic neurons and thereby increase the amount of serotonin available for neurotransmission. In fact, only a bare majority of studies have revealed low levels of 5-HIAA in the CSF of depressed patients, and this marker has not been a useful predictor of patient response to particular types of antidepressants.

3. Recently, studies of CSF GABA in depressed patients have found abnormally low levels in some series but not in others. While GABA levels may be lower in some depressed patients, this proves not to be a marker that is specific to depression, because low GABA levels have been found in groups of schizophrenic patients as well.

Single-transmitter theories of depression have not had great explanatory power. Research in this area has been complicated by the fact that there have been no antidepressants available that have purely serotonergic or purely noradrenergic effects, making single-transmitter hypotheses difficult to test empirically. Newer theories about the possible interactions of different transmitter systems look promising. For example, the "permissive" hypothesis of serotonin holds that defective serotonin dampening of other neurotransmitter systems (e.g., norepinephrine and dopamine) permits wide fluctuations in mood, which might account for excursions not only into depression but also into mania.

It must be emphasized that many people who are clinically depressed do not have demonstrable neurotransmitter deficiencies, nor do they necessarily respond to treatment with antidepressants. Thus, neurotransmitter deficiencies do not sufficiently account for all depressive syndromes.

Receptors

Researchers have been able to characterize many receptor sites for neurotransmitters and various psychotropic drugs in brain and peripheral tissue. They have found that long-term use of antidepressant medications and ECT tends to decrease the number of postsynaptic β-adrenergic receptors while enhancing neuronal response to serotonergic and α-adrenergic stimulation. Also, lithium tends to decrease β-receptors and serotonin receptors in some areas of the brain. Studies also suggest that α_2-adrenoreceptors in the platelets of some depressed patients are desensitized relative to those in normal control subjects. Precisely what these findings mean for our understanding of the pathophysiology of depression is not yet clear.

Neuroendocrine systems

Hypothalamic, pituitary, adrenal cortical, thyroid, and gonadal functions have been examined for possible clues to the etiology of mood disorders. The pituitary-adrenal axis has been of particular interest in recent years, especially the empirical finding that some depressed people cannot suppress cortisol production by the adrenal cortex when challenged with a dose of dexamethasone sufficient to suppress cortisol production in normal individuals. Hypercortisolism in depressed patients is one of the most consistently replicated findings in biological psychiatry, and so it was thought that the dexamethasone suppression test (DST), which measures the ability to suppress cortisol production, might be a specific test for medication-responsive depression. Unfortunately, this has not proved to be the case, since abnormal results from DSTs are common among patients with other psychiatric disorders, such as eating disorders. Thus, abnormal cortisol response to dexamethasone may be an indicator of certain types of psychiatric illness, but it is not specific to depression.

Other biological factors

Other important areas of research in the biology of depression include sleep, circadian rhythms, neuroanatomic measures such as ventricular-brain ratio (VBR) and sulcal width, and animal models of "kindling" and behavioral sensitization. Although abnormalities have been found in all of these areas, they lack diagnostic specificity for depression and are as yet of unclear significance.

Personality and psychodynamic factors

The literature on the *psychodynamics of depression* is vast. No single personality trait or group of traits that predisposes one to depression has been identified, nor has a single psychological mechanism by which depression comes about been elucidated.

Many psychodynamic theorists note that those prone to depression are characterized by low self-esteem and a high degree of self-criticism. Some conceptualize depression as anger turned inward. Others write about instability and insecurity in early mother-child interactions as laying the groundwork for later sensitivity to separations from loved ones and a resulting vulnerability to depression when faced with separation or loss.

In studying the roots of depression, much attention has been focused on the role of interpersonal loss. Freud and his followers examined the similarities (and differences) between normal bereavement and depression, noting that people commonly seek help for depressive episodes that seem to come on the heels of some setback in personal relationships (e.g., loss of a job, death of a loved one, breakup of a marriage or romance). Researchers have noted an increased incidence of depression among adults who suffered the loss (by death) of a parent in childhood. Such early losses may make individuals particularly sensitive to losses later in life and thus more vulnerable to depressive illness. But not all those who lose parents in childhood become depressed as adults, and there seem to be many variables that determine one's response to loss. The variety of psychological factors that contribute to depression is practically infinite.

While psychodynamic theory locates the vulnerability to depression in formative childhood experiences, cognitive-behavior theory deemphasizes the past and instead focuses on disturbances in the content and process of thought as leading to depressed mood and behavior. Depression is thought to result from cognitive distortions—unrealistically negative views of self, the world, and the future—that must be corrected in order to relieve affective disturbance. A similar model, that of *learned helplessness*, emphasizes the role of uncontrollable experiences in the patient's life that generate feelings of helplessness and result in depression.

Treatment

Optimism is usually justified in treating patients with depressive disorders. Currently available therapies have proved effective and afford depressed patients a good prognosis, particularly in cases of acute depressive episodes. A wide range of somatic and psychological treatment modalities are useful in depression. You must be ready to use varying combinations of treatments tailored to each individual patient's needs. Basic approaches to the treatment of depression are outlined below, and more detailed descriptions of various types of treatment are to be found in Chapters 17 and 18.

Treat emergencies first

Suicide constitutes the greatest danger to depressed people, and you must assess the suicide potential of every patient who complains of depressed feelings. Suicidal thoughts and actions may be obvious, or clues to self-destructive intent may be subtle. For example, drug abuse, reckless driving, and other "daring" activities often represent disguised suicidal wishes (for the assessment of suicide risk, see Chapter 15). Given that affectively ill patients constitute the largest group of people who commit suicide, you must be ever vigilant to this possibility. The danger of homicide must not be overlooked, since people with mania or depression may try to kill others on the basis of deluded beliefs—for example, the depressed mother who feels her children would be better off dead than growing up in a cruel and heartless world, or the manic who believes a traffic warden is trying to kill him.

Acute psychosis must be treated as an emergency, as must *severe starvation and/or dehydration secondary to anorexia*. All of the above conditions (see Table 6-5) should prompt you to consider immediate hospitalization to stabilize the patient medically and to keep the patient and others physically safe.

Table 6-5. General indications for hospitalizing a depressed patient

Significant risk of suicide

Significant risk of homicide

Loss of ability to care for oneself, either because of immobilizing symptoms or because of psychotic thinking

Acute medical conditions of life-threatening proportion that result from the depression (e.g., anorexia, dehydration)

Concomitant medical conditions (e.g., severe cardiac disease) that require special diagnostic and treatment considerations

Somatic therapies

Medications and ECT are particularly useful in treatment of depressive disorders that include psychosis and/or physical symptoms (particularly the classic vegetative signs noted above).

Tricyclic (or heterocyclic) antidepressants (TCAs). These antidepressants are the most widely used medications for unipolar depression. Their actions seem to be related to their capacity to potentiate the CNS actions of norepinephrine and serotonin. TCAs are used in the treatment of acute depressive episodes, in the alleviation of more chronic depressive syndromes, and as maintenance therapy to prevent the reoccurrence of depressive episodes. Between 50% and 85% of patients with unipolar depression improve when treated with TCAs. Classically, those with physical symptoms (anorexia, insomnia, psychomotor retardation) are more responsive to TCA treatment than those patients who have more "neurotic" or reactive depressions. The indications for the use of TCAs are discussed in detail in Chapter 18, along with the principles that physicians use in prescribing these medications. TCAs are less widely used to treat bipolar depressions because of the risk of precipitating mania (see below).

Lithium. This agent is most widely used as an antimanic drug, but recent studies have shown lithium to be effective in preventing the recurrence of depressive episodes in unipolar depressive patients. Lithium maintenance is now being used as an alternative to TCA maintenance for the prophylaxis of recurrent depression. Lithium has also been found useful in potentiating (i.e., enhancing) the effects of TCAs and monoamine oxidase inhibitors (MAOIs) in about half of those depressed patients who do not respond to an antidepressant alone. Adding lithium to the patient's regimen produces improvement in 7 to 10 days. Finally, lithium alone is often used to treat depression in bipolar patients who might become manic if treated with an antidepressant.

Monoamine oxidase inhibitors. The antidepressant action of MAOIs is thought to be related to their ability to block the metabolism of norepinephrine and serotonin in the CNS. MAOIs are generally the second-line drugs in treating depression pharmacologically, because they are somewhat less effective than TCAs and because adverse reactions are more common with MAOIs than with TCAs However, MAOIs are useful in treating depression in cases where TCAs are contraindicated or have not proved helpful. MAOIs are the treatment of first choice for patients with "atypical" depressions—that is, patients who do not have the classical neurovegetative symptoms but instead have high levels of anxiety, phobias, or obsessive-compulsive symptoms (see Chapter 18 for more details). Like TCAs, MAOIs can precipitate mania in bipolar patients and so must be used with caution in this population.

Electroconvulsive therapy. ECT (sometimes referred to as "shock treatment") involves the induction of a seizure by passing a controlled pulse of electrical energy through the brain. The seizure is induced while the patient is partly paralyzed by a muscle relaxant and under general anesthesia. The seizure itself is necessary for the antidepressant effect of ECT, although the operative mechanism is not known. Courses of treatment vary, but patients often receive between 6 and 20 treatments, given at a rate of 3 or 4 treatments per week. ECT is safe and highly effective. It has the advantage of being rapidly effective; response often occurs within days rather than weeks. Thus, ECT is frequently the treatment of choice when depressive symptoms are so severe as to be life-threatening and rapid improvement is essential (see Chapter 18).

Major tranquilizers. These tranquilizers, also called antipsychotics or neuroleptics, are very useful in treatment of depression that is complicated by psychotic symptoms or overwhelming anxiety. They are often used in combination with TCAs or with ECT, because psychotic depression does not generally respond well to antidepressant therapy alone. Symptoms likely to respond to treatment with antipsychotics include delusions, hallucinations, confusion, and overwhelming anxiety.

Sedatives and minor tranquilizers. Benzodiazepines, barbiturates, and other sedatives and antianxiety agents are sometimes used to treat anxiety, restlessness, insomnia, and irritability that are part of depressive syndromes. However, when depression is the basis for these symptoms, they frequently resolve with antidepressant therapy. Like all CNS depressants, these drugs can actually cause depression and thereby complicate, rather than alleviate, the illness. Minor tranquilizers can be used effectively on a short-term basis to alleviate anxiety and insomnia in depressed patients while they wait for antidepressant medication to take effect.

Note that insomnia associated with a depressive syndrome is best treated by treating the depression itself, not by the chronic use of sedatives or hypnotics.

Sleep manipulation. Manipulation of sleep is a technique recently developed to treat depressed patients who cannot tolerate or do not respond to medication or ECT. *Partial sleep deprivation* involves having the patient go to bed early (e.g., 9:00 P.M.) and awaken after 4 hours of sleep, thereby both shortening the duration of sleep and advancing the time of sleep. Studies have shown that up to two-thirds of depressed patients improve with this technique, but relapse occurs within 10 days to 2 weeks after it is stopped. *Phase advance* is a similar technique, in which patients are put to bed 4 hours early but are allowed to sleep until they naturally awaken. Sleep manipulation may be helpful to depressed patients while they are waiting the 1 to 3 weeks required for most antidepressants to take effect.

High-intensity light. This is a newly developed modality used to treat those depressed patients whose illness follows a seasonal pattern. Patients who regularly suffer from major depressive episodes during the late fall and winter are treated with exposure to several hours of bright artificial light during the days of shortened sunlight, and a majority of them improve rapidly. The light suppresses plasma melatonin secretion, which is thought to be associated with its antidepressant effect.

Psychological therapies

Individual psychotherapy. This modality based on psychodynamic principles is widely used, particularly for mild and chronic forms of depression. Psychodynamic psychotherapy emphasizes the importance of past experiences and unconscious motivation in determining human behavior.

Short-term therapy (roughly 5 to 20 sessions) is often aimed at support, crisis intervention, and symptom relief for acutely depressed people so that they may cope better with daily activities and in dealing with others. Long-term psychotherapy (several months to several years) allows patients to identify, examine, and resolve intrapsychic conflicts that impair their lives, and to explore ways in which important childhood experiences have served as inadequate models for current relationships. Patients who improve with short-term treatment may or may not need more extended psychotherapy. The decision to continue in long-term treatment is usually based on whether a patient's life is chronically hampered by emotional difficulties and the extent to which he or she is motivated to explore these difficulties.

Interpersonal therapy (IPT). This therapy, which was formulated by Klerman and Weissman, is a form of individual psychotherapy developed specifically for patients who have nonbipolar, nonpsychotic depressions. It is short-term (12 to 16 sessions) and emphasizes education about depression, as well as helping the patient to develop better strategies for managing current life situations. These include abnormal grief reactions, disputes with others, role changes with which the patient feels unable to cope, and impairments in social functioning. Unlike more classical forms of psychodynamic therapy, IPT emphasizes the present rather than childhood experiences.

Group psychotherapy. Psychotherapy in groups can help depressed people improve their social skills and self-esteem. A therapy group provides a mutually supportive environment in which patients can examine their styles of dealing with others and test out new ways of forming relationships.

Cognitive-behavior therapy. This therapy, which was developed by Beck, is a specific technique for treating depression and anxiety. It is based on the premise that distorted modes of thinking about oneself and the world in negative and pessimistic terms foster depression, and that by identifying such cognitive distortions and by teaching the patient to substitute more realistic and self-enhancing thoughts, painful feelings can be reduced. The therapy is short-term, and sessions are more structured than those in psychodynamic psychotherapy. Cognitive-behavior therapy aims to help the patient change his or her way of thinking by means of education about depression, identifying and testing maladaptive thoughts (e.g., "I am a worthless person"), and helping the patient develop new strategies for dealing with current life problems.

In clinical studies, cognitive-behavior therapy has been shown to be of value to many depressed and anxious patients. Clinicians debate whether the therapeutic effects are due to cognitive and behavioral techniques per se or to the trust and rapport that develop between patient and therapist. Equally controversial is the assumption in cognitive therapy that negative thoughts can actually cause painful feelings rather than simply result from them. Cognitive-behavior therapy continues to be a subject of active research (see Chapter 17).

Combining different treatment modalities

Used in combination, somatic and psychosocial treatments are generally more effective than either modality alone. Psychotherapy influences social effectiveness and personality functioning, while medications and ECT affect physiological functions such as sleep, appetite, and sexual drive.

Thus, many patients can benefit from both types of treatment.

Decisions about treatment must be based on the availability of resources, on the patient's willingness to comply with different regimens, and on the patient's motivation to engage in psychotherapeutic work. No one treatment for depression is universally effective, and none has been shown to be the treatment of choice for all types of depression. Ongoing clinical trials are now attempting to evaluate the relative efficacy of different treatments used alone and in various combinations.

BIPOLAR DISORDERS (MANIC-DEPRESSIVE ILLNESS)

Bipolar disorders are illnesses that are characterized by two extremes of mood: elation and depression. Stereotypically, the person with bipolar illness cycles from wild mania into deep depression and back into mania again. In reality, bipolar illness covers a variety of clinical pictures that will be discussed below.

Depressive episodes in bipolar illness are clinically indistinguishable from those seen in unipolar illness. Thus, the distinctive—and often most dramatic—feature of bipolar illness is elation. Like depression, elation encompasses a broad spectrum of moods, including normal states of euphoria and joy, as well as the pathological elations known as mania and hypomania. **Mania** denotes extreme elation, hyperactivity, agitation, and accelerated speech, often with disordered thinking. **Hypomania** refers to a syndrome similar to, but not as severe as, mania. Hypomania is defined in DSM-III-R as a condition including all of the symptoms of mania, but without marked impairment in social or occupational functioning and without suicidal or homicidal impulses that would necessitate hospitalization.

The term *elation* warrants an explanatory note. An individual's subjective experience of mania and hypomania can be pleasurable, involving feeling "high," happy, and euphoric, but these mood states are also characterized by extreme irritability, paranoia, and rage. Thus, it would be more accurate to speak of *excited* rather than elated mood states, since the manic person's subjective experience often varies from extreme euphoria to profound dysphoria.

The major syndromes included under bipolar disorders are *bipolar disorder* (also known as *manic-depressive illness*) and *cyclothymia*. The two are distinguished on the basis of the intensity and duration of symptoms. Further divisions of the bipolar group have been proposed, but none widely adopted. You may, however, hear about the category of *bipolar II*, recently used in some clinical settings to denote a syndrome of major depressive episodes and milder episodes of elation without frank mania.

Bipolar Disorder (Manic-Depressive Illness)

Bipolar disorder generally includes full-blown episodes of mania and depression. Manic episodes may alternate one-for-one with depressive episodes, or one mood extreme may predominate. While people who only experience depressive episodes are categorized as having unipolar illness, those who only experience manic episodes are included in the bipolar category. Such people are quite rare; the rule in bipolar disorder is a history of both depressive and manic episodes.

Symptoms of mania

The symptoms of depressive episodes have already been discussed at length. Because the diagnosis of MDI hinges on the recognition of manic episodes, it is essential that you learn to recognize the symptoms of mania and hypomania. The cardinal symptoms outlined in DSM-III-R are listed in Table 6-6 and described below.

Mood disturbance. The manic person commonly experiences euphoria, and this mood can be quite infectious. In fact, you may find yourself smiling and suppressing the urge to laugh when interviewing a euphoric patient—a reaction that should prompt you to suspect the diagnosis of mania. Those who know the person well usually recognize that the euphoria is uncharacteristic and excessive. Manic people have seemingly limitless enthusiasm for interacting with others, and commonly seek people out in an intrusive way (e.g., they may call friends to chat at 4:00 A.M. and be oblivious to others' wish to sleep). As noted above, the predominant mood in some manic individuals is irritability rather than euphoria. Particularly when their desires are in any way

Table 6-6. The symptoms of mania and hypomania

Mood disturbance (euphoria, irritability)
Hyperactivity (motor restlessness, overinvolvement socially, at work, or
 sexually)
Pressured speech
Flight of ideas
Distractibility
Inflated self-esteem
Decreased need for sleep
Lability of mood
Delusions and hallucinations (in mania)

thwarted, people who are manic can respond with extreme annoyance, even rage and violence (whence the term "maniac").

Hyperactivity. This includes motor restlessness and overinvolvement in sexual, recreational, occupational, and other activities. Manic individuals will plan and enter into a variety of projects, overcommitting themselves and using poor judgment. A patient may, for example, start to repaint his house, begin to write a novel, and rebuild his auto engine—all in one day. Along with poor judgment, manic people commonly demonstrate expansiveness, grandiosity, and unwarranted optimism, and these characteristics lead to many painful consequences. For example, someone in the throes of mania can give away an entire fortune, amass huge debts on a buying spree, take off impulsively on a trip around the world, drive recklessly, engage in uncharacteristic sexual behavior, or spend time on street corners and engage strangers in conversation.

Pressured speech. Manic people speak as if they are under pressure to get the words out. They speak loudly and rapidly and are usually difficult to interrupt. Their speech content may be normal, full of jokes and puns, or full of hostile accusations and angry tirades. Manic people often have a theatrical style and can be quite entertaining. Associations and word choice may be based on sounds rather than ideas, resulting in "clang" associations (e.g., "talk–tic-toc–what's up doc?").

Flight of ideas. This involves skipping from one idea to another in a continuous flow of accelerated speech. The speaker makes associations that are comprehensible but based on puns, extraneous stimuli, or other chance factors. If it is severe, flight of ideas can make the manic person's speech impossible to follow.

Distractibility. Manic people have difficulty in screening out extraneous stimuli. They often react to noises, sights, or smells, shifting their focus of attention rapidly from one irrelevant stimulus to another (hence, the use of seclusion in a quiet, unadorned room as a means of calming agitated manic patients).

Inflated self-esteem. An unrealistic sense of one's own merits and importance often accompanies an elevated mood. Some people simply become overconfident and less self-critical; others develop grandiose ideas of delusional proportions. They may come to believe, for example, that they have a special relationship with God, that they have a plan to save the universe from destruction, or that they have unparalleled gifts they must share with the world.

Decreased need for sleep. Almost all manic people experience a decreased need for sleep, feeling full of energy despite little or no rest. Some manic individuals actually go without any sleep for days at a time and do not report feeling tired.

Lability of mood. Some manic people move rapidly from euphoria to anger or depression. Mood swings may last for minutes or even several hours at a time, but rarely longer.

Delusions and hallucinations. The content of delusions or hallucinations is usually consonant with an elevated and grandiose mood. For example, a patient may believe that he or she is being persecuted by enemy agents because of possessing special powers. Another may believe he or she sees God and speaks directly with Him.

Diagnosis of mania

The diagnostic criteria outlined in DSM-III-R for a manic episode are essentially as follows:

1. A distinct period of elevated, expansive, or irritable mood.
2. During the mood disturbance, at least three of the following symptoms are persistent:

   - Increase in goal-directed activity or psychomotor agitation
   - Increase in talkativeness or pressured speech
   - Flight of ideas or racing thoughts
   - Inflated self-esteem
   - Decreased need for sleep
   - Distractibility
   - Excessive involvement in pleasurable activities that may have painful consequences (e.g., buying sprees, reckless driving, sexual indiscretions)

3. The mood disturbance is severe enough to cause marked impairment in functioning in social relationships or at work, or necessitates hospitalization to prevent harm to self or others.
4. Delusions or hallucinations are not present for longer than 2 weeks during a period of normal mood.
5. Symptoms are not due to another condition, such as schizophrenia or a paranoid disorder, or to an organic factor.

Manic episodes are usually classified as mild, moderate, or severe; occurring with or without psychotic features (delusions, hallucinations, or catatonia).

Differential diagnosis

Many clinical studies have concluded that bipolar disorder has been underdiagnosed in the United States in recent years because it is frequently mistaken for other mental illnesses, most notably schizophrenia. Although there are many causes of excited and elated states, only a small number of disorders are commonly confused with bipolar disorder.

Organic affective syndromes. Organic causes of elation and full-blown mania include the use of such drugs as steroids, alcohol, and amphetamines, as well as specific illnesses like cerebral tumors, multiple sclerosis, and dementia. The evaluation of a first acute manic episode should include a thorough physical examination, routine laboratory screening (complete blood count, routine blood chemistries, urinalysis), screening of serum and urine for toxic substances, and a thorough medical and drug history to rule out organic causes of mania (Table 6-7).

Schizophrenia. Mania and schizophrenia often appear very similar. In some cases it is almost impossible to distinguish between them on the basis of presenting symptoms alone. For example, hallucinations, paranoia, grandiose delusions, loose associations, bizarre behaviors, and irritability are common features of both illnesses. Thus, the clinician must frequently rely on factors other than the patient's mental status to make as accurate a diagnosis as possible. Table 6-8 outlines historical data that favor a diagnosis of bipolar disorder and those that favor a diagnosis of schizophrenia.

Schizoaffective disorder. This diagnostic category is used for people who exhibit symptoms of a mood disorder (mania and/or depression) but whose chronic impairment of thought and functioning is more consistent with schizophrenia. Many clinicians consider this a "wastebasket" diagnosis and believe schizoaffective disorder is a variant of bipolar disorder or schizophrenia rather than a separate disease entity. The diagnosis is usually made when it is impossible to categorize an illness as bipolar disorder or schizophrenia. Lithium and antidepressants are often used for schizoaffective patients, but generally with less success than in treating true bipolar or unipolar affective illness. Antipsychotic

Table 6-7. The medical workup of the manic patient

Medical history—including drug use
Physical examination
Routine laboratory screening
   Complete blood count (CBC)
   Blood chemistries (SMA-12)
   Urinalysis
   Thyroid function tests
Screening of blood and urine for toxic substances

Table 6-8. Features that help to differentiate between bipolar disorder (manic-depressive illness) and schizophrenia

Favors bipolar disorder	Favors schizophrenia
Previous episode of mania or depression	No previous history of affective disturbance
History of complete recovery between acute episodes of illness	History of residual impairment between acute exacerbations of illness
Good premorbid functioning	Gradual deterioration and poor premorbid functioning
Family history positive for a remitting psychotic illness	Family history negative for remitting psychotic illness
History of favorable treatment response to lithium and/or ECT	Poor response to treatment with lithium and/or ECT

drugs are also used to treat disordered thinking, and the combination of an antipsychotic and lithium or an antidepressant is very common in treating schizoaffective illness.

Cyclothymia. Essentially, this disorder involves periods of depression and hypomania, but with briefer mood swings and less severe symptoms than in bipolar disorder. This diagnosis will be discussed at greater length below.

Clinical course

People with bipolar disorder may initially present with either a manic or a depressive episode. Obviously, a patient who presents with a depressive episode and no history of mania may have either bipolar or unipolar illness. Only time will tell whether that person will go on to have manic episodes or only experience bouts of depression.

In bipolar illness, the first disturbance of mood is often manic. Manic episodes generally begin suddenly and escalate rapidly over a few days, but onset may be gradual. Mania may persist for several days or several months, but the episodes are generally briefer and occur more abruptly than major depressive episodes. Particularly if it is not treated early, mania generally goes through stages of severity, beginning with a mild syndrome and progressing to a much more dramatic and disorganized clinical picture. Initially, mood is predominantly euphoric, but the manic individual becomes increasingly irritable and finally panicked and/or enraged. What begins as mildly increased psychomotor activity develops into frenzied and bizarre behavior; initial suspiciousness, grandiosity, and racing thoughts give way to frank delusions, hallucinations, and flight of ideas. This increase in severity is followed by a gradual abatement of symptoms and ultimately a return to normal mood in the majority of manic people; but the rate at which they pass through these stages of mania is highly variable.

Almost everyone who has one or more manic episodes will eventually have at least one depressive episode. An episode of either type may be followed immediately by a brief episode of the other kind, but manic and depressive episodes are usually separated by an intervening period of normal mood and functioning. Some people go for many years after an initial mood disturbance without any recurrence; others have clusters of manic and depressive episodes; still others have increasingly frequent manic and/or depressive episodes as they grow older.

There is a subgroup of bipolar patients (estimates range from 10% to 35%) who do not return to normal moods or functioning between episodes, but have a chronic course with significant residual symptomatic and social impairment.

Before lithium, ECT, and antipsychotics were used in the treatment of mania, the average duration of a manic episode was 3 months; with these modalities, that time has been considerably shortened. Because there is marked variation in both the severity and the duration of manic and depressive episodes and the length of intervening periods of normal mood, you should develop a profile of mood cycles for each patient in order to plan for the most effective treatment.

While the most common presentation of bipolar illness is distinct periods of mania and depression, the disorder may present with fluctuations of the symptoms of mania and depression from week to week, or even hour to hour. Such people are called *rapid cyclers*. Bipolar disorder can also present with features of mania and depression together, presenting a picture of a *mixed disorder*.

The most common complications in the course of a manic episode are substance abuse and the consequences (personal, financial, etc.) of poor judgment.

Epidemiology

Between 0.4% and 1.2% of the adult population carry the diagnosis of bipolar disorder. The lifetime risk of developing bipolar disorder is roughly 1%.

Age. The first manic episode in bipolar disorder usually occurs before age 30. However, there is another group of patients who first develop mania in their 40s. A first manic episode in someone over the age of 50 is unusual, and in such cases you should strongly suspect an organic cause of mania (e.g., drugs, CNS tumor).

Sex. Bipolar disorder is roughly as common in men as in women, although studies suggest a slight preponderance of the disease among women (the male:female ratio is 1.0:1.2). This is in contrast to the unipolar depressive disorders, which are considerably more common in women than in men.

Socioeconomic status. Although there are no sharp distinctions on the basis of socioeconomic class, there appears to be a somewhat higher incidence of bipolar disorder in the higher socioeconomic strata.

Marital status. There is no appreciable difference in the incidence of bipolar disorder on the basis of marital status.

Family history. The frequency of bipolar disorder is markedly higher among the biological relatives of those who have the disease. Sixty to sixty-five percent of bipolar patients have family histories of major mood disorders.

Etiology

The cause of bipolar disorder is not known. As with unipolar depressive disorders, researchers have looked at a wide variety of biological and psychological variables.

The most substantial information we have to date is about the genetic basis of the illness. Twin studies, family studies, and surveys of the general population support the idea of a genetic predisposition to bipolar disorder. Most striking are twin studies that show the concordance rates for bipolar disorder to be 68% for monozygotic twins and 23% for same-sex dizygotic twins. (In other words, among identical twins, if one is bipolar, the other will be bipolar in 68% of cases. By contrast, among twins who are not genetically identical, the rate is only 23%.) It is possible that incomplete gene penetrance accounts for the fact that the concordance rate for bipolar disorder in monozygotic twins is less than 100%. However, it is also possible that other nongenetic factors operate in determining which individuals develop the clinical syndrome of bipolar disorder and which do not.

Recently, investigators have identified a specific gene location on the short arm of chromosome 11 which is linked to a form of bipolar disorder in a large Amish family. This research combined sophisticated epidemiology with modern molecular genetic techniques to yield the first clear localization of genetic material directly correlated with affective illness.

Neurochemical studies of bipolar individuals have shown decreased levels of urinary MHPG during depressive episodes, but no similar derangement of the levels of biogenic amines during manic episodes. Investigators have speculated that mania results from an increase in levels of dopamine in the brain, but this hypothesis has not been proved in research studies. Investigators have also hoped to solve the mystery of bipolar disorder by elucidating the mechanism by which lithium exerts its therapeutic effect; but to date we do not know how lithium works.

Treatment

Acute mania. Depending on its severity, an acute manic episode may constitute a mental health emergency. You must quickly assess the manic patient's propensity for self-destructive or violent behavior, and ability to care for himself or herself.

Self-destructive behaviors include not only overtly suicidal behaviors but also acts involving such poor judgment as to be potentially life threatening (e.g., reckless driving, "daredevil" stunts).

Particularly when paranoia is severe, manic people can be very violent and may even kill others because of a delusional belief that they are acting in self-defense.

In mania, a patient's inability to care for himself or herself often takes bizarre forms—for example, walking naked outdoors in freezing weather, giving away all one's money to strangers, going on wild spending sprees, not sleeping or eating for many days.

Any of the above warrant hospital admission. Hospitalization should also be considered for a first manic episode, to facilitate a complete medical workup and planning for adequate ongoing treatment.

Treatment of an acute manic episode generally involves both medication and setting limits on manic behavior (see Table 6-9). Severe mania is often terrifying to the patient insofar as it represents a loss of self-control. Hospital admission to a locked unit can therefore be reassuring, because it conveys the message that others will take control and keep the patient safe.

Similarly, many manic patients initially require locked-door seclusion and physical restraint to keep them from harming themselves or others; this, too, can be reassuring rather than punitive. Physical restraint should be used only when other measures have proved insufficient to calm the manic individual. Frequently, unlocked seclusion alone will have a significant calming effect. Manic people are highly excitable and

Table 6-9. Common therapeutic interventions in bipolar disorder (manic-depressive illness)

Acute mania
    Setting limits on manic behavior
        Seclusion
        Physical restraints
    Antipsychotic medications
    Lithium
    Anticonvulsants
    ECT

Acute depression
    Suicide precautions, assistance with self-care
    Lithium
    Antidepressants
    Antipsychotic medications
    ECT

Prevention of further episodes (maintenance)
    Lithium
    Antipsychotic medications
    Antidepressants
    Education about the illness for patients, families
    Psychosocial therapy

---

easily distracted, so the simple act of reducing sensory stimulation in a quiet, secluded room can help to ease severe agitation.

Pharmacological treatment is aimed at both the rapid amelioration of symptoms and long-term reduction in the frequency, severity, and duration of manic episodes.

Antipsychotics are the mainstay of rapid treatment. They have a marked antianxiety effect and can considerably reduce the manic person's terror, combativeness, and confusion. Manic people generally respond to adequate oral or intramuscular doses of neuroleptics (see Chapter 18) within a few hours to a few days, often eliminating the need for seclusion and restraint. Because lithium takes roughly 10 to 14 days to work, an antipsychotic such as chlorpromazine (Thorazine) is often the first-line medication. Lithium is started in addition to the neuroleptic as soon as the necessary preliminary laboratory work has been completed. In many cases, the antipsychotic may be discontinued once the patient has been stabilized on lithium.

Lithium produces a response in roughly 70% of acutely manic people in 10 to 14 days. It decreases both the severity and the duration of the acute manic episode, and dramatically reduces the rate of relapse. Because mood stabilization is related to the amount of lithium in the bloodstream, serum lithium levels are monitored to titrate the correct dosage of the medication. Bipolar patients who respond to lithium should be continued on it for 9 to 12 months. (For a more extensive discussion of indications, contraindications, and guidelines for the use of lithium, see Chapter 18.)

Anticonvulsants have recently been used to treat acute mania, either as an adjunct to the medications described above or as a substitute for them. Carbamazepine (Tegretol) has been shown to have antimanic effects equal to those of neuroleptics, working as fast as neuroleptics and possibly faster than lithium. Patients who are "rapid cyclers" and those who do not respond to lithium may be particularly responsive to carbamazepine. It also enhances the antimanic effects of lithium and chlorpromazine when used in combination with these medications. Clonazepam (Klonopin) also has antimanic properties and has the added benefit of sedation for those who need relief from excitation and irritability. Valproate is also coming into use as an antimanic medication.

Electroconvulsive therapy has been shown to be a safe and effective treatment for acute mania. It is often used as a second-line measure when antipsychotic treatment is either ineffective or, for some reason, contraindicated in a particular case. ECT and lithium should not be used concurrently (i.e., when ECT is administered, lithium should be temporarily discontinued), because there is evidence that this combination may diminish the therapeutic effects of each modality and increase the risk of neuropsychological side effects.

Acute depression. There is considerable evidence that lithium is effective in preventing depressive episodes in bipolar patients. However, acute depressive episodes do occur in people who are maintained on lithium, and these often require treatment with antidepressants in addition to lithium. The principles of treatment are the same for acute depressive episodes in bipolar depression and in unipolar depression (see Table 6-9). However, there is a critical distinction between bipolar and unipolar depression in the use of antidepressants, because these agents can precipitate mania in bipolar people. Whenever possible, depressive episodes of mild to moderate severity in patients known or suspected to have bipolar disorder should be treated first with lithium alone, adding an antidepressant only if the response to lithium is not adequate. Treatment with an antidepressant must be undertaken with caution, and patients must be carefully monitored for signs of developing mania. If mania develops, the antidepressant must be discontinued and the mania treated.

Prevention of further episodes (maintenance therapy). Lithium is the mainstay of long-term as well as acute treatment of bipolar disorder. It has been shown to prevent recurrent mania and depression with moderate efficacy. Anyone who has had two or three previous episodes of mania should be considered for maintenance therapy. Because such underlying conditions as kidney disease, heart disease, and organic brain syndromes can make lithium administration dangerous, a careful medical screening must be done whenever maintenance therapy is contemplated. In addition, serum lithium levels must be sampled on a regular basis (usually monthly or bimonthly) to ensure that the patient is on an adequate dosage. Certain laboratory tests, including measurement of serum creatinine levels (to assess kidney functioning) and white blood cell count, must be used every few months to monitor the patient in order to prevent possible toxic effects of lithium on the body. Thus, lithium can only be used safely in people who can comply with a precise treatment regimen (see Chapter 18).

In bipolar individuals who manifest residual thought disorder between episodes of mood disturbance, **neuroleptics** are commonly used on a long-term basis along with lithium.

For some bipolar individuals in whom recurrent depressive episodes are severe and frequent, maintenance therapy with an **antidepressant** may be necessary in addition to lithium. In such cases, the patient must be carefully monitored to ensure that the antidepressant does not precipitate a manic episode.

Management of breakthrough episodes of hypomania usually begins with increasing the lithium dose while monitoring blood levels carefully. If the maximum tolerable dose of lithium does not bring the patient back to a normal mood state, you should add a neuroleptic or an anticonvulsant. If mania comes on suddenly and severely, do not wait for the increased lithium dose to take effect, but also add a neuroleptic or anticonvulsant immediately. Breakthrough episodes of depression in bipolar patients are likewise treated by raising the lithium level. In addition, it is important to evaluate thyroid function and treat any chemical evidence of hypothyroidism. When these two steps have been taken and depression persists, you may consider adding an antidepressant (particularly an MAOI).

Education is important to help patients and their families recognize the signs and symptoms of incipient mania and depression so that they may seek treatment for acute episodes early and thereby increase the likelihood that a full-scale affective disturbance can be prevented or ameliorated. Patients must have a clear idea of what treatment is available (hospital, emergency room, outpatient clinic) and whom they are to contact when they experience affective disturbances.

There is a good deal of controversy over whether any *psychosocial therapy* is helpful for bipolar people. Certainly, supportive therapy can be useful in helping people to cope with the devastating social and occupational effects of severe affective illness and in promoting compliance in taking medications. But it has not been demonstrated that insight-oriented, exploratory psychotherapy is useful in treating bipolar disorder. This disorder can occur in an infinite variety of personality types; some bipolar patients in remission may be psychologically quite healthy and function well, while others may have significant underlying personality disorders. In general, patients who, in remission, manifest personality disturbances that impair their functioning are candidates for psychotherapy, along with routine pharmacological treatment of bipolar disorder.

Cyclothymia

Clinicians recognize the existence of bipolar affective disturbances that are milder and briefer than those in bipolar disorder (i.e., manic-depressive illness). Cyclothymia describes a syndrome of chronic mood disturbance of at least 2 years' duration, characterized by numerous periods of depression and hypomania that are less severe and less prolonged than those in bipolar disorder (Table 6-10).

Diagnostic criteria. The diagnostic criteria for cyclothymia outlined in DSM-III-R are as follows:

1. During the past 2 years, there have been numerous periods of hypomania (including all of the criteria for a manic episode except marked impairment of functioning), and numerous periods of depression or loss of interest that are not of sufficient severity or duration to meet the criteria for a major depressive episode.
2. During this 2-year period, the person is never without hypomanic or depressive symptoms for more than 2 months at a time.
3. There is no evidence of a full-blown major depressive episode or a manic episode during this 2-year period.
4. The syndrome is not superimposed on a chronic psychotic disorder (e.g., schizophrenia) and is not due to an organic factor (e.g., repeated alcohol or drug intoxication).

Epidemiology. Cyclothymia usually begins early in adult life, generally with an insidious onset and a chronic course. The degree to which the illness impairs social and occupational functioning is variable, but is by definition not as severe as the impairment involved in bipolar disor-

Table 6-10. Symptoms of depressive and hypomanic periods in cyclothymia

Depressive symptoms	Hypomanic symptoms
Insomnia or hypersomnia	Decreased need for sleep
Low energy level or chronic fatigue	More energy than usual
Feelings of inadequacy	Inflated self-esteem
Decreased effectiveness or productivity at school, work, or home	Increased productivity, often associated with unusual and self-imposed working hours
Decreased attention, concentration, or ability to think clearly	Sharpened and unusually creative thinking
Social withdrawal	Uninhibited people-seeking (extreme gregariousness)
Loss of interest in or enjoyment of sex	Hypersexuality without recognition of the possibility of painful consequences
Restriction of involvement in pleasurable activities, guilt over past activities	Excessive involvement in pleasurable activities and lack of concern for painful consequences, e.g., buying sprees, foolish business investments, reckless driving
Feeling slowed down	Physical restlessness
Less talkative than usual	More talkative than usual
Pessimistic attitude toward the future, brooding about past events	Overoptimism or exaggeration of past achievements
Tearfulness or crying	Inappropriate laughing, joking, punning

der. Cyclothymia was previously assumed to be rare, but as the syndrome has become more clearly defined in recent years, it has been recognized with increasing frequency, particularly among people seeking outpatient treatment. It appears to be more common among women than among men. It is also more prevalent among those who have biological relatives with major depression and bipolar disorder than it is in the general population.

Clinical course. The most common complication of cyclothymia is substance abuse. As in bipolar people, cyclothymic individuals tend to medicate their depression with stimulants and alcohol, and to abuse stimulants and psychedelic drugs during hypomanic periods.

Differential diagnosis. The differential diagnosis of cyclothymia disorder is essentially the same as that for major depressive and manic episodes. Also, bipolar disorder may be superimposed on an underlying, more chronic cyclothymia.

Treatment. The treatment of cyclothymia is similar to that of bipolar disorder. Many patients experience a stabilization of their moods when they are maintained on adequate amounts of lithium.

Seasonal Affective Disorder

While clinicians have for many years noted that mood disorders often occur in patterns that correlate with the seasons of the year, it is only recently that investigators have identified a syndrome of seasonal affective disorder with specific diagnostic criteria. Those who suffer from the disorder are most commonly female and exhibit episodes of depression and hypomania (bipolar II). The disorder usually begins in the teens or twenties. Depressive episodes commonly begin in October or November and end in early spring. They include many of the symptoms of depression noted above, in addition to "atypical" symptoms such as hypersomnia (rather than insomnia) and carbohydrate craving and weight gain (as opposed to loss of appetite). When depressive episodes end in the spring, they are often followed by periods of hypomania. The disorder has been linked to changes in the length of days and exposure to sunlight, and depressive episodes have been treated effectively with increased exposure to light during winter months.

A FINAL NOTE ON MOOD DISORDERS

Affective illness is now the subject of intense research in this country and abroad. Data are emerging that suggest the existence of "affective equivalents"—that is, symptoms that do not look like mood disturbances yet respond to antidepressant medications. Among the symptoms thought to be possible affective equivalents are those of panic attacks, obsessive-compulsive disorder, and eating disorders. You will undoubtedly hear more about syndromes thought to be related to affective illness in the coming years.

BIBLIOGRAPHY

American Psychiatric Association: Mood disorders, in Diagnostic and Statistical Manual of Mental Disorders, 3rd Edition, Revised. Washington, DC, American Psychiatric Association, 1987, pp 213–233

Ballenger JC: The clinical use of carbamazepine in affective disorders. J Clin Psychiatry 49 (No 4, suppl):13–19, 1988

Beck AT, Rush AJ, Shaw BF, et al: Cognitive Theory of Depression. New York, Guilford Press, 1979

Bibring E: The mechanism of depression, in Affective Disorders. Edited by Greenacre P. New York, International Universities Press, 1953, pp 154–181

Blehar MC, Weissman MM, Gershon ES, et al: Family and genetic studies of affective disorders. Arch Gen Psychiatry 45:289–292, 1988

Carlson GA, Goodwin FK: The stages of mania: a longitudinal analysis of the manic episode. Arch Gen Psychiatry 28:221–228, 1973

Childress AR, Burns DD: The basics of cognitive therapy. Psychosomatics 22:1017–1027, 1981

Egeland JA, Gerhard DS, Pauls DL, et al: Bipolar affective disorders linked to DNA markers on chromosome 11. Nature 325:783–787, 1987

Freud S: Mourning and melancholia (1917), in The Standard Edition of the Complete Psychological Works of Sigmund Freud, Vol XIV. Translated and edited by Strachey J. London, Hogarth, 1957, pp 237–258

Hirschfeld RMA, Goodwin FK: Mood disorders, in The American Psychiatric Press Textbook of Psychiatry. Edited by Talbott JA, Hales RE, Yudofsky SC. Washington, DC, American Psychiatric Press, 1988, pp 403–441

Isenberg PL, Schatzberg AF: Psychoanalytic contribution to a theory of depression, in Depression: Biology, Psychodynamics, and Treatment. Edited by Cole JO, Schatzberg AF, Frazier SH. New York, Plenum, 1978, pp 149–171

Klerman GL, Weissman MM, Rounsaville BJ, et al: Interpersonal Psychotherapy of Depression. New York, Basic Books, 1984

Lloyd C: Life events and depressive disorder reviewed, I: events as predisposing factors. Arch Gen Psychiatry 37:529–535, 1980

MacVane JR, Lange JD, Brown WA, et al: Psychological functioning of bipolar manic-depressives in remission. Arch Gen Psychiatry 35:1351–1354, 1978

Pope HG Jr, Lipinski JF Jr: Diagnosis in schizophrenia and manic-depressive illness. Arch Gen Psychiatry 35:811-828, 1978

Rosenthal NE, Sack DA, Gillin JC, et al: Seasonal affective disorder: a description of the syndrome and preliminary findings with light therapy. Arch Gen Psychiatry 41:72, 1984

Rothschild AJ: Biology of depression. Med Clin North Am 72:765–790, 1988

Schilgen B, Tolle R: Partial sleep deprivation as therapy for depression. Arch Gen Psychiatry 37:267–271, 1980

Weiner D: The psychiatric use of electrically induced seizures. Am J Psychiatry 136:1507–1517, 1979

7

Personality Disorders

THE DIVERSITY AND COMPLEXITY of human personality are highly celebrated in our society. It may seem presumptuous, therefore, to speak of "personality types" or "character styles"—to try to fit ourselves amd our fellow beings into categories according to the way we behave. Yet human beings are generally consistent in their ways of dealing with the world and particularly with other people. Our styles of thinking, experiencing, and behaving usually remain stable as we encounter a variety of new challenges in new settings—hence the concept of character.

Character is reflected in our attitudes, our interests, our intellectual inclinations, our job aptitudes, and our social affinities. We all know people who fit certain stereotypes of character styles: the hard-driving unemotional scientist who buries himself in his laboratory work and is oblivious to life around him, or the dazzling actress who is the "life of the party." It would be no surprise to hear that the scientist is fastidious and conservative in dress, or that the actress wears lavish and seductive clothing. Nor would it be surprising that the scientist enjoys complex puzzles and mathematical games, or that the actress has little interest in balancing her checkbook. Of course, these are stereotypes; fortunately, most people are flexible enough to have a variety of styles in their repertoire. But most of us have a major personality style that shows itself in many different settings during all sorts of activities—in everything from the hobbies we enjoy to the lovers we choose.

Certainly, the typing of personalities does not imply any abnormality. In fact, the traits associated with particular personality types are often highly useful and adaptive, for they allow us to tolerate anxiety, to solve problems, to be creative, and to cope with a variety of life's stresses. For example, students would be in trouble if they did not possess some "obsessional" capacities for organizing and concentrating on a variety of tasks. Yet labels like "obsessive-compulsive" and "hysterical" have taken on very pejorative connotations in our daily language, and it is fashionable to use such terms in a sort of diagnostic name-calling.

When do personality *traits* become personality *disorders*? The boundary is not clear, but, generally, when character traits are so maladaptive and inflexible that they significantly impair one's work life and social life, or cause major subjective distress, a diagnosis of personality disorder is warranted.

WHAT ARE PERSONALITY DISORDERS?

Personality disorders are common and difficult to treat. The people who have them typically end up being labeled "bad" or "deviant" by others—even by mental health professionals. With that ominous prelude, let us look at some general characteristics of all personality disorders. The following generalizations may not hold true in every case, but they are good rules of thumb to help you put this category of psychopathology into a larger context:

- Personality disorders involve inflexible and maladaptive responses to stress.
- Personality disorders are global; they affect nearly all areas of a person's life, so that he or she is severely handicapped in working and loving. By contrast, neurotic persons' problems are confined to discrete aspects of their lives, while other aspects remain relatively free of psychological conflict.
- People with personality disorders commonly feel the problem lies not within themselves but in their environment (e.g., "No one understands me!" or "Everyone thwarts my plans!"). Neurotic persons are more likely to locate the source of their problems within themselves.
- Personality disorders do not, for the most part, involve psychosis. Brief psychotic episodes occur, but florid lapses in reality testing

(see Chapter 4) are the exception rather than the rule. Most people with personality disorders are in touch with reality most of the time.

- People with personality disorders are often untroubled by their illness, for they fail to see themselves as others see them. In fact, they may feel themselves to be in the best of emotional health, while others are quite distressed by their behavior. They may be dragged to mental health care facilities by others; the vast majority never seek treatment.

- People with personality disorders have an uncanny ability to get under the skin of others. They are likely, therefore, to be rejected by those close to them. They invariably irritate the mental health professionals who try to treat them. Treatment is difficult and failure is common.

- The complications associated with personality disorders are many. The most common are depression, suicide, violence and antisocial behavior, brief psychotic episodes, and multiple drug abuse.

From this list of features, you may wonder whether the label of "personality disorder" is simply a technical way of saying that someone is obnoxious. Indeed, the diagnostic label is easy to misuse in this way, as an epithet for any patient you do not like. But, in fact, individuals with personality disorders have specific and often crippling illnesses, defined not by their unpleasantness but by their degree of social dysfunction and personal inflexibility. They are incapable of responding to life's varied stresses and challenges except in a very rigid manner. They are like musicians who can play only one note.

Etiology

Little is known about the causes of specific personality disorders.

Environmental factors have been assumed to play the dominant role in the genesis of these disorders. Psychoanalytic theorists have focused primarily on the significance of childhood experiences within the family. However, few good large-scale studies have correlated early deprived or traumatic childhoods with later personality disorders. To date, there are no hard data to answer the perplexing question of why some people who suffer early emotional trauma develop severe character pathology, while others, with equally unhappy childhoods, do not.

Genetic factors are under active investigation as possible contributors to the development of personality disorders. There is some evidence for the heritability of certain character traits—particularly for the heritability of introverted personality traits. Work is also being done on the heritability of obsessive-compulsive traits.

Other constitutional factors, such as physical illness, seem to play a role in the development of personality disorders in some people. Neurological disorders—particularly birth-related trauma, encephalitis, and temporal lobe epilepsy—have been found to increase both the incidence and the severity of personality disorders. In fact, a history of minimal brain dysfunction (a childhood syndrome that includes such symptoms as learning disabilities and "hyperactivity") or the presence of soft (nonspecific) signs of neurological dysfunction (e.g., abnormal movements of arms or legs, incoordination, left-right confusion) in childhood correlates with an increased incidence of personality disorders in adolescence and adulthood.

Course and Prognosis

Personality disorders usually become evident in adolescence, or sometimes earlier. Clinical lore holds that once you have a personality disorder, you have it for life. However, surprisingly little is known about the course of these illnesses. It may be, for example, that personality disorders seem intractable because such people frequently fail in psychiatric treatment. Also, it may be that personality-disordered people who "grow up" or "burn out"—or in some way get better—cease to require professional attention, leaving only the truly intractable population in treatment and in correctional facilities. More work needs to be done in charting the course of these illnesses.

Diagnosis

The diagnostic criteria for the personality disorders are described below. Diagnosis is often difficult. The following are points to keep in mind in your assessments:

1. Be suspicious of reports by family or friends that the patient's personality has changed abruptly. Personality disorders do not begin suddenly. A history of sudden change in character should alert you to the possibility of some other illness, especially a central nervous system (CNS) disorder (e.g., tumor, cerebral vascular accident), incipient psychosis, or drug or alcohol abuse. Any of these can mimic a personality disorder.
2. Be curious about why someone with a personality disorder comes to you at a particular time. Look for some change in

important relationships that upset the former balance and suddenly made the disordered personality obvious to the patient or others.
3. Pay attention to your feelings about the patient. A person who makes you feel intensely angry, helpless, powerful, or frightened in the first few minutes of the interview may be showing you the nature of his or her personality disorder.
4. Beware of overdiagnosing personality disorders in people who are ethnically and culturally different from you. Behavior is more likely to look abnormal outside its social context.

Eleven personality disorders are described in the revised third edition of the *Diagnostic and Statistical Manual of Mental Disorders* (DSM-III-R). Two more (sadistic personality disorder and self-defeating personality disorder) are included in an appendix of DSM-III-R as "proposed diagnostic categories needing further study." The delineation of the various personality disorders has been a difficult task. First, there is no clear boundary to separate personality disorders from less severe conditions; diagnosis involves a measure of subjectivity. Second, personality is too complex to fit neatly into 13 categories. Many people with personality disorders exhibit features of more than one personality type. Some theorists have suggested that personality disorders are more accurately seen as clusters of pathological traits that can occur in an almost infinite variety of combinations.

As you read through the following descriptions, remember that these are stereotypes—individual people will have highly individual presentations. DSM-III-R has sorted the personality disorders under three general groups of patients (see Table 7-1): 1) patients who appear odd or eccentric; 2) patients who appear dramatic, emotional, or erratic; and 3) patients who are primarily anxious or fearful.

PARANOID PERSONALITY DISORDER

Profile

"Paranoid" is a common term in our everyday language, used to describe anyone from a jealous boyfriend to politicians who believe in a heavy buildup of nuclear armaments. Paranoia refers to a pervasive and unwarranted suspiciousness and mistrust of others. Suspiciousness may be highly justified and adaptive in war and other stressful situations, but paranoid people cannot abandon their suspicions when presented with

Table 7-1. Categorization of patients with personality disorder

Patients who appear odd or eccentric

Paranoid personality disorder
Schizoid personality disorder
Schizotypal personality disorder

Patients who appear dramatic, emotional, or erratic

Histrionic personality disorder
Narcissistic personality disorder
Antisocial personality disorder
Borderline personality disorder

Patients who are primarily anxious or fearful

Avoidant personality disorder
Dependent personality disorder
Obsessive-compulsive personality disorder
Passive-aggressive personality disorder

convincing contradictory evidence. They remain constantly on guard, because for them there is always a war going on.

Paranoid people are keen observers. They search intently for some confirmation that they are in danger. By disregarding facts that do not confirm their suspicions, they invariably find the plots and threats they so ardently seek. They are hypersensitive, they expect trickery and disloyalty from others, and they try to avoid all surprises by anticipating them.

Paranoid individuals appear tense, guarded, and secretive; they are often litigious and highly moralistic. They are usually humorless and overly serious. They have difficulty expressing warm emotions and tolerating feelings of being dependent on others. Paranoid individuals appear cold and may be quite logical. They are often interested in electronics, mechanics, and communication devices. They are also keenly aware of power and rank.

Because paranoid people seize upon irrelevant details to confirm their suspicions, they generally do not see the forest for the trees. They have very poor judgment in matters relating to their fears. They may, under stress, become floridly delusional (e.g., believing themselves wanted by the FBI) or experience ideas of reference. As a rule, however, psychotic episodes are brief and transient. The paranoid individual relies heavily on the defense mechanism of projection to maintain a psychological equilibrium. Projection involves attributing one's motives, feelings, or drives to someone else because one finds them unacceptable in oneself. This all happens unconsciously—that is, individuals who use projection are unaware that the motives they see in others are really their own. They make their inner world safe by making the outer world dangerous. Not surprisingly, paranoid people often bear a striking resemblance to the "demons" they choose.

In an interview, paranoid people are likely to be very businesslike. They may tell you they see no reason why they were referred to you. They may scan the room anxiously and have great difficulty relaxing. Or their preoccupation with details and constant questions may be the only things that belie their fear and mistrust.

Diagnosis

DSM-III-R (p. 339) provides a list of the items that are characteristic of the paranoid person's current and long-term functioning. These diagnostic criteria are shown in Table 7-2.

Table 7-2. DSM-III-R criteria for the diagnosis of paranoid personality
disorder

A pervasive and unwarranted tendency, beginning by early adulthood and present in a variety of contexts, to interpret the actions of people as deliberately demeaning or threatening, as indicated by at least *four* of the following:

1. Expects, without sufficient basis, to be exploited or harmed by others
2. Questions, without justification, the loyalty or trustworthiness of friends or associates
3. Reads hidden demeaning or threatening meanings into benign remarks or events—for example, suspects that a neighbor has put out the trash early to annoy him or her
4. Bears grudges or is unforgiving of insults or slights
5. Is reluctant to confide in others because of unwarranted fear that the information will be used against him or her
6. Is easily slighted and quick to react with anger or to counterattack
7. Questions, without justification, fidelity of spouse or sexual partner

Occurrence not exclusively during the course of schizophrenia or a delusional disorder.

Etiology

The causes of this disorder are unknown. A genetic predisposition to paranoid personality disorder has been considered, but no conclusive data on the genetics of the disorder have yet emerged.

Some psychoanalytic theorists suggest that people who were the objects of irrational and overwhelming parental rage may come to adopt their parents' style and project onto others the rage they believed was once directed toward them. Others have characterized the families of paranoid individuals as overly constricted emotionally.

Epidemiology

Little is known about the incidence or prevalence of paranoid personality disorder, because many paranoid people never seek treatment. The disorder is more frequently diagnosed in men than in women. There is no known familial pattern, but the disorder occurs with increased frequency in the biological relatives of schizophrenic individuals and has a possible biogenetic link with other paranoid disorders.

Course and Prognosis

No good long-term outcome studies have been done on paranoid personality disorder. Some people apparently have the disorder throughout life, whereas others "grow out of it" as stress diminishes or other life circumstances change. Some people who are diagnosed as having paranoid personality disorder go on to develop schizophrenia.

Differential Diagnosis

There are several conditions from which paranoid personality disorder must be differentiated.

Paranoid disorders. These disorders are characterized by persistent psychotic symptoms (e.g., delusions, hallucinations) that are not present in paranoid personality disorder.

Schizophrenia. Like paranoid disorders, schizophrenia is marked by persistent psychosis, which does not characterize paranoid personality disorder.

Borderline personality disorder. Although borderline individuals may show some paranoid features, they tend to be overinvolved in chaotic relationships with people. Paranoid people, by contrast, remain aloof and distant from others.

Antisocial personality disorder. Both antisocial and paranoid personality disorders involve difficulty with intimacy, but paranoid individuals do not have the lifelong history of antisocial behavior that is found in individuals with antisocial personality disorder.

Impulse disorders. These may be distinguished from paranoid personality disorder because they are characterized primarily by difficulty with impulse control rather than by suspiciousness.

Treatment

Because paranoid people are so frightened of intimacy and so reluctant to trust, a relationship with a therapist may be both longed for and dreaded. You must be particularly careful to operate in as open and straightforward a manner as possible in dealing with such people. Use humor sparingly and with great care at the start, for paranoid people are prone to feel that others are laughing at them rather than with them.

You must be careful to assume a professional manner, not one that is overly warm; paranoid people will be suspicious of and frightened by overtures they do not understand. When paranoid patients develop false beliefs about you (e.g., that you are part of a conspiracy to harm them), their accusations can easily become threats. You must limit any threatening behavior, both for your own and for the patient's safety.

Among the most commonly used treatments, individual supportive psychotherapy is probably the treatment of choice, although no good controlled studies on the treatment of paranoid personality disorder have been done. A supportive relationship with a therapist, while difficult to establish, may help the paranoid person make sense of and manage stressful life situations. More exploratory or interpretive psychotherapy is rarely possible with paranoid people. A primary aim of exploratory work is to help paranoid patients see how they attribute their own unacceptable thoughts and feelings to others, and the ways in which this distorted perspective hampers their lives. Paranoid individuals have difficulty tolerating confrontation by others in group therapy. The directive techniques used in behavior modification may be reassuring insofar as they are relatively impersonal, but paranoid people fear being controlled by others and may come to see the behavior therapist as attempting to exert control over them. There has been little research on the use of medications in paranoid personality disorder, but some clinicians prescribe low doses of antipsychotic medications to alleviate anxiety. Suspiciousness of medication often makes compliance a problem for paranoid individuals.

SCHIZOID PERSONALITY DISORDER

Profile

The term *schizoid* has long been used to describe people who are socially withdrawn, introverted, eccentric, and uncomfortable with others. If you consider the schizophrenic disorders as a spectrum (see Chapter 5), then schizoid personality disorder occupies the healthier end of the schizophrenic spectrum along with paranoid and schizotypal personality disorders. Schizoid individuals resemble schizophrenic people in their odd and withdrawn manner, but whereas schizophrenic people have chronically disordered thinking, schizoid individuals do not.

The avoidance of human contact is a way of life for schizoid people, and they show little need or longing for emotional ties to others. Instead, they are likely to be quite absorbed in their own private fantasy worlds, in which they carry on relationships with imaginary friends. Their sex life may exist only in this world of make-believe. While schizoid individuals may have quite violent fantasies, they usually express little emotion to others.

Schizoid individuals actively pursue isolation and will therefore choose solitary jobs other people find difficult to tolerate. They are likely to work as night watchmen or to bury themselves in the stacks of a library. In fact, schizoid people can be quite absorbed in and successful at such pursuits as mathematics and astronomy, which demand little human contact.

In an interview, you will find the schizoid person to be uncomfortable with you and eager for the meeting to end. He or she will typically make infrequent eye contact, show little emotion, and offer little in the way of spontaneous comments—that is, answering your questions but not elaborating on answers at all. Occasionally, you may hear odd word usage, but speech and thought content do not generally appear to be abnormal.

Why does the schizoid person flee from other people? Although he or she is seemingly indifferent to others, the schizoid person usually feels quite vulnerable and finds human interaction confusing, frightening, and painful. The isolation is thus sought in self-defense. One schizoid woman described her situation as that of a tiny, naked baby locked inside a steel drawer (Guntrip 1973, p. 152).

Diagnosis

The diagnostic criteria given in DSM-III-R (p. 340) for schizoid personality disorder are shown in Table 7-3.

Table 7-3. DSM-III-R criteria for the diagnosis of schizoid personality disorder

A pervasive pattern of indifference to social relationships and a restricted range of emotional experience and expression, beginning by early adulthood and present in a variety of contexts, as indicated by at least *four* of the following:

1. Neither desires nor enjoys close relationships, including being part of a family
2. Almost always chooses solitary activities
3. Rarely, if ever, claims or appears to experience strong emotions, such as anger and joy
4. Indicates little, if any, desire to have sexual experiences with another person (age being taken into account)
5. Is indifferent to the praise and criticism of others
6. Has no close friends or confidants (or only one) other than first-degree relatives
7. Displays constricted affect—for example, is aloof, cold, rarely reciprocates gestures or facial expressions such as smiles or nods

Occurrence not exclusively during the course of schizophrenia or a delusional disorder.

Etiology

No one knows why some individuals become schizoid and others do not. In psychotherapy, schizoid patients commonly report bleak childhoods devoid of emotional warmth, but no prospective studies have been done to see which factors in childhood can be correlated with schizoid personality traits in adult life. There is also considerable speculation, but no clear evidence, of possible genetic factors in the genesis of schizoid personality disorder.

Epidemiology

The incidence, prevalence, and sex ratio of schizoid personality disorder have not been well studied. The disorder may be prevalent in as much as 2% of the population and is thought to be more frequent in males than in females. However, many schizoid people never seek treatment, and the population seen by clinicians may not be representative of those schizoid individuals in the community. With the advent of DSM-III diagnostic categories for personality disorders, the schizoid diagnosis has declined in use, having possibly been subsumed by the avoidant and schizotypal categories.

Course and Prognosis

Schizoid personality disorder generally begins in childhood and may last throughout life. Neither the frequency of remission nor the frequency with which schizoid people go on to develop schizophrenia is known.

Differential Diagnosis

Schizoid personality disorder must be differentiated from the following.

Schizophrenia. The presence of a thought disorder at some time during the course of schizophrenia differentiates it from schizoid personality disorder. Also, schizoid individuals usually function better than schizophrenic people in work situations.

Schizotypal personality disorder. The schizotypal and schizoid disorders both involve an odd and eccentric manner, but schizotypal personality disorder is closer to schizophrenia in the following respects: poor work history, oddities of perception and communication, and a high frequency of schizophrenic relatives.

Avoidant personality disorder. Individuals with avoidant personalities are similar to schizoid people in that they avoid most human interaction. Unlike schizoid individuals, avoidant individuals profess to long for relationships with others but hang back from them because of extreme sensitivity to rejection.

Paranoid personality disorder. This disorder involves a greater ability to engage others socially. Paranoid people are more verbally aggressive than schizoid people are, and they are less absorbed in fantasy.

Treatment

Individual psychotherapy with schizoid patients is difficult but by no means impossible. Such people engage in any human interaction reluctantly, and a therapeutic relationship is no exception. However, as schizoid people begin to trust the therapist, they begin to share their fantasy lives, as well as their intense fears about becoming close to the therapist.

The value of group psychotherapy in treating schizoid people has not been established, but some schizoid individuals manage to become involved in and use groups to develop social skills and experiment with interpersonal closeness.

No specific role for medication has been defined in the treatment of schizoid personality disorder.

SCHIZOTYPAL PERSONALITY DISORDER

Profile

Schizotypal personality disorder denotes a condition similar to schizoid personality disorder but characterized by additional symptoms; it is believed to be genetically linked to schizophrenia. Although it is not always easy to differentiate schizotypal from schizoid individuals, schizotypal individuals are likely to look more obviously strange and eccentric, even to those who meet them in passing.

People with schizotypal personality disorder suffer from clear disturbances of thinking and communication. Although they may never have a frank psychotic episode with hallucinations or bizarre delusions, they show milder forms of thought disorder, such as derealization, ideas of reference, and perceptual illusions (see Chapter 4). They are extremely sensitive to others and so retreat into a world of imaginary relationships and vivid fears and fantasies.

In an interview, you will find schizotypal people to be withdrawn and to have a great difficulty with face-to-face interaction. They show little feeling, and their affects are at times grossly inappropriate to the subject being discussed. Speech is usually peculiar, in that they use words in odd ways and express ideas unclearly; you may need to ask for clarification often. Although schizotypal individuals will be guarded about their inner worlds, they may admit to unfounded beliefs (e.g., that they have special powers or that they are the focus of special attention).

Diagnosis

The DSM-III-R diagnostic criteria for schizotypal personality disorder (pp. 341–342) are listed in Table 7-4.

Etiology

This disorder is more common among the biological relatives of schizophrenic individuals than among the general population, but no studies have clearly demonstrated particular causal factors. Twin studies suggest the importance of genetic factors in the development of the disorder.

Epidemiology

Estimates of the prevalence of schizotypal personality disorder in the general population range from 2% to 6%.

Table 7-4. DSM-III-R criteria for the diagnosis of schizotypal personality disorder

A pervasive pattern of deficits in interpersonal relatedness and peculiarities of ideation, appearance, and behavior, beginning by early adulthood and present in a variety of contexts, as indicated by at least *five* of the following:

1. Ideas of reference (excluding delusions of reference)
2. Excessive social anxiety—for example, extreme discomfort in social situations involving unfamiliar people
3. Odd beliefs or magical thinking, influencing behavior and inconsistent with subcultural norms—for example, superstitiousness, belief in clairvoyance, telepathy, or "sixth sense," "others can feel my feelings" (in children and adolescents, bizarre fantasies or preoccupations)
4. Unusual perceptual experiences—for example, illusions, sensing the presence of a force or person not actually present (e.g., "I felt as if my dead mother were in the room with me")
5. Odd or eccentric behavior or appearance—for example, unkempt, unusual mannerisms, talks to himself or herself
6. No close friends or confidants (or only one) other than first-degree relatives
7. Odd speech (without loosening of associations or incoherence)—for example, speech that is impoverished, digressive, vague, or inappropriately abstract
8. Inappropriate or constricted affect—for example, silly, aloof, rarely reciprocates gestures or facial expressions such as smiles or nods
9. Suspiciousness or paranoid ideation

Occurrence not exclusively during the course of schizophrenia or a pervasive developmental disorder.

Course and Prognosis

The course of people with schizotypal personality disorder is relatively stable, marked by long-term impairment of role performance, persistent symptoms, and social isolation.

Differential Diagnosis

The three major disorders from which schizotypal personality disorder must be distinguished are schizoid personality disorder, schizophrenia, and borderline personality disorder.

Schizoid people do not show the oddities of speech, perception, and behavior seen among schizotypal individuals. Schizotypal individuals are not frankly psychotic, unlike schizophrenic people, who have gross psychotic disturbances at some point in their illness. Although many of the cognitive and perceptual oddities of schizotypal personality disorder are also found in borderline personality disorder, borderline individuals are more likely than schizotypal persons to have intense, stormy interpersonal relationships.

Treatment

As with schizoid people, schizotypal individuals are absorbed in fantasy and private belief systems that they may share, with great difficulty, in psychotherapy. Therapy is aimed at establishing a relationship and weathering the difficulties these people encounter in dealing with another human being. Exploratory psychotherapy is often resisted; supportive treatment is less threatening to many of these people. Rehabilitation programs and social skills training may help patients improve their work performance and better manage social situations.

Antipsychotic medication in low doses may help to diminish disordered thinking, anxiety, somatization, and ruminations in schizotypal individuals.

HISTRIONIC PERSONALITY DISORDER

Histrionic personality disorder is really a descendent of hysteria, a term commonly used in clinical settings. It is one of the oldest psychiatric diagnoses in Western civilization and has acquired a bewildering variety of uses over the years.

The four most common uses of the term describe 1) a specific personality style, 2) a conversion reaction (e.g., hysterical paralysis), 3) a neurotic illness characterized by phobias and anxiety, and 4) certain pathological character traits. It has also been used in our culture as a term of disapproval, particularly toward women. We will focus here on hysteria as a normal personality style, and then look at histrionic personality disorder as a pathological exaggeration of that style.

Hysterical people are typically warm and imaginative, with well-developed intuition. They tend to look at the world in global, impressionistic terms rather than focusing on details (i.e., they are "headline readers"). They gravitate toward activities that do not require intense concentration on facts but allow for the use of intuitive faculties. Thus, hysterical individuals are less likely to be technicians and scholars than they are to be actors or artists. Hysterical people tend to see those things in life that are vivid, colorful, and immediately striking; they often overlook more subtle or more neutral details. They are emotive and often act as the life of the party in groups. Stereotypically, hysterical people are seductive and somewhat superficial in their relationships, getting carried away by exaggerated emotionality that is not founded on deep convictions.

Hysterical individuals characteristically rely on the defense of *repression* to maintain their psychological equilibrium. Repression is akin to forgetting, in that it involves banishing unacceptable ideas, feelings, or impulses from one's conscious awareness in order to decrease anxiety. Thus, the hysterical person might simply repress the fact of an upcoming examination and forget to arrive on time. This tendency to "forget" unpleasant facts often makes the hysterical individual appear to be more scatterbrained and less intelligent than he or she really is.

Now let us go on to look at histrionic personality disorder, in which hysterical traits are highly inflexible and maladaptive.

Profile

Although people with histrionic personality disorder may be colorful and outgoing, they are also highly excitable and have great difficulty maintaining deep and lasting attachments to others. They tend to use displays of emotion to control other people—to get attention, to avoid unwanted responsibilities, and to coerce others into taking responsibility for their welfare. Typically, these people can induce guilt in others by throwing temper tantrums or bursting into tears, and their control by these means can be quite powerful. Their affections and loyalties are extremely fickle, and this frustrates those who try to get close to them. While these people are often quite seductive, their purpose in attracting partners is not always sexual—for example, they may seduce lovers who will then satisfy their wishes to be taken care of and nurtured.

Diagnosis

The diagnostic criteria given in DSM-III-R for histrionic personality disorder (p. 349) are shown in Table 7-5.

Etiology

The causes of histrionic personality disorder have not been demonstrated in any prospective studies. Psychodynamic theorists posit that disturbances in the early parent-child relationship play a central role in the genesis of this disorder. New research points to a possible familial association between histrionic and antisocial personality disorders, and one theory holds that histrionic personality disorder and antisocial

Table 7-5. DSM-III-R criteria for the diagnosis of histrionic personality disorder

A pervasive pattern of excessive emotionality and attention-seeking, beginning by early adulthood and present in a variety of contexts, as indicated by at least *four* of the following:

1. Constantly seeks or demands reassurance, approval, or praise
2. Is inappropriately sexually seductive in appearance or behavior
3. Is overly concerned with physical attractiveness
4. Expresses emotion with inappropriate exaggeration—for example, embraces casual acquaintances with excessive ardor; uncontrollable sobbing on minor sentimental occasions; has temper tantrums
5. Is uncomfortable in situations in which he or she is not the center of attention
6. Displays rapidly shifting and shallow expression of emotions
7. Is self-centered, actions being directed toward obtaining immediate satisfaction; has no tolerance for the frustration of delayed gratification
8. Has a style of speech that is excessively impressionistic and lacking in detail—for example, when asked to describe his or her mother, can be no more specific than, "She was a beautiful person"

personality disorder (the latter being more common in men) are sex-linked expressions of the same underlying genotype.

Epidemiology

Little information is available on the prevalence of this disorder, because people with this condition previously were included in the larger and more ambiguous category of hysterical personality disorder. Histrionic personality disorder is diagnosed much more frequently in women than in men, but this may reflect sex-role bias on the part of diagnosticians.

Course and Prognosis

Little is known about the outlook for this disorder, but it is thought to improve with advancing age.

Differential Diagnosis

Histrionic personality disorder and borderline personality disorder are quite similar. However, borderline individuals generally feel chronically empty, lack a sense of identity, experience brief psychotic episodes, and engage in overtly self-destructive acts. Histrionic people do not exhibit these features with any regularity.

Individuals with histrionic personality disorder may also suffer from a somatization disorder (akin to the old category of conversion hysteria). (See Chapter 8 for further details on somatization disorder.)

Treatment

Psychodynamic, insight-oriented psychotherapy is the treatment of choice for histrionic personality disorder. Both individual therapy and group therapy have been found useful. The therapist must work on helping histrionic patients to clarify their genuine feelings, since the experience of deeply felt emotion is foreign to them. The therapist must help histrionic patients learn to take responsibility for the consequences of their actions, and to use their rational cognitive abilities rather than remaining "helpless" and "scatterbrained."

NARCISSISTIC PERSONALITY DISORDER

Narcissus, legend tells us, was a beautiful Grecian youth who fell madly in love with his own reflection when he happened upon a pool one day. Realizing that he could never possess what he so ardently desired, he killed himself.

Narcissism has come to represent many things in our culture, including self-centeredness and the ethos of the "me generation." In one sense, narcissism simply refers to self-love, and loving self-regard is both desirable and healthy. Only when self-absorption impairs one's ability to form lasting attachments to others do we term it pathological. Ironically, the crippling self-doubt and insecurity involved in pathological narcissism are a far cry from simple self-regard.

Profile

People with narcissistic personality disorder have severe problems maintaining a realistic concept of their own worth. They generally set goals and make demands of themselves that are utterly unrealistic, and then feel inadequate and helpless when they fail to meet these standards. They constantly crave love, attention, and admiration from other people as a means of bolstering their faltering self-esteem. Their demands for such love and praise can be insatiable, and they are likely to fly into a rage when these demands are not met. They are exquisitely sensitive to perceived slights from others and approach people expecting to be disappointed. Thus, the narcissistic person struggles to keep a tenuous balance between the intense need to be admired by an important person and the rage he or she experiences toward that person's disappointing qualities. This struggle makes intimacy difficult and threatening. The narcissistic individual often idealizes other people, only to come to devalue and despise them when they reveal themselves to be in some way imperfect.

Narcissistic people are preoccupied with fantasies of unlimited success and tend to overestimate their abilities and their own specialness. This inflated self-importance often coexists with an unrealistic sense of worthlessness. Fantasies of achievement may take the place of actual work, but some people with this disorder are highly successful, pursuing fame and power with a relentless driven quality, never feeling satisfied with their achievements.

People with narcissistic personality disorder have difficulty recognizing how other people feel. They usually expect special favors from others without feeling any need to reciprocate; in this respect, they have a characteristic sense of entitlement. Narcissistic individuals are more concerned with how they look to others than with genuine feeling. They often use other people for their own ends.

All of this, it must be remembered, is in the service of protecting the narcissistic person's very fragile self-esteem. Narcissistic individuals feel devalued easily, and they may react to perceived slights not only with inappropriate rage but also with emotional withdrawal, depression, and even suicide. The "insults" that trigger such rage and depression are often as minor as a misunderstood remark or a canceled appointment.

Diagnosis

The diagnostic criteria that DSM-III-R presents for narcissistic personality disorder (p. 351) are shown in Table 7-6.

Etiology

No specific genetic or environmental factors have been clearly demonstrated to cause narcissistic personality disorder. Many psychoanalytic theorists believe the disorder stems from early childhood experiences in which parents did not encourage or appreciate the child's efforts at self-assertion, and did not help the child take pride in accomplishments. The child is left emotionally hungry and unable to maintain a stable sense of self-worth without constant support from people who are important to him or her (see Chapter 2).

Table 7-6. DSM-III-R criteria for the diagnosis of narcissistic personality
disorder

A pervasive pattern of grandiosity (in fantasy or behavior), lack of empathy,
and hypersensitivity to the evaluation of others, beginning by early adulthood
and present in a variety of contexts, as indicated by at least *five* of the
following:

1. Reacts to criticism with feelings of rage, shame, or humiliation (even if not
   expressed)
2. Is interpersonally exploitative: takes advantage of others to achieve his or
   her own ends
3. Has a grandiose sense of self-importance—for example, exaggerates
   achievements and talents; expects to be noticed as "special" without
   appropriate achievement
4. Believes that his or her problems are unique and can be understood only by
   other special people
5. Is preoccupied with fantasies of unlimited success, power, brilliance,
   beauty, or ideal love
6. Has a sense of entitlement: an unreasonable expectation of especially
   favorable treatment—for example, assumes that he or she does not have to
   wait in line when others do
7. Requires constant attention and admiration—for example, keeps fishing for
   compliments
8. Lack of empathy: the inability to recognize and experience how others
   feel—for example, annoyance and surprise when a friend who is seriously
   ill cancels a date
9. Is preoccupied with feelings of envy

Epidemiology

No good data on the prevalence of narcissistic personality disorder are
available. Reports in the literature indicate that the diagnosis is made
more frequently in men than in women, but it is not yet clear whether
men are actually more susceptible to the disorder. The diagnosis is common in outpatient practices.

Course and Prognosis

No good data are available on the outlook for this disorder. The diagnosis is rarely made before young adulthood, and the disorder is found in all
stages of adult life.

Differential Diagnosis

Some theorists have questioned the validity of narcissistic personality disorder as a separate diagnostic category because many people with other disorders have prominent features of pathological narcissism. In particular, it may be difficult to differentiate narcissistic personality disorder from the following.

Histrionic personality disorder. Although both disorders involve seductiveness and self-dramatization, the person with a histrionic personality disorder is generally more playful and warm, while the narcissistic person is likely to be haughty, cold, and more obviously exploitative in dealings with others.

Borderline personality disorder. As a rule, borderline individuals show poorer impulse control and are more socially and occupationally dysfunctional than narcissistic people. Borderline individuals often appear to be very emotionally needy, while narcissistic people appear to be more self-sufficient.

Antisocial personality disorder. People with antisocial personality disorder are more impulsive than narcissistic individuals and show a constant calculated disregard for social standards. Narcissistic people either do not recognize their violations of social norms or else view themselves as deserving to be above society's rules.

Obsessive-compulsive personality disorder. Both obsessive-compulsive individuals and narcissistic people set high standards and pursue perfection with a driven quality. However, the narcissistic person is haughty and claims perfection to maintain an idealized self-image; the obsessive-compulsive individual strives for perfection in order to feel capable and in control.

Treatment

Individual and group psychotherapies are the treatments of choice. There is currently an active debate among psychodynamic theorists about the proper approach to the treatment of narcissistic personality disorder. Heinz Kohut and his followers see the disorder as a developmental defect that results from inadequate parenting (specifically, lack of parental empathy for the child) and from other childhood traumata. They see the therapist's task as encouraging the patient to reveal his or her untamed grandiose self-view and idealized view of the therapist, with the goal of learning to accept and tolerate the inevitable disappointments and narcissistic injuries that occur in the relationship with the therapist, thereby repairing the deficit in the ability to modulate self-esteem. The therapist's interpretations emphasize the patient's longings to be understood in a perfect relationship.

By contrast, Otto Kernberg sees the narcissistic individual's grandiose self-view and idealization of the therapist as defensive maneuvers designed to protect against the awareness of more dangerous underlying feelings of rage, envy, and inferiority. According to this view, the therapist needs to interpret grandiosity and idealization as defensive, instead of treating these feelings as part of a normal developmental phase.

Regardless of the psychotherapeutic strategy you choose, treatment is fraught with difficulties. Narcissistic patients will often idealize you at the outset of treatment and then find it difficult to tolerate later recognition that you are not all-giving, all-knowing, and all-caring. This disappointment may cause disruptions in treatment; you and the patient must weather the storms of rage and periods of haughty devaluing that ensue. In group therapy, the patient may act out this scenario with group members or the group leader. The aim of therapy is to provide a consistent, caring relationship in which narcissistic patients can gain insight into their difficulties and develop more realistic concepts of themselves and of other people as neither perfect nor worthless.

To date, no role has been demonstrated for behavioral or pharmacological approaches in the treatment of narcissistic personality disorder.

ANTISOCIAL PERSONALITY DISORDER

Profile

The term *antisocial personality disorder* may sound quite judgmental and pejorative, but it is in fact an accurate label for this illness. The most salient diagnostic feature is a long history of antisocial behavior in which the rights of others are repeatedly violated. This is not simply the medical term for criminality, but describes a long-standing illness that impairs the most important areas of the person's life. In clinical settings, you may also hear the more informal term *sociopath* used to refer to people with antisocial personality disorder.

People with this disorder are not usually patients—that is, they do not commonly appear in mental health care settings—but are more likely to end up in courts, prisons, and welfare offices. When they do appear in mental health clinics, it is often either because they were brought there unwillingly or because they are trying to avoid the legal consequences of some recent act.

By definition, the people with this disorder begin their antisocial behavior before age 15. In childhood, they typically lie, steal, fight, and have pervasive difficulties with authority. In adolescence, sexual behavior begins early and may be unusually aggressive, and there is generally excessive drinking and drug use. By the time they reach adulthood, these people are usually unable to hold a responsible job or maintain family ties; most of them habitually break the law. Alcoholism, vagrancy, and social isolation are common, and a substantial number of these individuals commit suicide. What is often striking and exasperating about sociopathic individuals is their apparent lack of anxiety or depression in situations where one might expect such emotions.

People with antisocial personality disorder often turn on their charm at will in order to subtly manipulate others. You may find yourself baffled in an interview with somebody who has an antisocial personality disorder, for they can present a charming and strikingly "normal" facade. In fact, if an interview discloses nothing that seems abnormal, think first about the possibility that your patient has no disorder, but then consider whether you may have been "conned" by a sociopathic patient.

Obviously the diagnosis of this disorder depends not on the mental status examination but on the person's history. You are more likely to get reliable historical data from the family or from law enforcement officials than from the patient. Despite a healthy facade, the sociopathic patient may show you some signs of stress in the interview—complaining of tension, of vague somatic symptoms, of feeling depressed, or of feeling (often correctly) that others are hostile toward him or her.

Diagnosis

The diagnostic criteria for antisocial personality disorder given in DSM-III-R (pp. 344–345) are shown in Table 7-7.

Etiology

Both environmental and genetic factors seem to play a role in the genesis of antisocial personality disorder. The main environmental factor seems to be the sustained deprivation in early childhood of any consistent emotional ties with a significant person. The classic example of such deprivation is parents who are inconsistently available to the child and who are impulsive and erratic in their behavior. It is therefore no surprise to find that antisocial personality disorder is frequently found in the parents (particularly among the fathers) of those who have the disorder.

The evidence for genetic factors in antisocial personality disorder

Table 7-7. DSM-III-R criteria for the diagnosis of antisocial personality
disorder

Evidence of conduct disorder with onset before age 15, as indicated by a
history of *three* or more of the following:

1) Was often truant
2) Ran away from home overnight at least twice while living in parental
   or parental surrogate home (or once without returning)
3) Often initiated physical fights
4) Used a weapon in more than one fight
5) Forced someone into sexual activity with him or her
6) Was physically cruel to animals
7) Was physically cruel to other people
8) Deliberately destroyed others' property (other than by fire-setting)
9) Deliberately engaged in fire-setting
10) Often lied (other than to avoid physical or sexual abuse)
11) Has stolen without confrontation of a victim on more than one
    occasion (including forgery)
12) Has stolen with confrontation of a victim (e.g., mugging, purse-
    snatching, extortion, armed robbery)

A pattern of irresponsible and antisocial behavior since the age of 15, as
indicated by at least *four* of the following:

1) Is unable to sustain consistent work behavior, as indicated by any of
   the following (including similar behavior in academic settings if the
   person is a student):

   a) Significant unemployment for six months or more within five years
       when expected to work and work was available
   b) Repeated absences from work unexplained by illness in self or
       family
   c) Abandonment of several jobs without realistic plans for others

2) Fails to conform to social norms with respect to lawful behavior, as
   indicated by repeatedly performing antisocial acts that are grounds for
   arrest (whether arrested or not)—for example, destroying property,
   harassing others, stealing, pursuing an illegal occupation
3) Is irritable and aggressive, as indicated by repeated physical fights or
   assaults (not required by one's job or to defend someone or oneself),
   including spouse- or child-beating
4) Repeatedly fails to honor financial obligations, as indicated by
   defaulting on debts or failing to provide child support for other
   dependents on a regular basis
5) Fails to plan ahead, or is impulsive, as indicated by one or both of the
   following:

Table 7-7. *Continued*

---

    a) Traveling from place to place without a prearranged job or clear goal for the period of travel or clear idea about when the travel will terminate

    b) Lack of a fixed address for a month or more

6) Has no regard for the truth, as indicated by repeated lying, use of aliases, or "conning" others for personal profit or pleasure
7) Is reckless regarding his or her own or others' personal safety, as indicated by driving while intoxicated, or recurrent speeding
8) If a parent or guardian, lacks ability to function as a responsible parent, as indicated by one or more of the following:

    a) Malnutrition of child
    b) Child's illness resulting from lack of minimal hygiene
    c) Failure to obtain medical care for a seriously ill child
    d) Child's dependence on neighbors or nonresident relatives for food or shelter
    e) Failure to arrange for a caretaker for young child when parent is away from home
    f) Repeated squandering, on personal items, of money required for household necessities

9) Has never sustained a totally monogamous relationship for more than one year
10) Lacks remorse (feels justified in having hurt, mistreated, or stolen from another)

Occurrence of antisocial behavior not exclusively during the course of schizophrenia or manic episodes.

---

comes from studies which show that having a sociopathic or an alcoholic father is a powerful predictor of developing a sociopathic personality, even among children who were adopted at birth and not raised by their biological parents. Twin studies suggest a genetic factor in the genesis of the disorder as well. There is also an empirical association between alcoholism and antisocial personality disorder.

    Contrary to what might be expected intuitively, antisocial personality disorder is not correlated with such factors as living in a high-crime area, keeping bad company, or being a member of a deviant subgroup in society.

Epidemiology

The prevalence of antisocial personality disorder in the United States is estimated to be roughly 3% for males and less than 1% for females.

The disorder is more common among lower socioeconomic groups, probably because 1) most people with antisocial personality disorder have very poor work records and, therefore, impaired earning capacity; and 2) the fathers of those who have the disorder frequently had it themselves, so many of these people grew up in impoverished homes. However, the disorder is found in all socioeconomic classes, including the most privileged. It is more prevalent in urban than in rural areas.

The prevalence of the disorder among prison populations is very high—perhaps as high as 75%.

Course and Prognosis

The disorder begins in childhood, and antisocial behavior reaches its peak in young adulthood. Two changes seem to occur among people with antisocial personality disorder as they enter their 30s and 40s. First, for some people, the disorder seems to remit. Among those who have the disorder, roughly 2% improve (i.e., stop their antisocial behavior) each year once they get beyond age 21. Second, many of those who stop their antisocial behavior in their adult years develop hypochondriacal concerns, depression, and chronic substance abuse.

Differential Diagnosis

There are several conditions from which antisocial personality disorder must be differentiated.

Criminality. As noted above, antisocial personality disorder is not simply another term for criminality. It is a disorder that impairs all aspects of the individual's life—social functioning, work capacity, and the ability to achieve and maintain intimate relationships. Many people with this disorder manage to keep their actions within the limits of the law but nevertheless violate social norms and harm others by their behavior. Conversely, some people who commit crimes may act with loyalty and a sense of responsibility toward others in their lives (e.g., spouses, parents) and thus cannot be accurately labeled sociopathic individuals.

Borderline personality disorder. Both borderline and antisocial personality disorders may involve impulsive and destructive behavior, directed at the self as well as others. However, borderline individuals are more likely than sociopathic people to behave self-destructively. Also, although sociopathic people often act aggressively toward others without anger or guilt, borderline individuals usually become hostile only when feeling deprived by people who are important to them, and they commonly feel guilty about their anger. Borderline personality disorder is more frequently diagnosed in women, whereas antisocial personality disorder is more frequently diagnosed in men.

Manic episode. Mania may involve antisocial behavior, but such behavior is clearly episodic rather than chronic and long-standing, and it accompanies a highly altered mood.

Substance abuse disorder. Drug and alcohol abuse can certainly result in global impairment of functioning and chronic antisocial behavior (stealing, lying, etc.) as the individual struggles to maintain and conceal an addiction. In these cases, antisocial behavior stops when the drug abuse stops. Often, however, substance abuse is simply secondary to an underlying antisocial personality disorder, and both diagnoses may be warranted in such cases.

Treatment

Sociopathic individuals look unreachable and untreatable in an outpatient setting. They appear to lack anxiety, to lack any motivation for change, and to learn nothing from experience. However, these are only the characteristics of a sociopathic person who is in flight. When people with an antisocial personality disorder are immobilized—that is, when they are held in a treatment or prison facility and can no longer act to avoid unpleasant feelings—a very different picture emerges. Sociopathic individuals begin to experience considerable anxiety and become convinced that this anxiety will be intolerable. The fear of getting close to others becomes much more apparent, as does the sociopathic individual's sensitivity to criticism and rejection.

Thus, actual control over the behavior of people with antisocial personality disorder is the cornerstone of treatment. They must be prevented from running away, or from hurting themselves or others, when feelings seem intolerable. This control is usually impossible to achieve on an outpatient basis and can only be achieved in prison or on a locked inpatient unit. The goal of treatment is to show these people that they and others can tolerate their anxiety. Sociopathic individuals often need much more support than is possible in individual therapy. Peer support groups of all kinds are probably the most effective treatment, because the sociopathic individual can use such groups to identify with others who struggle with similar problems.

You may be tempted to try to rescue charming sociopathic patients and to shield them from the consequences of their own behavior (e.g., legal proceedings, prison sentences). This is antitherapeutic. People with antisocial personality disorder cannot be treated without the clear understanding that they are responsible for whatever they do.

Medications are likely to be abused by people with antisocial personality disorder. To date, there is no clear role for psychotropic medication in the treatment of this disorder.

BORDERLINE PERSONALITY DISORDER

For many years, psychiatric thinkers taught that an individual could be either psychotic or neurotic, but not both. Yet therapists reported many cases in which people became transiently psychotic under stress, recompensated quickly, and in most situations remained completely in touch with reality. Some thought these people had a mild form of schizophrenia; others called them severely neurotic. Out of this confusion, contemporary theorists developed the concept of the borderline personality—borderline referring to the line between psychosis and neurosis.

Profile

Many borderline people do indeed move in and out of psychosis. When they lose touch with reality it may take the form of frank hallucinations and delusions, but more often the psychosis involves dissociative states, derealization, and depersonalization (see Chapter 4). These episodes are usually brief—lasting several minutes to several days—and generally occur in response to stress (e.g., a breakup with a lover).

But reactive psychosis is by no means the only prominent feature of the borderline syndrome. Intense and persistent anger is one of the hallmarks of this disorder. Borderline individuals are characteristically rageful and demanding, going to great lengths to get others to feel responsible for their woes and their welfare. They form chaotic relationships with others because they struggle with intense dependence upon and intense hostility toward those to whom they become attached. Borderline individuals are adept at manipulating others to do their bidding. But their use of emotional blackmail (e.g., suicide threats) and their angry outbursts ultimately drive away the people who are important to them.

The borderline individual is easily overwhelmed by anger and frustration, and generally acts impulsively when feelings become intolerable. This usually involves repeated self-destructive acts (e.g., wrist slashing, overdoses, car crashes) and may also include drug abuse, sexual promiscuity, and abrupt changes in job and living situations.

Borderline individuals usually possess a facade of sociability and adaptiveness that makes them quite engaging in superficial contact. Thus, many borderline people are very good at interviews but function erratically and below their apparent capabilities in work situations.

People with borderline personality disorder chronically experience feelings of emptiness and uncertainty about who they are. This disturbed sense of identity can be seen in a variety of areas—gender identity, personal goals, the difference between their own and others' feelings, their self-image, and their body image. When borderline individuals complain, "I don't know who I am," they generally reflect a profound sense of internal chaos and confusion. This is particularly acute when there is no one around from whom the borderline person can take his or her cues; therefore, the borderline individual has difficulty being alone, and, in order to avoid such a situation, will seek out companionship, at times frantically.

Diagnosis

The DSM-III-R diagnostic criteria for borderline personality disorder (p. 347) are shown in Table 7-8. In addition to the criteria listed in this table, borderline personality disorder may involve psychotic experiences that are brief, reversible, and stress-related.

Etiology

Most of the major work on the etiology of borderline personality disorder has come from psychoanalytic theorists. They focus on early childhood, particularly between the ages of 6 months and 2 years, when the child learns to separate from the mother and gains a sense of himself or herself as a separate being. Many psychoanalysts postulate that disturbances in the mother-child relationship during this separation-individuation phase of development can leave children with a poorly developed sense of self and render them extremely vulnerable to separations from important others. One theorist (Kernberg) has hypothesized that borderline individuals may have an inborn deficit in their ability to tolerate anxiety.

Borderline patients commonly come from families in which violence, physical and sexual abuse, and drug abuse have occurred. Inconsistent parenting seems to be an important predisposing factor to the disorder, and such inconsistency can come from a variety of factors, including parental illness and psychological impairment.

Empirical studies are now under way to try to validate the theories mentioned above, and to explore possible biological factors in the etiology of borderline personality disorder.

To date, studies have failed to show a genetic relationship of this

Table 7-8. DSM-III-R criteria for the diagnosis of borderline personality
disorder

A pervasive pattern of instability of mood, interpersonal relationships, and
self-image, beginning by early adulthood and present in a variety of contexts,
as indicated by at least *five* of the following:

1. A pattern of unstable and intense interpersonal relationships characterized
   by alternating between extremes of overidealization and devaluation
2. Impulsiveness in at least two areas that are potentially self-damaging—for
   example, spending, sex, substance abuse, shoplifting, reckless driving, binge
   eating—does not include suicidal or self-mutilating behavior covered below
3. Affective instability: marked shifts from baseline mood to depression,
   irritability, or anxiety, usually lasting a few hours and only rarely more
   than a few days
4. Inappropriate, intense anger or lack of control of anger—for example,
   frequent displays of temper, constant anger, recurrent physical fights
5. Recurrent suicidal threats, gestures, or behavior, or self-mutilating behavior
6. Marked and persistent identity disturbance manifested by uncertainty
   about at least two of the following:

   a) Self-image
   b) Sexual orientation
   c) Long-term goals or career choice
   d) Type of friends desired
   e) Preferred values

7. Chronic feelings of emptiness or boredom
8. Frantic efforts to avoid real or imagined abandonment—does not include
   suicidal or self-mutilating behavior covered above

---

disorder to schizophrenia, and the relationship of borderline personality
disorder to affective disorders remains unclear. However, there appears
to be an increase in the prevalence of other personality disorders and
alcoholism among the biological relatives of borderline patients.

Epidemiology

The prevalence of borderline personality disorder is estimated to be
between 2% and 4% of the general population. This disorder is diagnosed
in 15% to 25% of psychiatric patients (both inpatient and outpatient). In
recent years, roughly 10% to 20% of hospital admissions have been of
patients with this diagnosis. Women are diagnosed as borderline more
than twice as often as men, but it may be that clinicians underdiagnose
the disorder in men and overdiagnose it in women.

Course and Prognosis

Because many of the characteristics of borderline personality disorder are common to normal adolescents, the disorder cannot be diagnosed before the age of 16. The disorder is most commonly seen in older adolescents and young adults. Patients commonly show severe dysfunction at work and in relationships, and some require repeated hospitalization or emergency-room attention for self-destructive behavior for several years after the diagnosis is made. Follow-up studies indicate that many of the borderline individual's most disruptive behaviors wane with time, but that impairment later in life may take a "quieter" form such as alcoholism. While suicide risk is higher for borderline individuals than for the general population, it is not as high as in affective disorders.

Differential Diagnosis

Other personality disorders. Borderline individuals often have features consistent with other personality disorders—particularly histrionic, narcissistic, schizoid, schizotypal, and antisocial personality disorders. If someone meets the criteria for more than one personality disorder, more than one diagnosis is warranted.

Affective disorders. Because the person with borderline personality disorder has intense and highly changeable emotional storms, it is easy to confuse symptoms of the disorder with mood swings due to an underlying affective illness. Recent studies suggest that up to 50% of people with borderline personality disorder have a concurrent affective disorder; in such cases both disorders should be diagnosed and treated.

Treatment

While psychotherapy is the treatment of choice for borderline patients, treatment is extremely difficult for patient and therapist. Borderline individuals often cannot tolerate the intense feelings they develop for the therapist, and their responses range from abruptly breaking off treatment, to intense verbal abuse, to severe self-destructive acts. They frequently threaten and attempt suicide, using this and other maneuvers to try to elicit signs of the therapist's love and concern. This behavior is designed in part to manipulate others, but it is nonetheless quite dangerous. You may become overwhelmed by your own emotional responses to borderline patients. Intense anger is common, as is an unrealistic sense of responsibility for the patient's safety.

Two differing views of psychotherapy with borderline patients predominate. Some clinicians advocate intensive individual psychotherapy (two or more sessions per week) aimed at in-depth exploration of how patients relate to others in their lives and, most important, how they relate to the therapist. Another view is that such intensive work prompts the borderline patient to become irreversibly clinging and dependent on the therapist, so that treatment should instead be limited to weekly sessions that focus on "here-and-now" issues such as improving job performance and stabilizing the patient's living situation. Group therapy is often advocated as an adjunct to both intensive and supportive individual therapies, since groups can often confront borderline individuals with their manipulative behavior quite effectively. Treating borderline individuals in groups is very difficult because of their wish to have an exclusive relationship with the therapist.

Cognitive therapy may help borderline patients to become more aware of tendencies to see the world and other people in black-and-white terms (i.e., all-good or all-bad), and to develop more realistic attitudes toward themselves and others. Behavior therapy has been used to manage suicidal impulses.

There has been a recent burgeoning of research on the pharmacotherapy of borderline personality disorder. Studies have suggested a role for low doses of antipsychotics in relieving depressive and cognitive symptoms of this disorder, for monoamine oxidase inhibitors (MAOIs) in relieving depression, and for anticonvulsants in reducing impulsivity. However, the results of these studies are not conclusive, the therapeutic effects of all of these medications are modest, and side effects often outweigh the benefits of pharmacotherapy with these patients. Medication should be used with caution on a short-term basis to treat specific target symptoms, and only when patients are capable of using medication safely and responsibly.

Whatever treatment regimen is decided upon, it is crucial that the therapist have support. This should always include the option to hospitalize the patient when self-destructive activities or psychosis make it impossible to continue treatment on an outpatient basis. Supervision, peer group support, and consultation with other clinicians can also help the therapist to maintain some perspective on the treatment during particularly difficult periods.

AVOIDANT PERSONALITY DISORDER

Profile

The hallmark of avoidant personality disorder is extreme sensitivity to rejection. Avoidant individuals stay away from relationships—not because they want to, but because they are so afraid of rejection. Only when guaranteed uncritical acceptance can they feel safe enough to get attached to other people.

Avoidant people generally lack self-confidence, which they attempt to bolster by seeking out unusually supportive companions. They are often afraid to speak up, and feel uncomfortable in the limelight and in positions of authority. In the interview, people with avoidant personality disorder will be anxious about what you think of them. They may seem fragile and waiflike. If you attempt to clarify something they have said, they are likely to interpret your comments as critical even when you did not mean them to be.

Diagnosis

The diagnostic criteria for avoidant personality disorder given in DSM-III-R (pp. 352–353) are shown in Table 7-9.

Etiology

The causes of avoidant personality disorder are unknown. Childhood experiences and inborn temperament may exert some influence in the genesis of this disorder.

Table 7-9. DSM-III-R criteria for the diagnosis of avoidant personality disorder

A pervasive pattern of social discomfort, fear of negative evaluation, and timidity, beginning by early adulthood and present in a variety of contexts, as indicated by at least *four* of the following:

1. Is easily hurt by criticism or disapproval
2. Has no close friends or confidants (or only one) other than first-degree relatives
3. Is unwilling to get involved with people unless certain of being liked
4. Avoids social or occupational activities that involve significant interpersonal contact—for example, refuses a promotion that will increase social demands
5. Is reticent in social situations because of a fear of saying something inappropriate or foolish, or of being unable to answer a question
6. Fears being embarrassed by blushing, crying, or showing signs of anxiety in front of other people
7. Exaggerates the potential difficulties, physical dangers, or risks involved in doing something ordinary but outside his or her usual routine—for example, may cancel social plans because he or she anticipates being exhausted by the effort of getting there

Epidemiology

There is no information on prevalence, sex ratio, or familial patterns of the disorder, but it is apparently common. Many patients who fulfill the criteria for this disorder have another diagnosis that is primary.

Course and Prognosis

The course and prognosis for avoidant personality disorder are also unknown.

Differential Diagnosis

Avoidant personality disorder was not included in diagnostic manuals prior to DSM-III (1980). There is considerable disagreement about whether the avoidant personality constitutes a true personality disorder or merely represents a trait common to a variety of personality types.

The individual with an avoidant personality disorder longs for and responds to genuine attention and support from others; the person with a schizoid personality disorder expresses no desire for social relations.

Avoidant people share with dependent personality disorder individuals their longing for and insecurity in relationships, as well as low self-esteem. However, avoidant people have difficulty forming relationships, whereas dependent people cling to relationships and have difficulty ending them in cases where it would be in their interest to do so. Unlike people with dependent, borderline, and histrionic personality disorders, avoidant people suffer quietly and are not demanding of attention.

Treatment

Psychotherapy is the treatment of choice. In individual therapy, a strong alliance is difficult to form because it is so easy for the avoidant individual to feel rejected. However, once formed, this alliance can help the avoidant person learn to weather the storms inherent in human interaction. Insight-oriented therapy can help patients ease the harshness of their own self-criticism, and see the ways that they project their self-criticism onto others and so expect relationships to be fraught with pain and rejection. Cognitive therapy can focus on false assumptions about the self and others.

Group therapy can demonstrate to avoidant individuals the difficulties their hypersensitivity poses for other people, and help them overcome social anxiety. But avoidant individuals are likely to be very reluctant to take the risk involved in entering into group therapy in the first place. Assertiveness training may improve the avoidant person's interpersonal functioning.

Some clinicians feel that an important distinction between avoidant and schizoid personality disorders is that the avoidant individual is more inclined than the schizoid to seek and profit from psychotherapy.

While benzodiazepines have been used to treat anxiety in avoidant patients, such use should be limited to particularly stressful periods to avoid tolerance and dependence.

DEPENDENT PERSONALITY DISORDER

Profile

Clinicians disagree about whether extreme dependence is a trait common to many types of personality disorders or whether it is truly a unique disorder in its own right.

People with dependent personality disorder structure their lives so that other people will take responsibility for their welfare. They feel unable to function on their own and so seek out lovers, bosses, and friends who will allow them to be passive and who will tell them how to live their lives. They avoid making decisions whenever they can get others to do it for them—for example, whom to see socially, where to work, and even what to wear.

The person with this disorder will put up with a great deal from others in order to preserve a dependent relationship and avoid having to function autonomously—for example, the wife who puts up with verbal and physical abuse from her husband because she feels incapable of functioning without him. Dependent people lack self-confidence and are preoccupied with fears of being abandoned.

Diagnosis

The diagnostic criteria for dependent personality disorder given in DSM-III-R (p. 354) are listed in Table 7-10.

Etiology

Most theorists who write about the roots of extreme passivity and dependence emphasize early childhood experiences. One hypothesis is that parents can foster dependent personality traits by giving their children the implicit or explicit message that independent behavior is bad and will lead to abandonment.

Table 7-10. DSM-III-R criteria for the diagnosis of dependent personality disorder

A pervasive pattern of dependent and submissive behavior, beginning by early adulthood and present in a variety of contexts, as indicated by at least *five* of the following:

1. Is unable to make everyday decisions without an excessive amount of advice or reassurance from others
2. Allows others to make most of his or her important decisions—for example, where to live, what job to take
3. Agrees with people even when he or she believes they are wrong, because of fear of being rejected
4. Has difficulty initiating projects or doing things on his or her own
5. Volunteers to do things that are unpleasant or demeaning in order to get other people to like him or her
6. Feels uncomfortable or helpless when alone, or goes to great lengths to avoid being alone
7. Feels devastated or helpless when close relationships end
8. Is frequently preoccupied with fears of being abandoned
9. Is easily hurt by criticism or disapproval

Evidence has begun to emerge that suggests that dominant and submissive personality traits may be genetically transmitted. Researchers have found a higher rate of concordance for these traits among identical twins than among fraternal twins. However, submissiveness and dependence are not the same thing, and it is not clear whether these two traits usually coexist in the same person.

Epidemiology

The diagnosis is more often assigned to women than to men. Patients who meet criteria for dependent personality disorder often present with concurrent disorders, such as substance abuse, depression, or somatic symptoms.

Course and Prognosis

The patient's ability to function depends on the maintenance of dependent relationships. When these are disrupted in some way (e.g., the death of a spouse), a person who previously functioned well may seriously decompensate and seek mental health care.

Differential Diagnosis

Dependent traits are common in other personality disorders, particularly in borderline, histrionic, avoidant, passive-aggressive, and schizoid personality disorders. Some diagnosticians believe that masochism—that is, the pleasure obtained from pain, failure, and disability—is the more central trait in dependent personality disorder than dependence per se. The disorder may be difficult to distinguish from self-defeating personality disorder, as both involve submissiveness and putting others' needs above one's own (see below).

Agoraphobia (see Chapter 8) may be mistaken for dependent personality disorder, but the agoraphobic individual is much more active in demanding that others take responsibility for his or her life (e.g., the agoraphobic husband who insists that his wife drive him everywhere). Dependent individuals "can't" do things because of a sense of inadequacy and incompetence, whereas agoraphobic individuals "can't" do things because of overwhelming fear and anxiety.

Treatment

Insight-oriented psychotherapy can be very helpful for people with dependent personality disorder. In the relationship with the therapist, patients can begin to examine the effects of their passivity on themselves and others, and to recognize their own competence and self-worth. Fantasies about the consequences of independence and assertiveness can be explored and tested against reality. In the beginning, it is important that the therapist respect the patient's need for dependent relationships (even abusive ones) and not push the patient to give them up until he or she is ready.

Group therapy, assertiveness training, and cognitive therapy can all help dependent patients improve self-esteem, bolster self-confidence, and try out new and more adaptive behaviors.

OBSESSIVE-COMPULSIVE PERSONALITY DISORDER

The "obsessive-compulsive" is a character familiar to every hard-working student. We often use this label to lampoon ourselves or others for being too careful, too preoccupied with detail, and too diligent or perfectionistic. The terms *obsessive* and *compulsive* are used in three ways: 1) to describe a classic preoccupation with unwanted thoughts or behaviors (obsessive-compulsive disorder), 2) to describe a general personality style, and 3) to describe a specific personality disorder.

Obsessions are persistent unwanted ideas or images that seem as if they come from outside the mind and force themselves on the victim's thoughts against his or her will. One might, for example, be obsessed with the thought that one has accidentally hurt someone, or be terrified of being contaminated by touching a doorknob. People who suffer from this disorder may be hopelessly preoccupied with obsessions despite realizing that these preoccupations are absurd and irrational. They usually feel powerless to keep obsessive thoughts out of their awareness and become anxious when they attempt to do so.

Compulsions are the behavioral equivalents of obsessions—repetitive urges to perform acts that are contrary to one's ordinary wishes or standards. Common compulsive acts include hand-washing, counting (e.g., money), and checking (e.g., to be certain the stove has been turned off). The action usually seems senseless; performing the act is not pleasurable, but it does relieve tension momentarily. When the problem is severe, people may need to spend most of their waking moments carrying out compulsive acts (e.g., cleaning) to avoid massive anxiety.

According to psychodynamic theory, obsessive thoughts and compulsive acts serve as benign substitutes for more threatening unconscious ideas or impulses (e.g., the wish to kill one's parent).

True obsessions and compulsions (i.e., discrete and isolated symptoms) are classified as a particular type of anxiety disorder, *obsessive-compulsive disorder (OCD)*, and this entity is discussed at greater length in Chapter 8. While people with obsessive-compulsive personality disorder may also have OCD, the two diagnoses are discrete and a great many patients have one without the other.

Obsessive-Compulsive Style

Much more common than true obsessions or compulsions is the obsessive-compulsive personality style, which may be both normal and highly adaptive. Like hysterical traits, obsessive-compulsive traits can be very useful—for example, when studying for an exam, organizing a business venture, or even planning a wild party.

Obsessive-compulsive people have the ability to focus their attention and screen out distractions. They can be skilled at highly detailed work; many obsessive-compulsive individuals are technicians, academicians, and scientists. Obsessive-compulsive people are perfectionists and list-makers. They are usually intensely and continuously active at some kind of work. Their deliberateness makes them less open than others to spontaneous experiences. Obsessive-compulsive individuals rarely get hunches, and often immerse themselves so completely in small details that they cannot step back and see the "big picture."

In contrast to hysterical people, obsessive-compulsive individuals are characteristically serious. They generally apply great pressure to themselves to live up to high standards of performance and morality, for they live according to the dictates of a very demanding conscience. "I should . . ." is their motto. They are their own harshest taskmasters and never feel free. In fact, many obsessive-compulsive individuals are uncomfortable in situations where they are truly free (e.g., on vacation).

Decisions are the bane of the obsessive-compulsive individual's existence, and he or she will try to find a rule or moral dictum to avoid having to exercise free choice. Obsessive-compulsive people have difficulty when faced with decisions in which no duty is involved and they must act wholly according to their own desires, because they are generally unaware of their desires.

Obsessive-Compulsive Personality Disorder

Profile. As with other personality types, the line between what constitutes style and what qualifies as a disorder is not at all clear in the case of the obsessive-compulsive individual. This is a judgment call, based on the extent to which personality traits are inflexible and impair one's ability to love and to work.

Individuals with obsessive-compulsive personality disorder are very limited in their ability to express warm and tender feelings toward others. Feelings provoke anxiety, and obsessive-compulsive individuals focus on facts instead of feelings to overcome anxiety. They are preoccupied with the "right" way of doing things and often alienate others by their insistence on having their own way. They can be moralistic to the point of absurd rigidity and extreme insensitivity to the needs of others.

Lists and routines dominate their lives. They may focus on their bowel habits, for example, to the point that any irregularity leaves them unable to function at their usual daily activities. Decision making will often be reduced to a "science." When this is not possible, obsessive-compulsive individuals may be paralyzed by indecision and the fear of making a mistake.

Other obsessive-compulsive traits include parsimony, extreme cleanliness, and orderliness. At the healthier end of the spectrum, the individual with obsessive-compulsive personality disorder may have a stable marriage and hold a responsible job, but is constantly tense and driven, unable to have fun.

When you interview people with obsessive-compulsive personality disorder, you will most likely find them neatly and conventionally dressed. They may sit stiffly, and will be serious in demeanor. They are likely to drone on and on in a monotonous tone of voice as they give detailed and often circumstantial answers to questions. In fact, when you ask how they feel about something, they will usually give an answer consisting of facts and circumstances instead of emotions. They will be slow to "warm up" to you, and preoccupied with ideas about what you expect of them in the interview.

Diagnosis. The DSM-III-R diagnostic criteria for obsessive-compulsive personality disorder (p. 356) are listed in Table 7-11.

Etiology. Classic psychoanalytic thinking emphasizes the importance of the anal phase of development (age 2 to 4 years) in the genesis of obsessive-compulsive personality disorder. Toilet training is the standard metaphor for this stage: Children want to gratify their urges wherever and whenever they occur, but these urges conflict with the desires of parents and society. The tension, then, is between the assertion of autonomy and the development of self-control.

Many therapists write about the role of rigid, controlling parents in fostering obsessive-compulsive personality disorder in their over-disciplined offspring. However, these ideas have yet to be validated in long-term prospective studies.

Recent studies suggest that the heightened sensitivity to change that is exhibited by obsessive-compulsive individuals may be part of a genetically determined temperamental predisposition. The balance of inborn and environmental factors involved in the genesis of the disorder has yet to be clarified.

Epidemiology. The prevalence of obsessive-compulsive personality disorder is unknown, because much depends on where the diagnostician draws the line between the personality style and the disorder. It is common among outpatient populations, and it is more frequently diagnosed in men than in women.

Course and prognosis. The course of the disorder varies tremendously. Obsessive-compulsive individuals are quite vulnerable to unexpected life changes and are prone to bouts of depression. However, some obsessive-compulsive people appear to "loosen up" with age and exhibit fewer symptoms of the disorder as they grow older. Still others develop frankly compulsive behaviors, and a small number appear to adopt compulsive symptoms as a prelude to a schizophrenic break. Unfortunately, many severely obsessive-compulsive people continue to lead an emotionally barren existence throughout life.

Differential diagnosis. People with *obsessive-compulsive disorder* (OCD) report being plagued by obsessive thoughts, or feeling unable to resist performing compulsive acts, and these symptoms are disturbing to those who have them. By contrast, obsessive-compulsive personality disorder is not characterized by ego-dystonic obsessions or compulsions.

People who fulfill the criteria for obsessive-compulsive personality

Table 7-11. DSM-III-R criteria for the diagnosis of obsessive-compulsive personality disorder

A pervasive pattern of perfectionism and inflexibility, beginning by early adulthood and present in a variety of contexts, as indicated by at least *five* of the following:

1. Perfectionism that interferes with task completion—for example, inability to complete a project because own overly strict standards are not met
2. Preoccupation with details, rules, lists, order, organization, or schedules to the extent that the major point of the activity is lost
3. Unreasonable insistence that others submit to exactly his or her way of doing things, **or** unreasonable reluctance to allow others to do things because of the conviction that they will not do them correctly
4. Excessive devotion to work and productivity to the exclusion of leisure activities and friendships (not accounted for by obvious economic necessity)
5. Indecisiveness: decision making is either avoided, postponed, or protracted—for example, the person cannot get assignments done on time because of ruminating about priorities—not included if indecisiveness is due to excessive need for advice or reassurance from others
6. Overconscientiousness, scrupulousness, and inflexibility about matters of morality, ethics, or values (not accounted for by cultural or religious identification)
7. Restricted expression of affection
8. Lack of generosity in giving time, money, or gifts when no personal gain is likely to result
9. Inability to discard worn-out or worthless objects even when they have no sentimental value

disorder may also show features of other personality disorders—particularly schizoid and paranoid personality disorders.

Treatment

Psychotherapy is the treatment of choice for obsessive-compulsive personality disorder; medication has not proved to be effective in this disorder.

Obsessive-compulsive people differ from many others with personality disorders in that they often see themselves as troubled and seek help on their own. Psychodynamic therapy is a long and slow process, because the obsessive-compulsive sees therapy, like every other relationship, as a struggle for control. The therapist must carefully sidestep potential battles and point out the patient's extreme sensitivity to issues of power and authority. The focus must be clearly maintained on the patient's feelings, because the obsessive-compulsive individual tends to use his or her intellect to defend against feelings that are less controllable than ideas and therefore more threatening.

Group psychotherapy has also proved effective, either alone or in combination with individual therapy. Group members can have a powerful influence on the obsessive-compulsive person, by pointing out the maladaptive ways of dealing with others revealed in the group. They can also reward the obsessive-compulsive person with praise when positive changes are made.

Behavior therapy, while useful for specific obsessive-compulsive behaviors, has not been shown to be effective for more global personality traits. Cognitive therapy may be less threatening than exploratory therapy, because a cognitive approach would be consonant with the obsessive-compulsive individual's intellectualizing style. However, cognitive work can founder if the patient sees the therapist as attempting to control his or her thinking.

PASSIVE-AGGRESSIVE PERSONALITY DISORDER

Passive aggression is a powerful means of controlling other people. Hunger strikes, sit-ins, and work slowdowns are common examples of how "doing nothing" can be a highly effective means of gaining attention or power. Where more openly aggressive behavior is impossible, passive resistance may be the only reasonable course of action. For example, Gandhi made masterful use of this technique on a national scale in India. However, as a global and pervasive style of dealing with life, passive-aggressive behavior is usually self-defeating and self-destructive.

Profile

Individuals with passive-aggressive personality disorder spend their lives saying "yes" and behaving as if they had said "no." They fail to live up to demands made on them by their jobs and by people who are important to them. They do not fail directly or deliberately, but "by accident"—for example, by forgetting, procrastinating, or misplacing things. Typically, passive-aggressive individuals are largely unaware of their obstructiveness and feel that they are doing their best. They feel that no one appreciates how hard they try and how many difficulties the world puts in their way. They do not get angry at others directly, nor are they direct about their own needs and desires. People usually experience the passive-aggressive person's behavior as punitive; initial guilty acquiescence gives way to anger and even abandonment. Thus, passive-aggressive people are not only underachievers who infuriate their bosses, but they are also tyrants who hold captive those friends and lovers who remain close to them.

Diagnosis

The diagnostic criteria for passive-aggressive personality disorder given in DSM-III-R (pp. 357–358) are shown in Table 7-12.

Etiology

There have been no prospective studies of the causes of passive-aggressive personality disorder. Early childhood experiences seem to be of primary importance in the genesis of the disorder, particularly in conveying the message to the developing child that the direct expression of aggression is in some way taboo.

Table 7-12. DSM-III-R criteria for the diagnosis of passive-aggressive personality disorder

A pervasive pattern of passive resistance to demands for adequate social and occupational performance, beginning by early adulthood and present in a variety of contexts, as indicated by at least *five* of the following:

1. Procrastinates—that is, puts off things that need to be done so that deadlines are not met
2. Becomes sulky, irritable, or argumentative when asked to do something he or she does not want to do
3. Seems to work deliberately slowly or to do a bad job on tasks that he or she really does not want to do
4. Protests, without justification, that others make unreasonable demands on him or her
5. Avoids obligations by claiming to have "forgotten"
6. Believes that he or she is doing a much better job than others think he or she is doing
7. Resents useful suggestions from others concerning how he or she could be more productive
8. Obstructs the efforts of others by failing to do his or her share of the work
9. Unreasonably criticizes or scorns people in positions of authority

Epidemiology

The prevalence, sex ratio, and familial patterns of this disorder have not been well studied. This disorder is rarely the primary clinical diagnosis.

Course and Prognosis

People with this disorder are prone to depression and to alcohol and drug abuse.

Differential Diagnosis

Borderline and histrionic individuals may use a great many passive-aggressive maneuvers, but they are more flamboyant and more openly aggressive than people with passive-aggressive personality disorder.

Passive-aggressive personality disorder may overlap significantly with dependent and self-defeating personality disorders. Passive-aggressive behavior often has a self-defeating component to it, but the passive-aggressive person seems less active in choosing situations that lead to failure or mistreatment. Dependent personality disorder does not involve such systematic thwarting of perceived expectations.

Because passive-aggressive behaviors are used defensively in a wide range of disorders, many clinicians question the validity of passive-aggressive personality disorder as a separate diagnostic category.

Treatment

Psychotherapy is the treatment of choice for passive-aggressive personality disorder. Patients invariably attempt to put the therapist in the same bind that they put others in their lives: If the therapist gratifies the patient's covert demands for assistance, the patient will make further and more unreasonable demands. However, the patient will interpret a refusal to honor these requests as rejection. The therapist must constantly try to sidestep this dilemma by bringing the patient's covert aggression out into the open. This means confronting veiled threats and manipulative efforts, and asking what the patient hopes to gain by such tactics.

Assertiveness training may help passive-aggressive patients develop more adaptive ways to deal with frustration. Medication has not proved useful in the treatment of this disorder.

SADISTIC PERSONALITY DISORDER

Sadistic personality disorder is included in DSM-III-R as a "proposed diagnostic category needing further study." It was included based on the experience of forensic psychiatrists who report that the disorder is common in their practices.

Profile

People with sadistic personality disorder are typically cruel, demeaning, and aggressive toward others both at work and in social situations. They may use physical violence to dominate others in relationships, or may simply intimidate and humiliate others to exert control over them. For example, a husband may physically abuse his wife and be overly harsh and humiliating in disciplining his son. People with this disorder are commonly fascinated with violence, weapons, torture, and martial arts. They typically lack respect and empathy for others, but rather take pleasure in others' mental or physical suffering.

Cruelty and violence are not used to achieve some particular end (e.g., a military aim in wartime, or to rob someone), but rather serve to set up an unequal power relationship. The diagnosis is not made if domination and cruelty exist in one relationship only (e.g., between husband and wife), as the pattern must be pervasive. Also, the diagnosis is not made if sadistic behavior is used only for sexual arousal—this is more properly diagnosed as sexual sadism (see Chapter 13).

Diagnosis

The DSM-III-R diagnostic criteria for sadistic personality disorder (p. 371) are summarized in Table 7-13.

Etiology

The etiology of sadistic personality disorder is unknown. Abuse seems to "run in families," and clinical experience suggests that having been physically, sexually, or emotionally abused as a child predisposes one to the development of this disorder in adulthood. Similarly, having grown up in a family in which one spouse abused another, or in which other children were abused, may predispose to the disorder.

Table 7-13. DSM-III-R criteria for the diagnosis of sadistic personality disorder

A pervasive pattern of cruel, demeaning, and aggressive behavior, beginning by early adulthood, as indicated by the repeated occurrence of at least *four* of the following:

1. Has used physical cruelty or violence for the purpose of establishing dominance in a relationship (not merely to achieve some noninterpersonal goal, such as striking someone in order to rob him or her)
2. Humiliates or demeans people in the presence of others
3. Has treated or disciplined someone under his or her control unusually harshly (e.g., a child, student, prisoner, or patient)
4. Is amused by, or takes pleasure in, the psychological or physical suffering of others (including animals)
5. Has lied for the purpose of harming or inflicting pain on others (not merely to achieve some other goal)
6. Gets other people to do what he or she wants by frightening them (through intimidation or even terror)
7. Restricts the autonomy of people with whom he or she has a close relationship (e.g., will not let spouse leave the house unaccompanied or permit teenage daughter to attend social functions)
8. Is fascinated by violence, weapons, martial arts, injury, or torture

The behavior above has not been directed toward only one person (e.g., spouse, one child) and has not been solely for the purpose of sexual arousal (as in sexual sadism).

Epidemiology

Sadistic personality disorder is more common in men than in women. It is commonly seen among forensic populations (that is, among psychiatric patients suspected or convicted of criminal behavior), but is uncommon in general psychiatric practice. The prevalence of the disorder is unknown.

Course and Prognosis

Little is known about the course and prognosis of sadistic personality disorder. Substance abuse is a frequent complication. Sadistic individuals often get into marital, occupational, and legal difficulties. They rarely seek mental health care unless pressed to do so by legal authorities (e.g., when suspected of child abuse).

Differential Diagnosis

The disorder may be difficult to distinguish from antisocial personality disorder, as both involve interpersonal exploitation without apparent guilt. Some patients may meet the diagnostic criteria for both disorders. Antisocial people exhibit broadly based antisocial behavior, while the antisocial activities of sadistic people focus specifically on maintaining dominance in interpersonal relations.

Treatment

Most people with sadistic personality disorder are not distressed by their sadistic behavior and so will not seek treatment unless pressed to do so by a law enforcement agency, or under threat of abandonment by a spouse. Individual psychotherapy may be helpful, focusing on the motivations for sadistic behavior (e.g., unconscious retaliation for past abuses by caregivers). Couples therapy may be helpful in identifying ways in which a couple enacts sadomasochistic scenarios and in assisting them to find alternate ways of interacting. However, sadistic individuals are resistant to change and may promise better behavior but remain locked into an abusive role. Behavioral techniques may be of value if the patient desires alternate outlets for his or her aggressive impulses. No role for medication has been determined in the treatment of this disorder.

A note of caution: You should never attempt to shield people from legal or other consequences of their sadistic behavior, regardless of how contrite they appear or how well they rationalize their behavior. In some situations (e.g., when you suspect that a patient has abused a child), you may be legally obligated to report your patient's behavior to welfare or law enforcement agencies. Many sadistic people will only curtail their harmful behaviors when reprimanded by a more powerful authority.

SELF-DEFEATING PERSONALITY DISORDER

Self-defeating personality disorder is included in DSM-III-R under "proposed diagnostic categories needing further study." Often referred to as "masochism," this diagnostic entity has been used by clinicians under one label or another for nearly a century. Masochism, however, is a problematic term, in that it has been used historically to refer to certain supposedly normal aspects of female sexuality, and to denote unconscious pleasure derived from pain. Both of these usages are controversial, and the "self-defeating" label is meant to avoid these associations.

Profile

Self-defeating personality disorder describes individuals who habitually engage in self-defeating behaviors, including avoiding situations that lead to pleasure, choosing situations (lovers, jobs) that will involve suffering, and preventing other people from providing help even when it is offered. For example, a man may repeatedly choose lovers who are unfaithful to him and are abusive to him. A woman may choose work where she will be overworked and underpaid, when more rewarding employment is available to her.

People with this disorder react negatively to positive life events (e.g., getting a promotion, finishing college) and may even become depressed or preoccupied with guilt in response to such events. They consistently refuse others' offers of help, even when they need it, or they may undermine others' attempts to help them. Yet, self-defeating individuals may be self-sacrificing to the point of damaging their own welfare (e.g., the woman who exhausts herself taking care of friends, but who refuses to seek medical attention for her own illnesses). Such sacrifices may be completely unsolicited by others and may, in fact, make other people feel guilty.

People who try to help the self-defeating individual often become frustrated and angry. In addition, patients with this disorder may actively incite such angry responses, feeling hurt when these responses are elicited. In addition, self-defeating people commonly find uninteresting those individuals who treat them well (e.g., caring lovers as opposed to abusive ones).

This diagnosis is not made when self-defeating behavior occurs only in anticipation of or response to abuse (physical, sexual, or psychological). It is also not made if self-defeating behaviors occur only when the person is depressed.

Diagnosis

The DSM-III-R diagnostic criteria for self-defeating personality disorder (pp. 373–374) are summarized in Table 7-14.

Etiology

The etiology of self-defeating personality disorder is unknown. It appears that growing up in a family where physical, sexual, or psychological abuse occurred may predispose to the development of this disorder in adulthood.

Table 7-14. DSM-III-R criteria for the diagnosis of self-defeating personality
disorder

A pervasive pattern of self-defeating behavior, beginning by early adulthood
and present in a variety of contexts. The person may often avoid or
undermine pleasurable experiences, be drawn to situations or relationships in
which he or she will suffer, and prevent others from helping him or her, as
indicated by at least *five* of the following:

1. Chooses people and situations that lead to disappointment, failure, or
   mistreatment even when better options are clearly available
2. Rejects or renders ineffective the attempts of others to help him or her
3. Following positive personal events (e.g., new achievement), responds with
   depression, guilt, or a behavior that produces pain (e.g., an accident)
4. Incites angry or rejecting responses from others and then feels hurt,
   defeated, or humiliated (e.g., makes fun of spouse in public, provoking an
   angry retort, then feels devastated)
5. Rejects opportunities for pleasure, or is reluctant to acknowledge enjoying
   himself or herself (despite having adequate social skills and the capacity for
   pleasure)
6. Fails to accomplish tasks crucial to his or her personal objectives despite
   demonstrated ability to do so (e.g., helps fellow students write papers, but
   is unable to write his or her own)
7. Is uninterested in or rejects people who consistently treat him or her well,
   (e.g., is unattracted to caring sexual partners)
8. Engages in excessive self-sacrifice that is unsolicited by the intended
   recipients of the sacrifice

The behaviors above do not occur exclusively in response to, or in
anticipation of, being physically, sexually, or psychologically abused.

The behaviors above do not occur only when the person is depressed.

Epidemiology

The prevalence of self-defeating personality disorder has not been systematically studied, but the disorder is thought to be relatively common.
Many people with the disorder never come to psychiatric attention. The
disorder is more common in women than in men.

Course and Prognosis

Little is known. Some people with self-defeating personality disorder
maintain stable (if unhappy) relationships and work lives. Others can

come to serious physical harm in relationships. Depression and suicide are complications of this disorder.

Differential Diagnosis

Those who are victims of physical, sexual, or psychological abuse may appear to be self-defeating. For example, a woman may fail to seek support from friends while she is involved with a physically abusive lover. This may be in response to the threat of further violence from her lover if she were to disclose her predicament to others. A diagnosis of self-defeating personality would only be warranted if this person also had a history of engaging in self-defeating behavior in other distinct areas of her life.

Self-defeating behavior in depression may also mimic the personality disorder. However, in such cases, self-defeating behavior will not be present when the person is no longer depressed.

Self-defeating personality disorder may overlap with other Axis II categories, particularly dependent personality disorder and passive-aggressive personality disorder.

Treatment

Psychotherapy is generally the treatment of choice, but treatment of self-defeating personality disorder is fraught with difficulty. Self-defeating patients commonly feel that they do not deserve happiness. They may unconsciously thwart the therapist's efforts to help them improve their relationships and self-view. When progress does start to occur in treatment, they may react with guilt and depression (a so-called "negative therapeutic reaction"). The patient may arouse the therapist's own unconscious sadism and thereby recreate a subtly abusive relationship in the treatment. Or the therapist may simply become impatient with the patient's persistent self-defeating behaviors. In any case, the therapist may need to listen empathetically to the patient's calamities and establish a firm alliance before any productive work can be done on clarifying and understanding the patient's contribution to these unrewarding life situations.

Couples therapy can help when a patient plays out a self-defeating role with an abusive spouse. Cognitive interventions can help to minimize self-blaming and self-defeating cognitive styles. No role for medication has been determined in the treatment of this disorder. However, antidepressants may indeed be required when patients are concurrently depressed.

SOME FINAL THOUGHTS ON TREATMENT

People with personality disorders are notoriously difficult to treat. Their pathological ways of dealing with the world are deeply ingrained, yet they act as if the problem lies with the world and not with them. They are often angry, demanding, and abusive toward therapists and have an extraordinary capacity to home in on the weaknesses and vulnerabilities of those who try to help them. They will attempt to form the same type of pathological relationship with you that they form with others in their lives. They are generally reluctant to see their behavior as a problem and are likely to blame you when their wishes are not fulfilled in therapy.

You may become so angry at such patients that you will unwittingly retaliate when they are abusive. You may, for example, withdraw your emotional investment from your work with them in subtle ways, prompting them to feel increasingly worthless. Pay close attention to the hostile feelings that invariably arise toward the patient with a personality disorder; by being aware of these feelings and tolerating them, you can avoid acting on them. The following ground rules may be helpful to you in dealing with a personality-disordered patient, whether you are doing a single interview or embarking on long-term therapy:

1. Focus on the patient's behavior, not on his or her explanations of that behavior.
2. Do not listen to repetitious complaints. When patients recount the supposed injustices the world has dealt them, direct the focus to their own role in these events.
3. Maintain the stance that you and your patients are collaborating (i.e., that you are doing something with them rather than for them or to them).
4. Pay close attention to your own fantasies of "rescuing" the patient. You are bound to be disappointed.
5. Set limits on any behavior that threatens your safety, the patient's safety, or the future of the treatment. This may range from ending your meeting early to putting the patient in the hospital. When patients try to push you into the role of savior, friend, or co-conspirator, show them what they are doing.
6. Scoldings and guilt trips are of no use to your patients. You must simply hold them responsible for their behavior, rather than making any moves to shield them from its consequences.
7. Provide yourself with support. Seek supervision from a more senior person, or "let off steam" with a peer. Use all the help available to you to weather the difficult times that are unavoidable in treating people with personality disorders.

BIBLIOGRAPHY

Adler G: Psychotherapy of the narcissistic personality disorder patient: two contrasting approaches. Am J Psychiatry 143:430–436, 1986

Akhtar S, Thompson JA: Overview: narcissistic personality disorder. Am J Psychiatry 139:12–20, 1982

American Psychiatric Association: Diagnostic and Statistical Manual of Mental Disorders, 3rd Edition. Washington, DC, American Psychiatric Association, 1980

American Psychiatric Association: Diagnostic and Statistical Manual of Mental Disorders, 3rd Edition, Revised. Washington, DC, American Psychiatric Association, 1987, pp 335–358, 369–374

Chodoff P, Lyons H: Hysteria, the hysterical personality, and "hysterical" conversion. Am J Psychiatry 114:734–740, 1958

Cowdry RW: Psychopharmacology of borderline personality disorder: a review. J Clin Psychiatry 48(No 8, suppl):15–22, 1987

Frosch JP (ed): Current Perspectives on Personality Disorders. Washington, DC, American Psychiatric Press, 1983

Gunderson JG: Borderline Personality Disorder. Washington, DC, American Psychiatric Press, 1984

Gunderson JG, Singer MT: Defining borderline patients: an overview. Am J Psychiatry 132:1–10, 1975

Guntrip H: Psychoanalytic Theory, Therapy, and the Self. New York, Basic Books, 1973, pp 145–173

Kernberg O: Borderline personality organization. J Am Psychoanal Assoc 15:641–685, 1967

Kohut H: The Analysis of the Self. New York, International Universities Press, 1971

Lilienfeld S, Van Valkenburg C, Larntz K, et al: The relationship of histrionic personality disorder to antisocial personality and somatization disorders. Am J Psychiatry 143:718–722, 1986

McGlashan TH: The Chestnut Lodge follow-up study. Arch Gen Psychiatry 43:20–30, 1986

Shapiro D: Neurotic Styles. New York, Basic Books, 1965. (An excellent and highly readable discussion of personality styles.)

Siever L, Klar H: A review of DSM-III criteria for the personality disorders, in Psychiatry Update: The American Psychiatric Association Annual Review, Vol 5. Edited by Frances AJ, Hales RE. Washington, DC, American Psychiatric Press, 1986, pp 279–314

Torgerson S: Genetic and nosologic aspects of schizotypal and borderline disorders: a twin study. Arch Gen Psychiatry 41:546–554, 1984

Vaillant GE: Sociopathy as a human process: a viewpoint. Arch Gen Psychiatry 32:178–183, 1975

Waldinger RJ: Intensive psychodynamic therapy with borderline patients: an overview. Am J Psychiatry 144:267–274, 1987

Waldinger RJ, Gunderson JG: Effective Psychotherapy with Borderline Patients: Case Studies. New York, Macmillan, 1987

Widiger TA, Frances A, Spitzer RL, et al: The DSM-III-R personality disorders: an overview. Am J Psychiatry 145:786–795, 1988

8

Anxiety, Phobias, Dissociative Disorders, and Somatoform Disorders

ANXIETY DISORDERS

What is anxiety? Each of us has experienced it, and our era has been called the age of anxiety. Yet precise definition of the term is difficult, for it has been applied to a wide range of emotional responses.

Fear is a normal reaction to a consciously recognized external source of danger. It is appropriate to the source of danger, both in its intensity and in its duration, and it dissipates when action is taken that leads to escape or avoidance. Fear involves both subjective feelings of apprehension and objective physiological changes that usually include rapid heartbeat, rapid respiration, muscle tremor, and redistribution of blood from the skin and internal organs to the large muscle groups. These changes prepare the body for the violent muscular activity ("fight or flight") that may be necessary in responding to a threat.

Anxiety, by contrast, involves tension, apprehension, or even terror about danger, the source of which is largely unknown or unrecognized. Like fear, anxiety is accompanied by increased activity of the sympathetic nervous system, which is manifested by such physical signs as sweating, rapid heartbeat, tremor, rapid breathing, and gastrointestinal distress. But, unlike fear, anxiety stems from sources that are not obvious to the one who suffers, or that seem minor compared with his or her

199

intense emotional reaction. Anxiety is common and in many instances consists of an overreaction to mildly stressful events (e.g., excessive concern over a relatively unimportant examination). We regard anxiety as pathological when it interferes with daily functioning, the achievement of desired goals, or reasonable emotional comfort.

Situational anxiety occurs in response to a specific stress and ends shortly after the stress is removed. *Free-floating anxiety*, by contrast, involves apprehension that is not clearly linked to a specific situation. The DSM-III-R system for classifying anxiety disorders can be summarized in a decision tree (Figure 8-1).

Anxiety disorders are the most common psychiatric illnesses in the general population. Simple phobias are most common, but people with these disorders often do not seek treatment. Among those presenting for treatment, the most frequently encountered anxiety disorders are obsessive-compulsive disorder and panic disorder.

Panic Disorder

Panic disorder is a dramatic syndrome characterized by discrete spontaneous panic attacks—crescendos of fear and apprehension—associated with multiple physical symptoms. Attacks resemble the body's normal physiological response to a life-threatening situation or extreme physical exertion. However, in panic disorder, attacks come on suddenly and unpredictably without provocation.

Panic attacks are characterized by feelings of fear, extreme tension, and a sense of impending doom. Various physical symptoms accompany these feelings, most commonly:

- Shortness of breath
- Palpitations
- Chest pain or discomfort
- Choking or smothering sensations
- Dizziness, vertigo, or unsteady feelings
- Feelings of unreality (depersonalization or derealization)
- Paresthesias (tingling in hands or feet)
- Hot and cold flashes
- Sweating
- Faintness
- Trembling or shaking
- Numbness or tingling
- Fear of going crazy, dying, or doing something uncontrolled during an attack
- Nausea, vomiting, diarrhea

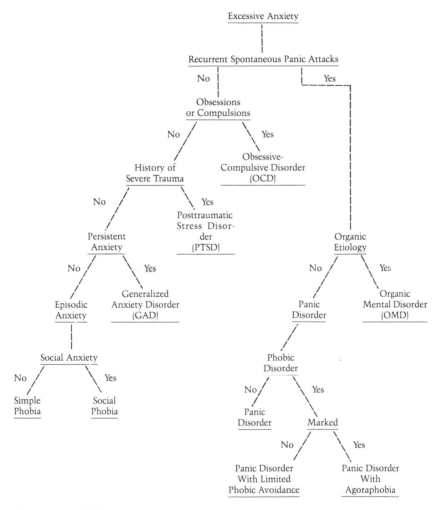

Figure 8-1. Diagnostic decision tree for the anxiety disorders. Note that patients may have more than one disorder and thus must be evaluated for each disorder. Reprinted, with permission, from Hollander E, Liebowitz MR, Gorman JM; Anxiety disorders, in *The American Psychiatric Press Textbook of Psychiatry*. Edited by Talbott JA, Hales RE, Yudofsky SC. Washington, DC, American Psychiatric Press, 1988, pp. 443–491. Copyright 1988 American Psychiatric Press.

Often, the first panic attack occurs when the patient is under significant stress—for example, a break-up with a lover, leaving home for the first time, the death of a friend, or the beginning of a new job. Attacks also commonly occur for the first time immediately postpartum and when people are under the influence of mind-altering drugs.

Patients are usually engaged in some routine activity (e.g., shopping or reading) when a panic attack begins. They suddenly feel an overwhelming sensation of fear, apprehension, and impending doom. Some describe feeling that they are about to die or that some nameless catastrophe is about to befall them. This sense of dread is accompanied by several of the physical symptoms listed above, all of which are consistent with massive autonomic nervous system discharge. Attacks commonly last for 5 to 20 minutes or, more rarely, for up to an hour. They recur with varying frequency.

Because many people experience an occasional spontaneous panic attack without significant impairment, the diagnosis of panic disorder is made only when attacks occur frequently (four in one month) or when the patient suffers from persistent fear of having another attack. Panic disorder may be limited to one brief period of illness lasting several weeks or months, it may recur several times, or it may become chronic. People with this disorder usually develop nervousness and apprehension between attacks; when this is severe, agoraphobia ensues.

Panic disorder is common; epidemiologic studies indicate that as much as 1.5% of the general population meet criteria for the disorder at some time during their lives. The disorder is diagnosed more often among women than men, and typically begins in late adolescence or early adulthood, but may begin as late as the fourth or fifth decade of life.

Agoraphobia. Agoraphobia denotes a fear of being in places or situations from which escape might be difficult or in which help might be unavailable in the event that one develops a symptom that could be incapacitating or embarrassing. Typical symptoms that agoraphobic patients fear include dizziness or falling, loss of bladder or bowel control, vomiting, palpitations, and chest pain. This fear causes the person to restrict his or her travel or to require a companion when away from home. Some people endure feared situations alone, but suffer intense anxiety. Being away from home alone, being in a crowd, crossing a bridge, and traveling by public transportation are among the common fears reported by agoraphobic patients.

Agoraphobia with panic attacks. Agoraphobia and panic attacks so frequently occur together that you are more likely to encounter them in combination than separately in your clinical work.

How do the two go together? Panic attacks routinely come first, and agoraphobia—the fear of being alone and/or in public places where help is unavailable—develops in response to these terrifying episodes of panic. People who experience recurrent symptoms of panic become preoccupied with a fear of developing subsequent attacks, and develop an increasing number of phobias about the settings in which they have experienced attacks in the past (e.g., in the supermarket, while driving a car). The number of situations they avoid increases until these individuals are considered truly agoraphobic. Between panic attacks, they develop chronic anticipatory anxiety about having another attack.

They often do not seek professional help until they have had symptoms for many years, and by that time they may have agoraphobia with multiple specific phobias, and chronic anticipatory anxiety in addition to the panic attacks themselves. Sadly, some people with this syndrome become shut-ins, unable to leave the house or stay alone even for short periods of time.

Etiology

Work on the etiology of panic disorder has accelerated in the past decade, and researchers continue to explore several promising theories about the biological basis of the disorder. None of these, however, has been proved.

The symptoms of panic attacks, such as palpitations, sweating, and tremulousness, lead naturally to the theory that they are the result of massive discharges from the β-adrenergic nervous system. This hypothesis has not been verified empirically, although some studies suggest that beta-blocking agents such as propranolol ameliorate panic attacks.

A second hypothesis is that panic attacks result from increased discharge in the *locus coeruleus* and increased central noradrenergic turnover. The locus coeruleus, located in the pons, contains more than half of all noradrenergic neurons in the central nervous system (CNS). While electrical stimulation of this structure in the brains of animals has been shown to produce fear and anxiety, the relevance of these animal models to anxiety disorders in humans is a subject of debate.

Investigators have found that intravenous infusion of *sodium lactate* will provoke a panic attack in most patients with panic disorder, but not in normal subjects. The mechanism by which this occurs is not clear, and investigators hope that its elucidation might provide a key to biochemical factors in the etiology of panic attacks.

Recent studies have yielded evidence for a *genetic predisposition* to panic disorder. Family history studies have found panic disorder to be as much as 10 times more frequent in the biological relatives of those with panic disorder as among normal control subjects. Twin studies show the concordance for panic disorder among monozygotic twins to be five times that among dizygotic twins. However, there are still confounding environmental variables—for example, the possibility that parents treat identical and fraternal twins differently.

Psychological theories of the etiology of panic disorder are discussed under generalized anxiety disorder, since the two disorders are commonly discussed together in the psychological literature.

Differential diagnosis

Psychotic disorders, medical illnesses (see Table 8-1), and substance abuse and withdrawal can all produce symptoms of panic and must be ruled out before you make this diagnosis. Conversely, because the symptoms of panic attacks mimic many organic disorders, people often consult internists for these symptoms and may have extensive medical workups and numerous consultations before the idea of a panic disorder is considered.

Panic attacks that are triggered only by specific social situations (e.g., urinating in public lavatories), by specific obsessive fears (e.g., being prevented from washing one's hands), or by specific phobic situations (e.g., seeing a snake) do not qualify for the diagnosis of panic disorder. Rather, they are categorized as other anxiety disorders, such as social phobia, obsessive-compulsive disorder, and simple phobia, respectively. Panic disorder is characterized by the unexpected nature of the attacks at some point in the illness.

Treatment

Treatment of panic disorder must be aimed at each of the three aspects of this syndrome: panic attacks, anticipatory anxiety, and agoraphobia. It begins with a careful history, a physical examination, and laboratory

Table 8-1. Somatic illnesses that are commonly accompanied by anxiety

Cardiovascular	Neurological
Angina pectoris	Partial complex seizures
Cardiac arrhythmias	
Mitral valve prolapse	Toxic metabolic
Hyperkinetic heart syndrome	Medication side effects
Recurrent pulmonary emboli	Substance abuse
	Withdrawal states
Endocrine	
Hyperthyroidism	
Pheochromocytoma	
Hypoglycemia	
Hypoparathyroidism	
Cushing's syndrome	

studies to rule out underlying organic illnesses. Panic attacks can be blocked effectively by maintaining patients on a tricyclic antidepressant, particularly imipramine, desipramine, or clomipramine. Monoamine oxidase inhibitors (MAOIs) are also effective and are commonly used as second-line medications when patients do not respond to a tricyclic. Once panic attacks have been effectively blocked with an antidepressant, the patient should be continued on the medication for 6 months before a taper is attempted.

Anticipatory anxiety and free-floating anxiety can be treated with selective intermittent use of a benzodiazepine (e.g., oxazepam). Some clinicians have advocated the use of the benzodiazepine alprazolam (Xanax) alone, because it both reduces anticipatory anxiety and blocks panic attacks. However, long-term use of alprazolam is sometimes complicated by tolerance and dependence, which prompts many clinicians to rely on alternative treatments. Clonazepam (Klonopin) is a newer benzodiazepine that is also thought to have antipanic properties, but it has not yet been well studied. Buspirone (Buspar), a nonbenzodiazepine antianxiety agent, is less sedating and less prone to be abused than are the benzodiazepines, but its efficacy in panic disorder has not been proved.

Agoraphobia may be treated with behavior therapy designed to expose patients gradually to feared experiences so that they can slowly master their fear of recurrent attacks in specific situations (e.g., in supermarkets, at parties). Dynamically oriented psychotherapy may be necessary when anxiety is due to conflicts over separation from important others or to reactions to the environment that must be explored before symptoms will resolve.

For example, there are patients who, despite effective treatment of their panic attacks, are resistant to behavior therapy and remain wary of asserting themselves. They may be able to face feared situations only when, in dynamic psychotherapy, they have explored unconscious conflicts about separation and addressed the unconscious meaning of independent behavior.

Generalized Anxiety Disorder

Generalized anxiety disorder is characterized by unrealistic or excessive anxiety and worry about two or more life circumstances for at least 6 months. For example, someone with this disorder may be unduly worried about finances and about the health of a friend who is quite healthy. A teenager who is popular with peers and doing well in school may be unrealistically anxious about academic performance and about social situations. The symptoms of anxiety vary greatly from person to person, but usually include the following manifestations:

- *Motor tension*: trembling, muscle aches and tension, easy fatigability, inability to relax, and restlessness
- *Autonomic hyperactivity*: sweating, palpitations, rapid respirations, rapid pulse, dry mouth, clammy hands, dizziness, paresthesias (tingling in hands or feet), nausea, stomach pain, frequent urination, diarrhea, hot or cold spells, flushing, pallor
- *Vigilance and scanning*: feeling on edge, exaggerated startle response, irritability, distractibility, difficulty concentrating, trouble falling asleep

Generalized anxiety often accompanies other psychiatric disorders, particularly depressive syndromes, schizophrenia, and various personality disorders. The diagnosis of generalized anxiety disorder is not made when another mental disorder or an underlying organic disorder is responsible for the patient's distress (e.g., when anxiety occurs only during a depressive or psychotic episode, or during drug intoxication).

People commonly attempt to medicate their anxiety by abusing such drugs as alcohol, barbiturates, and antianxiety agents. In such cases, substance abuse often stops when the anxiety disorder is treated. The extent to which anxiety interferes with work and social life varies greatly among individuals with this disorder, but impairment is usually mild. The epidemiology, natural history, and prognosis of generalized anxiety disorder have not been well studied, but research is currently underway to better document the prevalence and course of this disorder.

Etiology

Many **biological theories** about the etiology of generalized anxiety disorder involve the same anatomical and neurochemical factors postulated to play a role in the genesis of panic disorder (see above discussion). Thus, research strategies often aim to elucidate the biological underpinnings of both.

One area of research that may relate specifically to the etiology of generalized anxiety disorder involves the neurotransmitter *gamma-aminobutyric acid* (GABA). GABA is an inhibitory neurotransmitter—that is, it slows transmission of signals from one neuron to another—by binding to specific GABA receptors in the CNS. Investigators have discovered a benzodiazepine receptor in gray matter that is linked to the GABA receptor. Benzodiazepines bind to the receptor and facilitate the action of GABA in slowing neural transmission. In laboratory animals, acute anxiety can be produced by β-carbolines, which block benzodiazepine binding to the benzodiazepine receptor. This phenomenon has led to the hypothesis that in people with generalized anxiety disorder a substance is produced that interferes with the benzo-diazepine–GABA receptor complex and thereby produces anxiety. To date, however, no such substance has been found.

Numerous **psychological theories** of the etiology of anxiety have been advanced. Early psychoanalytic theorists postulated that anxiety stemmed from repressed sexual urges. Freud believed that psychic energy associated with these unacceptable sexual thoughts and impulses built up and, when it became too strong to be held back by repression, broke through to consciousness in the form of anxiety. Based on his clinical experience, Freud revised this theory to formulate the idea of "signal anxiety"—which remains a major operating principle of psychodynamic thought. This theory holds that anxiety is not the result of failed de-fenses (as was earlier believed), but rather is a signal that the individual is in some danger. Anxiety prompts the individual to mobilize defenses that aid in avoiding the dangerous situation and reducing the amount of anxiety.

A classic example is the danger posed by an intrapsychic conflict. When a young child's wishes come into conflict with parental expecta-tions and the realities of the world, the child may imagine being pun-ished for these wishes. (For example, a youngster who harbors murder-ous wishes toward her little brother may fear that she will be severely punished for these feelings.) These conflicts may be within a young child's awareness, but they are repressed as children grow up. In adult-hood, circumstances may reactivate an unconscious conflict and foster anxiety. Typical childhood fears that may be repressed and lead to anxi-ety disorders in adult life are the following:

- Loss of, or separation from, a parent or other caregiver on whom one depends
- Loss of love through anger or disapproval of an important person
- Damage to or loss of the genitals (also called *castration anxiety*)
- Loss of self-esteem when one fails to live up to one's moral stan-dards adopted from early caregivers

Psychodynamic therapy aims at understanding the nature of the anxiety and its childhood antecedents. For example, in therapy, a woman who becomes terrified when her husband leaves on a business trip may discover that this anxiety is not based on any actual danger to herself or her husband, but because the separation revives her early fears of separa-tion from parents.

Learning theory holds that anxiety is a response that has been condi-tioned by specific environmental situations and that therefore can be unlearned. For example, a combat veteran who experiences severe anxiety in the midst of a bombing raid may find that loud noises alone are sufficient to produce the same anxiety reaction long after the combat situation is over. Treatment would be aimed at uncoupling the stimulus of loud noise from the anxiety reaction through techniques such as systematic desensitization.

How do we make sense of the fact that there are such different approaches to the etiology of anxiety disorders? In fact, the biological, psychodynamic, and learning theory approaches are not mutually exclusive and may well be complementary. This is consistent with the clinical reality that no one form of treatment is effective for all patients who suffer from pathological forms of anxiety. Medication, dynamic psychotherapy, and cognitive-behavior therapy have all been used successfully with some patients, and combinations of these may well be more effective than any one alone.

Differential diagnosis

Differential diagnosis of generalized anxiety disorder may be complicated, as anxiety is a feature of many other psychiatric disorders. In particular, many depressed patients are also anxious, and many people with persistent primary anxiety become demoralized and depressed. However, patients with generalized anxiety disorder do not usually show the full range and intensity of vegetative symptoms (early morning awakening, loss of appetite, and diurnal mood variation), nor do they lose their ability to enjoy things and to be cheered up. Also, when anxiety is the primary disorder, anxiety symptoms usually precede a mood change, while the reverse holds when a mood disorder is primary.

The full range of medical disorders that underlie panic symptoms may also result in generalized anxiety (see Table 8-1), and so must be ruled out whenever generalized anxiety disorder is considered. Among people who come to health care facilities complaining of anxiety, medical illness is found in a minority of cases. Nevertheless, the possibility of underlying somatic disease must not be overlooked when you evaluate anxious patients, and everyone who is being evaluated for anxiety for the first time should have a thorough medical evaluation as well as a mental health assessment.

Treatment

The treatment of generalized anxiety disorder can include a variety of modalities.

Antianxiety medications. Antianxiety medications (e.g., benzodiazepines) are used to relieve symptoms and improve functioning. However, these medications are prone to abuse, and dependence on them is a common problem among anxious patients. Thus, you must closely monitor their use (see Chapter 18). Buspirone, the new nonbenzodiazepine antianxiety agent, is less sedating and has less potential for abuse than the benzodiazepines. Recently, investigators have begun to explore the use of tricyclic antidepressants for long-term maintenance therapy for generalized anxiety disorder.

Psychodynamic psychotherapy. This modality is effective in helping some people understand and master the underlying conflicts that prompt anxiety. A therapeutic relationship provides much-needed emotional support to anxious patients.

Cognitive-behavior therapy. Cognitive-behavior therapy can teach patients techniques of relaxation and imaging that they can use in anxiety-provoking situations to overcome fears and decrease symptoms, while systematic desensitization allows people to become less sensitive to anxiety-producing stimuli (see Chapter 17).

Phobias

A phobia is a persistent and irrational fear of a specific object, activity, or situation that results in a compelling desire to avoid what is feared. Even though the afflicted person recognizes the fears as excessive or unrealistic given the actual dangerousness of the object, activity, or situation, he or she nevertheless goes to some lengths to avoid it. If this avoidant behavior has no major effect on the person's life, the phobic behavior does not constitute a disorder (e.g., being afraid of spiders). However, when the phobia impairs one's ability to function at normal daily tasks, the diagnosis of a phobic disorder is warranted.

Phobias are generally divided into three major categories (Table 8-2):

Table 8-2. Major categories of phobias

Agoraphobia
Fear of being alone or in public places from which escape might be difficult or help unavailable in case of sudden incapacitation

Simple phobias
Fear of specific objects or situations (other than being alone, being away from home, or embarrassment in public)

Social phobias
Fear of embarrassment or humiliation in public situations

1. **Agoraphobia** involves fear of being alone, fear of leaving home, or fear of being in public places from which escape might be difficult (e.g., crowds or closed spaces) and where help might not be readily obtainable. As noted above, agoraphobia most commonly occurs in conjunction with panic disorder, usually beginning between ages 18 and 35. When it occurs without panic disorder, the clinical manifestations are the same as those described above.

2. **Simple phobias** involve fear of specific objects or situations other than being alone, being away from home, or embarrassment in public (e.g., fear of snakes, fear of heights). For most people with phobias, anxiety occurs not only when they are faced with the dreaded stimulus but even when they anticipate encountering it (anticipatory anxiety). Psychoanalytic theory holds that simple phobias begin as perceived dangers from within—that one's own fears of forbidden sexual or aggressive impulses become transposed onto some external object (e.g., snakes). Internal dangers cannot be avoided, but a danger in the external world can be; thus, by using the defense mechanism of *displacement*, the phobic person achieves a partial solution to the problem.

3. **Social phobias** involve a fear of embarrassment or humiliation in situations in which one must interact with other people (e.g., fear of speaking in public, using public lavatories, or eating in public). When forced into the situation they fear, people with this disorder experience profound anxiety with a variety of physiological symptoms, including tremor, palpitations, sweating, and faintness. Individuals with social phobias often report being very much afraid that others will notice their discomfort and ridicule them for it. This can lead to social isolation, particularly if more than one social phobia is present. Onset of this disorder usually occurs in the late teens or early twenties. While it may begin after a humiliating social experience, many people who develop social phobias recall no clear precipitant.

Treatment

Cognitive-behavior treatment of simple and social phobias is often quite successful in alleviating the symptom and restoring the patient's lost ability to function at daily tasks. *Systematic desensitization* is a widely used behavioral technique that involves the creation of a hierarchy of anxiety-producing stimuli (e.g., thinking about a snake, then looking at pictures of snakes, and finally watching a live snake). The therapist then uses this hierarchy of stimuli to desensitize the patient, presenting the stimuli to the patient gradually until they no longer produce anxiety (see Chapter 17). This kind of exposure to the feared situation is the treatment of choice for simple phobias. Patients often benefit from group therapy in which they can be supported by others in gradually facing the feared situation. Systematic desensitization is also useful in treating social phobias, along with cognitive therapy and social skills training designed to decrease anxiety in social situations. *Flooding* is another behavioral technique used to treat simple and social phobias. It involves repeatedly exposing the individual directly to the feared stimulus or situation until the anxiety response diminishes. Some patients tolerate this technique well, but others find it too stressful.

Psychodynamic psychotherapy that focuses on the childhood origins and symbolic meanings of the patient's fears has also been found to be helpful in some cases.

Pharmacotherapy with benzodiazepines and other antianxiety drugs can alleviate anticipatory anxiety, but these drugs are generally not suitable for long-term treatment. Some clinicians have found the phobic anxiety itself responsive to treatment with imipramine or phenelzine (see Chapter 18). Performance anxiety has been treated symptomatically with the beta-blocker, propranolol, 20 mg, orally administered 1 hour prior to the performance. At present, however, cognitive-behavior therapy is the mainstay of treatment for simple and social phobias.

Obsessive-Compulsive Disorder (OCD)

Obsessions are persistent, unwanted thoughts, impulses, or images that seem to the person to be senseless and intrusive, yet persist in his or her mind despite efforts to ignore them or neutralize them with some action. Common obsessions include thoughts of violence (e.g., hurting one's father), contamination (e.g., acquiring a dreaded disease by touching a doorknob), and doubt (e.g., the persistent fear of having left a door unlocked).

Compulsions are repetitive, purposeful, intentional behaviors that are meant to neutralize an obsession, usually according to some strict set of rules or in a stereotyped manner. People feel that they must perform these acts to avoid some dreaded situation, yet try to resist performing them because they recognize them to be unreasonable. Compulsive acts do not bring the person pleasure, but they do momentarily relieve tension and anxiety. When the person attempts to resist the compulsion, tension builds up and can be relieved when the compulsive act is performed. The most common compulsions are hand-washing, counting (e.g., numbers of cracks in the sidewalk), checking (e.g., to be sure the stove has been turned off), and touching (e.g., the objects in one's bedroom before going to sleep). Others include repeating, arranging, hoarding, and reassurance seeking. The array of behaviors that can be performed compulsively is practically infinite. Compulsive rituals result in slowed activity in daily living, and some patients have primary obsessional slowness, in which every activity becomes slowed down as part of a ritual.

People with OCD often struggle desperately to suppress unwanted thoughts and resist performing compulsive acts, only to suffer unbearable tension and anxiety. Most keep giving in to compulsive rituals and some cease all efforts to resist them. Depression is a common outcome of these struggles. Also, patients may become avoidant (even phobic) of feared situations. For example, a man with elaborate compulsive rituals around the removal of "dirt" after touching objects handled by others may become a recluse to avoid contamination. The diagnosis of OCD is made when obsessions or compulsions are so time-consuming, or cause so much subjective distress, that they interfere with social or occupational functioning.

Obsessive-compulsive disorder is seen in children, but most commonly begins in late adolescence or young adulthood. Onset is usually insidious, without any clear precipitating stressor. The disorder may be fluctuating or constant and progressive. The most common course is a chronic one, with waxing and waning of symptoms over months or years; an episodic or deteriorating course is not common. OCD appears to be much more common than was previously thought, with a prevalence of 1% to 2% of the general population. Men and women are affected in equal numbers, but among children OCD is up to three times more common in boys than girls. First-degree relatives of OCD patients show a higher than normal frequency of depression and obsessional character traits.

Etiology

Psychodynamic theory posits a continuum between obsessive-compulsive personality traits and the frank obsessions and compulsive rituals of OCD. Freud believed that OCD (or obsessional neurosis, as it was then called) develops when patients are unable to manage anxiety (e.g., about sexual or aggressive impulses) with more adaptive defense mechanisms, and return to the more infantile defenses of isolation, undoing, reaction formation, and displacement characteristic of the anal phase of development (see Chapter 2). However, epidemiological studies of OCD patients reveal that the disorder is distinct from obsessive-compulsive character—that is, that OCD patients do not necessarily have obsessive-compulsive character traits (as opposed to histrionic, schizoid, etc.) and that people with obsessive-compulsive character traits are more prone to depression and paranoia than they are to develop OCD. One essential distinction between OCD and obsessive-compulsive personality is that the former involves symptoms that are ego-dystonic, while the latter is a largely ego-syntonic character style.

Learning theory holds that OCD develops in two stages. First, the person links anxiety with a particular mental event, and, second, the person performs some ritual to lessen the anxiety. If this maneuver works, it reinforces the repetition of the ritual, and a compulsive behavior results. Some thoughts or images may also become associated with lessening of anxiety, resulting in cognitive compulsions.

Biochemical theories have focused on serotonin (5-hydroxytryptamine [5-HT]) and the serotonergic system. Clomipramine, a tricyclic antidepressant, has been found to have some antiobsessional effects, and it blocks serotonin reuptake at synaptic clefts more effectively than other tricyclics. Also supporting the role of serotonin in OCD is the finding that reduction of OCD symptoms is correlated with a reduction of platelet serotonin levels. However, the hypothesis that serotonin is implicated in the genesis of OCD remains unproved. Some investigators postulate that pharmacological blocking of serotonin reuptake corrects for abnormalities in some other (as yet unidentified) neurochemical system that is the real culprit in OCD.

Several *neurological findings* are of interest, including the fact that some patients develop OCD following head trauma, and that there is a subgroup of OCD patients who exhibit neurological "soft signs." However, to date, there is no substantive evidence for a neurological abnormality in the pathophysiology of OCD.

Differential diagnosis

Patients with *schizophrenia* may exhibit bizarre thoughts and rituals that can look like obsessions and compulsions. However, they commonly suffer from delusions that they believe to be real and of external origin, and that they do not resist; whereas people who suffer from OCD know that obsessions and compulsions are the creations of their own minds, and they experience them as ego-alien.

Patients with *depression* often develop obsessive rumination, and OCD patients frequently become depressed. The two disorders may be present concurrently. Usually, whichever disorder is primary precedes the other disorder in time.

Phobic disorders can present like OCD, and vice-versa, in that OCD patients often avoid certain feared situations (e.g., avoiding handshakes for fear of contamination). Phobic patients can usually successfully avoid what they fear (e.g., urinating in public lavatories), whereas OCD patients cannot so successfully avoid anxiety-provoking obsessions or the stimuli (e.g., potential contamination by germs) that give rise to their anxiety.

Treatment

Cognitive-behavior therapy is the best studied and, to date, most effective modality we have in the treatment of OCD. Behavior therapy employs two techniques: exposure and response prevention. Exposure may be gradual, as in systematic desensitization (discussed above under phobias), or more abrupt, as in flooding, which involves prolonged exposure to the anxiety-provoking situation (e.g., dirt) until the patient is less sensitive to it. Exposure techniques aim to decrease the patient's anxiety in the dreaded situation, while response prevention involves having the patient face the feared situation without giving in to the compulsive response. For example, the person exposed to dirt would not be allowed to engage in excessive hand-washing, and the pathological doubter would be taught techniques for stopping the ruminations about whether he or she has left the stove on. While the efficacy of cognitive-behavior therapy needs further empirical study, preliminary research suggests that a majority of OCD patients improve with these techniques.

Psychodynamic psychotherapy was once thought to be the treatment of choice for OCD, because obsessions and compulsions appear laden with unconscious symbolism and dynamic meaning. However, patients with this disorder typically do not respond well to exploratory psychotherapy, but can become "stuck" in endless ruminations about the meanings of their symptoms without any substantial behavioral change. Supportive therapy that provides reassurance to anxious and depressed OCD patients can be helpful, particularly when they are concurrently in anxiety-provoking behavioral treatments.

Pharmacotherapy for OCD patients is an area of intense research activity at the present time. A variety of psychotropic medications have been reported to be helpful in case reports and uncontrolled studies. But most promising are recent well-designed controlled studies of the tricyclic antidepressant clomipramine (Anafranil), which show it to be significantly more effective than placebo and other tricyclics, producing partial or complete remission of OCD symptoms in a majority of patients. New controlled studies have also suggested that newer serotonin reuptake blockers, such as fluoxetine (Prozac) and fluvoxamine, have specific antiobsessional effects, but their efficacy in OCD remains to be proved. No pharmacological treatment is standard for OCD at this time.

Posttraumatic Stress Disorder

Posttraumatic stress disorder (PTSD) occurs among people who have survived traumatic events that are outside the realm of normal human experience—for example, rape or assault, physical injury, military combat, bombings, torture, floods, or earthquakes. The afflicted person re-experiences the trauma through painful, intrusive recollections, day-dreams, or nightmares. Episodes may last from several minutes to several days. Less commonly, PTSD patients may have dissociative episodes (see below) in which they believe they are actually reliving the event.

This disorder also involves a kind of "psychic numbing" or decreased responsiveness to the environment, which may be experienced as decreased ability to receive pleasure from life's activities, or diminished capacity to feel interest in and tenderness toward other people. People with this disorder have persistent symptoms of increased autonomic arousal, including insomnia, irritability, difficulty concentrating, hypervigilance, and an exaggerated startle response. Anxiety and depression commonly occur with this disorder, and substance abuse is a common complication.

People who experienced traumatic events with others may also feel guilty about having survived when others did not (e.g., concentration camp survivors). Some people are only minimally impaired by this disorder, but others are severely incapacitated by phobic avoidance of all situations that might remind them of the traumatic event and trigger further episodes. PTSD victims may withdraw from any engagement in life, believing that it is futile to invest themselves in family or work life. This disorder has received increasing attention in the United States in recent years because of its prevalence among those returning from the Vietnam War. The syndrome is found in a high percentage of disaster victims (some estimates are as high as 30%). It is also common among people who as children were victims of sexual or physical abuse.

The disorder may begin with an exaggerated reaction to the trauma and a subsequent preoccupation with it. The diagnosis of PTSD is warranted if symptoms continue beyond 4 to 6 weeks after the event and include autonomic arousal and hyperreactivity, psychic numbing, avoidant behavior, and reliving of the trauma. Life becomes centered around the traumatic event, and the person's life-style and functioning at home and at work may begin to change. Finally, people who go on to develop chronic PTSD become preoccupied with the physical disability resulting from the trauma. They often develop somatic symptoms at this time, as well as chronic anxiety and depression. Substance abuse, inability to work, and deteriorating relationships with loved ones are all common.

Etiology

While the immediate cause of PTSD appears to be the specific stressor that is outside the realm of normal human experience, we do not know why some people develop this disorder following severe trauma while others do not. Inadequate social supports may increase the likelihood that a particular trauma victim will develop PTSD, but good data on this question are lacking. Similarly, the severity or frequency of the trauma may determine who is more likely to develop PTSD, but studies are needed to confirm this hypothesis. While serious preexisting psychopathology is thought to predispose people to PTSD, the evidence for this hypothesis is lacking.

The autonomic arousal seen in PTSD is similar to that seen in opiate withdrawal, which has led to the hypothesis that PTSD, like opiate withdrawal, may be mediated by noradrenergic hyperactivity. Clonidine, an α_2-noradrenergic agonist, has been shown to suppress the symptoms of opiate withdrawal, and preliminary trials suggest some promise for this medication in relieving the hyperreactivity, explosiveness, nightmares, and insomnia of PTSD patients as well.

Differential diagnosis

Posttraumatic stress disorder must be distinguished from *organic mental disorders* following acute trauma. In particular, you must rule out concussion, delirium, organic hallucinosis, and organic intoxication and withdrawal states, all of which can mimic PTSD.

Major depression and *dysthymia* are frequent complications of PTSD. While PTSD patients may avoid many situations that they associate with the original trauma and thus appear to have phobias, phobic patients do not have typical PTSD symptoms and, as a rule, do not have histories of severe trauma.

Generalized anxiety disorder includes many symptoms that are identical to those experienced by PTSD patients, but in generalized anxiety disorder there is no traumatic precipitant and the onset is usually insidious. PTSD patients sometimes meet the criteria for panic disorder and suffer from frank panic attacks.

It is also important to distinguish PTSD from *malingering*, since the secondary gain (unemployment benefits, etc.) from illness can be great. Malingering individuals usually give histories that are inconsistent and do not correspond to objective data. They also commonly have histories of antisocial behavior.

Treatment

Pharmacotherapy, psychodynamic psychotherapy, and cognitive-behavior therapy have all been reported to be useful in the treatment of PTSD. To date, however, no well-designed empirical studies of the efficacy of these modalities have been carried out.

Pharmacotherapy. Numerous medications have been used to treat PTSD patients. Antidepressants (e.g., imipramine, phenelzine) have been reported to decrease flashbacks, diminish forced recollections, and improve disturbed sleep. Beta-blocking agents (e.g., propranolol) have been used in small numbers of patients to diminish symptoms of autonomic arousal, as has clonidine. However, controlled trials of these medications are lacking.

Psychodynamic psychotherapy. This modality may be helpful in the acute aftermath of a traumatic event. Supportive therapy can help patients reduce stress and possibly prevent more chronic or delayed responses to the trauma. A model of long-term psychotherapy for people who develop the more chronic PTSD syndrome begins with supportive therapy and moves to more aggressive working through of the experience, including reappraisal of the traumatic event, and reframing patients' views of themselves and the world (e.g., exploring patients' assumptions that they are helpless and that the world is invariably hostile and dangerous). The mutual support of group psychotherapy can be particularly helpful for PTSD patients who feel the need to share their experiences with those who have survived similar traumatic events.

Cognitive-behavior therapy. This modality is particularly useful for PTSD patients who are phobic or become overwhelmingly anxious in certain situations. Systematic desensitization to dreaded stimuli (e.g., loud noises) or situations (e.g., crowded subways) can lessen anxiety and improve functioning in patients whose lives are limited by their fears. Less gradual and more intense exposure ("flooding") has been reported to be helpful, particularly in Vietnam War veterans, but many patients cannot tolerate this technique. Relaxation techniques can also be helpful in decreasing anxiety. Cognitive techniques such as thought-stopping can be useful in decreasing unwanted ruminations about the traumatic event and its sequelae.

DISSOCIATIVE DISORDERS

Dissociative disorders have fascinated students of the mind for centuries. Accustomed to thinking of the human psyche as an indivisible whole,

19th-century physicians were baffled by patients who demonstrated dissociative symptoms—who seemed to have removed clusters of mental elements from their conscious awareness and willful control. Freud's early theories of the unconscious were based largely on work with patients who appeared to have a "splitting of consciousness" that could be reintegrated via hypnosis or psychoanalysis.

Entire areas of memory, personal identity, or consciousness are literally dissociated from the rest of the mind in dissociative disorders, so that patients experience amnesia, fugue states, altered personality states, and episodes of depersonalization. Under the proper circumstances, these seemingly lost clusters of mental events can be recovered, sometimes quite suddenly.

Dissociative disorders are dramatic and have received much publicity in literature, in films, and on television. But, in fact, mild dissociative phenomena are normal features of everyday life. For example, people commonly become so absorbed in reading a book that they lose awareness of what is going on in the environment, or become lost in thought and fail to get off a bus at the proper stop. Hypnotic trances and certain types of religious experiences (e.g., speaking in tongues) are also examples of dissociation. Some individuals are more prone to dissociation and more hypnotizable than others, and some cultures sanction and encourage dissociation, while others pathologize it. DSM-III-R includes four types of dissociative disorders (also see Table 8-3), which are described below.

Table 8-3. Major categories of dissociative disorders

Psychogenic amnesia
  Sudden inability to recall important personal information

Psychogenic fugue
  Amnesia combined with sudden travel away from home, usually in flight from an intolerable situation

Multiple personality disorder
  The existence of two or more distinct personalities within an individual, each of which is dominant at a particular time

Depersonalization disorder
  Feelings of self-estrangement or unreality that impair social or occupational functioning

Psychogenic Amnesia

Psychogenic amnesia is a sudden inability to recall important personal information (e.g., name, occupation, family). This may be amnesia for one's entire life up until the moment of onset, or it may be amnesia for a circumscribed period of time (e.g., for the events surrounding a car crash). Amnesia may be selective: some events during a specified period of time are forgotten, while others are still subject to recall. Onset is often abrupt and follows a stressful or traumatic event.

People with this disorder usually first enter into an altered state of consciousness in which they may perform complex activities, may wander around, and are often confused and disoriented. This phase lasts from minutes to hours, followed by the awareness that they do not remember what has transpired over a period of time, and sometimes do not remember their own personal identities. In this stage, some patients are distressed by their amnesia, while others seem indifferent to it. Amnesia generally resolves abruptly, and recurrences are rare.

Etiology

Several types of trauma typically induce psychogenic amnesia. Life-threatening situations (war, disasters, physical and sexual abuse), the threatened or actual loss of an important other, and overwhelming ego-dystonic homicidal, suicidal, or sexual impulses are all commonly associated with the onset of the disorder. The psychological explanation for psychogenic amnesia involves the use of repression (see Chapter 2) to banish unacceptable or unbearable thoughts and feelings from consciousness. Disavowing whole areas of experience and even one's identity can be seen as a defense against acknowledging forbidden wishes or potentially overwhelming feelings. Clinicians have also speculated about a physiological predisposition to dissociation in response to stress.

Differential diagnosis

Unlike amnesia that is due to organic mental disorders, psychogenic amnesia usually has an abrupt onset following a traumatic or unusually stressful experience. The amnesia following head trauma is retrograde (amnesia for events prior to the trauma), whereas psychogenic amnesia is usually anterograde (for events after the traumatic event). Unlike multiple personality disorder, which involves prolonged and recurrent alterations of consciousness, psychogenic amnesia is usually a single isolated event.

Treatment

A high percentage of episodes of psychogenic amnesia recover spontaneously, and no specific treatment beyond support is necessary. Hypnosis has also been useful in helping patients to recover lost information. In cases where spontaneous recovery does not occur and hypnosis is not successful, use of an *Amytal interview* may be effective. This procedure involves intravenous administration of sodium amobarbital until the patient is sedated but not asleep, and then interviewing the patient under the influence of this medication. Gentle exploration will often help the patient to recall dissociated material. Ongoing psychotherapy may be necessary once recovery has occurred, to help the patient understand the conflicts that prompted such profound dissociation.

Psychogenic Fugue

Psychogenic fugue involves amnesia combined with physical flight, usually from an intolerable situation. The individual travels away from home, assumes a new identity, and is unable to recall his or her previous one. This is generally a short-lived phenomenon, involving a minimal amount of travel, but it may be quite prolonged and may result in the assumption of a whole new life in another locale (e.g., a man may leave his family, move to another city, get a new job, and make a new set of friends).

Little is known about the prevalence of this disorder, but it is believed to be uncommon. It has been reported most frequently among people exposed to major trauma such as natural disasters or war. Some clinicians report that preexisting psychopathology and a history of growing up in a dysfunctional family may predispose one to psychogenic fugue. Many patients with this disorder have intense separation anxiety and suicidal or homicidal impulses.

The disorder usually occurs in response to a stressor, and the fugue state usually lasts from several hours to several days. It is important to differentiate psychogenic fugue from organic mental syndromes (including drug intoxication), multiple personality disorder (which involves repeated shifts in identity), and malingering. Temporal-lobe epilepsy can involve dissociative experiences, including amnesia and travel, but does not involve assumption of a new identity.

Recovery is usually as abrupt as the onset, and recurrences are rare. Patients seldom remain in a fugue state by the time they come to the attention of a physician, but in such cases, hypnosis or an Amytal interview can be useful in retrieving information about the patient's identity. Once the baseline identity has been recovered, psychodynamic therapy may be needed to help the person understand the intrapsychic and interpersonal stressors that precipitated the fugue, and to develop more adaptive coping mechanisms.

Multiple Personality Disorder

Multiple personality disorder involves the existence within the individual of two or more distinct personalities, each with its own unique set of memories, attributes, and social relationships. Each personality is dominant and determines the individual's behavior at different times, and the transition from one personality to another is often abrupt.

The personalities are usually distinct and represent different unintegrated aspects of the person's identity. For example, an individual may have one shy and inhibited personality, another that is gregarious and promiscuous, and a third that is hostile and suspicious. The personalities may call themselves by different names. The personalities may have different voices, mannerisms, facial expressions, handedness, and even different allergies and responses to medications. They may have different findings on psychological testing. Each one may be unaware of the existence of the other personalities, only being aware of lost periods of time when the other personalities are dominant; or they may be aware of each other and wage battles or even cooperate. The transition from one personality to another is usually sudden. It may be triggered by particular environmental cues, by a stressful situation, or by an intrapsychic conflict.

Multiple personality disorder was thought to be rare, but in the last decade clinicians have begun to report making the diagnosis more frequently. This is probably due to a heightened awareness of the manifestations of this disorder, of its similarity to posttraumatic stress disorder, and of the high incidence of childhood sexual and physical abuse that are common elements in the histories of patients with multiple personality disorder. The incidence and prevalence of the disorder are unknown. In the majority of cases the manifestations of multiple personality disorder wax and wane over time, so that at any given moment, the prevalence of the disorder may appear deceptively low. More than three-quarters of patients are female. Most are diagnosed between late adolescence and early middle age.

Some patients with multiple personality disorder function well in the world, while others are severely impaired in work and social relationships by dissociation and frequent switches from one personality to another. Common complications of this disorder include suicidal ideation and attempts, self-mutilation, and substance abuse.

Interesting case studies of multiple personality disorder in the popular literature include *The Three Faces of Eve* and *Sybil* (see chapter bibliography).

Etiology

The overwhelming majority of patients with multiple personality disorder (up to 98%) have histories of childhood sexual and physical abuse. The disorder often runs in families, affecting multiple generations and siblings in the same generation. This appears to be due to the transmission of trauma from one generation to the next, as well as the inability of impaired parents to protect children from abuse by others. Many children identify with and adopt the abusive behavior of their parents, so that they grow up to be abusive adults. It may be that some children are congenitally predisposed to dissociate. This predisposition, in combination with inadequate environmental supports (e.g., people outside the home) and the lack of other defenses with which to cope with the trauma, may result in prolonged and extensive use of the dissociative defense to take flight from what is overwhelming and unacceptable.

Differential diagnosis

The diagnosis of multiple personality disorder is difficult to make. Patients with this disorder may present with a wide variety of psychological and somatic symptoms, but may not give histories of multiple personalities and are unlikely to manifest personality switches in an initial interview. Elements in a patient's history that should alert you to the possibility of multiple personality disorder include fluctuating symptoms and levels of functioning, amnesia for certain behaviors or periods of time, discovery of objects or handwriting in the patient's possession that he or she does not recognize, failure of psychiatric treatment in the past, and multiple prior diagnoses.

Many patients also hear voices that they recognize as coming from within their own heads but that are experienced as alien. Hearing voices may be mistaken for auditory hallucinations and result in a diagnosis of *schizophrenia*.

Altered states of consciousness and behavior in multiple personality disorder may be mistaken for *temporal-lobe epilepsy*, but in the latter condition, alternating separate identities do not exist. *Psychogenic fugue* and *psychogenic amnesia* are distinguished from multiple personality disorder by the fact that they do not involve repeated shifts in identity, but usually consist of single dissociative episodes. *Malingering* can be difficult to distinguish from multiple personality disorder; however, information from relatives, friends, police, and others will usually fail to corroborate the malingerer's story of dissociative phenomena and distinct personalities.

Symptoms of multiple personality disorder are similar to those found in *depression, anxiety disorders, posttraumatic stress disorder,* and *borderline personality disorder*. Indeed, the overlap of multiple personality disorder with each of these disorders is thought to be considerable. In many cases, patients present for psychiatric help manifesting symptoms consistent with one of these other disorders, and it is only during treatment that they reveal the existence of multiple personalities.

Treatment

Individual psychodynamic psychotherapy is usually the treatment of choice for multiple personality disorder, with the goal of helping the patient to integrate the different personalities into one cohesive self. Once patients begin to trust the therapist, they will allow various personalities to enter the treatment, and the concerns of each personality can be understood and attended to. Often, personalities are in conflict with one another, and these conflicts may be worked through in treatment. Reintegration of the personalities may occur abruptly or gradually. Experienced therapists report that, in many successful cases, the integrated personality remains stable once the patient has finished therapy.

To date, no medications have been found to be specifically helpful in the treatment of this disorder. Antianxiety agents can provide temporary symptomatic relief when anxiety is a prominent part of the clinical picture, and antidepressants may be useful when the patient suffers from a concurrent major depressive episode.

Depersonalization Disorder

Depersonalization disorder involves recurrent or persistent episodes of depersonalization, during which people feel that they are detached observers of their own mental processes or bodies, that they are automatons, or that they are in a dream. People with this disorder often report feeling as if they were watching a play rather than participating in real life, or as if they were watching themselves from a distance. They may feel that they are not in control of their actions and fear that they are losing their sanity. However, their ability to test reality remains intact (e.g., knowing that one is not literally an automaton). Episodes of depersonalization constitute a disorder only when they cause the individual marked distress. The disorder is often chronic, commonly waxing and waning as the person's degree of anxiety or depression increases or decreases.

There is considerable disagreement among clinicians about the validity of depersonalization disorder as a separate diagnostic entity. Episodes of depersonalization are reported by 30% to 70% of normal young adults, particularly during times of stress. Moreover, depersonalization is a symptom that is commonly associated with a variety of other mental disorders, particularly schizophrenia, panic disorder, depression, phobias, temporal-lobe epilepsy, substance abuse, and borderline personality disorder. Depersonalization disorder is a diagnosis of exclusion when other disorders have been ruled out through a careful history and physical examination, toxic screen, EEG, and other appropriate laboratory studies.

There is little information on the treatment of this disorder, in part because the diagnosis is made infrequently in clinical settings. No medication has been reported to be specifically effective in treating depersonalization. Some reports indicate favorable treatment results using hypnosis, dynamic psychotherapy, and cognitive-behavior therapy, but further research on the efficacy of these approaches is needed.

SOMATOFORM DISORDERS

The somatoform disorders are, quite literally, psychiatric disorders that assume the form of somatic illness. On the illness-disease spectrum illustrated in Figure 11-1 (see Chapter 11), these fall on the far end of the psychogenic spectrum, where emotional factors predominate in the origin of physical symptoms. As any internist will tell you, these disorders are very common in general medical practice. Like delirium, they form a prominent part of the consultation-liaison psychiatrist's practice, in both inpatient and outpatient medical settings.

Patients afflicted with somatoform disorders are often called "doctor-shoppers" or "hypochondriacs." They go from one medical facility to another, seeking help for an illness for which physicians can find no organic basis. It is a frustrating situation for patients, their families, and their physicians. They are told that there is nothing wrong, or that it is "all in their heads," yet they remain convinced that their pain and physical symptoms are real.

In fact, their symptoms and concerns *are* real—as real as if there were visible physical lesions to account for them. And patients with these disorders do not experience their symptoms as being within their control—that is, they do not feel that they have voluntarily produced these problems. Yet the symptoms are linked to psychological factors that these patients are generally reluctant to explore, and so the patients persist in searching for an organic cause.

The somatoform disorders fall into the five major categories outlined below (also see Table 8-4). All are characterized by physical symptoms that cannot be accounted for by any demonstrable physical findings or known physiological mechanisms.

Body Dysmorphic Disorder (Dysmorphophobia)

This disorder involves a preoccupation with some imagined defect in appearance in a person who, to others, appears normal. Patients with this disorder are most commonly troubled by aspects of the face, such as the shape of the nose, mouth, or jaw, wrinkles or moles, or facial hair. Less often, patients are distressed by the appearance of their hands, feet, breasts, or other body parts. In some cases, the person does have a slight physical anomaly, but the distress experienced from it is grossly out of proportion to the abnormality.

Patients with this disorder often make numerous visits to plastic surgeons and may have multiple operations to try to repair the supposed defect. They may avoid social and occupational settings because of anxiety about the defect, and they often develop depression or obsessive-compulsive symptoms in association with this disorder. It most com-

Table 8-4. Major categories of somatoform disorders

Body dysmorphic disorder
  Preoccupation with some imagined defect in appearance in a normal-
    appearing person

Somatization disorder
  Multiple recurrent somatic complaints of several years' duration that are
    not due to any physical disorder

Conversion disorder
  Sudden, dramatic loss of physical functioning that has no known
    pathophysiological cause and appears to be a manifestation of a
    psychological need or conflict

Somatoform pain disorder
  Pain in the absence of adequate physical findings or pathophysiological
    explanations, and in association with psychological factors that seem to
    play an etiological role

Hypochondriasis
  Unfounded fears of having serious illness

monly begins in the teenage years or 20s and may persist for several years.

Patients with body dysmorphic disorder are not delusional—that is, they can acknowledge the possibility that they might be exaggerating the extent of the defect or that there might not be a defect. When the belief is of delusional severity, the diagnosis of *delusional disorder, somatic subtype* is used instead. Patients with *anorexia nervosa* who have unfounded beliefs about body weight, and patients with *transsexualism* who are dissatisfied with their gender-related physical characteristics, are not given the diagnosis of body dysmorphic disorder.

Somatization Disorder

Somatization disorder, also called *Briquet's syndrome* or *Briquet's hysteria*, is characterized by multiple somatic complaints that are recurrent and of several years' duration, for which medical attention has been sought but for which no physical cause can be found. Complaints are often general, vague, and dramatically presented. Any or all body systems may be involved, but the most common complaints are pseudoneurological (e.g., pseudoseizures), gastrointestinal, gynecological, sexual, and cardiopulmonary. Chronic pain is generally present (e.g., back pain, joint pain), and abdominal pain is probably the most frequent specific complaint encountered among people with this disorder.

To differentiate symptoms of somatization disorder from general "aches and pains" and from those of panic disorder, the diagnostic criteria require that a symptom of somatization disorder be 1) associated with no known organic pathology or pathophysiological mechanism; 2) not present solely during a panic attack; and 3) distressing enough to cause the person to take medicine other than nonprescription pain relievers, see a physician, or alter his or her life-style.

Somatization disorder usually begins during teenage years and less often in the 20s, but by definition before age 30. It has a chronic course, usually involving consultation by many physicians and frequently complicated by multiple hospital admissions and unnecessary surgical procedures. Abuse of both prescribed and nonprescribed substances is common. Anxiety and depression often accompany the disorder. When afflicted individuals seek psychiatric help, it is often for symptoms of depression, or after suicide threats or gestures. The disorder is much more commonly diagnosed in women than in men, and the lifetime prevalence for women may be as high as 2%.

Before you make this diagnosis, you must rule out organic illnesses (e.g., multiple sclerosis, systemic lupus erythematosis) that can present with vague and diffuse symptomatology. Also, panic disorder patients experience numerous somatic symptoms, but these occur only in the context of panic attacks. Some schizophrenic patients suffer from somatic delusions as part of their illness (e.g., "my insides are rotting"); it is important to differentiate such psychotic patients from people with somatization disorder, who are, by definition, not psychotic and who do not benefit from treatment with antipsychotic medication.

Conversion Disorder

Also called *hysterical neurosis, conversion type,* this is the classic disorder that fascinated Freud and other pioneers in the field of psychoanalytic psychiatry. It typically involves the sudden and dramatic onset of blindness, paralysis, seizures, or other symptoms that seem to suggest neurological disease but that have no known pathophysiological cause. It is different from somatization disorder in that it generally involves a single symptom during any one episode, and this symptom results in the loss or alteration of a particular physical function.

In addition to the symptoms mentioned above, typical conversion symptoms include loss of speech, involuntary movements, inability to walk, loss of coordination, tunnel vision, and anesthesia or paresthesia of a body part. Although symptoms appear to be neurological, careful examination and tests reveal discrepancies between the loss of function and known anatomical distribution of motor and sensory nerves. For example, anesthesia of a hand typically occurs over a "glove" distribution, rather than along lines of anatomical sensory innervation. In some cases, symptoms suggest autonomic or endocrine disturbances, such as hysterical vomiting, and pseudocyesis ("false pregnancy").

Conversion symptoms are not under the patient's voluntary control, yet they appear to be the expression of a psychological conflict or need. These symptoms are thought to provide patients with two sorts of gains. The *primary gain* from the symptom is relief from an emotional conflict and the reduction of anxiety. The symptom actually represents the conflict and achieves a partial solution to it. In such cases, there is usually a temporal relationship between an event that provokes conflict and the onset of the symptom (e.g., conflict about expressing overwhelming rage at a spouse that results in loss of speech).

The *secondary gain,* common to all somatoform disorders, is that by assuming a sick role, the disabled patient can avoid unwanted responsibilities and get support from others that would not otherwise be forthcoming. Because the conversion symptom diminishes anxiety and intrapsychic conflict, patients may be blind or paralyzed and yet seem relatively unconcerned about their severe physical disability—a phenomenon called *la belle indifférence.*

Conversion disorder usually begins in adolescence or young adulthood, although it may occur for the first time later in life. Episodes of conversion begin suddenly during times of severe stress and often resolve abruptly. Episodes may be recurrent. Functioning is often greatly impaired, and the patient may develop physical complications (e.g., limb contractures) due to prolonged loss of function. Unnecessary medical procedures can also produce serious complications. Although it was more common several decades ago, the disorder is now relatively rare in clinical practice in industrialized nations.

Somatoform Pain Disorder

Somatoform pain disorder involves the predominant complaint of pain in the absence of any physical findings or pathophysiological explanation, or pain that is grossly in excess of what would be expected from a physical condition. It differs from somatization disorder in that pain, rather than a variety of symptoms, is the primary presenting complaint. Pain generally does not follow the anatomical distribution of sensory nerves, and laboratory studies reveal no underlying lesions. There is usually a relationship between the exacerbation of psychological conflict or need and the onset of or increase in pain. Secondary gain is generally an important motivating force in the illness (e.g., the man whose chronic back pain worsens every time his wife plans an outing with friends). However, the patient does not experience the pain as being within his or her voluntary control.

The disorder typically begins in the 30s or 40s, but it can occur at any age, and it may remit spontaneously or become chronic. Patients are typically incapacitated by the disorder to the extent that they may be unable to work, and assume a role as an invalid. The disorder is diagnosed twice as often in women as in men, but the reasons for this are not clear. As you might expect, frequent medical consultations, unnecessary surgery, and abuse of analgesics are common complications of somatoform pain disorder.

Hypochondriasis

Unlike the other somatoform disorders, hypochondriasis involves unfounded *fears* of having serious illness. It is based on a preoccupation with body functions and the unrealistic interpretation of physical signs or sensations as abnormal (e.g., an occasional cough may be interpreted as a sign of lung cancer). By definition, these concerns are not frankly delusional; the person can acknowledge the possibility that his or her fears are unfounded. However, patients cannot shake their fears of physical illness despite repeated reassurance from physicians and persistently negative physical and laboratory findings.

Hypochondriasis is equally common among men and women. It begins most frequently between the ages of 20 and 30, but may occur at any age. It is quite common in general medical practice, and its chronic course invites extensive workups and unnecessary surgery. Although some patients can continue to function with only mild impairment at home and work, others become invalids. One danger in treating people with this disorder is that real organic pathology may go unnoticed because of repeated "false alarms." Past experience with true organic illness seems to predispose some patients to this disorder.

Treatment of Somatoform Disorders

The treatment of somatoform disorders is difficult. Patients usually refuse to accept the possibility that the roots of their problems are psychological. Insight-oriented psychotherapy can help some patients explore and resolve conflicts that foster physical symptoms; with conflict resolution, symptoms often disappear spontaneously. However, many of these patients are particularly resistant to exploratory psychotherapy. Biofeedback and other behavior modification techniques can help patients to relax and control pain and anxiety.

Antianxiety medications are helpful for some patients on a short-term basis, but the potential for abuse and dependence on such medications limits their value in the treatment of these disorders. Antidepressants have been found to be helpful for patients who have prominent symptoms of depression along with somatic complaints.

One great service that a psychiatrist can provide patients who have somatoform disorders is to coordinate their medical care, so that "doctor shopping" ends and unnecessary surgical procedures are avoided. This requires a good working relationship between the psychiatrist and other physicians responsible for the patient's medical care.

BIBLIOGRAPHY

Ballenger JC: Pharmacotherapy of the panic disorders. J Clin Psychiatry 47 (No 6, suppl):27–32, 1986

Braun BG (ed): Treatment of Multiple Personality Disorder. Washington, DC, American Psychiatric Press, 1986

Dietch JT: Diagnosis of organic anxiety disorders. Psychosomatics 22:661–669, 1981

Fisher C: Amnesic states in war neuroses: the psychogenesis of fugues. Psychoanal Q 14:437–468, 1945

Freud S: Splitting of the ego in the process of defense (1940), in The Standard Edition of the Complete Psychological Works of Sigmund Freud, Vol 23. Translated and edited by Strachey J. London, Hogarth Press, 1964, pp 271–278

Herman J: Father-Daughter Incest. Cambridge, MA, Harvard University Press, 1981

Jenicke MA, Baer D, Minichiello WE: Obsessive-Compulsive Disorders: Theory and Management. Littleton, MA, PSG Publishing, 1986

Katon W: Panic disorder: epidemiology, diagnosis, and treatment in primary care. J Clin Psychiatry 47 (No 10, suppl):21–30, 1986

Kluft RP (ed): Childhood Antecedents of Multiple Personality. Washington, DC, American Psychiatric Press, 1985

Kluft RP: Multiple personality disorder: an update. Hosp Community Psychiatry 38:363–373, 1987

Perry JC, Jacobs DJ: Overview: clinical applications of the Amytal interview in psychiatry emergency settings. Am J Psychiatry 139:552–559, 1982

Putnam FW, Guroff JJ, Silberman EK, et al: The clinical phenomenology of multiple personality disorder: review of 100 recent cases. J Clin Psychiatry 47:285–293, 1986

Rasmussen SA, Tsuang MT: DSM-III obsessive-compulsive disorder: clinical characteristics and family history. Am J Psychiatry 143:317–322, 1986

Schreiber F: Sybil. New York, Warner Books, 1974. (An account of the psychotherapy of a woman with multiple personalities.)

Sheehan DV: Current concepts in psychiatry: panic attacks and phobias. N Engl J Med 307:156–158, 1982

Teicher MH: Biology of anxiety. Med Clin North Am 72:791–814, 1988

Thigpen CH, Cleckley HN: The Three Faces of Eve. New York, Popular Library, 1974. (A highly readable case study of a woman with multiple personalities.)

Torgerson S: Genetic factors in anxiety disorders. Arch Gen Psychiatry 40:1085–1089, 1983

van der Kolk BA (ed): Post-Traumatic Stress Disorder: Psychological and Biological Sequelae. Washington, DC, American Psychiatric Press, 1984

Part III

Special Populations

9 Geriatric Psychiatry 233
10 Children and Adolescents 271
11 Consultation-Liaison Psychiatry 325
12 Neuropsychiatry 345

INTRODUCTION

This section deals with special topics that are of increasing importance in the field of psychiatry. Chapter 9 is a discussion of geriatric psychiatry and the particular problems common among the elderly. This chapter covers some of the organic mental disorders that are especially relevant to older patients.

Children and adolescents are discussed in Chapter 10. The chapter begins with an overview of psychological and physical development, as these are always relevant to understanding mental illness in younger patients. The chapter then covers the basic diagnostic entities encountered among children and adolescents.

Consultation-liaison psychiatry is discussed in Chapter 11. The psychiatric consultant on a medical or surgical service may be your first contact with psychiatry in a clinical setting. You will want to become familiar with the uses of psychiatric consultation for medical patients. As part of a student rotation, you may be asked to perform a psychiatric consultation yourself, and this chapter will give you a framework for doing that.

Finally, an introduction to neuropsychiatry is provided in Chapter 12. As our understanding of the interface between psychological and neurological functioning increases, neuropsychiatry has become an important area of psychiatric medicine. In this chapter, you will be introduced to new technological tools that have already improved diagnosis and treatment of mental disorders and that promise to advance further our understanding of the functioning of the human brain. Chapter 12 also deals with those organic mental disorders that have not been covered in Chapter 9.

9

Geriatric Psychiatry

THE ELDERLY CONSTITUTE an ever-increasing proportion of our population. Improved quality of life and—more importantly—low birth rates in recent decades have changed the composition of our society, and this trend will continue into the next century. In 1900, only 3 million people in the United States were over the age of 65. In 1985, 28 million people were over 65, and by the year 2030 that number is expected to increase to 65 million. In 1900, 4% of Americans were over 65, compared with 12% in 1985 and a projected 21.2% by 2030.

As a physician, your average working life will be 35 years, and during that time the elderly will come to represent one-fifth of our population. This "demographic imperative" has prompted a burgeoning of interest in geriatric medicine in recent years, and with it, better research into what constitutes health as well as illness among the aged.

Organic mental disorders may occur at any age, but they are more frequent among the elderly. Because of their particular significance for this age group, these disorders are considered in this chapter.

MYTHS ABOUT AGING

In your medical training, much of your exposure to older people occurs in hospitals, providing a somewhat skewed view of this population and perpetuating myths about old age:

233

Myth: Most of the elderly live in nursing homes and other institutions for chronic care.

Fact: In 1980, only 5% of those over 65 lived in institutions, while 67% lived with family members (spouses, children, etc.) and another 28% lived alone or with individuals other than family members.

* * *

Myth: Most of the elderly are in poor health.

Fact: In 1984, 68% of the elderly living outside institutions rated their health as good or excellent. However, 47% were limited in activity because of a chronic condition.

* * *

Myth: Most of the elderly are poor.

Fact: In 1985, 12.6% of those over 65 lived below the poverty level, but that number reduces to 3.5% when food, housing, and medical benefits from unearned sources are included. In 1982, 71% of the elderly reported themselves as highly satisfied with their standard of living. This is a much higher rate of satisfaction than that reported by any other age group.

* * *

Myth: Sexual interest and activity wane in old age.

Fact: While some individuals become less sexually active because of illness or lack of a partner, many of the elderly maintain a strong interest in sex. In fact, 15% of those over 65 report an *increase* in sexual activity with aging.

Why the myths? We tend to see the elderly through distorted lenses for a variety of reasons. Many younger people are not intimately acquainted with individuals over 65. As social mobility increases, it is less likely that grandchildren and grandparents live near each other, and the resulting generational segregation fosters ignorance about late-life interests and concerns. This can be compounded by our own fears of aging and death. The elderly represent the late stages of life and, as such, may be shunned by younger people who wish to avoid reminders of their own mortality. As physicians we are dedicated to preserving life, and old age represents our ultimate inability to do that. Insofar as the elderly remind us of our parents, we may unconsciously cling to the common childhood fantasy that they are sexless, and thereby make the elderly feel that sexual concerns are inappropriate and unacceptable.

These myths can seriously affect the quality of care we give to our older patients. To the extent that we harbor unrealistic views of old age, we may fail to understand the concerns that the elderly bring to us, and inadvertently deprive them of psychological and somatic treatments that may be of considerable help.

NORMAL PROCESSES OF AGING

What really happens in the process of aging remains poorly understood. Many changes thought to be normal are in fact due to illnesses associated with old age. Our knowledge of nonpathological processes continues to grow as research in geriatrics intensifies.

Biological Changes

Some biological changes are particularly relevant to the mental health of older people. Decreased visual acuity, peripheral vision, and night vision may restrict activity in older patients, which may contribute to lowered self-esteem and depression. Decreased auditory acuity, speech perception, and auditory discrimination may hamper social interaction and contribute to suspiciousness and even paranoia among people who cannot hear what others say to them. Increased reaction time, decreased muscle strength, and impaired mobility reduce the scope and speed of activities that are possible for the elderly.

Our requirements for sleep decrease as we age. While young adults require an average of 8 hours of sleep per night, people over the age of 90 require less than 6 hours. Those over 65 experience more periods of waking that disrupt sleep, and the average elderly person lies awake for one-fifth of the night. By age 75, one-third to one-half of healthy people complain of insomnia.

Sexual interest may increase or decrease with age, depending on the person's health and social circumstances. Contrary to the prevalent myth, impotence in men is not caused by advancing age, but rather by physical, drug-related, or psychological problems. Normal men do experience slower sexual response as they age, along with decreased erection, seminal fluid volume, and excitatory pressure. Older women experience a delay and decrease in vaginal lubrication, and some experience briefer orgasms and painful uterine contractions during orgasm. Vaginal lubrication can be augmented by topical aids, and painful uterine contractions can be helped by estrogens.

As it ages, the normal brain changes with respect to the synthesis, turnover, and receptor binding of neurotransmitters. Levels of norepinephrine, serotonin, dopamine, gamma-aminobutyric acid (GABA), and acetylcholine decrease, and this results in increased sensitivity of receptor sites in areas of the brain associated with mood, cognition, and coordination. The clinical significance of these findings is not known, but one hypothesis is that these changes in neurotransmission are associated with increased anxiety and depression in response to stress or loss, and with progressive decline in memory function.

Cognitive Changes

Research on cognitive changes in the elderly has been fraught with difficulty. Most of it has been conducted in artificial laboratory settings, where elderly people may develop anxiety because of unfamiliar surroundings and fast-paced presentation of tasks. Learning can occur at a very advanced age. Short-term memory declines on experimental tasks, and memory for remote events is also diminished, but recall and recognition of past events remain high. Mild forgetfulness of names and dates is normal, and many older people need reassurance of this fact. However, more serious forgetfulness (leaving the stove on repeatedly, leaving doors open inadvertently, losing one's way in familiar surroundings) is not normal and requires a thorough evaluation.

Psychological Changes

Growing older is not, in and of itself, a crisis. Life is punctuated by normal points of transition, and old age includes many normative changes with which each person must cope. These include physical changes, retirement, marriage of children, birth of grandchildren, death of spouses and other important people, and the acceptance of one's own death. While much has been written about the losses sustained by the elderly, less attention has been focused on the freedoms afforded by advancing age, including freedom from a work routine, freedom from child-rearing responsibilities, and the freedom that comes with a sense of limited time to enjoy life. Neugarten (1979) notes that most people adapt well to life changes, provided they occur "on time" (i.e., when the individual expects that they will occur).

As during other periods in life, the older adult musters characteristic coping mechanisms and defenses in the process of adapting to change. These remain relatively constant through life. So, for example, the retired attorney who was highly organized in early life may cope with mild memory impairment by continuing to use her adaptive obsessional defenses (see Chapter 2) to make lists and use other aids to compensate for her forgetfulness. By contrast, the aging starlet who was never very attentive to details may cope with forgetfulness with characteristic repression and rationalization, taking little notice of her impairment and telling herself that those silly little details were not worth remembering anyway.

Not only coping skills, but psychological concerns and vulnerabilities persist into later life. The man who was always jealous of his wife's friendships with other men may continue to be preoccupied with sexual jealousy in his 80s. What's more, this man may become more suspicious if impaired hearing makes it harder for him to attend to social interactions as he ages. The woman whose fragile self-esteem fluctuated with the ups and downs of her academic career may continue to be plagued by self-doubt in retirement. These concerns often remain very much alive for older individuals, and may be exacerbated by the life changes that accompany aging.

ASSESSING THE OLDER PATIENT

The Psychiatric History

The format for a psychiatric history discussed in Chapter 3 applies to people of all ages. Geriatric patients are often referred by family members, health professionals, or friends. Because the patient may be largely unaware that there is a problem (e.g., in cases of dementia), it is important to obtain information about the concerns and observations of those who make the referral.

Explore current symptoms in depth. Common symptoms that warrant psychiatric evaluation include thoughts of suicide, depressed mood, crying, loss of appetite, weight loss, memory problems, loss of interest in usual activities, confusion, agitation, assaultiveness, irritability, delusions or hallucinations, loss of energy, and physical illness for which no organic basis can be found.

Take a careful history of the development of symptoms. It is important to note whether symptoms developed gradually over months or years, or whether the onset was abrupt. Particularly in cases of cognitive impairment, the course of the illness can tell you much about diagnostic possibilities. A slow, gradual deterioration of mental functioning over months suggests a dementing process such as Alzheimer's disease (see below), while more rapid onset suggests an acute confusional state with a potentially treatable cause. Similarly, rapid personality change suggests an acute organic cause (e.g., frontal-lobe tumor), while more longstanding personality problems may be due to a life-long personality disorder that has become more troublesome as the patient's social situation changes with age. As with younger patients, *always try to answer the question, "Why now?"* In particular, ask about any recent changes in the patient's medications and about any changes in the patient's life situation.

Take note of the past psychiatric history. Many psychiatric illnesses persist into old age, such as personality disorders and affective episodes. Mania and depression produce cognitive symptoms that can look similar to dementia, but require very different treatments. A history of a mood disorder in the past and rapid onset of the current symptoms would suggest recurrent mania or depression, rather than dementia.

Take a careful medical history. Confusional states and depression can be caused by a wide variety of organic illnesses, including tumors, thyroid disease, diabetes, electrolyte imbalances, congestive heart failure, subdural hematomas, and cerebral vascular accidents. *Medical illness commonly presents with psychiatric symptoms among the elderly.* Thus, you may be the first to hear about such illnesses in your capacity as a mental health care worker.

Pay special attention to the family and social history. Older people often manage quite well with considerable physical or cognitive impairment until a stable social situation is disrupted. For example, a man may appear to have become demented immediately after his wife's death, suggesting an acute onset. However, by taking a careful history you determine that he was in fact losing memory function for years prior to his wife's death, but that she compensated for his deficits. Such information will be important not only for diagnosis but also for treatment, because restoring necessary social supports is often an essential part of therapy with older individuals.

A Formal Mental Status Examination

The mental status examination described in Chapter 4 is an important part of the assessment of every patient. With older individuals, it is particularly important to assess cognitive functioning formally, even when patients give very coherent histories. This assessment includes questions about orientation, attention, calculation, recall, and learning of new information. Patients may be able to mask subtle memory difficulties in conversation, but these are more likely to emerge during formal questioning.

One note of caution: Some older individuals with cognitive deficits deny that they have any impairment. For such people, your detailed questions about names, dates, etc., may force them to confront their deficits abruptly, resulting in sudden flashes of anger or depression. Should this occur, you would be wise to postpone further formal assessment of mental functioning until the patient is more calm and more comfortable with you and the current surroundings.

A Thorough Physical Examination

A thorough physical examination, including a complete neurological examination and appropriate laboratory screening, is necessary. If it is not feasible for you to do this in the context of a psychiatric evaluation, you must be sure that a physical evaluation is done and that you are rapidly apprised of the results.

PSYCHOPATHOLOGY AND TREATMENT

The elderly are subject to many of the same mental disorders as are younger people. As you try to make sense of psychiatric symptoms presented by the geriatric patient, and as you develop a treatment plan, it is important to keep the following in mind:

1. *Do not assume that your patient has been properly diagnosed or treated in the past.* Many older individuals have not had adequate mental health care earlier in their lives. Moreover, psychiatric diagnosis and treatment have changed greatly in recent decades. For example, the elderly "chronic schizophrenic" man with a long history of delusions and hallucinations, maintained for many years on neuroleptic medication, may in fact suffer from manic-depressive illness. Thorough questioning of relatives may reveal a history of highs and lows, as well as the existence of affective illness among biological relatives.
2. *In developing a differential diagnosis, consider your patient's age.* Remember, for example, that schizophrenia seldom develops after age 45, whereas affective illness may begin at any time of life, and that the elderly are subject to a host of organic ailments that have psychiatric manifestations. Thus, a patient who develops delusions for the first time at age 60 is far more likely to suffer from a mood disorder or an organic brain syndrome than from schizophrenia. Among elderly men, the four most common mental disorders are severe cognitive impairment (dementia), phobias, alcoholism, and dysthymia. Among elderly women, the most common mental disorders are phobias, severe cognitive impairment, dysthymia, and major depression.
3. *Focus on treatable problems.* Your elderly patients are likely to have multiple problems. Whereas some symptoms are untreat-

able, other difficulties may respond dramatically to simple non-medical interventions. For example, an elderly man who suffers from paranoia may be considerably less symptomatic when a hearing aid improves his ability to make sense of his interactions with others. A woman with Alzheimer's disease who is severely agitated at night may improve her sleep if given regular daily exercise. Support for her exhausted family members (e.g., Meals-on-Wheels; a support group) can enhance the quality of the patient's life and that of her caregivers' lives.

Psychosis

Psychotic thinking without a major mood disturbance is found primarily in three conditions common to elderly people: 1) schizophrenia, 2) organic brain syndromes, and 3) delusional (paranoid) disorder, often called *paraphrenia*.

   Schizophrenia. This disorder is, for most patients, an illness that persists into old age. However, one-third of those with the disorder recover completely by age 65. The remaining two-thirds often experience a waning of "positive" symptoms—that is, active delusions and hallucinations become less troublesome to the patient. "Negative" symptoms such as apathy and blunted affect persist and may even worsen. Medication dosages can usually be reduced and sometimes discontinued as schizophrenic people become less agitated and more cooperative in old age. As noted above, some older individuals have been misdiagnosed as schizophrenic in their youth and in fact have a mood disorder. Every schizophrenic patient deserves a careful review of his or her history and records, to be sure that a more treatable psychotic illness has not been missed.
   Organically based psychosis. This disorder occurs as a manifestation of medical illnesses and drug-related conditions among elderly people. The most common physical causes of paranoia and delirium among geriatric patients include alcoholism, anticholinergic medications, steroids, hypothyroidism, malnutrition, and postoperative states. (Delirium is discussed later in this chapter.)
   Delusional disorder. This disorder (also known as *paraphrenia*) is similar to schizophrenia in that it includes paranoid delusions, and often hallucinations as well, and has no known organic cause. Unlike schizophrenia, delusional disorder comes on late in life, does not involve progressive deterioration, and does not impair the person's affect, intellectual abilities, or volition. This disorder comes on slowly and insidiously. Patients become preoccupied with the false belief that they are being

harrassed, assaulted, and intruded upon. They often respond to these delusions quite actively, complaining to the police about imagined intruders, striking out at neighbors verbally or physically in retaliation for supposed wrongdoing, or shrinking away from contact with others. People with this disorder may stop eating, shout at hallucinated persecutors, barricade themselves in their homes, sneak about at night, and even attempt suicide to escape their persecutors. They are generally unaware that they are ill, and are brought to treatment by relatives, neighbors, and other third parties.

When considering the diagnosis of delusional disorder, you should take care to rule out an underlying treatable dementia, delirium, or depression. Also, be sure to take a careful social history: many of the elderly *are* in fact victimized. A certain degree of suspiciousness may be realistic and adaptive among older people and must be distinguished from the florid delusions of the paraphrenic individual. Moreover, you can be of considerable help to an older patient simply by identifying and intervening to help change a social situation in which the patient is being abused or neglected.

Delusional disorder accounts for about 10% of psychiatric admissions after the age of 60. Its prevalence is thought to be less than 2% of the elderly population, but more than 3% of the elderly who reside in nursing homes. It is much more common among women than men, even when the greater proportion of women in the geriatric population is taken into account.

The etiology of delusional disorder is unclear. There is some suggestion that many who go on to develop this disorder had similar but milder traits as young adults—that is, they were less sociable, more easily offended, and less emotionally forthcoming than their peers. Chronic deafness is associated with the development of delusional disorder, usually after several decades of social impairment due to hearing loss. It may be that in vulnerable individuals who are by nature somewhat withdrawn and suspicious, an impairment such as loss of hearing precipitates the disorder by isolating them further and inhibiting reality testing in social situations.

Treatment of delusional disorder, like that of schizophrenia, relies on the use of antipsychotic medications. High-potency neuroleptics (e.g., haloperidol) are often the medications of choice, because they are less likely than their low-potency counterparts to produce orthostatic hypotension, urinary retention, and confusion. Dosages should be low initially, and they should be raised cautiously. A low-potency antipsychotic may be more useful for cases in which sedation would relieve the patient's severe agitation or anxiety. Preventive use of antiparkinsonian medications (e.g., Cogentin) is not recommended, as elderly patients are particularly sensitive to anticholinergic side effects. For patients who cannot comply with an oral medication regimen, depot fluphenazine can be given intramuscularly every 2 weeks. (For a more detailed discussion of the use of antipsychotic medications, see Chapter 18.)

The great majority of patients with delusional disorder will return to their premorbid state when treated with medication appropriately. Maintenance on medication is usually necessary to keep these patients symptom-free, but once symptoms have remitted, dosages can usually be lowered to less than half of what was given initially. All elderly patients on neuroleptic medications need to be maintained on the lowest possible dosages and should have medication-free trials every 6 months in order to minimize the risk of tardive dyskinesia.

Measures that improve hearing and decrease social isolation (e.g., through day treatment programs) can be invaluable in alleviating paranoia among patients with delusional disorder, as well as among those with other paranoid disorders.

Course and prognosis

The prognosis for psychotic elderly patients varies with the disorder that causes their loss of reality testing. As noted above, schizophrenic patients recover in as many as one-third of the cases, and the majority become more placid and less troubled by their psychotic symptoms as these individuals age. The course and outcome of psychosis due to organic and iatrogenic factors vary with the treatability of the underlying disorder. The prognosis for delusional disorder is good for those who comply with treatment, but poor for those who cannot be maintained on antipsychotic medication.

Mood Disorders

Depression

Depression in the elderly, just as in younger people, is commonly manifested by symptoms such as sadness, decreased appetite, insomnia, decreased energy and libido, and thoughts of suicide (see Chapter 6). When depression presents in this typical fashion, diagnosis is not difficult. However, many elderly people suffer from what are called *masked depressions*—depressive episodes that are in some way disguised. Two common forms of masked depression are somatic complaints and dementia syndrome of depression (pseudodementia).

Somatic complaints are sometimes the only symptoms that depressed elderly patients experience. These patients do not experience sadness, but rather they experience that they are physically unwell. They make repeated visits to their primary care physician with a variety of complaints, including backache, fatigue, gastrointestinal distress, and headaches.

Dementia syndrome of depression (pseudodementia) is a syndrome in which dementia is the result of depressive illness and not organic brain disease. It is discussed in the section on dementia below.

While *psychotic depression* may occur at any age, depressive delusions assume a characteristic form among the elderly. Patients commonly believe that they are physically ill (e.g., that they have cancer or that their viscera are rotting). Older people typically develop hypochondriacal concerns as they age, in part because they do, in reality, have more to worry about physically. However, somatic delusions differ from these less pathological concerns in that delusions are not amenable to reassurance, so medical examinations cannot allay the psychotically depressed person's fears. Similarly, many depressed elderly people develop delusions of poverty. Despite adequate resources, patients may believe they have no money for food, clothes, or shelter, and financial statements do little to reassure them. Delusions of guilt about wrongdoing in the past may have a core of reality yet be wildly exaggerated. Such distortions can put the patient at serious risk for suicide.

In evaluating an older patient who appears depressed, you must take care to distinguish depression from grief reactions. A normal grief reaction following the loss of a loved one may last up to 12 months and is characterized by many of the classic vegetative symptoms noted above. Often, such reactions resolve over time with support from others and particularly when the grieving person has the opportunity to mourn the loss by talking with others. However, if the grief reaction is severe and incapacitating, pharmacotherapy and/or psychotherapy may be necessary even before 12 months have passed.

Similarly, your differential diagnosis of depression in an elderly patient must include systemic diseases, central nervous system disorders, and medication reactions. Medical illnesses such as secondary carcinoma of the brain, hyperthyroidism, pernicious anemia, heavy-metal poisoning, and carcinoma of the head of the pancreas may present first with symptoms that look like depression. Among the medications that can cause depression in people of all ages are benzodiazepines, barbiturates, digitalis, L-dopa, antihypertensives, and anticonvulsants. Because the elderly are more likely than younger people to suffer from medical illness and to be taking multiple medications, these causes of depression are more common in the geriatric population.

Epidemiology. Until recent epidemiologic studies showed otherwise, it was assumed that depression was more common among the elderly than among younger adults. This was in part due to the fact that suicide is more common among the elderly. Also, the prevalence of depressive disorders (including major depression, atypical depression, and dysthymia) is approximately 15% of the general population over 65. However, the Epidemiologic Catchment Area (ECA) Study has determined that clinical depression is actually *less* common among the elderly than among younger adults. Major depressive episodes account for a large proportion of inpatient admissions among the elderly, while atypical and masked depressions are more common in outpatient settings.

Etiology. The causes of depression in the elderly are almost certainly multiple and involve both psychosocial and neurochemical factors. Life events such as the death of a loved one or physical illness and disability often precede the onset of depression. Social isolation, and in particular the absence of a confiding relationship with another person, seem to render elderly people less able to weather negative life events.

Neurochemical factors in the genesis of depression remain the subject of intense research interest. In the aging brain, monoamine oxidase activity increases, resulting in increased degradation of biogenic amines. Moreover, tyrosine hydroxylase activity decreases, reducing the rate at which biogenic amines are produced. The relationship between depression and lowered biogenic amine concentration at synapses is as yet only hypothetical but provides the rationale for the use of medications that affect the concentration of these substances in treating depressive disorders in older patients.

Treatment. Somatic therapies for depressed geriatric patients are the same as those available to younger people. The indications for their use are also similar—namely, in cases where the syndrome is incapacitating, where there are neurovegetative signs, where psychosis or suicidal ideation is present, and where the depressive episode does not appear to be a short-lived reaction to life events. In cases of masked depression, the target symptoms you treat will not be "depressive," but rather cognitive problems of dementia or somatic complaints such as back pain or headache. The elderly are more sensitive to side effects and are at risk for more of the medication complications of somatic therapies, so they must be more carefully evaluated and monitored when these therapies are used. The following discussion of medications and electroconvulsive therapy (ECT) is not meant to stand alone, but rather it is intended to supplement the discussions found in Chapter 6 (mood disorders) and Chapter 18 (somatic therapies) with information specifically relevant to geriatric patients.

Antidepressant medications are the mainstay of somatic therapy for depression in adults of all ages. The cyclic antidepressants, trazodone, and monoamine oxidase inhibitors (MAOIs) are all equally effective, and there are no clinical predictors of patient response that can help you decide which medication to use. Therefore, your decision will be based on side effects—those that will be best tolerated by your patient and may even be desirable, and others that must be avoided. The most common serious side effects of antidepressants are 1) orthostatic hypotension, 2) cardiac arrhythmias, and 3) anticholinergic effects. Orthostatic hypotension can be dangerous to older patients who are prone to falls and serious sequelae such as subdural hematomas and hip fractures. Ventricular arrhythmias and complete heart block are especially likely in elderly patients with preexisting arrhythmias who are given tricyclic antidepressants, as these medications exert quinidine-like effects on the heart. The secondary (demethylated) amines desipramine and nortriptyline appear to be the least cardiotoxic of the cyclic antidepressants. MAOIs, while not cardiotoxic, cause orthostatic hypotension.

Anticholinergic side effects are common with antidepressant medications. Dry mouth can cause dentures to become ill-fitted and make it more difficult for elderly patients to eat and speak. Constipation may be severe enough that patients stop taking their medication. Urinary retention is a problem in elderly men with enlarged prostates, and can predispose older patients to bladder and kidney infections. Geriatric patients are also prone to develop central anticholinergic delirium, which includes disorientation, hallucinations, restlessness, and agitation. Any patient who becomes delirious on antidepressants should be taken off the medication until the anticholinergic effects have cleared. The medication can then be restarted at a lower dose.

Sedation is a common side effect of antidepressants. This may be troubling to some elderly patients, whereas it may be helpful to agitated patients who are anxious or unable to sleep. Doxepin and amitriptyline are among the more sedating cyclic antidepressants and cause anticholinergic side effects. Among older patients, desipramine and nortriptyline are probably the best tolerated of the cyclic antidepressants. Trazodone is very sedating, but it has no anticholinergic activity. Phenelzine is mildly sedating, while tranylcypromine has activating effects (see Chapter 18), and both of these MAOIs have mild anticholinergic activity.

When prescribing antidepressants, start with a lower dosage than you would in younger adults (e.g., 10 to 20 mg per day of desipramine or nortriptyline) and increase the dosage slowly by small increments (e.g., by 10 mg per day every 5 days). In addition to the screening measures outlined in Chapter 18 for antidepressant treatment, you must monitor elderly patients for signs of cardiotoxicity with a pretreatment electrocardiogram (ECG) and subsequent periodic ECGs over the course of treatment. Similarly, monitor the patient's blood pressure by taking it both seated and standing before the medication is begun and after each dosage increase, looking for dramatic drops in pressure that might predispose patients to falls.

Electroconvulsive therapy is probably the safest, most effective, and fastest-acting treatment for severely depressed elderly patients. Particularly for patients who are suicidal, delusional, or so unable to care for themselves that their physical health is in jeopardy, ECT is often the treatment of choice in that it can produce rapid and dramatic improvement. Treatments are usually carried out on an inpatient basis, three times per week. Most elderly patients respond at least partially after three to six treatments, and they are then given an equal number of further treatments to complete the course. Patients with recurrent depressive episodes may be less likely to relapse if ECT is followed by maintenance on an antidepressant or lithium. (ECT is discussed in greater detail in Chapter 18.)

Psychotherapy is widely used in the treatment of depression in the elderly, either as an adjunct to somatic therapies or alone. For those older individuals who are mentally intact and amenable to psychotherapy, the techniques are the same as those used in younger patients. Exploratory therapy can help patients to explore the origins of unrealistic guilt and self-condemnation, and to understand their reactions to losses and other interpersonal stresses. Contrary to popular myth, older individuals are capable of insight that leads to growth, just as are younger people. Cognitive therapy can help patients uncover and correct distorted thinking that accompanies depression. Supportive techniques are quite commonly useful, especially for elderly people who have multiple physical and social problems. The therapist may be directive and explanatory, helping patients to deal with family and social situations and to develop practical solutions to problems resulting from cognitive impairment. Most important, psychotherapy can provide a warm and supportive relationship for older people who have lost or never had such relationships. Therapy may be complicated by the therapist's countertransference feelings about parents, about nurturing an older person, and about growing old. (For more information about psychotherapeutic techniques, see Chapter 17.)

Mania

Mania is much less common than depression in the elderly, and first manic episodes generally occur before the age of 65. (Bipolar disorder is discussed at length in Chapter 6.) However, on rare occasions, mania does occur for the first time in elderly patients, most of whom have histories of depressive episodes earlier in their lives. Mania certainly can recur in old age among people who have had previous manic episodes. The typical picture of elated mood, hyperactivity, decreased sleep, and flight of ideas may be as florid in the manic 80-year-old as it was when he or she was 20. Other elderly people present with atypical manic symptoms, including confusion, irritability, affective lability, increased paranoia, and mixed depression and elation. As in younger people, mania may be precipitated by antidepressant treatment in older adults.

Treatment. Treatment of acute mania commonly involves the use of neuroleptics and lithium or carbamazepine. ECT may also be useful in treatment of acute mania when patients do not respond to medication. Maintenance treatment with lithium or carbamazepine may help prevent further manic episodes. (Carbamazepine has been shown to be safe and effective for manic patients who do not respond to lithium, but it has not been systematically studied in the elderly.)

Lithium must be administered with caution in patients who have preexisting cognitive impairment, or cardiac or renal disease. Careful pretreatment screening is important and is outlined in Chapter 18. Lithium dosages must be considerably lower in the elderly than in younger people. This is because the elimination half-life of the medication is prolonged because of the decreasing glomerular filtration rate that is part of the normal process of aging. Start with a dose of 150 mg per day or less, increasing as tolerated to reach a blood level of 0.4 to 0.8 meq/l. Note that this is considerably lower than the level of 0.8 to 1.2 meq/l that is desirable in younger patients. In acute mania, some elderly patients may require lithium levels as high as 1.3 meq/l. The side effects of lithium are described in Chapter 18. However, older patients differ from younger ones in that the first signs of lithium toxicity in the elderly may be confusion, disorientation, and memory impairment. Thus, it is easy to confuse lithium toxicity with mania in the elderly.

A Word About Suicide

While suicide may be associated with a variety of mental states, it is often a complication of mood disorders, and so it is mentioned here. The rate of completed suicides increases with age for white men. While the suicide rate peaks at age 50 for white women and at 30 for blacks of both sexes, the high rate for elderly white men brings the rate for the entire population over 65 above that for any other age group. People over 65 constitute 11% of the population but account for 17% of all reported suicides. Suicide ranks among the top 10 causes of death in this age group.

Why the higher rate for elderly white men? The answer is not clear. Depression is actually less common in this group than among older women and younger adults. We do know that older men use more lethal means than younger people, such as shooting, hanging, or drowning, so the ratio of completions to attempts is higher in this population. Factors that put older people at increased risk of suicide are the same as for younger adults: living alone, failing health, alcoholism, and a history of previous suicide attempts. It is important to explore the possibility of suicide with all elderly patients. Do not assume that "frail" elderly people lack the wherewithal to put suicidal thoughts into action.

Anxiety Disorder

Anxiety is a fact of life, and as we age, realistic sources of anxiety often increase. Older people may be worried about problems with children and grandchildren, about failing health, about the impending loss of a spouse or friend, or about financial matters. Because the elderly often have fewer resources with which to adapt to changing circumstances in their lives, they may be more prone to situational anxiety than younger people. Often, you can manage anxiety that is based largely in real-world problems with support, encouragement, and practical assistance, rather than with specific psychiatric treatments.

Anxiety is classified as a disorder when it seriously interferes with daily functioning or a reasonable level of emotional comfort. Like younger people, the elderly are susceptible to generalized anxiety disorder, phobias, and panic disorder. The prevalence of anxiety disorders in the general population of people over 65 is about 10% for women and 5% for men.

Because they are more susceptible to physical ailments, the elderly are more likely to have accompanying physical illness when they present with anxiety. This can result in two very different problems: 1) it is easy to overlook physical illness when an elderly patient presents with classic symptoms of an anxiety disorder; and 2) if you find underlying physical illness, it is common to treat only the somatic problem and to neglect a concurrent anxiety disorder in an elderly person. When you evaluate an older patient whose chief complaint is anxiety, be alert to the possibility of underlying physical illness, but also be aware that physical illness and an anxiety disorder may coexist. A list of common physical conditions that are often accompanied by anxiety can be found in Table 8-1 (see Chapter 8).

Anxiety may accompany other psychiatric disorders as well, and you must include these in your differential diagnosis. Depressive disorders may present with anxiety, but will also include typical or atypical symptoms of depression. Anxiety usually resolves when the depression is treated appropriately with antidepressant medications or ECT. Schizophrenia and delusional disorder can also present with anxiety, but will be characterized by paranoia or other cardinal features (see the discussion of delusional disorder above). Antipsychotic medication will relieve both the primary symptoms and the secondary anxiety associated with these disorders. Finally, dementia and delirium may be associated with anxiety. Demented patients often improve with low doses of antipsychotic medication (but can become more confused on benzodiazepines), and delirium requires a workup for an organic cause (see below).

Once you have ruled out physical illness and other primary psychiatric disorders, you are in a position to think about treatment. The treatments for panic disorder, phobias, and generalized anxiety disorder in the elderly are essentially the same as those used in treating younger patients (see Chapter 8). Cognitive-behavior therapy, psychotherapy, and medication are all used effectively in treating anxiety disorders.

Benzodiazepines are effective in the short-term management of severe anxiety in the elderly. However, older patients are more sensitive to the effects and side effects of these medications. Elderly people are more likely to have reduced plasma protein levels, and because benzodiazepines bind extensively to plasma proteins, such patients will have higher levels of unbound drug on any given dose of medication. Hepatic metabolism decreases with age, and benzodiazepines with active metabolites (diazepam, chlordiazepoxide, flurazepam) will take longer to be eliminated by elderly patients. Liver disease can further compound this problem. This means that older patients are more likely to have unwanted and prolonged sedation, impaired motor coordination, confusion, disorientation, and apathy as a result of benzodiazepine use.

In choosing a benzodiazepine, it is therefore important to use the lowest dose that provides adequate relief, to watch carefully for subtle signs of toxicity, and to choose a medication based on the patient's particular needs and state of physical health. Long-acting benzodiazepines (e.g., diazepam or chlordiazepoxide) may be used in single daily doses to provide relief from anxiety throughout the day. They are less likely to cause withdrawal symptoms, but more likely to accumulate to undesirably high levels because of their prolonged elimination time. Short-acting benzodiazepines are often preferred in older patients because these agents are less likely to accumulate and cause toxic effects. However, prolonged use of these medications can result in tolerance, dependence, and withdrawal reactions. As a rule of thumb, consider low doses of short-acting benzodiazepines first, and limit their use to acute anxiety reactions whenever possible.

Insomnia. This is a frequent complaint among elderly people. As we age, we sleep fewer hours and have more interrupted sleep. Medications, physical illnesses, and anxiety can exacerbate this disruption. By age 75, one-third to one-half of elderly people complain of insomnia, and the typical elderly person lies awake one-fifth of the night. At age 90 people sleep an average of 6 hours per night, compared with 8 hours per night in young adults.

Sleeplessness is a common symptom of depression, and anyone presenting with this complaint must be evaluated for the presence of a mood disorder. It is important to treat any underlying mood disorder, physical condition, or substance use problem (e.g., alcohol or caffeine) that causes insomnia, rather than attempting to address the insomnia itself. But once possible underlying causes have been ruled out, you may consider using medication to relieve insomnia either on a short-term basis or intermittently when the problem is chronic. Benzodiazepines are the most widely used medications in the treatment of insomnia, and their use is discussed above and in Chapter 18. You might also consider a low-dose neuroleptic in a cognitively impaired or agitated patient who suffers from sleeplessness.

Dementia and Delirium

Dementia and delirium are conditions characterized by *global* intellectual impairment. People with these disorders commonly suffer from deficits in memory, in abstract thinking, in the ability to learn new tasks and solve problems, and in orientation to time, place, and person. These syndromes generally result from diffuse disease of the brain and consequent loss of function of large numbers of neurons.

Dementia, by contrast, is often called a *chronic organic brain syndrome*. Consciousness is not usually clouded in dementia until the end stages of the dementing process. The onset of dementia is usually insidious and the course is one of slow but persistent deterioration. The demented person is much less likely than the delirious person to manifest hallucinations or other signs of disordered thinking. The demented individual is not generally agitated or hyperactive; rather, motor activity is usually normal or slow.

Delirium is commonly referred to as an *acute organic brain syndrome*. It is characterized by a clouded state of consciousness, often with rapid onset, a fluctuating course, and short duration. In addition to diffuse intellectual deficits, the delirious person is likely to suffer from hallucinations, delusions, and increased motor activity (see Table 9-1).

Both dementia and delirium are included under the general diagnostic category of *organic brain syndromes*. But this term is not particularly useful, for it is nonspecific and conveys little information about the

Table 9-1. Comparison of dementia and delirium

Dementia	Delirium
"Chronic organic brain syndrome"	"Acute organic brain syndrome"
Consciousness unimpaired (until late in the course of disease)	Consciousness clouded
Normal level of arousal	Agitation or stupor
Develops insidiously over months or years	Develops rapidly
Often chronic, progressive	Often reversible
Common in nursing homes, psychiatric hospitals	Common on medical wards in general hospitals

conditions it is meant to describe. It is also somewhat misleading in that it implies that we can neatly separate disorders that have "organic" causes from other mental illnesses that are functional in origin. It makes more sense to refer to dementia and delirium, as well as other "organic" syndromes (such as those caused by drugs and alcohol), by their specific names.

Dementia and delirium are *not* diseases; they are conditions that can result from a large number of underlying organic processes affecting brain tissue. A vast array of underlying somatic illnesses can give rise to them. Stereotypically, delirium is reversible, whereas dementia is irreversible. However, there are remediable causes of both dementia and delirium, and you must diligently search for such treatable illnesses whenever someone presents to you with global cognitive deterioration.

You need not memorize all the possible organic causes of dementia and delirium, but it *is* important that you do the following:

- Learn to recognize the signs of dementia and delirium so that you will not overlook these syndromes.
- Be aware of possible underlying causes that are treatable.
- Understand the need for careful medical examination and laboratory workup of every patient who presents with altered cognitive functioning.
- Understand the course and treatment of those common syndromes that are not reversible.

Dementia

Dementia is defined as a deterioration in intellectual abilities that is of sufficient severity to interfere with social or occupational functioning.

The deficit involves many aspects of cognition, particularly memory and judgment. Higher cortical functions such as language, abstract reasoning, and the ability to follow directions are also commonly impaired. Although dementia is most common in the elderly, it is *not* synonymous with old age, nor is it a normal part of the aging process; rather, it implies diffuse disease of the brain that has impaired the functioning of large numbers of nerve cells in the cerebral cortex. The DSM-III-R criteria for the diagnosis of dementia are shown in Table 9-2.

Clinical picture. As noted above, dementia normally has an insidious onset, evolving over many months or even many years. It often begins with vague, nonspecific physical complaints, increased moodiness or irritability, and subtle withdrawal of interest from life. People often seem to be "not themselves," and their personalities appear to lose their sparkle. The early symptoms are so subtle that families often cannot identify any specific disorder and instead are likely to be hurt by the seemingly willful moodiness and emotional withdrawal of their loved one. Demented people begin to have trouble with any activity that requires new or original thought or learning. Dementia may thus be apparent earlier in those who are involved in more intense creative and intellectual endeavors.

Early memory loss may go unnoticed by the affected individual and his or her family. For example, demented people may begin to forget dates or telephone numbers but may compensate for this quite well by writing things down. They may forget instructions or directions and may need to ask that these be repeated several times before they can commit the information to memory. Some demented people notice such deficits in memory themselves, whereas others remain oblivious to them even when the deficits become obvious to family and friends. Demented people may even fabricate false details (*confabulation*) to fill in gaps in their memory. As the dementia progresses, demented individuals become increasingly distractible. They may, for example, begin tasks but forget to return to them after an interruption. People who live alone may forget to turn off the stove, and thereby put themselves in danger.

Demented people eventually begin to lose more skills, and their deficits become more obvious. They commonly become lost on their way to familiar places, and it is then that their condition may begin to seem more serious to those around them. Language initially remains unimpaired, but as other intellectual functions deteriorate, language usually begins to become more stereotyped and to convey less and less information. Demented individuals may perseverate in speech (i.e, repeat the same word or phrase over and over again), or they may continue to perform work, such as arranging chairs, long after the task has been completed. Although they normally become more quiet and socially

Table 9-2. DSM-III-R criteria for the diagnosis of dementia

Demonstrable evidence of impairment in short- and long-term memory. Impairment in short-term memory (inability to learn new information) may be indicated by inability to remember three objects after 5 minutes. Long-term memory impairment (inability to remember information that was known in the past) may be indicated by inability to remember past personal information (e.g., what happened yesterday, birthplace, occupation) or facts of common knowledge (e.g., past presidents, well-known dates).

At least one of the following:

1) Impairment in abstract thinking, as indicated by inability to find similarities and differences between related words, difficulty in defining words and concepts, and other similar tasks.
2) Impaired judgment, as indicated by inability to make reasonable plans to deal with interpersonal, family, and job-related problems and issues.
3) Other disturbances of higher cortical function, such as aphasia (disorder of language), apraxia (inability to carry out motor activities despite intact comprehension and motor function), agnosia (failure to recognize or identify objects despite intact sensory function), and "constructional difficulty" (e.g., inability to copy three-dimensional figures, assemble blocks, or arrange sticks in specific designs).
4) Personality change (i.e., alteration or accentuation of premorbid traits).

The disturbances described above significantly interfere with work or usual social activities or relationships with others.

Not occurring exclusively during the course of delirium.

Either one or the other of the following:

1) There is evidence from the history, physical examination, or laboratory tests of a specific organic factor (or factors) judged to be etiologically related to the disturbance.
2) In the absence of such evidence, an etiologic organic factor can be presumed if the disturbance cannot be accounted for by any nonorganic mental disorder (e.g., major depression accounting for cognitive impairment).

Criteria for severity of dementia:

Mild: Although work or social activities are significantly impaired, the capacity for independent living remains, with adequate personal hygiene and relatively intact judgment.

Moderate: Independent living is hazardous, and some degree of supervision is necessary.

Severe: Activities of daily living are so impaired that continual supervision is required—for example, unable to maintain minimal personal hygiene; largely incoherent or mute.

withdrawn, some demented people become more active in socially inappropriate ways, such as going on spending sprees or becoming physically assaultive.

When dementia becomes severe, people are unable to perform such simple tasks as feeding themselves, despite the fact that motor functions remain intact. They forget the names of friends, are unable to recognize even close relatives, and finally forget their own name and date of birth (although this information is usually the very last to be forgotten). They increasingly neglect their personal hygiene and begin to disregard normal rules of social conduct. More infantile behaviors such as incontinence and extreme emotional lability (fits of laughing and crying) may appear. Finally, many people become totally mute and unresponsive to the environment. At this stage, death often occurs within a few months, but people with end-stage dementia may linger on in this stage for several years.

Although dementia occurs most frequently in the elderly, the age at which it develops and the course it takes depend on the underlying cause. Demented people may remain unaware of and unconcerned by their growing deficits, or they may recognize them and react with anxiety, depression, or paranoia. When personality changes occur, they are usually exaggerations of preexisting character traits. (For example, a man who has always been somewhat suspicious by nature may become floridly paranoid as dementia progresses.) People with dementia sometimes develop hallucinations, delusions, hypochondriacal concerns, and even suicidal ideation as a result of such personality change and deterioration. All the symptoms of dementia can be exacerbated by stress, such as a move to unfamiliar surroundings, hospitalization, loss of a loved one, or concurrent medical illness. Dementia is not a lethal condition in and of itself, but the inability to care for oneself predisposes people to malnutrition, decubitus ulcers ("bed sores"), and pneumonia caused by inhalation of saliva, food, or stomach contents. (This type of pneumonia, called *aspiration pneumonia*, is the most common cause of death among patients with dementia.)

Irreversible causes. *Senile and presenile dementia (Alzheimer's disease)*, the most common form of dementia, accounts for roughly half of all cases. It is of unknown etiology and is associated with diffuse loss of brain tissue, specifically in the cerebral cortex. Clinicians have traditionally made a distinction between presenile and senile dementia, based on whether the disease began before or after age 65. While early onset cases tend to have a stronger genetic loading and pursue a more rapid and severe course, the disease is essentially the same whether the onset is at age 45 or 95. There is no apparent difference in neuropathology between early- and late-onset cases. The term *Alzheimer's disease* was once synonymous with presenile dementia, but you will now hear it used to describe dementia of unknown cause without reference to age of onset.

Alzheimer's disease usually begins after age 65, but it is seen as early as age 40. Estimates of the prevalence of Alzheimer's disease among those in the general population over age 65 range from 5% to 12%, and it is a leading (although often unreported) cause of death among the elderly. Most people who suffer from dementia live outside of institutions, although dementia is the most common reason for admission to a nursing home. Women develop Alzheimer's disease more frequently than men, but this is probably due to the fact that they live longer, and not to any predisposition to the illness. Men who survive to age 85 have a 1 in 3 chance of developing dementia in their lifetime.

The symptoms of Alzheimer's disease begin very gradually and progressively worsen, often over several years. At present, the disease process is irreversible. Afflicted individuals may live as long as 10 years after the onset of the disease, but they eventually require total care and succumb to secondary illnesses (e.g., aspiration pneumonia).

Physical findings are generally absent in Alzheimer's disease, or are present only in the end stages of the illness, when there may be changes in the person's reflexes on neurological examination (hyperactive deep tendon reflexes, positive Babinski reflexes, and snout, suck, and rooting reflexes—all signs of frontal-lobe release). People with Alzheimer's disease often have normal computed tomography (CT) scans of the brain, although these scans typically show some tissue loss in the cerebral cortex and enlargement of the cerebral ventricles, particularly if the disease is far advanced. Electroencephalographic, or brain wave, abnormalities are present in about 80% of patients (usually diffuse slowing and decreased alpha rhythm), but these changes are not diagnostic. Positron-emission tomography of Alzheimer's patients shows a substantial generalized decline in oxygen in the cerebral hemispheres and a decline in glucose utilization as the disease progresses. However, the significance of these findings is not yet clear. *There are no diagnostic laboratory studies; the clinical diagnosis of Alzheimer's disease is made only when the history, physical examination, and laboratory workup have ruled out other causes of dementia.*

At autopsy, people with Alzheimer's disease have characteristic changes in brain tissue that include the following:

- Senile plaques—microscopic abnormalities of the cerebral cortex, consisting of nerve cells tangled around a core of protein material called "amyloid."
- Neurofibrillary tangles—filaments tangled inside nerve cells throughout the cortex of the brain.

- Granulovacuolar degeneration of nerve cell bodies—under the microscope, brain cells appear to have "holes" in them.

Such changes occur in normal aging brains, but much less extensively than they do in the brains of people with dementia.

Despite recent intensive research into the causes and treatment of this devastating and common illness, its etiology remains a mystery. Several hypotheses about the cause of Alzheimer's disease have received a great deal of attention. In particular, investigators at autopsy have found aluminum in the neurofibrillary tangles and neuritic (senile) plaques of patients with Alzheimer's, and the level of silicon is elevated in the brains of these patients as well. The significance of these observations is as yet unclear. Research into a possible viral etiology (particularly a slow virus) has not yielded any conclusive results to date. Finally, researchers have found a 40% to 90% decrease in the enzyme choline acetyltransferase in the cerebral cortex and hippocampus of Alzheimer's patients. There is hope that a cholinomimetic compound could be developed that would help preserve memory function in Alzheimer's patients if the disease were caught in its early stages.

Pick's disease is similar to Alzheimer's in its clinical manifestations and pathology, but does not involve changes in the parietal lobes of the brain. Because this incurable familial disorder is rare and almost impossible to differentiate clinically from Alzheimer's, it need not be discussed in detail here.

Cerebrovascular dementia, or "hardening of the arteries" in the brain, was once thought to be responsible for most cases of dementia. Alzheimer's disease has since been recognized as the major dementing illness in the elderly, but cerebrovascular disease is thought to account for a significant number of cases as well (perhaps 15% to 25%).

Atherosclerosis, or "hardening" of blood vessel walls by the accumulation of fatty deposits, does not, in and of itself, result in dementia. Rather, it predisposes people to brain damage from *blood clots*, which block arteries and thereby starve brain tissue of oxygen; and from *hemorrhage*, or bleeding into brain tissue resulting in tissue death. In fact, it appears that multiple small clots and hemorrhages in brain tissue produce dementia, and the condition often has a fluctuating, "stuttering" course with stepwise deterioration in functioning (see Table 9-3). People with this disease commonly have high blood pressure or diabetes, two conditions that predispose people to atherosclerosis. Some people give a history of several strokes in the past, but many have had "silent" strokes and have no awareness of discrete episodes of neurological illness. There are usually specific neurological signs (e.g., weakness of one limb). In

Table 9-3. Differential diagnosis of cerebrovascular dementia vs. Alzheimer's disease

Cerebrovascular dementia	Alzheimer's disease
Sudden onset	Insidious onset
Stepwise deterioration	Gradual deterioration
Preservation of isolated functions	Global intellectual impairment
Focal neurological signs	Absence of focal signs
History of hypertension, diabetes	No characteristic history of systemic
History of stroke(s)	illness

some cases, cerebrovascular disease and Alzheimer's coexist, and both contribute to the picture of dementia.

Although atherosclerosis in major arteries (e.g., narrowing of the internal carotid artery) may be surgically correctable, much atherosclerosis occurs diffusely among smaller vessels and is therefore not treatable with surgery. High blood pressure can be controlled in most cases, and early treatment of hypertension in people who have no symptoms of dementia can help to prevent or arrest the development of cerebrovascular dementia. People who have had or are at risk for strokes may benefit from the administration of anticoagulants or aspirin, which may prevent abnormal formation of blood clots.

Treatable causes. *Tumors.* Most brain tumors cause specific neurological signs (e.g., weakness on one side of the body), and their diagnosis is therefore not likely to be confused with that of Alzheimer's disease. However, depending on their anatomical location, tumors may initially present with psychiatric symptoms and no other obvious disturbances, and so may be mistaken for signs of "senility." The most common forms of brain tumors are gliomas (which constitute 30% to 50% of all brain tumors), meningiomas (20%), and secondary metastases (20%), most often from lung or breast cancer or malignant melanomas. Tumors of the frontal lobe, thalamus, and corpus callosum, as well as olfactory groove meningiomas, are particularly likely to present with psychiatric symptoms but no neurological findings. Thus, it is generally recommended that every person with dementia (indeed, everyone who has undergone a major personality change) have a CT scan of the brain to rule out a tumor. Obviously, how treatable tumors are depends largely on the location of the tumor and whether it is malignant or benign, but in some cases intellectual impairment can be completely reversed by successful surgical intervention.

Brain trauma. Trauma to any part of the nervous system usually results in maximal impairment immediately after the event. Victims of brain injury continue to recover lost function for up to 1 year. Such obvious cases of trauma are not generally mistaken for Alzheimer's disease or other forms of primary dementia. However, *chronic subdural hematoma* is easy to confuse with Alzheimer's, and the consequences of failing to recognize this life-threatening problem may be disastrous.

Subdural hematoma denotes a collection of blood that is outside the brain but within the skull. It often results from head trauma, but, particularly in elderly people, the trauma may be minor or not recalled at all. When blood collects slowly and puts gradually increasing pressure on the brain, the person may become demented over days or even weeks without specific neurological signs or impaired consciousness. A CT scan will generally reveal these masses of blood (which are often on both sides of the head). Surgical evacuation of the hematoma may be life-saving and will frequently reverse the intellectual impairment.

Normal-pressure hydrocephalus (NPH). A small subgroup of people who present with dementia have been found to have hydrocephalus (excessive accumulation of cerebrospinal fluid [CSF] that enlarges the ventricles of the brain) with normal CSF pressure. The flow of CSF from the ventricles to its usual site of absorption in the subarachnoid space surrounding the cerebral cortex is somehow obstructed, so that fluid collects within the ventricles and causes the characteristic syndrome of *dementia, gait apraxia,* and *urinary incontinence.* (Gait apraxia is a particular type of abnormality of locomotion in which the person has normal strength and coordination, but literally loses the intellectual ability to organize the act of walking, and therefore has difficulty in lifting each foot in succession.)

Although some people with NPH have a history of meningitis, subarachnoid hemorrhage, or trauma that might account for the obstruction of the normal flow of CSF, in many cases there is no apparent cause for this abnormality. The syndrome develops gradually, often over 6 to 12 months. A CT scan reveals dilated ventricles, out of proportion to the degree of loss of brain tissue.

Treatment is surgical: a shunt allows CSF to flow from the cerebral ventricles to another body cavity, such as the abdominal cavity. In cases that are accurately diagnosed, this procedure can result in dramatic improvement in symptoms. However, in some cases no improvement ensues—perhaps because of misdiagnosis—and the shunt procedure has many complications. Although NPH occurs infrequently, it must be considered in the differential diagnosis of dementia because it is potentially treatable.

Dementia secondary to systemic illness. As noted above, a great many systemic illnesses—including metabolic disturbances, infections, and exposure to toxins—can present with gradual intellectual deterioration. These conditions run the gamut from porphyria to pellagra, from lead poisoning to tuberculous meningitis. It is therefore critical that each demented patient be carefully screened for these disorders so that you will not overlook treatable causes of dementia. These illnesses are well described in general medical texts. Table 9-4 lists some of the most common diseases that may present with dementia.

Table 9-4. Some diseases that may present with dementia

Metabolic disorders
    Hepatic encephalopathy (liver failure)
    Wilson's disease
    Uremia (kidney failure)
    Hypoxia (congestive heart failure, anemia)

Deficiency diseases
    Wernicke-Korsakoff syndrome (thiamine)
    Pernicious anemia (vitamin B_{12}, folate)
    Pellagra (niacin)

Endocrine disorders
    Thyroid disease (hypothyroidism, thyroid storm)
    Hypercalcemia (parathyroid disorders)
    Cushing's disease
    Pancreatic disease (diabetic ketoacidosis, hypoglycemia)

Toxins (exogenous)
    Drugs of abuse: amphetamines, cocaine, alcohol, LSD
    Prescription drugs: bromides, steroids, reserpine, methyldopa, L-dopa,
        propranolol, scopolamine, atropine
    Industrial toxins: lead, mercury, manganese, carbon monoxide, organic
        solvents

Infections
    Chronic meningitis (tuberculosis, cryptococcosis)
    Viral meningitis
    Syphilis (tertiary lues)
    Creutzfeld-Jakob disease (slow virus)

Neurologic diseases (often accompanied by movement disorders)
    Huntington's chorea
    Parkinson's disease
    Spino-cerebellar degeneration

Neoplasms

Dementia syndrome of depression (pseudodementia). Despite the implication of its name, this condition is a true dementia, but it is due to a functional psychiatric disorder depression. When dementia is seen in elderly people, it is assumed to be due to Alzheimer's disease. In fact, many older people who present with a deterioration in personality, retardation of thought and action, apathy, disorientation, sleep disturbance, and global loss of intellectual functions are not demented, but depressed.

It may be impossible to differentiate depression from dementia on the basis of clinical findings, but if you take a careful history from family or close friends, you are likely to find that people with dementia syndrome of depression (DSD) have not deteriorated over many months or years, but have been "demented" for only a few weeks. Moreover, you are likely to see that this deterioration is associated with feelings of sadness. Be particularly alert to DSD in anyone with a family history of depression or manic-depressive illness. Points in the differential diagnosis of DSD and dementia are summarized in Table 9-5.

Differentiating between dementia and depression is extremely difficult, because demented people who recognize their growing deficits may react with depression, and depressed people may also have mild dementia. The important point is that, whenever you suspect a depressive component to the illness, it is worth giving "demented" people a trial of antidepressant therapy or electroconvulsive therapy (ECT), for they may respond. In fact, some people who appear floridly demented recover all their lost mental abilities when the underlying depression is treated. If

Table 9-5. Differential diagnosis of dementia vs. dementia syndrome of depression (DSD)

Dementia	Dementia syndrome of depression
Insidious onset	Sudden onset
Slow progression	Rapid progression
Family history negative for affective illness	Family history positive for affective illness
Depressive symptoms absent or follow intellectual changes	Depressive symptoms present and precede intellectual changes
Patient is indifferent to or about deficits	Patient is concerned (even denies deficits)
Behavior is disoriented	Behavior is oriented
Treatment for depression relieves intellectual impairment	Treatment for depression does not affect intellectual impairment

DSD goes undetected, it may be fatal, because the person may lapse into total self-neglect or attempt suicide.

Interview and evaluation. Demented people are often brought to physicians by family members when they can no longer tolerate such symptoms as increased emotional outbursts, socially embarrassing or dangerous behavior, and suspiciousness. Demented people are less likely than delirious ones to be psychotic or to appear medically ill. They are often quite alert, neatly dressed, and socially appropriate when they meet you. Evidence of dementia in the course of conversation may be difficult to find and may only take the form of an apparent hesitancy in answering questions. People may cover their memory deficits by dismissing a question as unimportant (e.g., "I don't need to know the date any more since I retired") or by giving a tangential answer.

Only by performing a careful mental status examination (MSE) will you pick up early signs of dementia. People with dementia will have difficulty with tests of recent memory and so be unable to remember three unrelated objects (e.g., apple, bicycle, chair) several minutes after they are given the task. Their interpretations of proverbs will be concrete if their abstract thinking is impaired, and they will have difficulty naming objects, doing simple calculations, following directions, or copying geometric patterns.

If dementia is more advanced, signs of memory impairment, distractibility, and other cognitive difficulties will be readily apparent in conversation before you get to the MSE.

A word of caution in interviewing demented people: It is important to be particularly gentle in testing cognitive functioning. A person who is suddenly forced to confront his or her intellectual deficits during the interview may become acutely embarrassed, anxious, depressed, or agitated. Such "catastrophic reactions," as they are called, can sometimes be avoided if you proceed slowly, respectfully, and with tact in conducting an MSE.

Taking a history. As you do a general evaluation, keep the following in mind:

1. *Document the course of the illness.* When did problems first begin? What were the earliest changes noted? What intellectual functions seem to have deteriorated? Was deterioration rapid or slow, stepwise or gradual? Has the patient become unable to care for himself or herself, and in what ways?
2. *Note any accompanying symptoms of mental illness.* Have there been mood changes (depression, sadness, elation)? Has the patient shown signs of disordered thinking (e.g., hallucinations, paranoia)?

3. *Note accompanying physical symptoms.* Have there been vegetative signs (sleep disturbance, weight loss) or other signs of
systemic illness (e.g., fever)? Has the patient suffered from headaches, seizures, or paralysis? Has he or she begun to make any
involuntary movements?
4. *Take a medical history.* Note major medical or neurological
illnesses. Be sure to document any history of mental illness as
well (e.g., affective illness, psychotic episodes).
5. *Note all medications, drug use, and possible exposure to toxins
at home or work* (and their relationship to the onset of symptoms). Do not forget over-the-counter preparations.
6. *Obtain a careful family history.* Has anyone else in the family
been demented or suffered from other neurological disease? Is
there a family history of depression or mania?
7. *Pay attention to the patient's social supports.* How much can
the patient do for himself or herself? How much assistance is
required? Who is available to assist? Have the patient's support
systems been stressed beyond their limits, or can the patient
continue to receive adequate care at home if the condition is not
reversible?

The mental status examination. Take particular care in doing an
MSE on a person who presents with suspected dementia, for it is essential
that you document the nature and extent of the existing cognitive deficits. (The MSE is discussed at length in Chapter 4.)

In examining demented people, be sure to proceed gingerly, to minimize anxiety as you ask about intellectual impairment. Focus on cognitive functions, particularly the following:

- Orientation
- Memory—immediate, recent, and remote. (Be careful to test con-
centration as well, and note attention span.)
- Fund of information
- Calculations
- Abstraction
- Judgment
- Language—spontaneous speech, naming objects, reading and
writing

You might consider using a structured instrument such as the Mini-
Mental State Exam (a standardized set of MSE questions), which will give
you a more quantitative assessment of your patient's cognitive functioning. This can be useful both in grading the extent of the patient's cogni-

tive impairment and in monitoring change in cognitive function over time.

Physical examination. A physician should perform a thorough physical examination on every patient who presents with intellectual deterioration. This should include particular attention in the neurological examination to the following:

- Focal neurological signs (weakness, sensory loss)
- Papilledema (swelling and blurring of the borders of the optic disc)
- Frontal-lobe release signs (snout, suck, palmomental, and rooting reflexes)
- Hyperreflexia, Babinski reflexes

Laboratory studies. Basic laboratory studies should include the following:

- Urinalysis
- Chest X-ray
- Blood studies, including complete blood count (CBC) with differential, metabolic screening battery (e.g., electrolytes, glucose, blood urea nitrogen [BUN], creatinine, liver function tests, serum calcium), serological test for syphilis, thyroid function tests, serum B_{12}, and folate
- CT scan of the brain
- Electrocardiogram

Other studies that may be indicated on the basis of the patient's history and physical examination include the following:

- Lumbar puncture
- Toxic screen
- Arterial blood gases
- Electroencephalogram

Treatment of dementia. Treatment is likely to be most successful when there is an underlying remediable cause. Whether or not treatment will result in reversal of the cognitive deficits depends on the underlying illness, and on how far the illness has progressed before the initiation of therapy.

In more than three-quarters of all cases of dementia, no treatable cause exists, and therapy is designed to provide symptom relief and support. Such therapy can be remarkably effective in helping patients and their families deal with the stresses of dementing illness. Individual psychotherapy and family therapy can help clarify many of the problems the illness presents, and help patients and families find ways of dealing with this chronic debilitating illness. Intervention in the patient's environment may be necessary (e.g., arranging for home care by professionals or for care in a nursing home).

Drug treatment has been helpful in treating specific symptoms in many cases of progressive dementia. Depressive symptoms often respond to treatment with antidepressants (e.g., a tricyclic such as desipramine). Anxiety, insomnia, and agitation are commonly alleviated by minor tranquilizers (particularly the benzodiazepines), although these drugs may cause paradoxical agitation in some people. In cases of severe agitation and psychosis, antipsychotics (e.g., haloperidol) are often effective. Drug treatment in elderly patients must be undertaken with caution, for these patients generally require smaller doses than do younger adults, and are more prone to such side effects as postural hypotension (a drop in blood pressure that occurs with postural change). However, medication need not be avoided, for it can provide elderly patients with considerable relief from the symptoms that accompany the dementing process.

You may do the initial evaluation on an outpatient basis, but hospitalization often allows for a more thorough workup and enables you to monitor the patient more carefully if a trial of medication is indicated. The decision to hospitalize a patient who presents with dementia will depend on the severity of the condition, the social supports available to the patient, and whether serious systemic illness is suspected.

A word about aging. The notion that "senility," or dementia, is an inevitable part of the aging process pervades our youth-oriented culture. In reality, among more than 25 million Americans over the age of 65, only 1 to 2 million suffer from significant intellectual impairment. The overwhelming majority of the elderly care for themselves and live outside of institutions.

The majority of older people maintain their intellectual competence as they age, although the speed with which they perform mental functions (e.g., recalling names or dates) declines somewhat. While mild or "benign" impairment in memory is common among the elderly, this is easily compensated for by keeping notes and establishing routines. The notion that dementia is synonymous with old age is a myth. Dementia is a pathological state, *not* a part of the normal human life cycle.

Delirium

Delirium is a syndrome in which consciousness is clouded, the attention span is shortened, sensory misperception is common, and thinking is often disordered. Like dementia, delirium involves global cognitive deficits, but, in addition, there is a change in the person's level of arousal and marked disorientation. Delirious people often present to emergency rooms or on hospital wards with extreme agitation and disordered thinking, whereas demented people more often come to medical attention in less dramatic ways and hide their deficits rather well in the early stages of the condition.

Delirium develops over hours or days rather than over months or years. Sometimes the syndrome begins as a "quiet delirium" of insidious onset, with mild symptoms of sleeplessness, anxiety, depression, irritability, forgetfulness, nightmares, or incoherent speech. More severe delirious states often include florid hallucinations, rapid or slowed thoughts, severe agitation or stupor, extreme distractibility, and fits of uncontrollable crying or laughter. The DSM-III-R criteria for the diagnosis of delirium are shown in Table 9-6.

Underlying medical illness is almost always identifiable in cases of delirium. Illnesses that can produce delirium include virtually all of those listed as causes of dementia. Such acute medical conditions as infection, anemia, hypertensive encephalopathy, cerebral edema, and dehydration and fluid and electrolyte imbalance commonly cause delirium. The cumulative effects of hypnotics, sedatives, tranquilizers, antidepressants, diuretics, and over-the-counter remedies—especially in the presence of renal, hepatic, or cardiac disease—can result in clouding of consciousness as well as frank psychosis. In addition, mild organic brain disease lowers the threshold of tolerance for most medications. A long list of street drugs (see Appendix B) can cause this condition, not only through intoxication but also during withdrawal. Alcohol withdrawal resulting in delirium tremens is discussed in Chapter 14.

Delirium often occurs in hospitalized patients, particularly among patients in intensive care units. Alterations in sensory input are common in these settings: patients are exposed to noises of machines, to sounds of other patients, to unfamiliar lighting, and to the comings and goings of many staff. The elderly are more prone to develop delirium than are younger people. Nearly one-third of those over 65 who are hospitalized for any reason become delirious at some point during their stay. You are likely to encounter this on general medical wards, where older people often experience transient confusion at night. This phenomenon, referred to as "sundowning," is believed to be related to the combined effects of sleep medication, decreased stimulation by a reduced nighttime staff, anxiety or depression from loneliness, and faulty perception (often the result of impaired sensory organs).

In the past, almost all patients undergoing open-heart surgery with cardiac bypass became at least temporarily delirious sometime after they

Table 9-6. DSM-III-R criteria for the diagnosis of delirium

Reduced ability to maintain attention to external stimuli (e.g., questions must be repeated because attention wanders) and to appropriately shift attention to new external stimuli (e.g., perseverates answer to a previous question).

Disorganized thinking, as indicated by rambling, irrelevant, or incoherent speech.

At least *two* of the following:

1) Reduced level of consciousness—for example, difficulty keeping awake during examination.
2) Perceptual disturbances: misinterpretations, illusions, or hallucinations.
3) Disturbance of sleep-wake cycle with insomnia or daytime sleepiness.
4) Increased or decreased psychomotor activity.
5) Disorientation to time, place, or person.
6) Memory impairment—for example, inability to learn new material, such as the names of several unrelated objects after 5 minutes, or to remember past events, such as a history of the current episode of illness.

Clinical features develop over a short period of time (usually hours to days) and tend to fluctuate over the course of a day.

Either one or the other of the following:

1) Evidence from the history, physical examination, or laboratory tests of a specific organic factor (or factors) judged to be etiologically related to the disturbance.
2) In the absence of such evidence, an etiologic organic factor can be presumed if the disturbance cannot be accounted for by any nonorganic mental disorder —for example, manic episode accounting for agitation and sleep disturbance.

awakened from anesthesia. However, recent attention to medication and anesthesia, and improved electrolyte management, have reduced the incidence of this complication. Similar preventive measures with renal dialysis patients have decreased the frequency of delirium in this population as well.

The treatment of delirium usually involves discovering the underlying causes and remedying them. A thorough history is essential to your evaluation. Often this must be obtained from those who accompany the patient. Be sure to ask in detail about medications, including over-the-counter preparations, as these are common culprits. Careful physical examinations and MSEs are also part of the workup. You may learn a great deal about the patient's condition by simply observing at the bedside. Nurses' notes are often helpful in calling attention to subtle behavioral changes. Be careful to distinguish between a "troublesome" patient and a delirious one. Some patients who appear to become "cantankerous" or uncooperative for no reason are actually delirious and need medical attention.

If the cause of the condition is not obvious, laboratory studies (as noted for dementia above) are indicated and should include a toxic screen. An EEG, when it shows generalized slowing, is presumptive evidence of an organic brain syndrome and can be used serially to monitor changes in the patient's condition. Not all delirium is reversible, but a great many cases resolve completely when the acute medical condition is effectively treated.

Managing the delirious patient. You may encounter delirium in a wide variety of clinical situations (e.g., in a hospital, in a nursing home, or in an outpatient clinic). Regardless of the setting and the underlying cause of the syndrome, there are certain interventions that can help ease a delirious patient's agitation and disorientation:

1. *Establish structure for the patient.* Delirious people are confused and often combative. They may tend to wander from place to place, particularly in unfamiliar locales. Therefore, set clear physical boundaries for the patient so that he or she feels contained (e.g., in one particular room). Physical restraint may be necessary for safety with the patient who is combative, and may be a relief to the patient who feels out of control.

2. *Orient the patient to time, place, and person.* Disorientation can be quite frightening to delirious people. Introduce yourself and all other staff members by name and professional title, stating the purpose of your interaction with the patient. Address the patient by name and remind the patient of where he or she is, what day it is, and what time it is. Your repeated reminders to the patient of this information will, in and of itself, help him or her calm down.

3. *Control the patient's sensory input.* Disorientation can be made worse by too much or too little sensory input. The sights and sounds of a busy clinic or emergency room may overwhelm a distractible patient. Conversely, the silence and darkness of a hospital room at night may add to the confusion of a delirious person. Therefore, it is important to work with delirious people in relatively quiet, secluded places where there are a limited number of staff, but where there are constant visual and verbal reminders of time, place, and person.

4. *Stay with the acutely disoriented person at all times.* Someone should remain with the acutely delirious patient at all times to prevent the patient from harming self or others, from wandering off, or from becoming more disoriented and frightened.

5. *Present your treatment plans firmly and repeatedly.* Remind the patient of what you are doing and why. Enlist the help of accompanying family and friends in this endeavor.

A word of caution: Delirium may look like an acute episode of a functional psychosis (e.g., a schizophrenic or a manic episode). *Anyone who presents with an acute psychotic episode and no prior history of psychotic illness must have a thorough medical workup.* Otherwise, you may miss life-threatening and potentially treatable medical conditions that masquerade as mental disorders.

BIBLIOGRAPHY

Adams RD, Fischer CM, Hakin S, et al: Symptomatic occult hydrocephalus with "normal" cerebrospinal fluid pressure. N Engl J Med 273:117–126, 1965

Albert ML (ed): Clinical Neurology of Aging. New York, Oxford University Press, 1984

American Association of Retired Persons: A Profile of Older Americans. Washington, DC, American Association of Retired Persons, 1985

Berezin MA, Liptzin B, Salzman C: The elderly person, in The New Harvard Guide to Psychiatry. Edited by Nicholi AM Jr. Cambridge, MA, Harvard University Press, 1988, pp 665–680

Blazer DG, Bachar JR, Manton KG: Suicide in late life: review and commentary. J Am Geriatr Soc 34:519–525, 1986

Caine ED: Pseudodementia: current concepts and future directions. Arch Gen Psychiatry 38:1359–1364, 1981

Hoffman RS: Diagnostic errors in the evaluation of behavioral disorders. JAMA 248:964–967, 1982. (A survey of patients on medical and surgical wards who develop behavioral disturbances. Many of these are of organic etiology but are misdiagnosed as primary psychiatric disorders.)

Karlinsky H, Shulman KI: The clinical use of electroconvulsive therapy in old age. J Am Geriatr Soc 32:183, 1984

Katzman R: Alzheimer's disease. N Engl J Med 314:964–973, 1986. (A good review of recent thinking about the pathophysiology and possible etiologies of the disease.)

Kaufman DM: Clinical Neurology for Psychiatrists. New York, Grune & Stratton, 1981, pp 89–111. (A clear and highly readable textbook of neurological disorders, including a discussion of the neurological aspects of dementia.)

Lipowski ZJ: Organic brain syndromes: overview and classification, in Psychiatric Aspects of Neurologic Disease. Edited by Benson DF, Blumer D. New York, Grune & Stratton, 1975, pp 11–35

McAllister TW: Overview: pseudodementia. Am J Psychiatry 140:528–533, 1983

Myers WA: Dynamic Therapy of the Older Patient. New York, Jason Aronson, 1985

Neugarten BL: Time, age, and the life cycle. Am J Psychiatry 136:887–894, 1979

Robins L, Holzer J, Weissman M, ct al: Lifetime prevalence of specific psychiatric disorders in three sites. Arch Gen Psychiatry 41:949–958, 1984

Vaillant GE: Adaptation to Life. Boston, MA, Little, Brown, 1977

Wells CE: Chronic brain disease: an overview. Am J Psychiatry 135:1–12, 1978

10

Children and Adolescents

THE IMPORTANCE OF DEVELOPMENT

Growth and change are an integral part of human existence. Each person is involved in a life-long process of development, and each of us continually attempts to master developmental tasks, whether we are 8 months or 80 years old. It is easy to forget the fact that development does not stop in adulthood, because change in adult life is less dramatic, less rapid, and more easily overlooked than change in the childhood years.

Child development proceeds with incredible speed. Consider, for example, the difference between a 3-month-old child who has just begun to laugh and roll over, and a 3-year-old who runs, pedals a tricycle, speaks in full sentences, and follows complicated verbal directions. Given the rapidity with which children change, mental health cannot be evaluated outside of the context of development. The child's physical, emotional, and intellectual capabilities are in constant flux, and with them, our expectations about what is normative and what constitutes pathology.

Behaviors that are the norm in one age group become worrisome when we see them in another. For example, the child who wets the bed repeatedly at age 3 years is not considered abnormal, but the 7-year-old who exhibits the same behavior is likely to be given a diagnosis. Separation anxiety and panic at mother's departure is normal in a 15-month-old, is more worrisome in an 8-year-old, and is considered to represent severe psychopathology in an adolescent.

Similarly, psychiatric symptoms that seem rather mild in one age group may be much more ominous in another. The well-trained 4-year-old who, during a stressful time, reverts back to bedwetting and soiling, is usually suffering from a mild reaction to disturbing events. However, the appearance of bedwetting and fecal incontinence in an adult is a troubling sign that often suggests severe mental illness (e.g., psychosis).

The clinician who works with children not only must understand what is normative for a child at a given age but also must look at the child's unique developmental pace and judge the presence and severity of symptoms against the child's own developmental standard. Growth does not occur along a single line. In fact, children develop intellectually, physically, emotionally, and socially at varying rates. The boy who is ahead of his peers in physical growth may be several months behind in cognitive development; the girl who is intellectually precocious may throw tantrums that are more common among children 2 years her junior. Moreover, development does not follow a straight path forward, but involves both progression and regression. For example, a toilet-trained 3-year-old may regress to bedwetting temporarily when a sibling is born, and such short-lived backsliding is expectable and normal.

Anna Freud (1965) is noted for her concept that each child grows along different developmental lines. She described six such lines of psychological development:

1. The move from total dependency on caregivers to participation in adult relationships.
2. The shift from suckling to rationally controlled eating.
3. The progression from wetting and soiling to bladder and bowel control.
4. The progression from lack of responsibility for care of one's own body to voluntary endorsement of principles of health and hygiene.
5. The shift from egocentricity to the capacity for companionship, sharing, and empathy.
6. The progression from play with one's own body to play with toys, to the capacity for work.

Many schemes of physical, intellectual, and emotional development have been devised by those who study children. The following are brief summaries of several of the most widely discussed developmental models. Each describes growth along a particular developmental line. While the table of motor milestones given below is fairly straightforward and noncontroversial, the schemes of psychological development included here represent particular views of individual theorists. They are not meant to be taken as "gospel," but are presented in order to familiarize you with concepts that you are likely to hear about in the course of your clinical work, and to give you a sense of the many variables that must be taken into account in assessing the mental health of children.

MOTOR AND BEHAVIORAL DEVELOPMENT

Table 10-1 contains a summary of normative behavior for infants and children at specific ages. These data are the result of empirical work by observers of child development. Remember that children do not grow according to any rigid timetable, so the information in this table consists of averages.

PSYCHOLOGICAL DEVELOPMENT

The following are three theories of how human beings develop psychosocially. These theories are not mutually exclusive, but, rather, are in many respects complementary schemes. Mahler's ideas about separation and individuation focus on the experience of infants and toddlers, while the developmental stages of Freud carry the child into adolescence, and Erikson's stages encompass birth through old age.

Mahler's Concept of Separation-Individuation

Margaret Mahler has made major contributions to our understanding of infant development. Her ideas are based on data she has gleaned from years of careful observation of infants and mothers in the nursery. She hypothesizes that each child goes through stages of separation and individuation from the mother or other primary caregiver, and that the way in which children negotiate these stages influences the development of personality traits such as the capacities for trust, empathy, and emotional stability in interpersonal relationships.

Normal symbiotic phase (age 0 to 5 months). The infant starts out in a state of total helplessness and lives in what Mahler has called a "symbiotic" relationship to the mother (or other primary caregiver). Mahler (1974) defines mother-infant symbiosis as the human infant's

Table 10-1. Normative motor and behavioral development

Age	Motor behavior	Learning and adaptive behavior	Language	Self-care and social behavior
Under 4 weeks	Makes alternating crawling movements Moves head to one side when placed in prone position	Responds to sound of rattle and bell Regards moving objects momentarily	Small, throaty, undifferentiated noises	Quiets when picked up
1 month	Can hold head erect for a few seconds	Shows no interest and drops objects immediately	Beginning vocalization such as cooing, gurgling	Regards faces Responds to speech
4 months	Holds head balanced Rolls over	Follows a slowly moving object visually Reaches for objects	Laughs aloud Sustained cooing and gurgling	Spontaneous social smile Begins to recognize familiar people
7 months	Sits steadily, leaning forward on hands	One-hand approach and grasp of toy Bangs and shakes rattle Transfers toys from hand to hand	Vocalizes "m-m-m" when crying Makes vowel sounds such as "ah"	Pats mirror image Expectantly awaits feeding
10 months	Sits alone with good coordination Pulls self to standing position	Attempts to imitate scribble	Says "da-da" or equivalent Responds to name	Responds to social play such as "pat-a-cake" and "peek-a-boo" Feeds self cracker and holds own bottle
1 year	Walks with one hand held Stands alone briefly		Uses one or two words Gives a toy on request	Cooperates in dressing

Age				
18 months	Walks unassisted, seldom falls Throws ball	Builds a tower of three or four cubes Scribbles spontaneously and imitates writing motion	Says 10 words, including own name Names a ball and carries out two directions with it—for example, "give to daddy," "put down"	Feeds self in part, spills Pulls toy on string Carries or hugs a special toy, such as a doll
2 years	Runs well, no falling Kicks large ball Goes up and down stairs alone	Builds a tower of six or seven cubes Imitates vertical and circular strokes	Uses three-word sentences Carries out four simple directions	Puts on simple clothing Refers to self by name
3 years	Rides tricycle Jumps Alternates feet going up stairs	Builds tower of 9 or 10 cubes Copies a circle and a cross	Gives sex and full name Uses plurals Describes what is happening in a picture book	Puts on shoes Unbottons buttons Feeds self well Understands taking turns
4 years	Walks down stairs, one step per tread Jumps over a rope Catches ball in arms	Copies a square Repeats four numbers Counts three objects with correct pointing	Names colors, at least one correctly Understands prepositions (e.g., "on," "under," "in,") and adjectives (e.g., "cold," "tired")	Washes and dries own face Plays cooperatively with other children
5 years	Skips, using feet alternately Usually has complete sphincter control Catches a bounced ball	Draws a recognizable man with a head, body, limbs Counts 10 objects accurately	Names the primary colors Names coins: pennies, nickels, dimes Asks meanings of words	Dresses and undresses Prints a few letters Plays competitive exercise games

Source. Reprinted, with permission, from Waldinger RJ: Fundamentals of Psychiatry. Washington, DC, American Psychiatric Press, 1986, pp. 222–223.

prolonged, absolute dependence on the mother that results from the infant's biological unpreparedness to maintain his or her life separately.

Differentiation (age 5 to 10 months). As the infant begins to be less physically tied to the mother (developing the ability to crawl), and as the sensory apparatus matures, the infant achieves a growing awareness of being separate from the mother. The infant begins to compare the familiar (mother) with the unfamiliar (other people), and in this phase "stranger anxiety" first appears.

Practicing (age 10 to 15 months). The infant uses increasing motor skills to practice leaving mother's side. The infant crawls and then walks away from mother but repeatedly comes back to her for "emotional refueling," to be reassured of her continued presence.

Rapprochement (age 15 to 22 months). The toddler's increasing motor and cognitive abilities prompt further recognition of separateness from the mother. This awareness becomes surprising and frightening, particularly in times of stress (e.g., when the toddler falls down and mother is not nearby to respond to the cry for help). The toddler struggles with the desire to be autonomous and the equally intense desire to have mother always available to magically fulfill the child's every wish. Thus, the toddler's behavior in this phase often alternates rapidly between rejecting mother and clinging to her.

Object constancy (age 2 years and beyond). The infant develops the ability to evoke a memory of mother's comforting presence even when she is not physically nearby. This allows the infant to comfortably leave the mother's side.

Mahler's work has been particularly important in thinking about older children and adults who show marked difficulty in forming stable, trusting relationships with others, and whose capacity to separate from important others is limited. It has been hypothesized that people with borderline personality disorder suffered severe disturbances in the mother-child relationship during the rapprochement subphase of the separation-individuation process. However, as with most psychiatric disorders, no prospective studies of development have been able to adequately operationalize these concepts to demonstrate a causal connection between such early developmental disturbances and subsequent manifestation of severe personality disorders.

Freud's Psychosexual Stages

Freud's scheme of psychosexual development (see Figure 10-1 for summary), which underlies so much of psychodynamic thinking, has been described in Chapter 2. It is based on a theory of sexual and aggressive

Age	Freud	Erikson
1	Oral	Trust vs. mistrust
2	Anal	Autonomy vs. shame/doubt
3	Phallic	
4	Oedipal	Initiative vs. guilt
5		
6	Latency	Industry vs. inferiority
7		
8		
9		
10		
11		
12	Adolescence	Identity vs. role confusion
13		
14		
15		
16		
17		
18		
Early Adulthood		Intimacy vs. isolation
Midlife		Generativity vs. self-absorption
Old Age		Integrity vs. despair

Figure 10-1. The developmental theories of Freud and Erikson.

drives, and it limits itself primarily to the influences of the nuclear family on the child's emotional growth.

Erikson's Developmental Tasks

Erik Erikson brought Freud's psychosexual stages out of the confines of the family and took into account the interaction between the child and the society in which he or she lives. Moreover, whereas Freud's psycho-sexual stages focus on pathology and follow the process of development only through puberty, Erikson's theories start with psychological health and the idea that the human personality continues to change and to be molded by the environment throughout life into old age.

Erikson focuses his attention on the ego (see Chapter 2) as the primary agent through which we organize perceptions, govern actions, and adapt to the environment. He writes that the ego is in a state of well-being when we live as we both wish to and feel we ought to. The pull between wishes (e.g., for instant gratification) and the internalized re-strictions of parents and society (what we "ought" to do) constantly forces the ego to negotiate between conflicting demands. The ego grows stronger when it can meet new life situations in such a way as to find creative and adaptive ways of bringing personal wishes and social expec-tations into harmony.

The following sections summarize Erikson's developmental stages.

Sensory-oral stage: trust versus mistrust (age 0 to 18 months). If the child's needs for care and sensory stimulation are met by the mother, the child develops basic trust in the self and the world. However, if the mother-child interaction is disturbed (e.g., if the child is deprived or unduly frustrated, or if care is inconsistently available), the child devel-ops a fundamental mistrust of the world and the sense that he or she will lose what is wanted or needed. Weaning can take place without great trauma to the child's sense of well-being if the child has developed the basic trust that his or her needs will be met.

Muscular-anal stage: autonomy versus shame and doubt (age 18 months to 3 years). As the child learns to develop control over more aspects of life, including bladder and sphincter muscles, the choice be-comes whether to keep or to let go. If parents allow the child to function with some autonomy around issues such as toilet training—if they are supportive without being overprotective or punitive—the child gains confidence in his or her autonomy by age 3, feeling the capacity to control the self and, to some extent, the environment. However, if the child is overrestrained and made to feel ashamed and foolish, he or she mistrusts his own rightness and becomes plagued by self-doubt.

Locomotor-genital stage: initiative versus guilt (age 3 to 6 years). The child's new-found capacities for locomotion and learning increase curiosity about the outside world. The child can now initiate physical and intellectual activity. The child's independent initiatives are reinforced if the environment allows for physical freedom and satisfaction of curiosity, but initiative is stifled when the child is made to feel bad about new behaviors and interests. The child begins to develop an intense interest in the parent of the opposite sex and may compete with the same-sex parent and siblings for affection. In forming the superego, parental values and societal values are gradually internalized as self-guidance. If the child incorporates rigid and punishing standards, initiative is inhibited and guilt predominates.

Latency stage: industry versus inferiority (age 6 to puberty). The child develops confidence in abilities to function in the adult world—to master physical tasks, to reason deductively, and to use intellectual skills in comprehending the world outside of the home. Peer relationships and school become important. Peers comprise a reference group in which the child can test ideas and behaviors, and competence relative to others takes on new importance. The child can become confident of his or her industriousness and capacity to function in the adult world, or if mastery is thwarted, he or she can come to feel inferior.

Puberty and adolescence: ego identity versus role confusion (teen years). In the struggle to develop a personal identity, the teenager falls in love with heroes, ideologies, and members of the opposite sex. The adolescent is "suspended between" the morality learned as a child and the ethics to be developed as an adult. In this confusion, adolescents cling to each other, and peer groups become of central importance. Teenagers must undergo further psychological separation from parents in order to prepare for intimate relationships with peers, and, as part of this process, children commonly "deidealize" parents who were once thought to be "perfect" or "heroes." Blos has described this period as the second separation-individuation phase of development (see Mahler 1974, p. 225).

Young adulthood: intimacy versus isolation (age 18 to 34). The young adult who has successfully weathered the identity crisis of adolescence emerges with a sense of self that is firm enough to make intimacy possible without the fear of losing one's own identity. Emotional and sexual closeness involves mutuality. The person who is not capable of sharing love and friendship in long-term relationships becomes self-indulgent and isolated.

Adulthood: generativity versus stagnation (age 35 to 60). During the middle years, adults choose between becoming involved in meaningful and socially useful tasks, and the stagnation of satisfying only personal needs or pursuing personal pleasures. Generativity refers not to bearing children, but to the investment of the self in an endeavor outside of the home; parents can stagnate, and people who have no children can be generative.

Maturity: ego integrity versus despair (age 60+). According to Erikson's schema, the person who, in old age, can look back on a life in which intimacy has been achieved and generativity expressed, feels a sense of satisfaction and ego integrity. By contrast, those who have never developed beyond narcissistic self-absorption look back in despair upon a life that has been lived to little purpose.

Figure 10-1 is a comparison of the developmental stages of Freud and Erikson. (Mahler's developmental schema ends at age 2 years.)

THE "NORMAL" CHILD AT VARIOUS STAGES OF DEVELOPMENT

What do children look like at various phases of development? The following are brief descriptions of what is considered normative. Keep in mind, however, that the "normal child" is a fictional character and that these descriptions are only meant to serve as crude guides to what is to be expected in healthy children.

Early Infancy (Birth to 4 Months)

The infant's main task during these early months is to adjust to extra-uterine life. The child is born with sucking and crying reflexes, and is programmed to respond positively to human stimuli. The infant at first only stares at the surroundings, but by the age of 4 months he or she can follow moving objects visually, reach for objects, and roll over. By age 3 to 4 months, the baby can smile when talked to, will babble and coo, and can respond to human sounds by turning the head and vocalizing socially. Interest in people is generalized; the baby does not differentiate among individuals.

The healthy baby copes well with the mechanics of life, including eating and sleeping. Bodily needs are urgent. The baby is totally dependent on caregivers and has a low tolerance for frustration. Over this period, the infant cries less, develops increasing periods of wakefulness, and responds to feeding and oral sensations, as well as to sound, light, and touch. The baby begins to develop trust in the caregiving adult and to respond expectantly to caregivers. Minor problems at this stage include feeding and digestive difficulties, sleep problems, and excessive crying or irritability. More extreme problems include an inability to be comforted when crying, extreme lethargy (often secondary to deprivation of care and affection), failure to gain weight, and infantile autism.

Infancy (Age 4 to 18 Months)

The infant must begin to differentiate himself or herself from the mother and to develop some degree of self-reliance and self-control (including self-feeding and self-soothing). This age range is a period of growing social attachment.

As the sensory organs mature, the baby begins to have coordinated movements, including binocular vision and hand-to-mouth coordination. Over this period, the baby learns to sit up, to crawl, and to pull up. Many children walk unassisted by age 10 to 14 months. Grasp becomes much more precise, and the baby can manipulate objects by age 10 months. Infants at this stage put any object they can find into their mouths.

Babbling resembles one-syllable words by age 6 months. At 10 months the infant can respond to his or her name and shows signs of understanding some words and simple commands. By 12 months, the child can usually say one or two words.

Socially, the baby begins to recognize familiar people and is more responsive to them than to strangers. During this period, playful reciprocal interactions between the infant and primary caregivers foster the development of a deep emotional bond.

The typical 7-month-old plays with toys and feet, and expectantly awaits feeding. By 10 months, the baby can play simple nursery games (peek-a-boo) and feed himself or herself a cracker. Self-feeding continues to improve over this period. The infant also learns to cooperate in dressing by age 12 months. He or she begins to have more patience (e.g., while a bottle is heated), develops "stranger anxiety" at 6 to 10 months, and has a strong selective tie to the mother. The infant demonstrates joy in play during this period and begins to show outbursts of negativism and anger.

Minor problems at this stage include excessive crying, anger, and irritability. Finicky eating and disturbed digestion and elimination are also common, as is sleep disturbance (failure to sleep through the night). More serious problems include tantrums, obsessive head-banging or rocking, extreme apathy and lack of interest in the environment, anorexia with failure to gain weight, lack of social discrimination or tie to the mother, and wariness of all adults.

Toddler (Age 18 to 36 Months)

The toddler's tasks during the second 18 months of life include further development of motor capacities, toilet training, differentiating the self from others and developing a secure sense of autonomy, tolerating separations from caregivers, beginning cooperative relationships with peers, and learning gender distinctions.

Maturation of the infant's nervous system allows the toddler to achieve sphincter control and to improve fine motor movements and gait. Children can climb stairs and run unsteadily by 2 years of age, and by 2½, they can jump and possess good hand and finger coordination. Speech includes a definite repertoire of words and marked increase in understanding (e.g, "no" and "come here") by 18 months. By 2 years, the child spontaneously puts together two-word phrases to communicate needs and wishes (e.g., "want mommy"). By 30 months, the toddler can make three-word sentences, understands most of what is said to him or her, and ceases babbling so that all speech has communicative intent. During toddlerhood, the child develops what Piaget calls *object constancy* (i.e., the capacity for mental representation of objects).

The toddler continues the process of separation-individuation (see discussion of Mahler above), so that the child's sense of individuality is consolidated around 24 months of age. The toddler may meet parents' efforts at toilet training and discipline with marked resistance and may throw temper tantrums when wishes and aims are frustrated by others.

Toddlers learn to play "in parallel" with other children (as opposed to engaging in truly cooperative play), and they usually play with great energy. They are constantly "on the go" and strongly resist any interference from others. They are very concerned about power and "who-bosses-whom," as is evident in their play. Toddlers show dependence on their caregivers and are anxious about separations from them. They also demonstrate marked ambivalence, showing extremes of love and anger toward those who care for them. They get pleasure from exercising their new motor skills. Masturbation is common among 3-year-olds, as are imaginary companions. By 3½, the child talks appropriately of self and others, and learns to take turns with others.

Minor problems in this age group include poor motor coordination, speech difficulties (e.g., stammering), timidity, night terrors, sleep disturbance, difficulty with toilet training, difficulty weaning, anxieties, temper tantrums, inability to leave mother without panic, lack of interest in other children, and temporary regression to more infantile manners (e.g., bedwetting). Major problems include extreme lethargy, uncommunicative speech or no speech, desparate clinging to mother, impulsive destructive behavior, lack of play, psychosis, and autism.

Preschool (Age 3 to 5 Years)

The preschool child learns to master internal impulses and social skills, as the focus of life begins to shift away from parents toward peers and life outside of the home. Motor coordination continues to be refined, so that by age 4 most children can catch a ball in their arms, jump over a rope, walk a line, and copy a square. Five-year-olds can balance on one foot and catch a bounced ball, while six-year-olds can tie a knot in a piece of string. Speech becomes almost entirely intelligible. By age 4, language is well established, including comprehension of adjectives (cold, tired) and prepositions (under, over).

The preschooler's relationships with parents change with the development of sexual feelings for the parent of the opposite sex. The child's close physical attachment to the opposite-sex parent is given up to some extent, and the same-sex parent is seen as both a rival and as someone to be emulated (see Chapter 2). Resentment of the same-sex parent is often displaced to less threatening people (e.g., siblings, teachers). Relationships with other children become more important than in previous periods, dependence on the mother lessens, and the child spends increasingly long periods of time in activities away from the mother. Separation anxiety is finally mastered to the extent that the child can attend school.

Preschoolers typically shift back and forth between aggressive and regressive behavior as they struggle with conflicting wishes to be dependent and independent. Little boys and girls often appear confident, but these bold fronts collapse easily, particularly in the face of perceived threats or criticisms. Play is physically active, and boys may have particularly violent and cruel fantasies incorporated into their play. Children are inquisitive and imaginative at this age and ask many questions (e.g., "Where do babies come from?"). Children commonly identify with and imitate parents, teachers, and peers in their behavior as they attempt to try on new roles (e.g., sex roles). Minor problems at this age include those listed above for toddlers. In addition, reluctance to go to school is common at this age but normally resolves quickly. Major problems are also similar to those encountered among toddlers, but, in addition, prolonged school phobia and school refusal indicate significant emotional distress (see discussion of school refusal below).

Latency (Age 6 to 10 Years)

The latency period, which encompasses the primary-school years until the onset of puberty, is marked by greater awareness of the world at large, increased importance of peer relationships, and the mastery of new physical and intellectual skills. This is the period that Erikson characterized as representing a crisis of industry versus inferiority, as the child's sense of self is increasingly bound up with his or her developing competence at physical, intellectual, and social tasks.

Maturation of the central nervous system allows the child to perform complex motor movements and more complex mental operations. Language is fully developed by this period.

Social relationships are characterized by same-sex groups and clubs. The child identifies strongly with the same-sex parent and turns to others (e.g., teachers) as role models. Parents are no longer seen as all-knowing or all-powerful, and the ideas and behavior of people outside the home take on new interest and importance for the latency-age child. Aggression is channeled into healthy competition at school and at play. Latency-age children are preoccupied with mastering sexual and aggressive impulses, and hence their play commonly involves games with an abundance of rules. Fair play is of paramount importance.

Children in this age group develop pride and self-confidence as they master new tasks, and become less dependent on their parents. They are very concerned with sex roles and strongly identify with children of the same sex. Peer interaction and organized play are very important, as is exploration of the environment (school, community, nature). Children achieve better control of their impulses during this period and are better able to channel their energies into learning.

Minor problems at this stage include anxiety and oversensitivity to new experiences (at school, with peers, around separations), learning difficulties, lying, and temper tantrums. Children are often afraid of illness or bodily injury, and somatic complaints (e.g., stomachaches) may be expressions of emotional distress, as in school phobia. More serious problems include social withdrawal, failure to learn, speech difficulties (especially stuttering), uncontrollable antisocial behavior (e.g., chronic bullying, lying, or stealing), or self-destructive behavior (frequent "accidents," self-mutilation, suicide attempts). Other serious problems encountered in this age group include obsessive-compulsive rituals (e.g., severe hand-washing), phobias, anorexia or severe obesity, complete absence or deterioration of peer relationships, and inability to distinguish fantasy from reality.

Adolescence (Age 11 to 18 Years)

The onset of puberty brings about dramatic physical, emotional, and intellectual changes. No longer a child and not yet an adult, the adolescent must negotiate the transition into adult life. This involves coping with body changes and markedly increased sexual drives, consolidating one's sexual and personal identity, and struggling for emancipation from the child's role in the family. This is a time when the teenager develops more collaborative peer relationships, begins heterosexual relationships, and prepares for major educational and occupational choices.

Puberty initiates adolescence. The physical changes of puberty almost always occur in the same sequence, but their onset, speed, and age of completion vary considerably from one person to another. For girls, the spurt in height may begin at age 9 or age 15, but on average starts at age 10½. Similarly, menarche begins anywhere from age 10 to age 16½, with average onset at age 12½. Breast development may start at age 8 or at age 18. The sequence of changes for girls is as follows: breast enlargement, appearance of straight pubic hair, growth spurt, appearance of kinky pubic hair, menarche, growth of axillary hair, and maturity of full reproductive function.

For boys, the developmental timetable may also vary greatly. Testes enlarge at anywhere from age 9½ to age 17, with the average onset at age 11½. Similarly, a boy's height spurt and penis enlargement may begin at age 10½ or 16½, but on average begins at age 12½. The sequence of pubertal changes for boys is as follows: growth of testes, appearance of straight pubic hair, penile enlargement, early voice changes, first ejaculation, appearance of kinky pubic hair, growth spurt, growth of axillary hair, marked voice changes, and beard development.

Physical development is not confined to sex characteristics and height. Musculature develops rapidly during this period—more for boys than for girls. Thus, for example, boys are on average twice as strong at age 16 as at age 12. Cognitively, adolescents develop the capacity to deal with abstract concepts such as moral values and political ideals.

This is an exciting and tumultuous time, in which the adolescent pushes more rapidly for independence from parents and becomes keenly interested in other adults as role models and "heroes." The adolescent's primary allegiance shifts from parents to peers, as peer group values and ideals take on a new importance. Peers help validate the adolescent's push for separation from home, and in negotiating this shift, the adolescent commonly engages in battles with authority figures. Aggression may be channeled into destructive rebellion against parental figures, or into more constructive means of achieving independence from parents and into healthy competitive activities (e.g., sports, academics).

In the struggle between the wish to satisfy new sexual urges and the wish to control them, adolescents often vacillate between hedonism and asceticism. Their capacity for self-observation and insight becomes much greater, and the adolescent begins to think about who he or she is in new ways.

Adolescents are often inconsistent, moody, and unpredictable. This is evident in work, at play, and in their relationships with peers and adults. They try on a variety of roles and experiment with themselves and the world. They are eager for peer acceptance and approval, as evidenced by clothing fads and hero worship. They can be highly critical of themselves and others (particularly parents), as they struggle to develop moral and ethical ideals. They are at once anxious about losing their parents' nurturance and eager to be independent of parental ties. Confusion and insecurity are often covered over by false bravado, particularly in early adolescence. Teenagers fall in and out of love rapidly, and constant experimentation in peer relationships helps the adolescent to form his or her own identity. In later adolescence, the hold of the peer group loosens, and the adolescent moves toward taking his or her place in adult society.

Minor (and common) problems seen in adolescence include the following: apprehensions, fears, and guilt about sex, health, peer relationships, and school; defiant, impulsive, and depressed behavior; frequent physical complaints; dysmenorrhea; sexual preoccupation; excessive masturbation; poor relationships with peers or adults; unwillingness to assume greater responsibility or autonomy; unresponsiveness to parental discipline; and experimentation with drugs or alcohol. Major problems include the following: complete social withdrawal, major depression, delinquency, phobias, persistent hypochondriasis, anorexia nervosa (see Chapter 14), the complete inability to function at school or work, suicide attempts, drug or alcohol abuse and/or addiction, and psychosis.

Factors Influencing Development

The above developmental schemes and descriptions attempt to describe a fictional creation known as the "normal child." In reality, each child's development is unique, because development is a constantly changing relationship between a highly particular set of variables within the child and another equally individual set of variables in the child's environment. Prenatal influences on the child's intrauterine growth, genetic endowment, and inborn temperament are but a few of the "constitutional" variables that each child brings to the world. Environmental variables include the temperaments and expectations of parents, the quality and quantity of caregiving the child receives, the socioeconomic group into which the child is born, life events, and the child's constellations of siblings. Biological and environmental variables influence each other reciprocally.

Psychopathology in children may be thought of in terms of failures in development. How is it possible to take so many variables into account in determining what has gone wrong in the growth of a particular child? It is easiest to think of the child's development in terms of systems, as follows.

Inborn characteristics. The child's inherited traits, including everything from intelligence to eye color, from shape of the nose to temperament, will affect the child's acceptance by parents and within various cultural groups. This, in turn, affects self-image and self-esteem. Inborn traits also affect the child's ability to adapt to the environment into which he or she is born. In recent years, work has been done on characterizing types of inborn temperament among newborn infants. Thomas, Chess, and Birch (1968; see also Thomas and Chess 1984) are among the most prominent researchers in the area of inborn temperament. They have looked at variables such as distractibility, activity level, persistence, and adaptability in newborns. Most newborns can be described as having particular temperaments, such as "easy," "slow-to-warm up," or "difficult." It is not so much the inborn characteristics of the infant that are crucial determinants of later development, as the "fit" between the temperament of the child and the temperaments and expectations of the parents.

Organic impairment. Children who are born with or acquire physical conditions that handicap their functioning will almost always have psychological reactions to such impairment, and the impairment (e.g., an obvious handicap) will elicit reactions from the environment. Consider, for example, the child with an attention deficit disorder, a condition with a neurological basis that involves difficulty paying attention to tasks. Such a child is often labeled "bad," "disruptive," or "stupid" by exasperated parents and teachers, and these labels have a profound effect on the child's sense of self. Learning disabilities, seizure disorders (epilepsy), and other conditions with neurological components may prompt the child to receive and process environmental stimuli abnormally, and there is a high correlation between such organic disorders and emotional and behavioral symptoms. Chronic ailments such as asthma, and physical deformities, affect the child's ability to function in and be accepted by the world, as well as the child's self-image.

Family environment. Freud was intensely concerned with each person's "family drama" as a means of understanding individual development. Indeed, family members are the center of the young child's world prior to his or her going to school, and in this respect an understanding of the child's home life is essential to any assessment of psychological distress. Caregiving by parents or others will have a profound influence on the child's development. Caregiving refers not only to whether the child is fed, clothed, and sheltered, but also to the provision of sensory stimulation and the creation and maintenance of an emotional bond between the primary caregiver and the child. Infants who are offered an adequate diet but deprived of love and affection commonly "fail to thrive," and may literally die because they are unable to grow and gain weight.

Parental expectations of the child and parental values play a formative role in all aspects of development. Because they are dependent on parents for physical survival, love, and protection, children both consciously and unconsciously pay close attention to parents' signals about what they expect and value. Even a process that seems "biologically programmed," such as the acquisition of motor skills, may be greatly enhanced or inhibited, depending on the parents' comfort with a child's physical assertiveness and initiatives in exploring the environment. Similarly, children may develop language skills precociously or late, depending on the extent to which their parents value verbal ability and how parents react to the child's attempts at verbal mastery.

Children develop some personality traits and suppress others based on what is reinforced by parents. For example, a little girl whose father sees her as dainty and ultrafeminine may suppress her wishes to engage in rough-and-tumble play with boys. A boy who is named after a much-loved grandfather may be subtly encouraged by parents to take on grandfather's traits (e.g., an "artistic temperament" and interests). While these influences occur in every parent-child relationship, the self-fulfilling prophecies that result can sometimes be quite destructive. Consider, for example, the father who was himself quite an impulsive adolescent and who "fears" that his son will grow up to be a "hoodlum." By treating his son with suspicion and taking an intense interest in any mild misbehavior, the father communicates to his son that he is not trustworthy, and also that father will be attentive and intensely interested whenever the boy misbehaves. Such a situation encourages a child to act out a parental wish of which the parent may be totally unaware. (For an excellent discussion of this process, see Johnson and Szurek 1952.) Families who need to see one member in a certain way (e.g., as the one with all the bad traits, or as the "little angel") may stereotype a child in an attempt to maintain some emotional balance within the family system. Such stereotyping usually has a stifling effect on a child, as it fosters the suppression of some aspects of the self and exaggerates others.

Relationships with siblings are of central importance to a child's development, although this is a somewhat neglected area of research. Children spend at least as much time with their siblings as they do with parents. Siblings vie with one another for parental time and attention, and it is generally with siblings that the child first learns to share and to compete. Older siblings may actually parent younger ones or may introduce younger children to the world outside of the family (e.g., school, peer relationships). Siblings can be important sources of learning as well as nurturing in a child's development.

Major life events. Both intellectually and emotionally, children have limited resources with which to cope with and make sense of major life events. Thus, changes such as the birth of a sibling, illness of the child, separation from or death of a parent, or even a move to a new neighborhood may affect the child more profoundly and adversely than the same events would affect an adult. For example, the birth of a sibling may be both exciting and troubling to a young child. A newborn infant demands total care, and so the child must compete with the new arrival for parents' time and attention. Prolonged separation from one or both parents can exert a profound effect on the child. Death, divorce, separation, or the illness of a parent leaves the young child both bereft of a parent and confused about why this event came about. Because young children make sense of the world in egocentric terms, they commonly blame themselves for traumatic life events (e.g., "If I had been a better boy, daddy would not have gone away"). When children are seriously ill and require hospitalization, the trauma of medical procedures, combined with periods of separation from parents, can profoundly disrupt the child's sense of well-being and his or her body image.

Peers and community. Children are strongly influenced by the communities, cultural groups, and economic groups into which they are born. This influence is mediated by the parents in the first years of life, but as the child reaches school age and spends much of each day outside of the home, the influence of the larger community becomes more direct. School functioning is of central importance in assessing any older (age 6 and up) child's state of psychological health. The child's occupation is as a student, and like an adult who is having problems at work, the school-age child's problems in school should be taken very seriously. School performance not only gives an indication of possible learning disabilities and cognitive deficits, but gives some indication of emotional health and social development, particularly as reflected in the child's relationships with teachers and peers. For this reason, it is essential that you obtain information from the school about every child whom you see for psychiatric assessment.

THE DIAGNOSTIC EVALUATION OF THE CHILD

If we think of mental illness in children as a failure of growth and development, or a loss of attained developmental steps, then an initial goal of a psychiatric assessment is to determine where the child should be developmentally and where he or she deviates from this. Making accurate and informative psychiatric diagnoses is even more difficult with children than it is with adults. There are several reasons for this. First, children develop so rapidly that symptoms may not remain stable over even a very short time, and diagnoses may change. Second, each child develops at a unique pace, and so what may seem like a developmental "failure" (e.g., a child who does not walk at 18 months of age) may in fact be a developmental lag that will be followed by a "catch-up" period of rapid development. Finally, the diagnostic systems used for children are imprecise and inadequately developed, although vigorous efforts continue to be made toward making our diagnostic nomenclature clearer and more precise. In particular, the section of DSM-III (1980) devoted to the psychiatric disorders of children represented an important attempt (continued in DSM-III-R) to base diagnostic categories on observable empirical phenomena.

How Do Children Come to the Attention of Mental Health Professionals?

Unlike adults, children rarely ask directly for mental health care. They will usually show the world that they are in distress through some aspect of their dealings with family and peers, or in their school behavior. Achenbach (1966) found that most children who come to the attention of mental health professionals can be grouped into three categories. These are listed in order of the frequency with which children in these categories are referred for treatment:

1. Undercontrolled children who are impulse-ridden, create behavioral disturbances, and act with undue aggression toward others.
2. Pathologically detached children who lack interest in things around them, seem confused and withdrawn, and/or manifest bizarre forms of thinking.
3. Overcontrolled children, who are inhibited, shy, and anxious.

Boys more commonly show their distress in undercontrolled ways, by acting on their environment (e.g., by throwing tantrums, behaving destructively), whereas girls more often manifest emotional difficulties by becoming more withdrawn or inhibited. Not surprisingly, undercontrolled children cause more distress to their parents than do overcontrolled children, so boys are referred for mental health care over girls by a ratio of nearly 4 to 1. In addition to parents, others who commonly request mental health care for children include siblings, teachers, pediatricians, and court officials. Adolescents are often referred by others as well, but they will sometimes seek help on their own initiative. In adolescence, when referrals occur based on self-report in addition to behavior, the referral pattern changes. More overcontrolled and depressed adolescents are seen, and more girls than boys are referred.

Children do not come alone to mental health facilities. They are usually accompanied by parents, guardians, or some other person who wishes the child to have treatment. A mental health assessment should involve family members as well as others who care for, observe, and work with the child. This means that multiple interviews are usually involved—interviews with the child, with the entire immediate family (when possible) to observe family interactions, with parents as a couple or individually, and with teachers or other professionals.

INTERVIEWING PARENTS

Parents are likely to approach you with some guilt, for they have invariably asked themselves, "What did we do wrong?" They will usually be concerned about what you think of them as people and as parents, and may be reluctant to expose "family secrets." You must try to enlist the parents as allies from the beginning, preferably by informing them of how the evaluation process works, of the way in which recommendations are likely to be made, and about ways that they can help you in your work.

You may want to interview the child's parents prior to your first meeting with the child so that you can get some sense of why the child has been brought to you and what the parents' concerns are. Your task during the evaluation is not only to gather information from the parents about the child's past and present life, but also to learn more about the parents—their personality styles, their own family backgrounds, and their ways of interacting with their child. These parental qualities are being internalized by the child during each period of development.

Taking a History

You can use the outline for a psychiatric history found in Chapter 3 to organize the information you gather about the child, for the basic data you need is essentially the same for children as it is for adults. However, you will want to pay special attention to the following areas in the child's life.

Developmental phases. Ask about phases of infancy and childhood in greater detail than you might in taking the history of an adult. Focus specifically on each of the major periods of childhood: prenatal events, birth history, infancy, toddlerhood, preschool, elementary school, puberty, and adolescence. Ask about the child's temperament at each stage, motor and intellectual milestones (see Table 10-1), as well as social and emotional development that would be appropriate for each stage (see discussion above).

Specific symptoms and behaviors. You may want to ask about the child's fears and inquire about the presence of tics, obsessions (e.g., handwashing), head-banging, nightmares, tantrums, or violent outbursts. You might also want to note whether the child has had unduly prolonged separation anxiety from parents (often around starting school), or whether there have been problems with bedwetting (enuresis) or retention and incontinence of feces (encopresis). School performance and behavior, and relationships with peers should be explored in detail. Drug and alcohol use should be carefully documented. (Do not forget to ask about this, even in children of primary-school age.) Also, be sure to ask about eating problems, such as anorexia, bulimia, or obesity (for a discussion of anorexia and bulimia, see Chapter 14).

Medical history. This should be detailed, and in those cases where physical abnormalities are suspected or in cases where it appears that routine medical care has been neglected (e.g., no physical examination in the previous year), the child should be referred to a pediatrician. Pay attention to chronic illnesses, hospitalizations, and surgery. In particular, note whether there have been any major separations from parents due to hospitalization, and the child's reactions to illness and treatment. Be sure to ask about any medications the child is taking, as these can have side effects that mimic psychiatric disorders.

Home environment. You should spend a considerable amount of time obtaining a picture of the child's home and family life. This will involve taking a family history that is more detailed than that usually documented in adult cases. Try to obtain information about three generations of the family—that is, the grandparents, the parents and their siblings, and the child and his or her siblings. It is often helpful to draw a family tree when you record this information. For each person, try to document the following:

- Age
- Marital status
- Living situation (with the child or elsewhere)
- School and work history
- Physical health (including all medical problems)
- Mental health (pay special attention to depression and substance abuse)

- Relationship with the child (quality and quantity of time spent together)
- Death or other separations from the child

In addition, inquire about who have been the primary caregivers for the child, what the child's relationships to these people are like, and what changes have occurred in these relationships over time (e.g., a transition from full-time care by mother to participation in a day care program). Also, ask about other problems in the child's home life (e.g., concerning neighbors, other relatives, step-siblings from parents' previous marriages). Be sure to ask parents what they think are the possible causes of their child's difficulties. (Often, as you establish rapport with parents, much of this information will emerge spontaneously without your needing to ask long lists of specific questions.) Finally, remember to get an idea of the family's financial resources and social supports (e.g., availability of relatives, community agencies, church facilities), as these will be important factors to consider in developing a treatment plan for the child.

INTERVIEWING THE CHILD

The basic principles of clinical interviewing described in Chapter 1 apply to children as well as adults. However, work with children often requires an additional set of tools for understanding clinical material, because children will usually rely more heavily than adults on nonverbal modes of showing you their concerns, and will be likely to display their troubles in their play activities and in their behavior with you. Play is both a diagnostic and a therapeutic tool in working with children. Thus, an hour-long interview with a troubled 4-year-old might involve drawing a picture, playing "house" with a set of dolls, or making up stories using animal puppets.

Your first meeting with a child will most likely occur in a waiting room with the parent or other responsible person who has accompanied the child. Note how the child behaves with the parent and how he or she separates from the parent. Great difficulty in leaving the parent to go into your office may suggest some specific fears about the meeting with you or more general problems with separation.

The child needs to understand who you are and why he or she is seeing you. Even small children can understand that your office is a "place to talk about worries." Notice how the child deals with you in the first few minutes of the interview. Does the child warm up to you easily?

Can you engage him or her in conversation or play easily, or does the child remain aloof, guarded, or withdrawn? You may want to start talking with the child about something that he or she is likely to be interested in—for example, pets, sports, hobbies, or favorite foods. Or particularly with older children and adolescents, you might begin with a direct question about what has been on the child's mind or what the child understands about why he or she was brought to see you.

The Importance of Play

Young children cannot be expected to sit still and talk throughout an interview. In fact, you would not want them to, because in most cases the child provides you with invaluable information by being active with you and with toys and other objects in your office.

Play allows children to live out and rework problems that are bothering them, to recreate family situations, and to express feelings and impulses that might be "forbidden" in real life. In the stories they create, children can tell you what is on their minds even when they do not have the capacity to verbalize these concerns. For example, a boy of 5 may not be able to tell you how angry he is at his father (the conscious experience of anger at a loved and needed father may be too threatening), but he may play out scenes over and over again in which big abusive fathers are beaten by small but powerful little boys. A girl of 7 is not likely to be conscious of her belief that her parents got a divorce because she was a bad little girl, but in her play she might create stories about bad girls who get punished and daddies who come home again.

This process of using other figures in lieu of direct depiction of real-life figures is called *displacement.* Displacement is used by children, adolescents, and adults (see Chapter 2). However, the use of displacement by children is not a pathological defense, as it is in adults, but rather a normal developmental necessity. Conversely, the child who tells you directly during the first interview that he hates his father is likely to be the victim of trauma (e.g., child abuse at the hands of the father) and may be overwhelmed by it.

Your office should be equipped with materials that will allow for fanciful play—for example, drawing materials, clay, dolls and a doll house, puppets, and other toys that might interest children of various ages. Children will often begin to play with toys in your office spontaneously. You may invite a child to play, and then watch for a time, joining in when you feel it is appropriate.

The interpretation of the form and content of play is a complicated and fascinating skill that is well worth study. However, a discussion of this aspect of child psychiatry is beyond the scope of this chapter. It is best learned by watching experienced clinicians play with children (often with the use of a one-way mirror) and then talking to these clinicians about their understanding of what transpired.

In addition to toys, you can use verbal techniques to help children warm up to you and engage in fantasy and play. You can, for example, make up stories together. Or you might ask the child which animal he or she would most like to be. The choice of animal, and what the child describes about the creature, will give you information about self-image. Similar information can be obtained by having the child draw a person and then tell you about the person in the drawing (what the person is feeling, doing, etc.). You might also ask the child to make three wishes (e.g., to change something, to be something, and to do something). Asking the child to discuss his or her concerns directly may be too anxiety provoking and may disrupt the interview.

The term "play therapy" is often misunderstood to convey a sense of frivolousness or unimportance. The above discussion is meant to show you that with children of certain ages, play is the only developmentally appropriate means of communicating about their affective life, including joys, sorrows, and conflicts.

Be sure to give children the opportunity to talk about their strengths. Such information is important in assessing the child's self-esteem, but also in helping to convey the message that you are an ally who wants to hear about what the child feels proud of as well as those aspects of life that are more troublesome. You might get at strong points with a question like, "What things are you good at?" or "What do you like most about yourself?"

Remember that in dealing with children, you may have to be more parental than you would with an adult. For example, children need to know where the bathroom is, and you may have to escort them there during the session. You must set limits on destructive and disruptive behavior in your office, as this will reassure the child that you will not allow his or her impulses to get out of control, and will allow the session to proceed.

The above discussion about play may not apply to older elementary-school children (e.g., age 10 and up) and adolescents, who may wish to sit and talk as an adult might, or who may prefer to talk over a game such as checkers. Children in these age groups can often be quite open and direct in the expression of their concerns.

When interviewing adolescents, it is especially important to respect their autonomy and their right to decide whether to participate in the interview with you. Some adolescents will be very reluctant to talk. In such cases, a passive stance on your part is not as likely to be as helpful as active attempts to engage in discussion. Initially, you might ask about neutral topics of interest such as sports, music, or clothes.

Adolescents are likely to have concerns about controlling their impulses, about their sexuality and sexual identity, about intimacy, and about peer relationships. Many teenagers will be worried about some aspect of their sexuality ("Am I developing right?" "Am I gay?"). You might open the way for discussion of these matters with a general comment such as, "Many kids your age have questions about sex and their sexual feelings. Have you had any questions like that?" Since peer relationships are of the utmost importance during this period, you will definitely want to discuss friendships and the adolescent's concerns (if any) about social acceptance as part of your assessment interview.

The psychiatric evaluation of the child is recorded in much the same way that it is in the case of adult evaluations. Thus, in preparing a written case report, you can follow the format outlined in Chapter 3. Moreover, your observations of the child in your office should be recorded in the mental status examination, according to the format discussed in Chapter 4.

PSYCHIATRIC DISORDERS OF CHILDHOOD

Children suffer from many of the same disorders that are found in the adult population. Some disorders such as schizophrenia, bipolar illness, and depression are less frequently encountered among children; others (e.g., phobias) are just as common in children as in adults. Disorders such as attention-deficit hyperactivity disorder and functional enuresis are diagnosed more frequently among children than adults. And still others, like antisocial personality disorder, are by definition not diagnosed in children at all.

One of the best predictors of psychiatric problems in adulthood is a severe behavior disturbance in childhood. However, mental disorders in childhood do not invariably lead to the same disturbances in adult life. Moreover, some emotionally disturbed children grow up to have no diagnosable mental disorders whatsoever. Thus, for example, personality disorders are diagnosed infrequently and conservatively in children and adolescents, because the plasticity and instability of the personality during these developmental phases make it impossible in most cases to see any personality patterns as enduring and stable. Despite active research efforts in recent years, we still know very little about the relationship between psychopathology in childhood and mental illness in adult life.

What follows are brief discussions of the disorders that are most commonly encountered among children and adolescents. Some disorders listed in DSM-III-R are not included here because of the infrequency with which these diagnoses are made. For more detailed discussions of various clinical syndromes, you might wish to consult DSM-III-R and a general child psychiatry text.

As noted in the first section of this chapter, you must be sure to assess the presence and severity of psychiatric disorders in the context of what is developmentally appropriate for each individual child.

Attention-Deficit Hyperactivity Disorder

Attention-deficit hyperactivity disorder (ADHD) has been known by a variety of other names, most notably *hyperactive child syndrome* and *minimal brain dysfunction* (MBD). Estimates of the prevalence of ADHD range from 3% to 10% of elementary-school children, and ADHD is as much as five times as common in boys as in girls. The impulsivity and the difficulty in paying attention to tasks, both of which are usually involved in this syndrome, are frustrating for parents, teachers, and children alike. The disorder usually appears by age 3, but often goes undiagnosed until the child enters school.

The hallmark of ADHD is *inattention*, which usually involves the child's failing to finish things that he or she starts (e.g., school work, household chores, play activities), not seeming to listen to others, and easy distractibility.

The second major characteristic of ADHD is *impulsivity*. These children act before thinking, have difficulty organizing their work, shift excessively from one activity to another, often call out in class or have trouble waiting their turn in group situations, and require more supervision than other children.

The third major characteristic, *hyperactivity*, is seen in a great number of ADHD children, but not all of them. Symptoms include excessive running and climbing, difficulty sitting still, moving about excessively during sleep, and being always "on the go" as if driven by a motor.

Children with ADHD commonly throw temper tantrums and generally have a low tolerance for frustration. They are often socially immature, and, although sociable, lose the friends they make because of a need to dominate play situations. They often end up with compliant friends who are younger than they. Relationships with adults also tend to be poor, because behavior problems cause these children to be labeled "bad" or "unruly." Needless to say, ADHD usually results in academic difficulties, as children who are of normal intelligence cannot pay attention to tasks and organize their work, thus becoming underachievers. Many of these children also have specific learning disabilities (see below). The severity of the ADHD syndrome varies from one child to the next.

ADHD children commonly suffer from low self-esteem, secondary to their difficulties in relating to adults and peers, and secondary to school failures. This can result in significant emotional problems, and many of these children begin to exhibit antisocial behavior (e.g., lying, stealing, drug abuse) in adolescence if untreated in childhood.

The etiology of ADHD is an area of active research in child psychiatry. Maternal deprivation, environmental toxins (e.g., lead poisoning), genetic predisposition, severe early malnutrition, and intrauterine or postnatal brain damage are among the factors that have been implicated as possible contributors to the development of the syndrome. The course of the disorder is variable. As they move through puberty into adolescence and adulthood, some people retain all of the symptoms of ADHD, whereas others become free of the disorder completely. In a third group, the symptoms of hyperactivity disappear, but the attention deficit and impulsivity persist.

Diagnosis

The symptoms described above are listed in DSM-III-R (pp. 50–53). Signs of inattention, impulsivity, and hyperactivity must be judged on the basis of what is developmentally appropriate for a child at any given age. It is important to rule out other conditions that might be mistaken for ADHD. The differential diagnosis includes 1) medical illnesses such as constipation and hyperthyroidism; 2) neurological conditions such as behavioral syndromes resulting from trauma, infection, or lead poisoning; and 3) other psychiatric conditions, including anxiety disorders, parental abuse or neglect, major depression or mania, and manipulative behavior.

History. In many cases, the most reliable reports of abnormalities come from teachers rather than the child's parents, because teachers have greater familiarity with age-appropriate norms and a much larger comparison group on which to base their judgments.

Neurological examination. The presence of "soft" neurological signs (e.g., poor coordination, left-right confusion) is often a clue to ADHD, although only about 50% of children with the disorder have neurological abnormalities. Electroencephalograms are usually normal.

Psychological testing. Children with ADHD show standard patterns of deficits on routine psychological tests, particularly in areas of sustaining attention and organizing information. In addition to standard psychological tests including IQ tests, the child should be tested for specific learning disabilities, as these often coexist with ADHD.

Treatment

The treatment of ADHD involves not only the child but also the child's family and school. Family members need to be educated about the disorder and about what to expect from their child. Parents who feel frustrated and guilty about their problems in dealing with their child often find supportive psychotherapy helpful both in alleviating some of their own distress and in teaching them to respond to their child in ways that promote better functioning and less family strife. Individual psychotherapy is often useful for older children and adolescents to help the child with the secondary problems of ADHD, such as low self-esteem, depression, and poor social skills.

Children with ADHD commonly benefit from reducing sensory and emotional stimulation in their environments. This can be done with simple measures, such as creating quiet spaces with subdued colors and simple furniture in which the child can play, putting toys away in a closet when they are not in use, allowing only one friend to visit at a time, avoiding crowded places like supermarkets, and putting the child in a small classroom.

Special academic placement is often indicated for children with ADHD if they disrupt the learning process for others and cannot learn well in a traditional classroom setting. Consultation with teachers is especially important, both to determine what sort of academic program would be most helpful to the child and to enlist the teachers' help in monitoring the child's behavioral responses to the various treatment interventions.

ADHD is one of the few mental disorders of childhood for which the use of medication is clearly indicated in many cases. Roughly 75% of children with ADHD and hyperactivity respond to some form of somatic treatment. Chemotherapy is not curative but suppresses the symptoms of the disorder (particularly behavioral impulsivity), and many children benefit from the medication for as long as 10 years or until they reach puberty.

The most commonly used medications are stimulants, particularly amphetamine and methylphenidate (Ritalin). These medications exert a seemingly paradoxical effect, in that they do not heighten most children's level of arousal, but instead tend to improve concentration and performance, calm restlessness, improve impulse control, and make the child more responsive to reward and punishment. The mechanism by which stimulants produce these effects in children is not known. Side effects may include loss of appetite, irritability, headache, gastrointestinal distress, and insomnia. Also, many children experience some reversible growth retardation during the first year or two in which the medication is administered. "Drug holidays" (e.g., medication-free periods) during school vacations allow the child time to catch up in growth, and give the clinician an opportunity to observe whether medication is still necessary for the child.

Tricyclic antidepressants have also been found useful in treating ADHD, but early reports of cardiac side effects have made clinicians conservative about their use. Recent studies point to the relative safety of these medications. Baseline electrocardiograms and monitoring of serum levels of the medication generally are sufficient precautions to address the infrequent incidence of cardiac side effects.

Recently, much attention has been paid to diet as a possible aggravating factor in ADHD. Sugar, food dyes, milk, chocolate, and artificial additives are among the many substances cited as possible contributors to the ADHD syndrome. However, elimination of various foods has been found to be helpful in only a minority of cases.

Conduct Disorders

The category of conduct disorders covers a broad range of conditions found among children. These disorders all are characterized by a repetitive and persistent pattern of violating either the basic rights of others or major age-appropriate societal norms or rules. The term "conduct disorder" describes behavior but says nothing about underlying causes. There is considerable overlap between conduct disorders and ADHD—that is, many children with ADHD also have a conduct disorder. Further, some children with conduct disorders have soft neurological signs but do not exhibit behaviors characteristic of ADHD.

Conduct disorders are divided into three subcategories in DSM-III-R: group type, solitary aggressive type, and undifferentiated type. Conduct disorders of the *group type* denote behavior problems that occur mainly as a part of group activity with peers. This activity may or may not involve physical violence. Disorders of the *solitary aggressive type* denote aggressive physical behavior initiated by the individual child rather than as part of a group activity, usually toward both adults and peers. Children with a conduct disorder are classified as having the *undifferentiated type* when the features of their disorder cannot be classified as either solitary aggressive or group type.

Children with conduct disorders typically blame someone else for their problems and are mistrustful of others. They often hide low self-esteem under a veneer of "toughness." They may be sexually precocious and promiscuous, and often become involved in smoking and substance abuse. They are underachievers, and the socialized types often join gangs that engage in antisocial activities. The disorders are much more common in boys than in girls and are more common among the children of adults with antisocial personality disorder and alcoholism.

While a vast number of factors have been proposed as etiologies of conduct disorders, no causal relationships have been demonstrated to date. Poor impulse control, lack of parental care and limit setting, excessive inborn aggressive drives, cultural norms, and parental role modeling could all contribute to unusually aggressive behavior. Lack of social bonding appears to be associated with maternal deprivation, harsh or inconsistent treatment by parents (including physical abuse), parental rejection, and ADHD. Clearly, children with these disorders come from a wide variety of biological and environmental backgrounds.

Whereas habitual antisocial behavior in childhood and adolescence is associated with elevated risk of serious mental illness in adult life (depression, schizophrenia, antisocial personality disorder), many children with conduct disorders grow up without such serious disturbances. This is particularly true for children who exhibit group-type disorders. They often learn from experience, and many can be helped by various forms of psychological treatment. Moreover, some antisocial acting out in relatively healthy youngsters occurs transiently in response to environmental stresses and disappears when the children's situations change.

Juvenile delinquency is a widespread and serious problem in our society. More than 40% of people arrested for serious crimes are under the age of 18, and adolescents commit half of all rapes and murders reported in this country each year. Delinquent behavior peaks in adolescence, and mental health professionals are commonly called upon to assess and treat delinquent teenagers for emotional disorders that often underlie their antisocial behavior.

Many problems of adolescence contribute to delinquency. Some teenagers who suffer from organic brain damage (e.g., congenitally or as the result of later trauma) have poor impulse control, and the emotional and biological stresses of adolescence push them to the limits of their capacities for socialized behavior. Teenagers who have suffered severe physical and emotional deprivation (e.g., from frequent foster home changes, parental abuse and violence, or parental psychopathology or alcoholism) discharge tension in ways that have been modeled for them by their caregivers. Adolescents may behave violently or promiscuously in attempts to combat feelings of inadequacy. Delinquent behavior may be a call for help in response to family strife, or it may be the result of parents' encouragement of such behavior (e.g., the father who subtly encourages a son to act out the father's own destructive impulses).

Substance abuse is increasingly common among adolescents (see Chapter 14). In evaluating adolescents who abuse drugs, it is important to consider the possible contributing factors noted above. Moreover, it is particularly important to rule out depression, since some depressed teenagers will attempt to medicate themselves with drugs or alcohol.

Treatment of conduct disorders cannot be outlined in any standard way, because this diagnosis covers behavior problems that have multiple determinants. One child may come from a home in which parents are unconsciously encouraging him to lie and steal, another child may throw tantrums and behave antisocially secondary to an ADHD, and a third "delinquent" may be proving his manhood in a subculture that prizes and encourages defiance of authority. Thus, treatment strategies must be based on a careful diagnostic assessment, including consultation with family, school, and those legal or social service agencies, if any, involved with the child, as well as comprehensive pediatric and neurological evaluations.

Severely behaviorally disturbed youngsters whose behavior cannot be controlled effectively by parents and teachers may need placement in a residential treatment setting where limits can be enforced, children can be consistently held responsible for their actions, and constructive relationships with peers can be encouraged. Unfortunately, these settings are in short supply, and too few youngsters have access to them. In outpatient settings, many children and their families can be helped by therapy that focuses on the consequences of behavior and accepting responsibility for one's actions. Also, many of these children suffer from low self-esteem and serious depression, and therapy can provide a setting in which these children are valued and respected by the therapist and can in turn learn to appreciate their own strengths.

Specific Developmental Disorders

Specific developmental disorders describe impairment in one particular cognitive area of maturation: reading, arithmetic, language, or speech. These disorders are diagnosed in children who may otherwise function well, but who, based on their age and educational backgrounds, have obvious difficulty in one area of learning. Developmental reading, arithmetic, and language disorders correspond to what educators call learning disabilities, and these disorders are often not treated in mental health settings at all but are worked with in the educational system. These disorders are quite common; they are estimated to be present in 10% to 20% of elementary-school children. They are diagnosed twice as commonly in boys as in girls, probably due to a combination of actual increased frequency among boys and greater attention paid in some families and schools to the educational performance of boys and to their greater propensity for acting out.

These disorders are often seen in conjunction with others, particularly with ADHD and conduct disorders. In some cases, a child who performs poorly in school secondary to a specific developmental disorder will act out his or her distress by being truant or engaging in antisocial behavior, and in this way warrant the diagnosis of conduct disorder. In most cases, children with specific developmental disorders are not simply lagging behind their peers and do not catch up to them in time. Rather, most children with these problems continue to have signs of these disorders into adolescence and adulthood, although they may compensate quite well for their difficulties.

Developmental reading disorder. This disorder is often referred to as "dyslexia." It involves impaired development of reading skills that cannot be accounted for by the child's mental or chronological age or poor schooling. Assessment of poor performance is based on standardized reading tests (compared with the child's overall intellectual abilities as measured by IQ tests) as well as reading skills observed in the classroom. An example of the disorder is a 14-year-old eighth-grader of normal intelligence from an adequately stimulating home and school environment who reads at the level of a third-grader.

Developmental reading disorder often involves some difficulty in integrating and organizing visually derived information. Reading errors include omissions, additions, and distortions of words, and writing errors are often numerous and bizarre. Children with this disorder usually read slowly and comprehend what they read poorly. Soft neurological signs are often present, suggesting some organic basis for the disorder.

Developmental arithmetic disorder. Although not as common as a reading disorder, developmental arithmetic disorder is diagnosed by the same means (performance on standardized tests of math skills and performance in class compared with scores on IQ tests). Children with this disorder may also have reading problems.

Developmental language disorder. This disorder refers to delayed development of language skills, unrelated to hearing impairment or mental retardation. There are two types: expressive and receptive. The *expressive disorder* involves difficulty with vocal expression ("getting the words out") despite good comprehension. Articulation is generally immature, vocabulary is severely restricted, and sentence construction is poor. The *receptive disorder* is more serious than the expressive type in that it involves failure to develop both comprehension and expression. Children with this disorder have reading and spelling difficulties, and often show some auditory impairment.

Developmental articulation disorder. A type of speech disorder that is quite common, developmental articulation disorder is thought to occur in roughly 6% of boys and 3% of girls. It involves failure to develop articulation of later-acquired speech sounds such as r, sh, th, f, z, l, or ch. This is a less serious disorder than the language disorders described above in that the child's abilities to comprehend and express language are normal.

Developmental expressive writing disorder. This disorder refers to the impaired ability to develop writing skills despite normal intelligence, adequate schooling, and the absence of any visual, hearing, or neurological impairment. This disorder interferes with academic achievement or activities of daily living that require composition of written texts. The writing of individuals with this disorder is usually marked by spelling, grammar, and punctuation errors, as well as difficulty organizing paragraphs.

Developmental coordination disorder. This disorder denotes impairment in the development of motor coordination (e.g., clumsiness, poor performance in sports, and delayed motor milestones such as riding a bicycle) in the absence of any physical disorder or mental retardation. Obviously, the child must be measured according to what constitute appropriate skills for his or her age.

Treatment of specific developmental disorders is largely educational, and many children can make major improvements in their skills with special educational assistance. Learning disabilities are relative discrepancies in skills. Thus, a learning-disabled child may be quite bright and capable of devising strategies to compensate for the disability and thereby function quite well (e.g., the child with a reading disability who learns to remember everything he or she hears in class). However, children with these disorders may lose motivation to learn and give up in the face of repeated failures, so a major part of treatment is to support their self-esteem by putting them in situations (e.g., special classes or special tutoring) in which they can experience some success at their level of ability. When learning disorders are accompanied by coordination difficulties, special physical education programs may be helpful and may enhance the child's self-esteem and ability to interact with peers. Articulation disorders often respond well to speech therapy given in the schools.

Educational remediation is usually the treatment of choice, but psychotherapy may be needed when undermotivation, low self-esteem, or undue dependency has resulted from the presence of a developmental disorder.

Mental Retardation

Mental retardation is considered in this chapter because the disorder, though generally lifelong, is by definition present before the age of 18. (Similar conditions that begin after age 18 are classified as dementia.) The hallmarks of the disorder are intellectual functioning that is significantly below average (as measured on IQ tests) and resultant deficits or impairment in the person's adaptive behavior (e.g., ability to work, care for self, function socially). Low IQ alone is not sufficient for the diagnosis of mental retardation, but must be accompanied by evidence of poor functioning. The prevalence of mental retardation is thought to be about 3% among school-age children. Among the rest of the general population in nonacademic settings, the prevalence decreases to roughly 1%. Mental retardation may coexist with a wide variety of other psychiatric disorders, such as autism, ADHD, and hyperactivity. Also, severe mental retardation is often associated with multiple neurological abnormalities involving neuromuscular function, vision, or hearing. Seizures are common among severely mentally retarded people.

The organic causes of mental retardation are too numerous to list here. The most common (accounting for 25% of cases) are inborn chromosomal and metabolic abnormalities such as Down's syndrome (trisomy 21) and phenylketonuria (PKU). Prenatal infections such as rubella and toxoplasmosis, as well as heavy maternal alcohol consumption, are among the influences in utero that can result in mental retardation. Trauma during delivery (e.g., mechanical injury to the brain or transient loss of oxygen to brain tissue) can also result in mental retardation. Postnatal causes of mental retardation, including infection, hyperbilirubinemia, head trauma (including that resulting from child abuse), brain tumors, and lead poisoning, account for a sizeable proportion of cases.

Psychosocial causes of mental retardation are thought to include deprivation of social, linguistic, and intellectual stimulation. For example, this deprivation may result from parental neglect or from parental deficits in the ability to stimulate children (e.g., when parents are themselves retarded). Mental retardation due to known biological factors is as likely to occur in upper as in lower socioeconomic groups, but retardation without known organic cause is more commonly found among lower socioeconomic groups.

Subtypes of mental retardation

The population of mentally retarded individuals is divided into two large groups, consisting of those with *mild and borderline mental retarda-*

tion (IQ greater than 50) on the one hand, and of those with *moderate and severe retardation* (IQ less than 50) on the other. The vast majority of mentally retarded individuals fall into either the borderline or mild category.

Those with an IQ of 50 or above tend to live in underprivileged neighborhoods and may have siblings who are mildly retarded. They usually have no obvious neurological abnormalities or physical handicaps, and so appear normal. Usually, the diagnosis of mental retardation is made only after these individuals start school. In this group, psychosocial and hereditary factors seem to be of roughly equal importance in determining intelligence, as they are in determining intelligence in normal individuals.

By contrast, those who have IQs below 50 more commonly show obvious physical and neurological abnormalities and so look "retarded." They are more likely to live in institutional settings, to require special educational programs, or to work in sheltered workshops. Biological factors generally play a more prominent role than environmental ones in the development of mental retardation in this group. The diagnosis of mental retardation is made earlier than among those with milder impairment—often in the preschool years.

Mental retardation is classified by IQ (average = 100), and on this basis mentally retarded individuals are classified in one of four groups:

1. *Mild (IQ 50–70).* Roughly 2.5% of the population have IQs between 50 and 70. These people are termed "educable," and they make up about 80% of the population of mentally retarded individuals in this country. They develop social and communication skills before age 5 and are not distinguishable from normal children until after age 5. They can usually learn up to a sixth-grade level. As adults, they can usually develop social and vocational skills that allow them to be self-sufficient, but they may need assistance from others in times of stress.
2. *Moderate (IQ 35–49).* These people are termed "trainable" and comprise about 12% of the population of the mentally retarded. They can learn to communicate as preschoolers but are only poorly aware of social conventions. During school age, they do not often progress beyond a second-grade level academically, but can profit from training in social and occupational skills. As adults they can often care for themselves with moderate supervision, and perform unskilled or semiskilled tasks in supervised ("sheltered") workshops.
3. *Severe (IQ 20–34).* These people comprise roughly 7% of the

mentally retarded population. During the preschool years, they show poor motor development and little or no communicative speech. They may be able to learn to talk and perform elementary self-care (e.g., personal hygiene) during school age, but they do not profit from vocational training, and require a great deal of supervision in living throughout their lives.

4. *Profound (IQ below 20)*. The profoundly mentally retarded constitute 1% of the population of retarded individuals. Throughout life, they require a highly structured living environment with constant supervision. Speech and motor development are usually very limited; some people in this category can learn minimal self-care skills (e.g., personal hygiene).

The category of *borderline mental retardation*, also called borderline intellectual functioning in DSM-III-R, has boundaries that are less clear than those of the categories described above. This category includes people in the IQ range of 71 to 84. People whose intellectual functioning falls into this range may or may not be classified as retarded, depending on how well they adapt to their life circumstances. For example, the man who has an IQ of 80, who is self-supporting, and who, like his father, functions well at a job requiring semiskilled manual labor may never come to the attention of an educator or mental health professional. Another man with the same IQ, who is raised in an upwardly-mobile intellectual family, may develop low self-esteem based on an inability to keep up with peers and low status within his family, resulting in behavior problems and an eventual diagnosis. Retardation in this range is highly context-dependent.

Treatment of mental retardation begins with identifying and treating somatic causes, such as nutritional deficiencies and seizure disorders. Increased environmental stimulation is sometimes sufficient to assist children with mild or borderline retardation in their intellectual and social development when a deprived home environment has retarded the children's growth. Most treatment is habilitative—that is, it is designed to help the retarded maximize their potential for self-care and social and occupational functioning with 1) socialization programs to teach speech, hygiene, academic, and interpersonal skills, and 2) vocational training with sheltered employment opportunities.

Increasingly, emphasis has been on keeping even the most severely mentally retarded people in the community and out of institutions to maximize their socialization and ability to function in society. Some retarded children may need residential schools to cope with severe behavior problems, and some profoundly handicapped children may need nursing-home care. Otherwise, treatment is aimed at family care (in the child's own home or in foster care) and community-based education and training. The psychiatrist is apt to provide service to them indirectly via consultation with families and social service agencies, as well as more directly by prescribing medications for poor impulse control. In some patients who have some verbal capacity, psychotherapy can be useful.

The mentally retarded are an underserved population in this country. Mental health professionals are often called upon to help the mentally retarded and their families understand the problems the retarded person faces, and to plan for adequate training and assistance. The greater your knowledge about the resources and services available for the mentally retarded in your community, the more effective you will be in providing these patients with the help they deserve.

Pervasive Developmental Disorder (Autism)

Children with *pervasive developmental disorder*, or *autistic disorder*, show distortions in the development of multiple basic psychological functions such as attention, perception, reality testing, and movement. Unlike children with specific developmental disorders, who are impaired in one area of cognition but are otherwise normal, these children are globally and severely impaired in their abilities to function intellectually, motorically, and socially.

Autism is a condition in which the child is extremely unresponsive to other people (i.e., autistic), has gross impairment in communication skills, and shows bizarre responses to various aspects of the environment. Autistic children fail to develop normal interest in and attachment to others. Infants do not generally cuddle and are indifferent or averse to physical contact and affection. Older children fail to develop cooperative play and friendships. Some older children gradually develop some awareness of and attachment to parents; however, many autistic children treat human beings as though they were inanimate objects.

A profound language disorder is the clinical hallmark of autism. Autistic children who can speak usually exhibit immature grammar structure, echolalia (mimicking sounds made by others), reversals of pronouns, difficulty naming objects, and inappropriate nonverbal communications (e.g., bizarre facial expressions and gestures).

Autistic children may respond bizarrely to the environment in a variety of ways. Many of them appear to be "obsessed with sameness" and may react violently to minor changes in their environment, such as new clothes or a change in the child's place at the dinner table. They are often fascinated by motion, and stare at fans or other spinning objects, or at water running down the drain. The child may engage in ritualistic behavior (e.g., hand-wringing or hand-clapping) and compulsively self-destructive behavior (e.g., head-banging) with apparent imperviousness to pain.

Only 30% of autistic children have an IQ above 70. The disorder is chronic. Only one child in six grows up to make an adequate social adjustment and can work regularly; another one in six of these children makes only a fair adjustment, and two-thirds of autistic children remain severely handicapped and unable to lead independent lives. Many of these children develop seizure disorders in adolescence or early adulthood.

Childhood onset is specified in the diagnosis for children who are grossly impaired in social relationships and show bizarre communication and behavior, but who begin to show signs of the disorder after age 36 months. This disorder, too, occurs more frequently among the mentally retarded, but some children may have "islands" of unusual ability (so-called "idiot savants"). By contrast, children suffering from childhood schizophrenia are usually diagnosed above age 5 and show hallucinations, delusions, or other forms of thought disorder in addition to bizarre speech and behavior. These children are diagnosed by the same criteria used for adults (see Chapter 5).

The causes of autistic disorder are not known. However, some factors that are thought to predispose children to the development of infantile autism are maternal rubella (German measles), PKU, encephalitis, and meningitis. The prevalence of autism is 50 times as great in siblings of children with the disorder as it is in the general population. Previously, it was thought that "refrigerator mothers" who deprived the child of affection fostered the development of pervasive developmental disorders. However, recent research does not support this notion, but instead suggests that genetic and organic factors probably play a prominent role.

Treatment of these disorders is long and difficult. Medication has been of use in treating specific medication-responsive symptoms such as hyperactivity and seizures. Educational and habilitative approaches are most important to help remedy speech and learning disorders and incoordination. Behavior modification programs can help shape some children's behavior along more socially appropriate lines. Children who are severely retarded and behaviorally disturbed may require institutional care, whereas others can remain at home. Parents need a great deal of support and counseling, both to help them deal with their feelings about their child's difficulties and to help them preserve time and energy for themselves and other children in the family.

Functional Enuresis (Bedwetting)

Enuresis is one of the most common problems of early childhood. It is defined as the involuntary voiding of urine at least twice a month in 5- and 6-year-olds, and at least once a month in older children. The "accident" most commonly occurs at night in bed during non-REM sleep so that the child has no memory of wetting the bed. Enuresis occurs in at least 10% of 4-year-olds, and at age 5 this problem still affects 7% of boys and 3% of girls.

Eighty percent of enuretic children suffer from primary enuresis— that is, they have never achieved complete bladder control. Many children in this group lag behind their peers in the development of the inner neurological and psychological organization of bladder control. In some cases, difficulty over toilet training or conflict between parents is so upsetting to the child that he or she manifests distress through sphincter accidents. Twenty percent of enuretic children suffer from secondary enuresis, which occurs after a year or more of being "dry." Psychogenic factors are more commonly implicated in the genesis of secondary enuresis than the primary form, and typical contributing factors include such stressors as the birth of a sibling, parental conflict, starting school, or hospitalization. It is not uncommon for children to develop secondary enuresis temporarily due to regression along the developmental line of sphincter control in response to a specific stressor, and most episodes are so short-lived as to require no treatment. Most enuretic children become completely "dry" on their own by age 10.

Whenever a child presents with enuresis, it is always important to rule out an organic problem such as genitourinary tract abnormalities or infection, seizure disorder (with accidents occurring during seizures), and diabetes. The child should always be examined by a physician as part of your evaluation.

When enuresis is the presenting symptom of an underlying emotional disorder, psychotherapy and family therapy can often resolve the symptom by easing emotional stress in the child's life. A variety of behavior modification techniques have been effective with enuretic children, including charts and systems of reward with gold stars for dry nights, as well as bladder stretching with fluid forcing and holding of urine during the day for as long as possible. Mechanical devices such as buzzers that wake the child up at the first appearance of moisture on the bed have also been used with good results. Imipramine has been found to be helpful in many cases, although the mechanism by which this antidepressant exerts a therapeutic effect is not understood. The potentially toxic effects of imipramine on the heart make it a treatment to be used with caution. Parents need to be supported by the therapist so that they can be supportive of their child rather than punitive.

Functional Encopresis (Incontinence of Feces)

Encopresis, or incontinence of stool, involves voluntary or involuntary soiling at least once a month after age 4 that is not the result of an organic cause (e.g., bowel dysfunction). Encopresis is five times as common in boys as in girls and may be either primary (if continence has never been achieved) or secondary (when previously achieved continence is lost). Commonly, soiling results from a cycle of hard, painful stools that the child holds back as long as possible, and leakage around the impacted feces, followed by pain when the child finally defecates, and then holding back of the next stool to avoid further pain. This can be treated with stool softeners and suppositories that help the dilated rectum resume its normal size, along with a supportive and educative approach to the problem with the child and the parents. Rectal examination revealing the presence of hard stool in the rectum is sufficient to rule out the presence of Hirschsprung's disease (congenital megacolon).

Behavior modification techniques have been used effectively with some encopretic children. Children set goals with the therapist (e.g., learning not to retain feces, or having one bowel movement per day), and when these goals are achieved, the behavior is reinforced with rewards such as gold stars or a special privilege. Behavioral techniques can be particularly helpful in conjunction with psychotherapy when underlying personality problems play a major role in the etiology of the disorder.

More often, encopresis is part of a passive-aggressive, hostile, withholding relationship that the child has formed with the parents. This requires psychotherapeutic treatment of the parents and the child to explore underlying family conflicts, to help parents learn to respect the child's autonomy, and to help the child learn other avenues for the expression of anger and resentment. As with enuresis, encopresis sometimes occurs transiently when the child is under stress, as when a sibling is born or the child starts school. In such cases, the problem often resolves spontaneously when the stressful time is past. In a few instances, encopresis results simply from parental neglect when no one has bothered to toilet train the child.

Separation Anxiety Disorder

Separation anxiety is normal in infants and toddlers. Moreover, difficulty separating from parents and anxiety about being away from home are normal for brief periods when children take major developmental steps such as starting preschool, going to camp for the first time, and even leaving home to go to college. However, when separation anxiety is prolonged and severe in older children, it often disrupts the child's life in the way that agoraphobia disrupts an adult's (see Chapter 8). The essential feature of *separation anxiety disorder* is excessive anxiety on separation from primary caregivers or from home or other familiar surroundings, causing major symptoms of physical or emotional distress for at least 2 weeks.

Children with this disorder have prolonged and unremitting difficulty being away from home to attend school or camp, to sleep over at another child's house, or even to go on errands. Anxiety does not resolve after a few days or a few tries at a new activity, but persists and remains severe. Children may cling to parents and follow them around the house. Often children with this disorder have physical complaints such as nausea, vomiting, and headaches when separation is about to occur. Adolescents may experience dizziness, faintness, and palpitations at such times.

These children generally fear that some accident or illness will befall them or their parents if they are separated from them. Some children have explicit fantasies of particular dangers, while others experience vague anxiety when separated from parents but do not know what they fear. Concerns about dying and exaggerated fears about robbers, muggers, and monsters are common. Some children do not express fears at all, but become intensely homesick to the point of panic when away from home. Difficulty going to sleep, requests to sleep in the parents' bed, and nightmares about separation themes are common among these children. When separated from important people, these children often experience withdrawal, apathy, sadness, and difficulty concentrating.

School refusal

School refusal is often a symptom of separation anxiety disorder. A child's persistent refusal to attend school and insistence upon staying home with mother or some other primary caregiver (rather than simply wishing to "play hookey" or being kept at home by a parent) is a symptom that you should take very seriously, for it usually indicates distress of major proportions and often reflects a problem in the parent-child bond. In many cases, the child's fear of being separated from mother is related to mother's anxiety about the child's welfare and about being a good mother, with a need for the child's approval. School refusal may be a symptom of other psychiatric illnesses as well, most notably depression, psychosis, or a severe personality disturbance. Less frequently, the child's avoidance of school is due to a phobia about some element of the school situation rather than difficulty in separating from home. The cause of the child's refusal to attend school will in part determine your treatment strategy.

Treatment of school refusal begins with crisis intervention. When psychological assessment of the child and medical evaluation of the child's physical complaints do not reveal psychosis or some other psychiatric or medical reason to keep the child at home, the child should be returned to school immediately. Family members should be involved in evaluation and treatment. You should make clear to the child and family that there is no reason for the child to stay at home and that the only way to begin solving the problem is for the child to be back in school. A responsible person in the family needs to be sure that the child gets to school each day and stays there. (This often requires the cooperation of teachers as well.) The child may cling to mother and cry and throw tantrums in response to the expectation that he or she return to school. Nevertheless, after a few days of firm limits, the child becomes convinced that the parent intends for him or her to be in school, and the protest behavior ceases. When school refusal is due to separation anxiety, the family needs to be offered therapy, and, in particular, it is often the mother who must have psychotherapy in order to help her uncover her own difficulties in allowing the child to separate and lead an independent life. Systematic desensitization may help children who have developed phobias about particular aspects of the school situation. Antidepressants have been used effectively with some school-phobic children who experience panic symptoms, although we do not know the mechanism by which antidepressants alleviate panic (see Chapter 8).

School refusal has a relatively good prognosis in younger children, but it is much more serious in the small percentage for whom the disorder recurs in high school. Nearly half of high school children who experience separation anxiety disorder have an underlying psychotic illness and may need hospitalization.

Gender Identity Disorder

Gender identity disorder involves persistent and intense distress about one's assigned sex. Children desire to be the opposite sex, and some even insist that they *are* the opposite sex. The disorder is diagnosed before puberty and is often manifest as early as the third or fourth year of life.

Girls with this disorder are usually averse to wearing typically feminine clothing (e.g., dresses) and insist on wearing male clothing such as boy's underwear. They commonly repudiate their female anatomy, insisting on urinating while standing up, insisting that they have or will grow a penis, and insisting that they do not want to grow breasts or menstruate. They often have male companions and enjoy rough-and-tumble play but have no interest in more feminine pursuits like dolls or playing "house."

Boys with the disorder are preoccupied with activities that are stereotypically feminine (e.g., playing with dolls), and often shun male companions and games (e.g., sports). They may show a preference for cross-dressing in feminine clothing. Like girls with this disorder, boys commonly repudiate their gender-linked anatomy. They may insist they are girls or will grow up to be a woman, or that their penises are disgusting and ought to disappear.

Boys in particular face social ostracism during the latency years, as peers ridicule their feminine behaviors. Studies show that from one-third to two-thirds of boys with this disorder show a homosexual orientation after puberty. Girls may or may not be socially ostracized and may give up some of their insistence on stereotyped male dress and behavior during school years, and only a minority go on to a homosexual orientation after puberty. Very few boys or girls with this disorder go on to transexualism (see Chapter 13) in adult life.

Treatment for this disorder is psychotherapy. Most commonly, family problems and tensions foster the disorder by weakly or negatively reinforcing the child's normative gender role. Family therapy is often used to elucidate the sources of the problem and to help to remedy them. Individual psychotherapy is the mainstay of treatment for many children with this disorder. For example, a boy with this disorder who has an absent father and a close-binding mother may be able to form a healthy identification with a male psychotherapist and gradually feel safer to "try on" more typically masculine behaviors.

Identity Disorder

Identity disorder may begin at any time of life, but most commonly begins in late adolescence when people attempt to separate themselves psychologically (and often physically) from their families. This disorder involves severe subjective distress due to uncertainty about a variety of personal concerns relating to identity, including long-term goals, career choice, friendship patterns, sexual orientation, religious identification, moral values, and group loyalties. While most of us question some or all of these areas of our lives from time to time, people who have this disorder are so distressed by their uncertainty that their functioning in social relationships, at work, or at school is significantly impaired. The disorder is diagnosed if the impairment has lasted for at least 3 months.

People with identity disorder feel unable to resolve conflicts over life choices. For example, someone with this disorder may be preoccupied with the choice between a life dedicated to the pursuit of wealth and one dedicated to public service, or between participation in the Catholic Church or conversion to Judaism. People with this disorder feel so uncertain about who they are that they do not have the sense of a coherent identity. They are often mildly depressed or anxious as a result of this disturbance. They may try on a variety of identities, exhibiting widely divergent behaviors that are confusing to others. The disorder may be acute or chronic, and some adolescents with the disorder go on to develop personality disturbances such as borderline and narcissistic personality disorders.

Psychotherapy is at present the most widely used treatment for identity disorder.

Psychological Factors in Physical Illness

Physical illness is common among children and is always stressful. Children often develop physical symptoms (or consciously feign illness) as a response to emotional distress. Moreover, medical illnesses and their consequences (pain, restrictions, hospitalizations) present children with emotional challenges with which they must cope. Mental health professionals are often called upon to evaluate and treat children who suffer from psychosomatic disorders and emotional reactions to medical illness. Illness may be "faked" deliberately by a child, or emotions may be channeled into physical symptoms when direct expression of distress seems impossible or too threatening. Complaints such as stomachaches and headaches are extremely common in children and adolescents, and often are reactions to separation anxiety, phobias, and family strife. (For example, in a home where the father physically abuses the mother, a child may develop stomach pain so as not to have to go to school and leave mother alone.) Often, chronic stomachaches and headaches run in families, where children who communicate their emotional difficulties through physical symptom formation seem to learn such behavior from their parents. When children are brought to health care professionals complaining of nonspecific symptoms for which no organic basis can be found, it is important to consider depression, anxiety, and family crisis as possible causal factors.

Major medical illnesses are difficult for any child to cope with, and the extent to which illness can be tolerated and adapted to by the child depends on his or her stage of development, on the nature of the illness and the extent to which it interferes with the child's activities, on the child's relationships to his or her parents, and on the parents' reactions to the illness and their willingness to assist the child in efforts at coping.

Most young children react to illness with regression. They may, for example, revert to bedwetting, thumb sucking, or clinging behavior. This is expectable and usually resolves when the stress of the illness has passed. Younger children often do not understand their condition and interpret illness as a punishment for having been bad. Hospitalization is a major stress for almost any child, particularly for younger children who may have difficulty tolerating separation from parents, frequent encounters with strangers, new routines for dressing and eating, and painful medical procedures.

When illness touches on the special vulnerabilities of a child's developmental struggle at a particular phase of life, the child's anxiety about the illness may be greatly increased. For example, a surgical procedure may greatly exacerbate a 5-year-old's castration fears. Similarly, an adolescent immobilized with an injury may have heightened concerns about passivity and loss of self-control. Adolescents may use medical illness as a vehicle for acting out rebellion toward parents and other authorities (e.g., the diabetic teenager who refuses to take his insulin). Some children and adolescents do not express emotional distress during the course of a medical illness, but symptoms such as fears and night terrors may appear after the illness has passed.

Chronic illness poses particular problems for the developing child. Five percent of children and adolescents suffer from some form of chronic illness, with asthma and epilepsy the most common conditions in this age group. Chronic illnesses usually require adherence to some long-term treatment regimen, including special diets, medications, and/or restriction of activity. Young children may be confused by their illness and may develop frightening fantasies about it. Children may suffer self-esteem problems if they come to feel significantly different from their peers who do not have such conditions (as is common, for example, among hemophiliac children). Also, children are likely to be influenced by their parents' and siblings' reactions to their illness. Family members may be unduly anxious, depressed, or angry about the illness and the stresses it places on the entire household. Parents of children with potentially life-threatening illnesses such as asthma and congenital heart disease often behave overprotectively toward their children, fostering prolonged dependency and a lack of autonomy in the child.

The mental health professional is often called upon to determine the extent to which a physically ill child's emotional stress is due to the child's difficulties, to family tensions, and to the medical condition itself. You can do a great deal to help children and their families cope with illness by educating them about the illness, by giving parents and children a place to share their fears and frustrations about the condition, by working with families on responsible management of the illness, and by helping to minimize the trauma of medical procedures and hospitalizations. The latter can be done by helping the child to anticipate what he or she is likely to encounter in the hospital and by promoting frequent visits between parents and child when the child is in the hospital.

Depression

Depression occurs in children and adolescents as it does in adults, and the depressive disorders are discussed in Chapter 6. However, symptoms of depression in children vary somewhat from those commonly seen in older people, and what follows is a brief discussion of these differences.

There is controversy about what constitutes manifestations of depression in younger children. Many clinicians have advocated the concept of "masked depression"—depression that manifests in a variety of symptoms that are not typically associated with a depressed mood. Depressive equivalents in children are thought to include antisocial behavior (lying, stealing, running away from home), proneness to accidents, chronic boredom and fatigue, irritability, and escape into fantasy worlds (e.g., preoccupation with fantasy games like "Dungeons and Dragons") to the exclusion of participation in family and school life. Many depressed youngsters will not report depression or sad feelings, but will simply look sad most of the time, be inactive, and lack curiosity.

Children often become depressed after some loss, such as the death of a parent or friend, the death of a pet, parental divorce, or a failing grade at school. In some cases, a child becomes depressed in identification with a depressed parent or in reaction to the loss of parental care that results when a parent becomes depressed. Depressive symptoms may be short-lived and self-limited when they occur in reaction to a life event (in which case, the syndrome is diagnosed as an adjustment reaction), or symptoms may persist for many months.

Depression in adolescents often occurs without the unhappy, withdrawn presentation we usually associate with depressive disorders. Teenagers may deliberately hide their depression. Moreover, they may be unaware of feeling depressed, yet manifest their distress in symptoms such as headache, school failure, school refusal, hyperactivity, promiscuity, antisocial behavior, or drug abuse. Vegetative symptoms may or may not be present. Whereas some depressed teenagers lose weight, others gain. They may binge or starve, sleep long or little, be aggressive and boastful or withdrawn and self-deprecating, be outgoing or isolative. Depression is complicated by the considerable extent to which adolescents may make use of reaction formation (see Chapter 2). Factors contributing to depression in teenagers are similar to those thought to affect adults: biological, psychological, social. Adolescents may be particularly prone to depression when their attempts at separation and independence from parents generate feelings of loss and fears of abandonment.

While symptomatic behaviors may mask depression in children and adolescents, a skillful interview can readily unmask the underlying mood disturbance. In play interviews with children, their make-believe characters will often times be hopeless or exhibit murderous or suicidal feelings. Children may be able to tell you when their mood changed if they are asked in a developmentally appropriate way (e.g., "Did you begin to lose energy before Christmas or after?"). Similarly, they can tell you about such subtle symptoms as diurnal variation if asked in relation to their daily routines (e.g., "Do you usually have less energy before recess or after?").

In addition to meeting with the child or adolescent along with their families, the patient must be interviewed alone as part of a thorough examination of mood disturbance and suicidal feelings. It is reported that up to 70% of suicidal children and adolescents will deny such severity of upset when asked in front of their parents.

Treatment

Most children and adolescents respond promptly to psychosocial treatment. For children, interventions with parents and other family members are the first priority, particularly when the child needs parental help in weathering a crisis and accepting a loss, or when a parent is depressed. Play therapy is often helpful in allowing younger children to play out and rework problems and conflicts that are troubling them. Older children and adolescents can be greatly helped by psychotherapy, which allows them to verbalize and understand feelings, and provides them with experiences that enhance their self-esteem. This may occur individually or in groups.

Some adolescents with vegetative signs who do not respond to psychotherapy will respond to antidepressant medication. Younger children have also been shown, in some cases, to benefit from antidepressant therapy. Because prepubertal children are more sensitive to the cardiovascular side effects of tricyclics, these medications should be used with caution by experienced child psychiatrists. Intensive psychotherapy continues to be the mainstay of treatment for depression in children and adolescents.

Suicide

In recent years, the media have given increasing attention to the problem of suicide among adolescents. Suicide is one of the leading causes of death among teenagers and is increasing in this age group. Equally alarming is the dramatic increase in suicides among younger children; the rate of suicide among children ages 5 through 12 has more than doubled in the last two decades. Suicide is almost certainly underreported in children and adolescents, as it is among adults. Many suspicious deaths are recorded as "accidents."

Factors that prompt children and adolescents to attempt suicide are many and varied. Suicidal behavior commonly occurs around family losses such as separation, divorce, or death of a parent. Suicide by a parent or suicidal behavior and depression in a parent seem to predispose children to suicidal thoughts and behavior. Adolescents and children commonly report making suicide attempts out of anger or desperation at a family or social situation that seems hopeless and intolerable. Very often, suicide attempts represent a call for help, when the child or teenager is in severe emotional distress yet cannot ask for assistance more directly. Depression can prompt suicidal behavior, as can psychosis (e.g., in response to an hallucination). Younger children may be unable to grasp the concept of death as irreversible and think only of joining a loved person in heaven, or they may view death as a pleasant place to which they can escape when real life seems unbearable.

Treatment involves taking suicidal thoughts, threats, or gestures very seriously. Even when it appears that suicide threats are clearly manipulative or an expression of anger, the child should be given psychiatric attention immediately, and the extent of the child's distress should be acknowledged clearly. Hospitalization is often necessary when children cannot negotiate a "no suicide" contract, when depression or psychosis requires intensive treatment, or when the home situation seems to encourage further suicidal behavior (e.g., when family members give the child the message that he or she is expendable). Psychotherapy is usually indicated for the child and often for parents as well, and the focus is often on dealing with precipitating losses or finding more appropriate ways to express anger. Antidepressants are used less often with suicidal children and teenagers than they are with suicidal adults; but where serious depression is a contributing factor, these medications may be an important part of the treatment plan. As with suicidal adults (see Chapters 15 and 18), antidepressants must be used with great caution in treating suicidal children and adolescents. These medications are potentially lethal in overdose, so access to them must be carefully controlled by the prescribing physician and the child's parents.

Child Abuse

In the past two decades, there has been increasing recognition that child abuse has reached near epidemic proportions in our society. Like suicide, child abuse is underreported, and only a fraction of abused children get professional help. The term "abuse" covers a wide range of maltreatment, including neglect and deprivation of food, clothes and shelter, emotional neglect, verbal thrashings, actual physical assault, sexual activity, and murder.

Many parents who physically abuse their children were abused themselves as children, although no causal relationship has been demonstrated. Mothers are more likely than fathers to be child batterers, presumably due to the greater responsibility that mothers bear for child-rearing in most households, and the resulting greater intensity of the mother-child relationship. In cases of maternal abuse, the father often contributes to the problem in important but less obvious ways, through absence from the home and/or abuse of the mother. Fathers often abuse children directly as well.

There is a high correlation between a child's premature delivery and low birth weight, and subsequent child abuse, presumably because parents have difficulty coping with the child's extra needs and slower development. Also, premature babies are often separated from their mothers for long periods of time immediately after delivery, which may disrupt the normal process of maternal-child bonding. While child abuse occurs in all types of families and cuts across all socioeconomic lines, families in which abuse occurs are typically plagued with unemployment and financial problems, drug and alcohol addiction, divorce, and mental illness. Child batterers are often socially isolated, lacking peers who can suggest ways of handling parenting and disciplinary problems.

Children who are not obviously physically battered but who show signs of parental neglect and deprivation are considered to suffer from a maltreatment syndrome. Emotionally and physically deprived infants commonly show signs of failure to thrive (i.e., failure to grow and gain weight at age-appropriate rates), malnutrition, poor hygiene, minor cuts and abrasions, emotional withdrawal, retarded intellectual development, and apathy. As they get older, these infants often become children whose physical and intellectual growth has been stunted as a result of chronic parental deprivation.

Physical abuse is often difficult to detect, because children fear retaliation by parents if they report abusive behavior and because children love and fear the loss of the abusive parent. Battered children are sometimes brought to professionals for medical care with injuries that are the result of "accidents." Physical abuse should be suspected when the parents' history of what happened does not fit with the child's injuries, when families make multiple hospital visits to different hospitals (to avoid discovery of a pattern of injuries), and when parents are reluctant to share information about what happened. Moreover, when physical examination reveals multiple bruises above the waist, and when X-ray studies show multiple old fractures, physical abuse is highly likely.

Sexual abuse is even more difficult to detect than physical abuse. The term "sexual abuse" refers to a variety of situations in which a child under 18 years of age is used for the sexual purposes of another person. This includes any sexual contact with an adult, a nonfamilial older child or adolescent, a sibling (usually 5 years older or more), or involvement of the child in prostitution or pornography. Sexual abuse may occur among children close in age if threats or bribery is used to make a child participate in sexual acts. It most often occurs between fathers or stepfathers and latency-age daughters, but it can occur between mothers and sons, fathers and sons, and between adults outside the home and children of either sex. When incest occurs between parent and child, it is usually in the context of a disturbed marital relationship.

Sexually abused children often tell no one of their participation in sexual activities. They usually know that such behavior is wrong even before they have the words to describe it, but keep silent out of shame, fear, guilt, and a wish to protect the participating adult. No single sign is evidence that a child has been sexually abused. However, the following should lead parents and clinicians to consider the possibility of sexual abuse:

1. Unexplained injuries or pain in the child's genital area, including blood stains in underwear. (Such physical signs are present in less than 10% of sexual abuse victims.)
2. Sudden changes in behavior, such as fear of a familiar person or place.
3. More general signs of upset, including loss of appetite, nightmares, increased irritability, school difficulties, or abdominal complaints for which no physical cause can be found.

Children often come to the attention of educators and mental health professionals for failing grades or symptoms of depression but with no stated complaints of sexual abuse. A careful and thorough family evaluation, along with the development of a trusting relationship with the child, is essential in uncovering sexual abuse.

Abused children are in great physical and psychological danger, and abuse constitutes an emergency. If the child has any physical complaints, he or she must be given medical attention at once to rule out and treat physical injuries. Physicians and other health care professionals are legally obligated to report instances of abuse and suspected abuse to the relevant child protection agency in the community, and immediate intervention is necessary to assure that the child comes to no further harm. If possible, the perpetrator should be removed from the home in order for the child to remain with the family while the evaluation is conducted. The child's safety must be guaranteed. Extensive family treatment is essential if the child is to be allowed to remain at home, and foster care may be necessary. Whenever you suspect that a child has been physically or sexually abused, you must be sure that a thorough medical and psychiatric evaluation is done and that the child's family is involved in exploring the child's current situation. When in doubt, consult a supervisor or someone experienced in working with abused children. Do not leave your suspicions unexplored.

BIBLIOGRAPHY

Achenbach T: The classification of children's psychiatric symptoms: a factor-analytic study. Psychological Monographs 80(7):entire no 615, 1966

American Psychiatric Association: Diagnostic and Statistical Manual of Mental Disorders, 3rd Edition, Revised. Washington, DC, American Psychiatric Association, 1987, pp 27–95

Dugan TF, Coles R (eds): The Child in Our Times: Studies in the Development of Resiliency. New York, Brunner/Mazel, 1989

Erikson EH: Childhood and Society. New York, Norton, 1954

Fraiberg S: The Magic Years. New York, Scribner's, 1959

Freud A: Normality and Pathology in Childhood: Assessments of Development. New York, International Universities Press, 1965

Johnson AM, Szurek SA: The genesis of antisocial acting out in children and adults. Psychoanal Q 21:323–343, 1952

Lewis M: Clinical Aspects of Child Development, 2nd Edition. Philadelphia, PA, Lea and Febiger, 1982

Mahler MS: Symbiosis and individuation: the psychological birth of the human infant. Psychological Study of the Child 29:89–106, 1974

Mahler MS, Pine F, Bergman A: The Psychological Birth of the Human Infant: Symbiosis and Individuation. New York, Basic Books, 1975

Noshpitz J, Cohen RL (eds): Basic Handbook of Child Psychiatry. New York, Basic Books, 1979

Pfeffer CR: The Suicidal Child. New York, Guilford Press, 1986

Rutter M, Hersov L (eds): Child and Adolescent Psychiatry: Modern Approaches, 2nd Edition. Oxford, UK, Blackwell Scientific Publications, 1985

Thomas A, Chess S: Genesis and evolution of behavioral disorders: from infancy to early adult life. Am J Psychiatry 141:1–9, 1984

Thomas A, Chess S, Birch H: Temperament and Behavior Disorders in Children. New York, Brunner/Mazel, 1968

11

Consultation–Liaison Psychiatry

Don R. Lipsitt, M.D.
Robert J. Waldinger, M.D.

PSYCHIATRY, IN ITS DERIVATION from the Greek, is the art of healing (*iatros*) the mind (*psyche*). Modern psychiatry recognizes the intimate relationship between the mind, the brain, and the body, as well as their responsiveness to both narrow and broad environmental influence. Today's psychiatrist studies the total person and attempts to avoid the pitfall of either-or approaches to medicine; rarely is disease or illness totally "physical" (organic) or totally "emotional" (nonorganic). For example, the 38-year-old business executive with a high-stress job and several physiological risk factors for heart disease not only may sustain a heart attack under the pressure of mounting psychological tension but also may react with intense emotions to the experience of life-threatening illness. Moreover, his family's high level of anxiety about his illness may heighten his own anxiety and prolong his rehabilitative course.

This synthesis of biological, psychological, and social factors in all disease has spawned the term *biopsychosocial medicine* to emphasize the totality of the person's ailments. Earlier attempts to counteract reductionistic mind-body splits in diagnosis and treatment gave rise to *psychosomatic medicine*, a subdivision of medicine believed in the 1950s to apply only to a few particular diseases. Referred to as "the holy seven," these diseases were duodenal ulcer, ulcerative colitis, essential hypertension, bronchial asthma, rheumatoid arthritis, neurodermatitis, and hyperthyroidism. These seven syndromes were thought to be psychophysiological responses to excessive affects like fear, anger, rage, resentment, grief, and disgust. The psychosomatic approach was unique in its attention to the subjective nature of mental processes as well as to the objective signs of physical alterations.

Physicians trained in psychoanalytic investigation contributed extensively to our early understanding of mind-body relationships. With new, more comprehensive knowledge of behavioral responses to psychological stimuli, psychosomatic medicine expanded its scope to include virtually the entire realm of disease and illness. Recent laboratory investigation has dispelled some of the mystery of how psychological stimuli result in physiological response, with the discovery of neurotransmitters, peptides, and immune reactions that, collectively, have sometimes been referred to as the "biochemistry of the emotions."

The application of the psychosomatic approach to medical and surgical illness of all kinds paved the way for the evolution of *consultation-liaison psychiatry*, a specialized field of psychiatry that focuses on treatment of the whole person in the hospital setting and more recently in outpatient clinical sites. Consultation-liaison psychiatry brings psychiatric principles of diagnosis and treatment to nonpsychiatric health care systems. *Psychosomatic medicine* is an approach to understanding disease onset, formulating diagnosis, and instituting treatment, which integrates both physical and emotional factors. *Behavioral medicine* draws upon techniques of behavior modification to promote psychological health and to foster adaptation and rehabilitation. All three approaches encompass the popular theories of stress-related illness mediated through physiological variables such as neural, neuroendocrine, and immune processes, and the ability of the individual to cope effectively with the medical diseases caused by these processes.

AN ILLNESS-DISEASE SPECTRUM

The difficulties of integrating mind and body have permeated medical education and practice for centuries. New discoveries in neuroscience will help to bridge this dualistic gap but will never totally close it. Thus, the clinician must maintain an openness and fluidity in thinking about people whose ailments are multidetermined, in order to be able to shift between two polarities of physicality and emotionality without being confined to one or the other.

Physical and emotional experiences can be represented as two poles of a continuum (see Figure 11-1). If "illness" is defined as a subjective experience of distress without physical disorder, and "disease" is defined

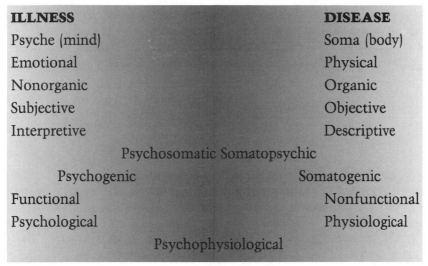

ILLNESS	DISEASE
Psyche (mind)	Soma (body)
Emotional	Physical
Nonorganic	Organic
Subjective	Objective
Interpretive	Descriptive
Psychosomatic Somatopsychic	
Psychogenic	Somatogenic
Functional	Nonfunctional
Psychological	Physiological
Psychophysiological	

Figure 11-1. An illness-disease spectrum. The more darkly shaded areas indicate regions of overlap; the more lightly shaded areas indicate polarities.

as malfunction of the body with or without conscious awareness, then most conditions for which people seek medical help fall somewhere toward the middle of this illness-disease continuum. Psychiatric nomenclature tries to avoid the either-or dilemma by referring almost exclusively to "disorders."

The psychiatrist who works in medical settings assesses clinical problems using a variety of conceptual frameworks, including psychosocial, psychodynamic, biomedical, psychoneuroendocrinological, psychoneuroimmunological, and psychopharmacological frameworks. The goal is to arrive at a useful synthesis of the data while living under the shadow of varying degrees of uncertainty and ambiguity.

In common parlance, polarized words referring to mind and body convey emphasis on one or the other. Realistically, all states involve both aspects in varying degrees; thus, the words "psychosomatic" and "somatopsychic" are the most accurate descriptors of all disordered states.

To illustrate, using schizophrenia as an example, our attention is drawn primarily to mental symptoms and their treatment, although we know that there are genetic, physiological, and anatomic abnormalities in this disorder. Irritable bowel disease, on the other hand, presents with prominent physical signs and symptoms, but treatment must also attend to psychological factors.

Signs and symptoms can be misleading. For example, a young woman who develops paralysis of her legs just prior to her wedding day has dramatic physical signs, yet she may be suffering from a conversion disorder caused by psychological conflict. On the other hand, a 50-year-old man who has become irritable and demanding with his loved ones over the last 6 months appears to have developed a personality disorder, but these personality changes may be early manifestations of a frontal lobe tumor.

CONSULTATION-LIAISON PSYCHIATRY

How can patients' emotional concerns be more than secondary issues compared to life-threatening physical conditions? If you look closely, you will see that emotional symptoms appear in almost everyone seeking medical care. Without sensitivity to this component, your best efforts at physical diagnosis and treatment will be totally ineffective with some patients.

The psychiatric consultant is often asked not only to make a diagnosis and recommend treatment but also to find out "what has gone wrong" when the plans of the medical staff seem to have gone awry (e.g., when a patient who is in urgent need of medical care refuses it). The consultation-liaison psychiatrist is somewhat irreverently called the "panic patrol," or the "troubleshooter," or the "fire brigade." He or she is called upon not only for expert advice about psychiatric diagnosis and treatment but also for an understanding of human behavior, an ability to communicate, and a capacity to synthesize data from multiple sources. To the extent that you learn to incorporate these skills into your care of patients, your effectiveness as a physician will be enhanced.

Your first contact with psychiatry is likely to be with consultation-liaison psychiatry as a part of the daily activity of a medical ward. This section will therefore describe in some detail that subspecialty's contribution to patient care, and the techniques used to enhance that care.

"Consultation" has traditionally referred to the psychiatrist's role as consultant in the assessment and treatment of medical and surgical patients and their families. "Liaison" refers to the psychiatrist's role as an educator who helps medical staff understand the psychosocial stressors and repercussions of disease and hospitalization. In reality, these two functions are inseparable in modern medicine.

Clinical Approaches

The following case examples may help you get a feel for what the consultation-liaison psychiatrist does in a clinical setting. When a psychiatric consultation is requested on a medical ward, the psychiatrist may concentrate on any one or on a combination of the following approaches.

Patient-oriented approach. A patient who was admitted for surgical exploration of an acute abdomen found herself unable to sign the necessary consent forms for surgery to take place. The psychiatrist, in taking a personal history, learned that the patient's mother died during surgery 5 years ago on the day the patient was admitted. Her anxiety was related to her private belief that she might experience the same fate and to her revived grief over the loss of her mother. Exploration of these concerns and acknowledgement by her surgeon of their importance made it possible for her to consent to the necessary operation. This approach required little more than sensitive history taking and minor psychotherapeutic intervention.

Consultee-oriented approach. A surgeon called for a consultation because a patient on whom he performed a mastectomy 2 days previously seemed to have forgotten his report that her breast mass was determined to be malignant. He was concerned that she was losing her memory and that the apparent memory deficit was the result of a stroke that might have occurred during her surgery. The psychiatric consultant interviewed the patient and determined that the woman's mental status was within normal limits. He learned that she was extremely frightened prior to surgery and now denied the information given her by the physician (i.e., that the tumor was malignant) because she was not yet ready to hear it. Moreover, she was angry at her physician for insisting that she "face facts." In discussing the situation with the physician, the psychiatrist explained how the psychological defense of denial worked in this case, and made suggestions about how and when to give the patient information so that she would not be overwhelmed by it but could engage in meaningful discussion about her follow-up care and prognosis.

Situation-oriented approach. The charge nurse on a medical ward requested a psychiatric assessment of a situation that was creating turmoil and dissension among her staff. A young female patient behaved in a demanding and surly manner most of the time, but with certain staff members she seemed compliant and "sweet." The psychiatrist held a case conference with the staff and from their reports determined that the patient was "splitting" the team—that is, she viewed some staff as good and some as bad. In response, the "bad" staff members saw the patient as angry and difficult, while the "good" staff found her charming. Not surprisingly, each group felt the other misunderstood this patient, and they disagreed on how best to provide nursing care. By suggesting to the staff that they were the objects of a process of splitting that is typical of borderline personality disorder, the psychiatrist helped them to get some distance on the situation, to have an intellectual appreciation of the problem, and to avoid taking it personally. The psychiatrist interviewed the patient in front of the staff and in doing so illustrated many features of her personality disorder and showed them techniques for setting limits on the patient's verbal abuse of her treaters. He also suggested ways to provide structure to her days in the hospital and enhance her compliance with necessary nursing and medical interventions.

Crisis-oriented approach. Early one morning, a house officer called for an emergency psychiatric consultation, indicating that an elderly foreign-born man had "gone psychotic" during the night. The man was threatening to sign out of the hospital because, in his words, "the little girls were trying to hold me down." When the psychiatrist arrived, he found the patient lying in bed with his trousers on. He was agitated and insisted on leaving. The nurse described how he got up during the night to urinate, even though he was supposed to be on bed rest. Two or three student nurses were enlisted to urge him back to bed, whereupon he became so angry that he smashed his glass urinal on the floor, cutting the leg of one student and frightening them all. On examination, the psychiatrist found that the man was not psychotic. In broken, accented English, he reported with embarrassment that he had recently undergone a prostatectomy and orchidectomy for prostate cancer. While he had difficulty communicating because of the language barrier, he nonetheless could make himself understood. As he relaxed in talking with the psychiatric consultant about his life, he told tales of achievement and bravery in his native land. He revealed a sense of humiliation that, in his view, the surgery had deprived him of his manhood. Once he was given an opportunity to tell his story and discuss his feelings about his illness, he became calm. He agreed to remain in the hospital for the necessary treatment and was assigned a male nurse who could talk to him "man to man." The crisis dissolved and the misapplied label of "psychotic" was deleted from his diagnosis.

The usual consultation involves variations of all these approaches, and liaison with hospital staff is almost always a part of each consult. Before any approach can be effective, it is essential that the psychiatrist establish an alliance with both patient and staff. The role taken by the psychiatric consultant in an individual case will depend upon several factors: the stated (and unstated) reasons for the consultation request; the types of individuals involved in the patient's care; the unique characteristics of the patient; and the nature of the problem.

The above examples illustrate the psychiatrist's role as interpreter, translator, and communicator. The psychiatrist can, just as readily, be called on to be a peacemaker in a tense situation, or a facilitator of doctor-patient relationships and patient care. Not infrequently, the psychiatrist is called on when ethical issues confront the staff with seemingly impossible dilemmas. In the face of highly ambiguous circumstances, physicians (and others) can become very anxious about decision making. For example, an elderly alert woman who had been admitted to the hospital following upper gastrointestinal bleeding refused to have a diagnostic gastroscopy. The woman shared with the new intern on the medical ward a copy of her living will to emphasize her right to refuse further examination. The intern, angry at being made to feel helpless, requested a psychiatric consultation. There was no psychiatric problem except to help the intern understand his anxiety at allowing a patient to leave the hospital without a complete assessment. It also became clear to the intern that his reason for requesting psychiatric consultation was based on the unreasonable expectation that the psychiatrist would talk the patient into a procedure she did not want. In such instances, the psychiatrist must take special care not to appear critical of either patient or physician in clarifying the issues.

The Consultation

Request for consultation

Psychiatric consultation may be requested by medical personnel when they encounter problems in the diagnosis, management, treatment, or outcome of the patient's disease. Recognition of the need for consultation depends upon a variety of factors, including the extent to which the patient's behavior or response interferes with treatment; the quality of relationships the patient has with the staff; the presence of identifiable psychopathology; medicolegal concerns; lack of response to usual treatments; and suspicion that the patient may be suicidal.

It is not unusual for obvious psychiatric disturbances in medical or surgical patients to go unrecognized and undocumented by medical staff. Studies of primary-care physicians' ability to diagnose depression have shown marked underrecognition and undertreatment. Because of recent changes in health care delivery, including rapid discharge of hospitalized patients, psychiatric consultation is often omitted from hospital care except when psychiatric illness interferes with medical treatment.

The reason stated for psychiatric consultation may be just the tip of an iceberg. For example, a medical resident requested a consultation on a patient who refused to sign a consent form for a barium enema. Discussion with the physician, examination of the patient's record, and an interview of the patient raised questions about the indications for the procedure and suggested that it had been ordered by the resident physician and resisted by the patient because there was some covert anger between them.

In pursuing the matter, the psychiatric consultant learned that the patient was resisting discharge on a very busy medical service, the attending physician was pushing the resident to "do something" with the patient, and the resident physician was in a quandary about how to justify the patient's continuing presence on the ward. Although the diagnosis was uncertain, the patient's admitting complaint of chronic diarrhea had been quiescent for several days. On morning rounds, the suggestion of a barium enema was presented, accompanied by some high-spirited laughter. In talking with the resident, the psychiatrist pointed out how frequently we all are unaware of ways in which we try to deal with our own and our patients' feelings. The consultant took care not to focus on the individual resident's behavior. The resident's wish to punish his patient probably had deeper personal roots, but these did not need to be explored for the purposes of this consultation. Such intervention calls for the utmost respect and colleagueship in addressing the problem.

Determining the reasons for a consultation request

In order to understand the covert as well as the overt reasons for a consultation request, the psychiatric consultant scrutinizes the patient's medical chart and solicits staff input about the patient.

Chart review. The medical record reveals a great deal of social and demographic data about the patient. It often contains staff opinions about the patient's treatment, along with the indications for consultation. Laboratory tests, vital signs, and a complete review of medication history are useful, particularly when the patient's mental status is in question. As a psychiatric consultant working in a medical setting, you must be alert to the presence of organic contributors to what medical staff have labeled "behavioral problems." Knowledge of those somatopsychic illnesses that are accompanied by mental symptoms will equip you for this challenge (see Table 11-1).

Familiarity with the patient's chart should not preclude asking patients to describe their own perception of their illness and treatment. On occasion, a patient may ask why the consultant is taking a history when "it's all in my chart." Often, you can reassure the patient and strengthen your alliance with a response such as, "I know I can read your record, but I would prefer to hear your story directly from you." Patients are usually grateful for such an expression of personal interest.

Patients sometimes express curiosity about what appears in their records and may ask to see them. In this situation, it is best to suggest that they discuss the matter with their primary physician. Patients have the legal right to read their medical records. All notes in the chart should be carefully written to respect the patient's confidentiality. They should be free of offensive or critical comments. This is especially important in cases where negative staff attitudes toward the patient or other staff have prompted the request for a psychiatric consultation.

Staff comments. Important information about the patient can be gleaned from the collective impressions of nurses, house officers, and attending physicians. For the psychiatric consultant, what sounds like anecdote or even gossip may be very revealing of an individual's character, behavior, or symptomatology. The input of nurses is especially useful, because they spend much of their working day (and night) with the patient, responding to the patient's needs and demands, and observing the patient interacting with other patients, friends, and family. These observations are sometimes more instructive than formal notes entered into the patient's chart. Information about changes over time, as in a delirium caused by medication, is more reliable from someone whose observation of the patient is more episodic. Keep in mind, also, that inviting input from staff immediately includes them in the diagnostic and therapeutic team that will help to carry out recommendations for the psychosocial care of the patient; you can begin this process following the patient interview by sharing your findings and impressions with interested staff. It is also advisable to share your impressions, formulation, and recommendations with the person who requested the consultation even before the formal note is written.

Consultation-Liaison Interviewing

The setting of the interview

The conditions for interviewing a patient in a medical hospital are seldom ideal. The patient is often in pain, or there are others in the room, so that privacy is not possible. Nurses, physicians, and other members of the army of caregivers in a hospital often dart in and out during an interview with important medications, questions, or instructions; there is almost inevitably distracting noise. The presence of other patients in the room, separated only by a curtain, can be expected to foster self-consciousness, embarrassment, and restraint in the person being interviewed. Patients who persist in telling their stories in this inhospitable environment do, indeed, want to be heard.

Table 11-1. Somatopsychic conditions and their mental symptoms

Disease	Mental symptoms
Endocrine	
Hyperthyroidism	Anxiety, depression
Hypothyroidism	Lethargy, anxiety, irritability, thought disorder, somatic delusions, hallucinations
Hyperparathyroidism Hypoparathyroidism	Anxiety, hyperactivity, irritability, apathy, depression, withdrawal
Hyperadrenalism (Cushing's Disease)	Depression, anxiety, thought disorder, somatic delusions
Hypoadrenalism (Addison's Disease)	Depression, negativism, apathy, thought disorder, suspiciousness
Hypoglycemia (insulinoma)	Anxiety, fear, dread, depression, fatigue
Metabolic	
Uremic encephalopathy	Apathy, fatigue, depression, delirium
Hepatic encephalopathy	Restlessness, tremor, agitation, delirium
Hepatolenticular degeneration (Wilson's disease)	Mood swings (sudden and changeable), explosive anger, psychosis
CO_2 intoxication (e.g., COPD)	Lethargy, disorientation, hypersomnia
Infectious	
AIDS	Depression, anxiety, disorientation
Pneumonia	Depression, delirium
Infectious mononucleosis	Severe anxiety, depression
Tuberculosis	Personality changes, irritability, apathy, lethargy, depression
Viral hepatitis	Depression, lethargy, weakness, irritability, late psychosis

Table 11-1. *Continued*

Disease	Mental symptoms
Syphilis—general paresis	Personality change, dementia, mania, psychosis
Nutritional	
Pellagra	Depression, confusion, psychosis
Wernicke's encephalopathy	Depression, altered awareness, psychosis
Korsakoff's syndrome	Retrograde amnesia, inability to learn, confabulation, psychosis
Pernicious anemia	Depression, feelings of guilt, worthlessness
Collagen/Vascular	
Systemic lupus erythematosus	Depression, psychosis, delirium
Cranial arteritis	Malaise, lassitude, irritability, mood changes
Cerebrovascular disease	Similar to dementia
Neoplastic	
Intracranial tumors	Varied according to site: personality changes, depression, anxiety, memory loss, psychosis
Pancreatic tumor	Early depression, sense of imminent doom without guilt
Other	
Multiple sclerosis	Personality changes, mood swings
Porphyria	Severe sudden anxiety, mood swings
Steroid psychosis	Hallucinations, delusions
Head injury	Personality change, anxiety, irritability, rage, psychosis
Pheochromocytoma	Anxiety, panic, fear, apprehension, trembling

Note. COPD = chronic obstructive pulmonary disease.

Introducing yourself

In spite of these drawbacks, the psychiatric consultant can do much to put the patient at ease. Introduce yourself by name and specialty: "Hello. I'm Dr. Fields from the Psychiatry Department." If this provokes a startled or hesitant response from the patient, you may need to state the reason for your visit: "Your doctor, Dr. Albert, asked me to come by and see you. Did you have some discussion with him about this?" Try to learn *from your patients* what they have been told or what they imagine to be your reason for coming; it is possible to give reassuring explanations only if you know what fears, distortions, or expectations the patient has. Simple clarification may be all that is needed: "Dr. Albert thought you were having a difficult time with your (pain, operation, hospitalization, etc.)." For most patients, this is usually sufficient to prompt further comment from them and to overcome any initial apprehension about talking with you. Should a patient continue to be apprehensive, you might explain that emotional care of the patient is a regular part of treatment in your hospital.

To promote further interaction, it is helpful to situate yourself so that the patient can make eye contact with you. Sitting on the patient's bed or using first names in attempting to put the patient and yourself more at ease will frequently have the opposite effect.

Time

It is usually not possible or even desirable in the consultation-liaison role to set definite time limits on each contact with a patient. Some patients will welcome the opportunity to talk and will need long interviews, whereas others who are reluctant to discuss emotional matters may be discomfited by your visit and cut it short or postpone it. As a consultant, you may have several consultations to perform in a single day, and you might begin by stopping by to introduce yourself to the patients and assess the urgency of each situation. You can then attend to the most pressing matters first and return to the others at a time of greater leisure. In some cases, you will be able to answer the questions raised by the consultee after only a few minutes at the patient's bedside. More complicated cases may require several visits with the patient as well as discussions with members of the treatment team.

Interviewing techniques

Consultation-liaison psychiatry requires specialized interviewing skills. Unlike a psychiatric evaluation performed in an outpatient clinic or inpatient psychiatric ward, where the patient expresses a wish for psychiatric help, the interview of a medical patient usually takes place because someone other than the patient has requested a consultation. Patients usually do not identify themselves as having a psychiatric problem. Nor has the usually brief preparation given them by their physician alleviated fears, distortions, and resistances commonly associated with a visit from a psychiatrist.

At the bedside of a medical patient, the psychiatrist uses an interviewing style that is at once more psychosocial and psychodynamic than routine medical history taking, yet less intensely focused on psychopathology than that used in a typical psychiatric evaluation. This technique involves a synthesis of two languages of the two conceptual worlds of psyche and soma.

Use the patient's physical condition as a starting point. The patient is focused on physical illness, because that is what prompted admission to the hospital. Medical or surgical patients in the hospital may be puzzled by questions that refer too persistently to feelings or the nature of important relationships. Questions that flow most naturally from, and use the language of, the medical condition will generally put the patient most at ease. While obtaining pertinent data about the patient's physical condition, the psychiatrist listens for clues to troublesome areas in the person's social and psychological life that may have bearing on the etiology, symptomatology, or outcome of the medical situation.

Balance interest in the patient's physical condition with attention to emotional concerns. As you gather information about a patient's medical condition, feelings may spontaneously emerge. Acknowledging their presence (e.g., by a simple "That was upsetting to you?") is usually sufficient to express understanding and acceptance. Because patients with physical disorders may have difficulty expressing themselves in the language of feelings, your insistence that they tell you about their feelings may disrupt and prematurely terminate an interview.

If the interview is "too medical," the patient may assume that you are there to answer questions about his or her illness. Should this happen, it is best to explain the consultant's role and not to attempt to provide medical answers even if you think you may have them. If the patient's lack of information turns out to be part of the explanation for anxiety or fear, you can discuss the situation with the person requesting the consultation and recommend ways to remedy the situation.

Pay attention to the patient's resistances. It is important to remember that the medical patient in a hospital setting seldom requests a psychiatric consultation and might never consider it outside the hospital.

It is a setting, therefore, in which the consultant must be especially alert to the patient's possible fear of psychiatrists and rejection of the consultation. If you approach patients tactfully and sensitively, you will usually receive a comfortable and welcoming response from the patient. Most hospitalized patients respond eagerly to an interested, attentive, empathic physician.

You can help diminish resistance by avoiding common pitfalls during the interview, such as:

1. Being too aggressive about your own agenda at the expense of the patient's (e.g., ignoring the patient's mention of a recent death in the family in order to pursue a history of an old quiescent ulcer)
2. Being overly passive in exploring personal issues (e.g., reluctance to ask about a man's sex life when discussing his recent prostatectomy)
3. Being too zealous in pursuit of feelings out of proportion to facts (e.g., asking a patient repeatedly how he felt about his dog's death when he makes it clear that he wants to change the subject)

Assess the patient's coping mechanisms. Physical illness usually involves a loss of physical function and with it, a loss of self-esteem. It is especially important, therefore, to assess patients' strengths, including their patterns of response to earlier losses and traumas. Even during a single interview, you can bolster defenses and give reassurance based on what the patient has told you about effective coping styles in the past. For example, a patient is seen who is so depressed that she believes she cannot ever adapt to her recent diagnosis of multiple sclerosis. As the history unfolds, she reports many previous instances of hardship, all of which she coped with successfully. Underscoring this patient's prior experience and calling attention to strengths she has temporarily "forgotten" result in immediate improvement in her attitude.

Learn to recognize when enough is enough. At a certain point in the interview, you will have sufficient data to answer questions posed by the consultee even though the history you have taken is incomplete. The beginner will always feel uneasy with this incompleteness and uncertainty, but experience will demonstrate the appropriateness of an abbreviated approach. For example, a physician requested a psychiatric consultation on a patient who appeared depressed, asking if an antidepressant was indicated. In a relatively brief time, the psychiatrist determined that the patient had a history of sadness since the death of his wife 5 years ago. He manifested the "vegetative triad" of depression—loss of appetite, constipation, and insomnia—and exhibited traits of a passive-dependent personality. The consultant does not have to learn all about the patient's early life, his schooling and occupational history, and the nuances of the patient's interpersonal relations to be able to answer effectively the consultee's questions and to recommend a trial of antidepressant medication.

Closing the interview

At the end of an interview, you may need to spend a few minutes helping the patient regain composure if he or she has become very distressed or tearful. The way that you end each encounter is as important as your introduction, especially since you may see this patient only once. In closing, it is often helpful to offer an empathic summary of your discussion such as, "This operation has frightened you because you're accustomed to being strong and active, and right now you feel weak." You can then assure the patient of the relevance of your encounter by indicating that you will be talking with his or her doctor; this highlights the continuity of treatment and enhances the patient's relationship with the primary physician. It is, of course, important to heed the patient's wish to maintain confidentiality about any specific revelations.

Writing the Consult Note

Most patients are so receptive and eager to tell their story that you will be impressed with how much information you can acquire in even a brief interview. It is the task of the consultant to prune and organize this data into a lucid, jargon-free, relevant note, addressing the specific questions of the consultation request and other relevant issues you may identify in your interview. The patient will tell you much that is of interest and helpful in your comprehensive evaluation. However, great discretion must be exercised in deciding how much of what you know needs to be written in the record. Unfortunately, this document will never be a foolproof keep-safe for the patient's confidential remarks.

A useful summary will state the following:

- The nature of the consultation request
- The reason for the patient's hospitalization
- A brief summary of the hospital course
- The meaning of the illness experience to the patient
- Findings of a mental status examination
- A description of the patient's characteristic pattern of dealing with stress or trauma
- A formulation of the problem and its etiology, diagnostic impressions, and a list of recommendations

If your recommendations include the use of psychopharmacological agents, both generic and trade names as well as proper dosages should be included. If you find that the patient is suicidal, provide explicit directions for promoting the patient's safety. Even though you may have discussed the patient with the physician and other staff, all recommendations must be very clearly stated in the note.

PSYCHOTHERAPY WITH MEDICAL-SURGICAL PATIENTS

Sometimes attending physicians and house officers forego asking for psychiatric consultation on the mistaken assumption that psychotherapy is always a time-intensive enterprise. This misconception often deprives patients of necessary and useful help. The stereotype of the 50-minute psychotherapeutic "hour" is nowhere more challenged than at the bedside of the hospitalized nonpsychiatric patient. The psychiatrist can develop an alliance with a patient within minutes and make an effective psychotherapeutic intervention even during one bedside visit. For example, the depression that sometimes occurs as a reaction to an acute physical disorder may be adequately treated during the patient's hospitalization. Personality disorders, on the other hand, do not lend themselves to brief treatment, but psychologically informed therapeutic interventions with staff and patient can minimize the negative effects of the patient's dysfunctional relationships on his or her medical condition. Brief interventions can, as well, alleviate conversion disorders, acute anxiety reactions, acute grief reactions, delirium, psychosis, and atypical pain reactions.

Basic psychotherapeutic principles include clarification, explanation, situational manipulation based on psychological knowledge, and reassurance based upon definition of fears, fantasies, distortions, and anxieties. Patients in the hospital are usually very receptive to such simple anxiety-allaying approaches as empathic listening, information sharing, and nonjudgmental history taking.

Identifying the patient's characteristic normal personality style provides a framework for understanding individual reactions to illness. As Kahana and Bibring (1964) have pointed out, for the hospitalized patient, illness takes on meaning and coloration based on the personality variables unique to the individual (see Table 11-2). Recognizing these characteristics helps the caregiver shape the treatment plan to the patient's needs and capacity to comply.

These characteristic personality types, which usually overlap, are as follows:

Table 11-2. Personality types in medical management

Personality type	Psychodynamic descriptor	Illness behavior	Treatment approach
Dependent, overdemanding	Oral, needy	Urgent requests	Show signs of caring, but with clear limit setting
Orderly, controlled	Compulsive	Self-disciplined	Use "scientific" approach; share information
Dramatizing, emotional	Hysterical	Flighty, teasing	Calm "professional" approach
Long-suffering, self-sacrificing	Masochistic	Help-rejecting	Avoid excessive reassurance; acknowledge pain
Guarded, querulous	Paranoid	Suspicious, wary	Acknowledge, but do not reinforce perceptions; do not argue or withhold information
Superior, grandiose	Narcissistic	Exaggerated self-confidence	Do not challenge patient's "expert" status
Uninvolved, aloof	Schizoid	Seeks isolation	Accept "unsociability," but avoid complete withdrawal

Source. Adapted from Kahana and Bibring 1964.

- Dependent, demanding type
- Orderly, controlling (obsessive-compulsive) type
- Dramatizing, histrionic (hysterical) type
- Long-suffering, self-sacrificing (masochistic) type
- Guarded, suspicious (paranoid) type
- Superior, special (narcissistic) type
- Seclusive, aloof (schizoid) type

It is important that these "types" not be used pejoratively to stereotype patients, but rather as guides to tailoring treatment for optimal results. For example, the obsessive-compulsive patient may respond best when information about the patient's condition is shared in great detail and when the physician invites the patient to participate actively in treatment planning. The self-sacrificing patient, on the other hand, may respond best to framing treatment as something that "will help you to be able to take better care of your family."

The alliance between caregiver and patient exerts a powerful healing effect in and of itself. The understanding conveyed by the interested, accepting, noncritical physician creates a context in which the patient attributes to the physician those characteristics needed to promote well-being; this is, in fact, the essence of the placebo response. For example, a middle-aged woman patient who had ambivalent feelings about the death of an abusive father assumed that her young resident therapist was 20 years older than he was and referred to him as "the kindest man in the world." In this fantasied context, she could experience a new and different kind of relationship with an "older" man.

Although much can be accomplished therapeutically in a single visit with the patient, follow-up visits during the patient's hospitalization will be useful in some cases. Supportive care for a patient who is especially vulnerable will help sustain him or her through an anxiety-provoking illness or surgery. Informing nursing staff and others of the therapeutic strategy also helps them to build this into their nursing care plan, another way of providing support for the patient. Acute grief following an amputation, mastectomy, or disfiguring illness may benefit from several consecutive psychotherapeutic visits by the psychiatrist, the social worker, or the psychiatric liaison nurse. The impulse to save time by administering medications for such crises should be resisted, because pharmacological intervention for acute grief is often a deterrent to coping effectively with this condition.

There is, of course, a time and place for judicious use of medications. The importance of a thorough review of all medications taken by an individual patient cannot be overemphasized, because many conditions that appear to be psychiatric illnesses are in fact due to multiple drug interactions, polypharmacy, or side effects of properly administered medications. Exploring the patient's attitudes about drug taking, and his or her previous experiences with, fears of, and knowledge of medications, will help to assure compliance with medical recommendations.

Remember that the consultant never writes orders for psychoactive or other medications unless requested to do so by the primary physician. As consultant, your job is to offer suggestions and their rationale to the consultee for integration into the patient's treatment plan. (For more detailed discussion of the use of psychoactive agents, see Chapter 18.)

SUMMARY

Many studies have shown that physical illness and psychiatric morbidity have a strong association. Understanding and appreciating the consultative and educational value of consultation-liaison psychiatry can greatly enhance the comprehensiveness, coordination, and continuity of all medical care. Many opportunities exist for the collaboration of the primary physician and the psychiatrist in the patient's best interest.

BIBLIOGRAPHY

Hackett TP, Cassem NH (eds): Massachusetts General Hospital Handbook of General Hospital Psychiatry, 2nd Edition. Littleton, MA, PSG Publishers, 1987

Hales RE: The benefits of a psychiatric consultation-liaison service in a general hospital. Gen Hosp Psychiatry 7:214–218, 1985

Kahana RJ, Bibring GL: Personality types in medical management, in Psychiatry and Medical Practice in a General Hospital. Edited by Zinberg NE. New York, International Universities Press, 1965, pp 108–123

Leigh H, Reiser M: The Patient: Biological, Psychological, and Social Dimensions of Medical Practice, 2nd Edition. New York, Plenum, 1985

Lipowski ZJ: Consultation-liaison psychiatry: the first half century. Gen Hosp Psychiatry 8:305–315, 1986

Lipsitt DR: The difficult doctor-patient encounter, in Office Practice of Medicine, 2nd Edition. Edited by Branch W. Philadelphia, PA, WB Saunders, 1989, pp 1348–1356

Reiser MF: Mind, Brain, Body: Toward a Convergence of Psychoanalysis and Neurobiology. New York, Basic Books, 1984

12

Neuropsychiatry

Sheldon Benjamin, M.D.

MODERN PSYCHIATRY HAS BENEFITED greatly from recent advances in the neurosciences. New neurodiagnostic technology has allowed psychiatric diagnosis and treatment to become more specific, while providing a means for testing neurobiological hypotheses. In the past, the term *organic brain dysfunction* was used to describe conditions that were largely outside the purview of the psychiatrist. These same conditions, with organically based psychiatric symptoms, are now the subject of intense study as possible avenues toward further understanding of the pathophysiology of major psychiatric disorders. As research demonstrates, all symptoms of mental illness are the product of an individual's experience filtered through his or her unique neural substrate. Thus, the term *organic* no longer describes syndromes outside the psychiatric realm.

Neuropsychiatry uses diagnostic techniques drawn from neurology, behavioral neurology, and neuropsychology in combination with traditional methods of interviewing and mental status evaluation to study psychiatric conditions associated with brain abnormalities (Table 12-1). The emphasis in neuropsychiatry is on the interplay of neurological, psychodynamic, genetic, and environmental factors. An enhanced neuropsychiatric understanding of psychiatric symptomatology allows treatment—whether psychopharmacological, psychotherapeutic, be-

Table 12-1. Clinical and neuroscience areas related to neuropsychiatry

Basic sciences	Clinical sciences
Neuroanatomy	General psychiatry
Neurochemistry	Psychopharmacology
Neurophysiology	Behavioral neurology
Neuropathology	Neuropsychology
Neuroimmunology	Neuroendocrinology
Behavioral genetics	Neuroimaging

havioral, or rehabilitative—to be more precisely tailored to the individual patient.

THE NEUROPSYCHIATRIC EVALUATION

The neuropsychiatric evaluation should determine the following:

- The level of dysfunction in the nervous system
- The degree of reversibility of the dysfunction
- The nature of the interplay of relevant psychodynamic, environmental, genetic, and neurological factors
- Any special interventions that might make it easier for a patient or family to live with those aspects of the dysfunction that are not reversible

History

Neuropsychiatric evaluation begins with a thorough history that follows the outline described in Chapter 3.

In eliciting the history of the present problem, it is important to establish whether the problem is static or progressive, constant or episodic, focal or diffuse, and how the condition has altered the patient's premorbid level of functioning. To determine this, the following information should be obtained:

- The identifying data section includes a statement about the patient's handedness (e.g., a 32-year-old right-handed, married bricklayer), because atypical handedness can occasionally offer a clue to the presence of congenital neurodevelopmental abnormalities.
- Information on the patient's premorbid educational, occupational, and social adjustment to allow comparison with the

present. Important areas to review include the patient's continence, skills at activities of daily living (e.g., cooking, cleaning, dressing, shopping, driving), and hygiene.

- Note any changes in the patient's coordination or gait.
- Too often overlooked is the patient's level of sensory input. Cataracts, hearing loss, diminished olfaction, and neuropathy, so commonly associated with the aging process, should be carefully considered, because sensory deprivation can exacerbate conditions such as psychosis, delirium, and dementia.

Frequently, the patient is unaware of changes that are apparent to his or her employer and family. The family is often the best source of information about a patient's personality changes. In many cases family members initiate a neuropsychiatric evaluation because their relative has developed behaviors that are disturbing to them.

In addition to past psychiatric history, the details of any past neurological illness are included in the medical history. Of particular interest are history of head trauma, loss of consciousness, seizures, central nervous system (CNS) infections, or sudden neurological events (e.g., strokes). Note should also be made of any history of atypical reactions to psychoactive medications, history of substance abuse, or family history of psychiatric or neurological disorders.

It is sometimes difficult to determine whether a given behavior truly represents a deterioration from a higher level of functioning or whether the patient has always behaved in this way and a change in circumstances has suddenly called this behavior to attention. Sufficient premorbid functional data must be gathered to determine whether a congenital encephalopathy, learning disorder, or behavior disorder was present prior to the onset of the current problem. In the evaluation of what appears to be an early onset of dementia, for instance, it may be discovered that a patient with borderline intellectual functioning had been able to get along in society only in the context of a rigid activity structure supervised by a parent. Following the loss of that parent, the patient may not be equipped to function independently. Until the recent loss is discovered, the patient may appear to have social, occupational, and intellectual abilities characteristic of a dementing illness.

Standard psychiatric syndromes may present differently when they are expressed by an abnormal nervous system. For example, a mentally retarded patient who is unable either to express feelings verbally or to display appropriate affect may develop self-abusive behavior such as head-banging as a symptom of depression.

You may find evidence supporting congenital brain abnormality in the patient's birth history, developmental milestones, and early educational history. A history of dyslexia or other learning disorders, repeating grades in school, or conduct or attentional problems may indicate a long-standing neuropsychiatric disorder. Sometimes, just inquiring what the patient's best and worst subjects were can be revealing. If a patient had a great deal of difficulty with reading, writing, and foreign languages, the physician should consider the possibility that the patient may have been dyslexic. If learning problems surfaced in visuospatial tasks, there could have been a right-hemisphere learning disability. Further inquiry as to the specific problems a patient had with these subjects could help clarify the question.

In taking the occupational history, it is useful to have the patient explain exactly what his or her job entailed. For example, it is far more revealing to learn that a shipping clerk was continually being reprimanded for slowness at transcribing orders than to learn that he was fired for "doing a poor job."

Examination

The neuropsychiatric examination consists of a neurological examination with attention to neurodevelopmental signs that may be increased in congenital encephalopathies (Table 12-2), and a thorough mental status evaluation. (The mental status examination [MSE] is outlined in Chapter 4.) Because of the neuropsychiatric emphasis on the interaction between cognitive substrate and psychiatric symptomatology, you will want to devote more time to testing the sensorium and intellectual functions than in the general psychiatric MSE. When the patient understands that your detailed MSE is for the purpose of understanding as clearly as possible how the patient experiences his or her condition, an empathic bridge is built between you and your patient, and the alliance is enhanced. If you do not take care to help the patient understand the reasons for this detailed evaluation, it will be difficult to obtain a complete examination.

Successful neuropsychiatric mental status evaluation depends on your ability to be flexible. Regardless of whether formal testing is utilized, you must satisfy yourself that each of the major areas of mental functioning (see Table 12-3) has been evaluated. To select appropriately from the many available bedside tests of cognitive function, you need a working hypothesis as to the possible cause of the behavior in question. For example, if you suspect the presence of a syndrome following head trauma, delirium, pseudodementia, drug or metabolic effects on mental status, or attention deficit disorders, you will want to emphasize tests of attention. If you are considering the diagnosis of dementia, you will want to determine whether there has been deterioration of all major cortical functions, as is seen with Alzheimer's disease, or whether the deficits are more focal, as is seen with vascular dementias. Sometimes, an area of mental status can be evaluated adequately on the basis of the interview and observation of other task behaviors without further testing. For instance, the silly, shallow, impulsive, easily distractible, socially inappropriate behavior of a patient with an orbitofrontal syndrome often betrays the diagnosis before the examiner has begun to test individual frontal functions.

The Written Report

The examiner's assessment should list any deficits found on neurological and mental status evaluation, as well as the level, locus, or type of dysfunction suggested by the deficits. A differential diagnosis should follow, with suggestions for any tests needed to exclude possible diagnostic alternatives. Often, you will make both a psychiatric and a neurological diagnosis. Appropriate neurodiagnostic testing may be ordered to confirm or refute the hypotheses suggested by the examination. The following is a sample assessment of a patient evaluated for deterioration of neurological deficits during stroke rehabilitation:

> **Assessment:** This 56-year-old, right-handed bank teller, 6 weeks post right middle cerebral artery infarct, has a left homonymous hemianopsia, left spastic hemiparesis of arm greater than leg, left-sided hyperreflexia with left Babinski response, and a left hemisensory loss on elemental neurological examination, all of which appear to have worsened in the past 3 weeks after initial improvement. Findings on mental status evaluation include flat affect, irritability, expressive aprosodia (loss of melodic qualities of speech used to convey emotion), left hemi-inattention, denial of the significance of his deficits, denial of symptoms of depression, and constructional apraxia. Discussion with nursing staff reveals that the patient's appetite and sleep have been poor since admission. His family informs us that his job performance had fallen off and he had been more irritable at home ever since losing his mother 6 months prior to his stroke.

> The patient's deficits are consistent with involvement of the entire right middle cerebral artery bed territory in his recent stroke. Information gathered from family and nursing staff suggests that the patient also suffers from an endogenous depression that may have already been extant at the time of his stroke. The patient's flat affect, expressive aprosodia, and denial of deficits, including depressive symptoms, have masked his depression.

> Other neurological conditions to be considered as reasons for this patient's clinical deterioration would be extension of the infarction or development of a right-hemisphere seizure focus. A noncontrast head computed tomography scan will rule out the former possibility. A sleep-deprived EEG could

Table 12-2. Neurodevelopmental signs

Sign	Examination	Localizing value
Neurodevelopmental signs of little localizing value		
Dysarthria	Slurring of spontaneous speech	Many possible causes
Inability to move eyes without head motion	Difficulty following finger with eyes alone during extraocular muscle exam	Many possible causes
Nystagmus	To and fro, up and down, or rotary movements of eyeballs observed during extraocular movement examination	Brain stem/cerebellum
Clumsiness or incoordination	General motor observation	Many possible causes
Drooling	Observation	Many possible causes
Overflow movements (including mirror movements)	Movements of tongue or fingers observed when patient concentrates on moving a different body part. Mirror movements are overflow movements of the homologous contralateral body part.	Extrapyramidal motor system
Increased jaw jerk	Exaggerated response to tap of chin with mouth slightly open	Upper motor neuron
Unsustained clonus	Several quick repetitive jerks occur in response to a single deep tendon reflex tap or a quick passive movement of the tendon (usually seen at ankles or knees).	Contralateral corticospinal tract
Neurodevelopmental signs of potential localizing value		
Asymmetric size of face or extremities	One side of face, one extremity or digit smaller than corresponding area on other side of body	Contralateral hemisphere
Slow or irregular fine finger movements	Slow or incoordinated movements when patient asked to touch each finger with thumb of that hand or tap toes regularly on floor	Contralateral pyramidal tract
Slow or irregular rapid alternating movements	Slow or incoordinated movements when patient asked to alternately slap palm and dorsum of hand	Ipsilateral cerebellum

Table 12-2. *Continued*

Sign	Examination	Localizing value
	on knee or tap heel on floor	
Motor impersistence	Inability to follow sustained motor commands (e.g., prolonged arm extension or tongue protrusion) without being continually reminded of the command	Right frontal
Asymmetric deep tendon reflexes	Unilateral increase in deep tendon reflexes	Contralateral corticospinal tract
Asymmetry of involuntary/ spontaneous smile but not voluntary smile	Weakness of corner of mouth observed with smile in response to a joke but not with smile in response to the command "smile"	Contralateral temporolimbic
Dystonic posturing of hands	Hand clenches, extends, or twists while walking, especially during tandem gait examination	Contralateral pyramidal or extrapyramidal motor system
Extinction to visual double simultaneous stimulation	Patient sees only one stimulus when stimuli (e.g., wiggling fingers) are presented to both visual fields at once.	Contralateral parieto-occipital
Extinction to tactile double simultaneous stimulation	Inability to recognize touch on both sides of body at once despite intact primary sensation	Contralateral parietal
Agraphesthesia	Inability to distinguish numbers traced on palm of hand with eyes closed despite intact primary sensation	Contralateral parietal
Astereognosis	Inability to distinguish objects placed in one hand with eyes closed despite intact primary sensation	Contralateral parietal

Note. Neurodevelopmental signs have frequently been referred to as "soft signs" and are said to be increased in any type of congenital encephalopathy. However, many of them (see bottom half of table) have distinct localizing value and should be treated as any other neurological sign.

Table 12-3. Major areas of mental functioning that should be covered in the mental status examination

Mental status areas	Cognitive status areas
Appearance (dress, behavior, idiosyncrasies)	Attention
Affect	Memory
Thought process	Language
Thought content	Visuospatial skills
Potential dangerousness	Calculation
Movement	Higher intellectual functions (insight, judgment, problem-solving skills, other prefrontal functions)

be used to seek evidence of the latter. Because there has been a low-grade fever on a few occasions recently, occult infection should also be ruled out with appropriate studies. A trial of tricyclic antidepressants should then be instituted. Because of his left hemi-inattention and left homonymous hemianopsia, it is recommended that the patient's bed be placed so that his right side faces toward the middle of the room and his hemianopsic side toward the wall to maximize stimulation. Ward staff should be alerted to always approach him from his right side to maximize his ability to attend to the interaction.

NEURODIAGNOSTIC METHODS

Neurodiagnostic techniques are used to evaluate brain structure, physiology, and cognitive function. Structural information is obtained from computed tomography (CT), magnetic resonance imaging (MRI), and specialized neurodiagnostic procedures such as cerebral angiography. Physiological information is obtained from electroencephalography, evoked potentials (EPs), positron-emission tomography (PET), single-photon–emission computed tomography (SPECT), and specialized neurophysiological techniques such as brain electrical activity mapping (BEAM). Neuropsychological testing is used to describe and quantitate cognitive function.

Structural Imaging

Computed tomography scanning. This involves computerized reconstruction of multiple X-ray images to visualize serial anatomic "slices" through the head. A CT scan of the head without the use of a special contrast medium is usually sufficient to diagnose changes in brain structure such as hydrocephalus, atrophy, or mass effect. Calcifications and blood appear as areas of increased density. Edema, necrotic areas (e.g., postinfarction), fatty tissue, and cerebrospinal fluid (CSF) collections appear as areas of decreased density. Tumors may be of increased, decreased, or mixed density depending on their composition. The administration of an intravenous contrast agent can help visualize vascular anomalies such as arteriovenous malformations or aneurysms, or lesions producing abnormalities of the blood-brain barrier, such as certain tumors, abscesses, or demyelinating lesions. The CT scan is quite useful for the diagnosis of skull fractures that may be hard to visualize on simple X-rays. CT scanning has been widely used in neuropsychiatric research for the calculation of ventricular-brain ratios as an indication of possible tissue loss. The most significant limitation of cranial CT is its inability to visualize structures immediately adjacent to bone because of artifact. The inferior surfaces of the frontal and temporal lobes, as well as the entire posterior fossa, are much better visualized with MRI technology.

Magnetic resonance imaging. Magnetic resonance images, like CT images, are computer-reconstructed serial brain "slices," but they are derived by an entirely different method. The subject's head is placed in a magnetic field that forces protons (hydrogen atoms) in the brain to align. A series of radio frequency pulses are then applied perpendicular to this field. These pulses cause the protons to change their alignment briefly, then emit energy as they relax back to their previous alignment. The energy emitted during proton relaxation is used to construct the brain images.

Magnetic resonance imaging relies on three parameters: the spin (proton) density, T_1 or spin-lattice relaxation time, and T_2 or spin-spin relaxation time. Proton density reflects the number of protons (hydrogen nuclei) present in the tissue sample. T_1 and T_2 values are tissue-specific. Imaging sequences can be varied to highlight the T_1 or T_2 components of the signal.

The two most common sequences in clinical use are known as inversion recovery and spin-echo. *Inversion recovery sequences* rely heavily on the T_1 component. They produce the best gray-white resolution and are therefore best for visualizing anatomic detail. *Spin-echo images* offer less anatomic definition, but are much more sensitive to differences between normal and abnormal tissue. Although the sequence can be manipulated to reflect more of the T_1 component, spin-echo sequences are usually T_2-weighted. These images are best for detecting small focal lesions (like multiple sclerosis plaques). Increased signal intensity or image brightness is associated with increased proton density (i.e., water content), decreased T_1 values, and increased T_2 values. Water content tends to increase with most brain pathology, resulting in increased T_1 and T_2 signals, the high T_1 signals appearing black (as CSF does on a CT scan) and the high T_2 signals appearing white. Some tissue components appear almost the same with either T_1- or T_2-weighted images. Air, calcium, and bone all have low proton density and appear dark in either type of image. Fat, with its short T_1 and long T_2 values, appears bright in either type of image. What may appear at first to be skull bone surrounding the brain on MRI is actually fat in the bone marrow that causes a bright signal.

Computed tomography imaging is superior for detection of calcifications and bone abnormalities. It can be done rapidly to rule out hemorrhagic conditions. MRI involves no ionizing radiation exposure for the patient and is superior for the detection of demyelinating lesions, posterior fossa lesions, and small infarctions. It is also the better imaging procedure for seeking temporal-lobe lesions in most cases (Figure 12-1). However, MRI can be an extremely anxiety-provoking procedure, especially for claustrophobic patients. At the current state of technology, the patient must lie in a narrow tunnel for 45 to 60 minutes with an intermittent knocking noise during image collection. It is important to explain the procedure thoroughly to the patient in advance. You may consider giving the patient a benzodiazepine to allay anxiety prior to the procedure.

Physiological Information

Neurophysiological testing

The scalp electroencephalograph measures the electrical activity of cortical areas beneath electrodes placed in standardized locations on the scalp. It can reflect damage to cortical, subcortical, or brain-stem structures, because normal electroencephalographic rhythms are dependent not only on intact cortical function but also on a subcortical pacemaker presumed to be in the diencephalon, and on the brain-stem reticular activating system.

The electroencephalogram (EEG) can be affected by structural abnormalities such as stroke, tumor, or trauma, and by metabolic abnormalities such as hypoxia or hypoperfusion. It is often affected by

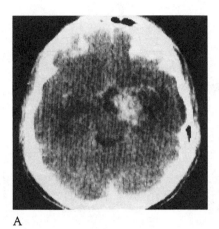
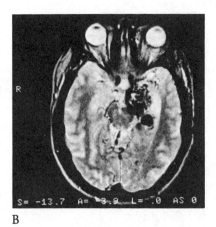

A   B

Figure 12-1. Comparison of a contrast-enhanced computed tomographic scan (A) and magnetic resonance imaging (B) of a deep left temporal lobe arteriovenous malformation. The patient is a 22-year-old male who has complex partial seizures with secondary generalization, and who has a history of interictal behavior syndrome, recurrent suicide attempts, and alcoholism.

drug toxicity and can be altered by certain medications such as benzodiazepines, even at therapeutic levels. The principal clinical use of the electroencephalograph in neuropsychiatry is the investigation of seizures, delirium, and dementia.

The normal electroencephalogram. The normal adult waking EEG is characterized by predominantly alpha activity (8 to 13 Hz) in parieto-occipital leads with the patient's eyes closed. Alpha activity attenuates with stimulation or eye opening. The anterior background may contain some beta (>13 Hz) and theta (4 to 7 Hz) activity, but should not contain delta activity (<4 Hz) except during Stage 3 and Stage 4 sleep or during hyperventilation. Figure 12-2 illustrates the appearance of the four basic electroencephalographic rhythms. The electroencephalographic pattern in childhood is slower and less organized than that found on an adult EEG, with the pattern gradually changing as the child matures from infancy through adolescence.

Electroencephalographic technique. The electroencephalographic tracing (i.e., the EEG) is a record of voltage differences either between two scalp electrodes or between a scalp electrode and a reference electrode, which is most commonly placed on the ear. To facilitate visualization and localization of abnormalities, the electroencephalographer examines activity recorded by several different electrode montages or recording patterns.

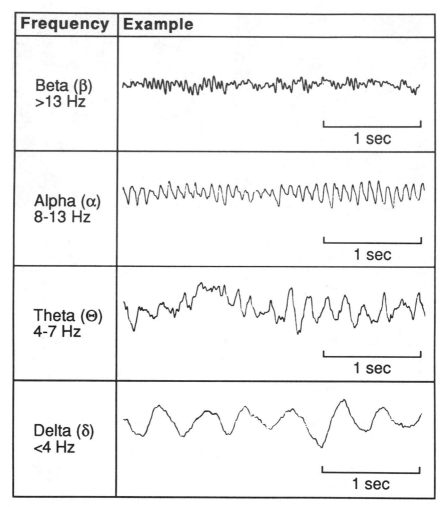

Frequency	Example
Beta (β) >13 Hz	1 sec
Alpha (α) 8-13 Hz	1 sec
Theta (Θ) 4-7 Hz	1 sec
Delta (δ) <4 Hz	1 sec

Figure 12-2. Basic electroencephalographic rhythms.

      Activating procedures are used to bring out latent abnormalities in the EEG. Common activating maneuvers include hyperventilation, photic stimulation with a strobe light, and recording the electroencephalographic pattern during sleep. In order to assure that the patient will sleep during a sleep electroencephalographic recording, the patient stays awake all night prior to the study and refrains from consumption of stimulants. Chloral hydrate sedation may be used to induce sleep if necessary. A sleep electroencephalographic recording is crucial to the evaluation of a suspected seizure disorder.

Temporolimbic seizure foci can be difficult to detect on the standard scalp EEG. Additional special electrodes are therefore often employed. Nasopharyngeal (NP) leads, inserted through the nostrils to the posterior pharyngeal wall, can increase detection of medial temporal abnormalities by an experienced technician. However, these leads can be uncomfortable and may be difficult to tolerate, especially for anxious or paranoid patients. In addition, swallowing with NP leads in place creates an artifact on the EEG. Sphenoidal leads, inserted through the soft tissue of the face below the zygomatic arch so that the electrode tip lies near the base of the skull in the region of the foramen ovale, can aid in localizing inferior temporal-lobe foci, but are too invasive for use in routine seizure evaluations. In some laboratories, noninvasive special electrodes such as extra temporal leads or "minisphenoidal" leads are available. The clinician should consult with the electroencephalography laboratory for help in selecting appropriate special leads.

Ordering an electroencephalogram. When requesting an EEG, it is important to explain on the requisition the specific symptoms that prompted you to order the test. If the study is being done as part of the workup for delirium or dementia, no sleep deprivation or special electrodes need be used. If the study is part of the evaluation of a possible seizure disorder, a sleep-deprived study is preferred. If a temporolimbic seizure focus is suspected, special electrodes can be requested (see above).

The interictal EEG is often normal even in well established seizure disorders. Activating procedures, special electrodes, and repeating the EEG increase the chance of detecting an epileptiform abnormality. Even with careful study, some foci elude electroencephalographic detection. *Epilepsy is a clinical diagnosis.* If there is a clear history of seizure activity, the diagnosis of seizure disorder can be made regardless of electroencephalographic findings. Similarly, if epileptiform abnormalities are detected in a routine EEG in a patient without any clinical evidence of seizures despite a carefully obtained history, that patient should not be diagnosed as epileptic.

Electroencephalographic abnormalities. Because the EEG reflects function rather than structure, identical electroencephalographic abnormalities may have widely varying etiologies. Slowing, for example, is seen over abnormally functioning brain tissue due to structural, metabolic, or degenerative causes. Diffuse slowing is most consistent with encephalopathic processes, but focal slowing is more consistent with structural abnormalities. Table 12-4 lists several conditions that can cause slowing in the EEG. Excessive beta activity is most commonly caused by sedative drugs. Spikes, sharp waves, and paroxysmal activity suggest a seizure disorder. Figure 12-3 shows sections of EEGs recorded during the three major types of seizure activity: generalized activity, complex-partial activity, and absence.

Table 12-4. Causes of slowing in the scalp electroencephalogram

Diffuse slowing	Lateralized (focal) slowing
Metabolic encephalopathy	Subdural hematoma
Dementia	Tumor
Medication effect (e.g., phenothiazines, lithium, barbiturates, tricyclic antidepressants, phenytoin)	Tuberous sclerosis
Normal drowsiness	Early Creutzfeldt-Jakob disease
Normal pressure hydrocephalus	Progressive multifocal leukoencephalopathy
Neurosyphilis	Neurosyphilis
Addison's disease	Infarction/hemorrhage
White matter diseases (multiple sclerosis, metachromatic leukodystrophy, progressive multifocal leukoencephalopathy)	Abscess
Parkinson's disease	Any focal brain lesion
Lacunar state (multiple small-vessel lacunar infarcts)	

Evoked potentials

Evoked potentials (EPs) are a computerized average of recorded electrical potentials generated by the brain in response to the repeated application of a simple stimulus. Somatosensory, visual, and brain-stem auditory EPs are the most common EPs in clinical use. Somatosensory EPs are obtained by delivering an electrical stimulus to either the tibial nerve at the ankle, the common peroneal nerve at the knee, or the median nerve at the wrist. EP wave forms are then recorded from electrodes placed over specific sites along ascending sensory pathways. The visual EP is measured by electroencephalographic electrodes over occipital cortex while the patient looks at a shifting checkerboard pattern on a screen. Brain-stem auditory EPs are measured from the acoustic nerve, the cochlear nucleus, the lateral lemniscus, and the inferior colliculus in response to a stimulus (a series of clicks) delivered to the ear. The early waves of an EP are related to the activity of specific anatomic landmarks along the

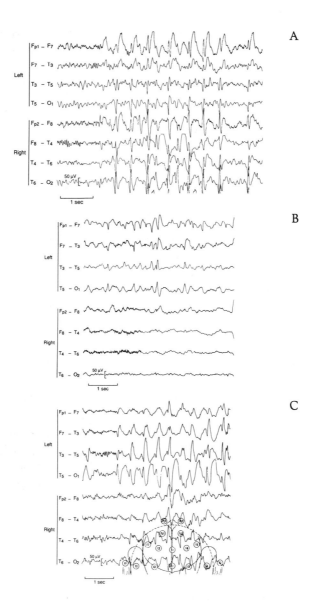

Figure 12-3. Appearance of seizures on an electroencephalogram (EEG). A. Generalized tonic-clonic seizures in an 11-year-old male. B. Complex partial seizure originating from the left temporal lobe in a woman who presented in a fugue state and was found to be in complex partial status epilepticus (continuous complex partial seizures). C. Generalized absence seizure (3-Hz spike and wave) in a 9-year-old girl. All EEG samples were recorded using a bipolar montage. Lead abbreviations: FP = frontal pole, F = frontal, T = temporal, O = occipital.

sensory pathway, while the later waves are thought to be related to cognitive processing of sensory information. By observing the wave form, amplitude, and latencies of EPs, the electrophysiologist can infer damage along the pathway being tested from sensory receptor to cortex.

Evoked potentials are often used in the evaluation of multiple sclerosis. The diagnosis of multiple sclerosis depends on the clinician being able to document CNS lesions in several locations that have occurred at different times. From the history or neurological examination the clinician may be able to infer one or more lesions. An abnormal delay in the transmission of an evoked potential can provide evidence of a lesion that was not obvious from the history or neurological examination. A unilaterally prolonged visual EP, for example, may be due to a past episode of optic neuritis that was unknown to the patient.

Event-related slow potentials (ERSPs), long-latency EPs, or cognitive EPs constitute a category of EPs used in neuropsychiatric research. The most commonly measured ERSPs are the P300 wave, the contingent negative variation (CNV), and the readiness potential. The amplitude of the P300 wave, a positive wave occurring 300 to 500 milliseconds following a sensory stimulus (in any sensory modality), appears to be related to the unexpectedness of the stimulus. In the P300 paradigm the subject is typically instructed to discriminate a particular stimulus from a series of like stimuli. Changes in the P300 potential are being investigated in aging and dementia studies. The CNV is evoked by giving the subject a warning stimulus followed shortly thereafter by another stimulus that requires a response, producing a slow negative wave in vertex and frontal electrodes. It is felt to be related to attention and motivation, increasing with increased interest in the stimulus and with degree of certainty that a stimulus will occur. It is decreased by attentional problems, boredom, and distraction sensitivity. The readiness potential (also known as the Bereitschafts potential) is also a slow negative wave deflection, but it occurs prior to voluntary muscle movements. The readiness potential has been used to compare voluntary and involuntary movements. This potential should theoretically be absent in a purely involuntary movement.

Computerized topographic brain mapping

Brain electrical activity mapping (BEAM or "brain mapping") utilizes a computer to perform spectral analysis of electroencephalographic data, giving the relative quantity of each brain-wave frequency detected by each recording electrode. It then converts the results into a topographic map that allows visualization of the distribution of the various brain-wave frequencies throughout the brain. The results can be compared to brain mapping data for normal age-matched subjects or patients with various neuropsychiatric conditions. While the standard EEG allows the electroencephalographer to determine the location of abnormal brain-wave frequencies, the BEAM technique calculates the amount of each brain-wave frequency at each topographic location, bringing out patterns that may be too subtle to appreciate on a routine EEG. Brain mapping technology may prove more useful in studying encephalopathies than seizure disorders, which are best evaluated by serial EEGs. It has been used in psychiatric research primarily to study schizophrenia. Although brain mapping technology has become widely available as powerful computers have become more ubiquitous, this procedure remains largely a research tool at this stage.

Positron-emission tomography and SPECT scanning

Positron-emission tomography (PET) scanning is perhaps the most promising neuropsychiatric research tool available today. It allows imaging of brain function based on differences in metabolism or biochemical differences among different anatomical areas. A specially prepared organic substrate containing a positron-emitting element (e.g., ^{18}F-labeled 2-deoxy-D-glucose) is injected into the patient. This compound emits gamma rays at the site at which it is utilized, allowing detection by gamma detectors surrounding the patient's head. Computer reconstructions of cross-sectional brain images are done that resemble those used in structural neuroimaging techniques such as CT scans. Areas of hypometabolism or hypermetabolism show up as decreased or increased uptake of the positron-emitting compound. PET can be used to visualize the brain areas that are activated for a given motor, sensory, or cognitive task by injecting the tracer while the subject performs the task. The function of specific brain areas in neuropsychiatric diseases can be compared to that in normal control subjects. Although PET findings among neuropsychiatric disorders vary, some characteristic PET changes, like the parietotemporal hypometabolism of Alzheimer's disease or the caudate hypometabolism of Huntington's disease, have been repeatedly demonstrated. Positron-emitting compounds have been developed that bind to specific neurotransmitter receptors. Dopamine-receptor–binding ligands, for example, have been used to study dopamine receptor density in Parkinson's disease and neuroleptic blockade of dopamine receptors in schizophrenia. Apart from cost, the major factor limiting availability of PET technology is that a cyclotron must be available on site to manufacture the needed tracers because of their short half-lives. Figure 12-4

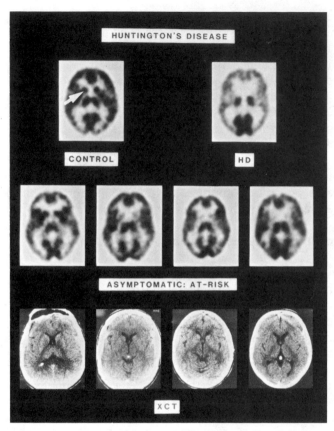

Figure 12-4. Positron-emission tomography (PET) and X-ray computed tomography (XCT) in Huntington's disease. The upper-left image demonstrates the typical, normal appearance of glucose metabolism at a tomographic level that passes through the heads of the caudate nuclei (arrow), the thalamus, and the visual cortex in a control subject. The upper-right image is from a symptomatic patient with Huntington's disease (HD). Note the marked reduction in metabolism in the caudate nuclei. The middle and bottom rows of images are from four subjects, all of whom were asymptomatic (chorea-free) but at risk for Huntington's disease. CT studies (bottom row) were normal for all four subjects. The metabolic activity of the caudate nuclei, as determined with PET (middle row), demonstrates graded changes ranging from a normal appearance (leftmost image) to one that closely resembles that seen in symptomatic patients (rightmost image). All PET studies were performed with use of the NeuroECAT device. Reprinted, with permission, from Mazziotta JC, Phelps ME, Pahl JJ, et al: Reduced cerebral glucose metabolism in asymptomatic subjects at risk for Huntington's disease. *New England Journal of Medicine* 316:357–362, 1987. Photo courtesy of John C. Mazziotta, M.D., Ph.D., Reed Neurological Institute, UCLA School of Medicine.

illustrates the advantage of PET over CT scanning in the search for brain abnormalities in very early cases of Huntington's disease.

Single-photon–emission computed tomography (SPECT) is a way of obtaining PET-like metabolic data using a standard gamma camera (like that used in bone scans) found in most nuclear medicine departments. It is thus much more affordable and practical than PET for clinical use, especially in hospitals where PET scanning is not available. The slightly poorer resolution of SPECT compared to that of PET is balanced by the lack of need for an on-site cyclotron because the tracers used have longer half-lives than do PET tracers. Using injected ^{123}I-labeled iodoamphetamine or inhaled xenon-133, regional cerebral blood perfusion can be measured by SPECT. Cerebral blood flow is related to metabolism, so data approximating those from PET can be obtained. As in PET, changes during motor or cognitive tasks can be measured. SPECT methods have been applied to the study of schizophrenia, mood disorders, seizure disorders, cerebral vascular disease, migraine, and dementias. Neuroreceptor ligands like those used in PET scanning are being developed. In the future, SPECT may be used to rule out neurological (e.g., traumatic, ischemic) causes for psychiatric symptoms when structural imaging is unrevealing.

Neuropsychological Testing

Neuropsychological testing is used to further evaluate cognitive functioning once the examiner has formed a clinical hypothesis about the nature of the patient's problem. The neuropsychologist administers a group of cognitive tasks to the patient based on the questions asked by the clinician requesting the consultation. A screening battery may be administered to evaluate each major brain function before focusing on problem areas with more specific tasks. The testing battery may take several hours. Common reasons for ordering neuropsychological testing include the following:

- To gather additional data in support of a possible diagnosis
- To localize cognitive deficits picked up on a screening MSE
- To determine a cognitive baseline against which future testing can be compared to document improvement or deterioration
- To determine the severity of an injury or deficit
- To facilitate rehabilitation planning
- To assess treatment effect
- To determine whether preexisting deficits could be contributing to a current clinical problem

The neuropsychological evaluation is most clinically useful when a specific question for the neuropsychologist to address is posed in the consultation request. Table 12-5 lists neuropsychological tests commonly used.

Neuropsychologists differ in their approach to testing and interpretation. The most frequently cited difference in approach is the battery versus the process approach. The battery approach relies heavily on the use of standardized tests to differentiate normal from abnormal behavior. The process approach tends to be less focused on whether right or wrong answers are obtained and more interested in the process by which the patient arrives at the answer. In reality, many neuropsychologists draw from both schools in formulating their clinical approach.

In reading the neuropsychological testing report, you should be alert to a few general findings:

- The presence of a verbal/performance IQ split on the Wechsler Adult Intelligence Scale (WAIS-R). A verbal/performance split refers to a difference of greater than 15 between the verbal IQ and the performance IQ that the neuropsychologist calculates from the language-related and motor/construction-based subtests of the WAIS-R. Care must be taken to allow for known primary sensory or motor deficits in interpreting these results. A verbal/performance IQ discrepancy may point to the presence of congenital or acquired focal brain damage.
- The presence of intertest scatter on the WAIS-R subtests. Intertest scatter refers to marked discrepancies among the IQ subtest scores. This nonuniform performance can be consistent with a decline from a previously higher level of cognitive function or can reflect focal damage. Again, you should be cautious in interpreting this finding in isolation, since variable attention and motivation can also be responsible.
- The presence of more than one neuropsychological abnormality in a given cognitive area.
- Any neuropsychological testing observations that appear to replicate the patient's psychiatric symptoms.

A neuropsychologist's finding of focal brain dysfunction is more robust if more than one test administered points to the same abnormality. It is even more meaningful if the neuropsychiatric history and examination have identified the same area of dysfunction. In such cases, focal brain dysfunction may be assumed even in the absence of a clear abnormality on structural imaging tests.

Table 12-5. Common neuropsychological tests used in the evaluation of adults

Intelligence	**Calculation**

Intelligence

WAIS-R
Stanford-Binet

Achievement

Wide Range Achievement Test

Attention

Serial 7's
WAIS-R Arithmetic, Digit Span, Coding
    subtests
Stroop Color-Word Interference Test
Cancellation tasks
PASAT
Halstead-Reitan Trail Making Test
Continuous Performance Task

**Abstraction/Concept formation and
    shift**

Wisconsin Card Sorting Test
Halstead-Reitan Category Test
Porteus Maze Test
Raven Coloured Progressive Matrices
Proverbs Test

Memory

Wechsler Memory Scale—Revised
Benton Visual Retention Test
Rey-Osterreith Complex Figure Test
California Verbal Learning Test
Selective reminding techniques
Paired Associate Learning Task

Language

Boston Diagnostic Aphasia Examination
    (BDAE)
Multilingual Aphasia Examination
Boston Naming Test (part of BDAE)
Token Test
Verbal Fluency Test
F-A-S Test (Controlled Oral Word
    Association Test)
Peabody Picture Vocabulary Test

Calculation

Wide Range Achievement Test
WAIS-R Arithmetic subtest

Visuospatial

Rey-Osterreith Complex Figure Test
Draw-a-clock task
Facial Recognition Memory Test
Line orientation
WAIS-R Block Design and Object
    Assembly subtests
Benton Revised Visual Retention Test
Bender Visual Motor Gestalt Test (Bender-
    Gestalt)

Body schema/somatosensory

Finger recognition
Right-left discrimination
Halstead-Reitan Tactual Performance Test

Motor

Purdue Pegboard Test
Halstead-Reitan Finger Tapping Test
Thumb-finger opposition
Motor impersistence

Note. PASAT = Paced Auditory Serial Addition Test. For further reading on specific
neuropsychological tests, see Lezak 1983. WAIS-R = Wechsler Adult Intelligence Scale—
Revised.

COMMON NEUROPSYCHIATRIC DISORDERS

Although neuropsychiatric evaluation techniques may be applied to any diagnostic problem arising in psychiatry, neuropsychiatrists are frequently called on to see patients with certain conditions. Two of the most common conditions evaluated, dementia and delirium, have been dealt with in Chapter 9. Several other common conditions are reviewed below.

Atypical Psychiatric Disorders

Neuropsychiatrists are often called on to evaluate atypical presentations of major psychiatric syndromes. Although there are many reasons why a psychiatric syndrome may be described as atypical, many atypical presentations have elements in common (see Table 12-6). A late age of onset for major mental illness should alert the examiner to do a careful evaluation for medical or neurological factors that could be contributing to the symptoms. Absence of prior personal psychiatric history and absence of a positive family history do not rule out primary psychopathology, but they do add weight to the argument in favor of an organic etiology. Electroencephalographic abnormalities and increased ventricular-brain ratios on cranial CT imaging or MRI increase the chances of congenital abnormalities having predisposed the patient to psychopathology. Patients with neurodevelopmental signs on exam, CT or electroencephalographic abnormalities as above, and a negative family history, may have developed their psychiatric condition as a result of gestational or perinatal injury combined with the effects of environmental stressors and experience. The more typical presentations of psychopathology are often associated with a genetic predisposition.

Table 12-6. Characteristics of atypical psychiatric syndromes

Late age of onset (>45)

Lack of personal history typical of the disorder

Lack of family history of the disorder

Neurodevelopmental signs on exam

Electroencephalographic abnormalities

Computed tomography scan/magnetic resonance imaging abnormalities (typically increased ventricular-brain ratios)

Organic Personality Syndromes

The term *organic personality syndrome* refers to a marked personality change related to an organic factor. The DSM-III-R criteria specify 1) that there be affective instability, recurrent explosive outbursts, impaired social judgment, apathy, or undue suspiciousness; 2) that the behavior not occur exclusively during delirium; and 3) that the patient not be demented. In order to make the diagnosis of an organic personality syndrome, you must obtain a premorbid history from someone close to the patient. Many types of brain insult can give rise to the general DSM-III-R organic personality syndrome. In addition, several diseases have been alleged to be associated with specific personality traits. However, the two main syndromes of organic personality change are the frontal-lobe syndrome and the interictal behavior syndrome of temperolimbic epilepsy.

Frontal-lobe syndrome

The most common organic personality syndrome is the frontal-lobe syndrome. Some authors (c.f. Cummings 1985a) distinguish among behaviors caused by damage to three major anatomic areas within the frontal lobes: the orbitofrontal cortex, the dorsolateral convexity, and the medial frontal lobes. In practice, most frontal-lobe syndromes consist of a mixture of symptoms arising from these three areas. One of the main causes of acquired frontal-lobe dysfunction is head injury, discussed separately below. The symptoms and principal causes of damage to each of the three frontal areas are reviewed below (see Table 12-7).

Orbitofrontal cortex damage. Damage to the orbitofrontal cortex gives rise to what has been called "pseudopsychopathic" behavior. This includes disinhibited, impulsive, immature behavior, with affective lability, shallow mood, and facetious humor known as "Witzelsucht." The disinhibition may include socially inappropriate comments, sexual behaviors, or explosive outbursts, but the patient's rage is less intense, planned, and prolonged than, for example, the interictal rage of some temporal-lobe epileptic patients (see below). If one considers the major connections of orbitofrontal cortex to limbic areas like the amygdala that are concerned with regulation of biological drives, the orbitofrontal syndrome can be seen as resulting from loss of higher level control over biological drives.

Dorsolateral convexity lesions. Lesions in the dorsolateral convexity give rise to "pseudodepressed" behavior. The patient may show psychomotor retardation similar to that seen in depression, but lack the

Table 12-7. Causes and symptoms of frontal lobe syndromes

Signs and symptoms	Common etiologies
Orbitofrontal cortex damage	
Disinhibited/impulsive (pseudopsychopathic)	Trauma
	Tumor
Inappropriate jocular affect, euphoria	Anterior cerebral artery aneurysm
Emotional lability	Pick's disease
Poor judgment and insight	Encephalitis
Distractibility	Psychosurgery
	Multiple sclerosis
Dorsolateral convexity lesions	
Apathetic (with occasional outbursts)	Trauma
Indifference	Hydrocephalus
Psychomotor retardation	Tumor
Motor perseveration and impersistence	Alzheimer's disease
Loss of set[a]	Multiple sclerosis
Stimulus boundness[b]	Psychosurgery
Discrepant motor and verbal behavior[c]	
Motor programming/sequencing deficits[d]	
Poor word-list generation[e]	
Poor abstraction and categorization	
Segmented approach to visuospatial analysis[f]	
Medial frontal syndrome	
Akinetic (paucity of spontaneous movement and gesture)	Vascular
	Deep medial tumors
Sparse verbal output	Hydrocephalus
Lower-extremity weakness/numbness	
Incontinence	

[a]Inability to keep rules or goal of a task in mind. For example, on the serial 7's subtraction task, the patient responds 100, 93, 83, 73, 63 instead of 100, 93, 86, 79, 72, 65.

[b]Inability to overcome automatic pull to most salient stimulus available. For example, the patient draws hands pointing to the 10 and the 11 instead of to the 11 and the 2 when asked to draw a clock with hands pointing to "10 after 11."

[c]Difficulty maintaining linkage between verbal output and motor task. For example, the patient might be able to repeat "knock, cut, slap" but be unable to perform the appropriate simultaneous hand movements in sequence when being taught the Luria three-step motor sequence.

[d]Inability to perform a series of motor tasks in the correct order. For example, the patient may perform all three hand movements of the Luria three-step motor sequence but in the wrong order.

[e]Difficulty coming up with more than a few words in a given category. The patient is given one minute to say all of the words he or she can think of that begin with a given letter, or is told to list as many members of a category (e.g., automobile models) as possible in 1 minute. Most high school graduates should be able to list at least 12 words.

[f]When asked to copy a complex figure, the patient will proceed one segment at a time rather than noticing the overall outline of the figure.

Source. Adapted from Cummings 1985a.

hopelessness, rumination, and depressive content of true depression. The most striking feature is the patient's apathy, coupled with loss of initiative, motivation, and spontaneity. These patients may have difficulty keeping up with the neurological exam because of a combination of difficulty moving from one task to the next (difficulty shifting set) and psychomotor slowing. They may also show motor impersistence, demonstrated by the inability to sustain a task such as holding the eyes closed and the arms extended for several seconds without constant repetition of the command by the examiner. The dorsolateral convexity is connected to motor areas and to parietal areas that are thought to alert the brain for appropriate motor response to sensory stimuli, thus laying the foundation for the apathy found in patients who have sustained damage to this area.

Medial frontal syndrome. This syndrome includes incontinence, akinetic mutism, and gait disturbance, which is due to motor and sensory deficits of the legs. When the medial frontal syndrome is due to hydrocephalus or tumor, appropriate treatment may reverse some of these symptoms. The medial frontal cortex is connected to accessory cortical motor areas and to the basal ganglia, thus explaining the akinesia central to this syndrome.

Head injury

Head injury is a major reason for neuropsychiatric evaluation and can cause a host of neuropsychiatric syndromes and focal deficits. Damage may be caused by focal lesions at the sight of impact (coup) or at a locus opposite the point of impact (contracoup). These lesions may include cerebral contusion, intracerebral hemorrhage, subdural hematoma, and epidural hematoma. Head injuries may also cause anoxic damage to brain tissue because of edema. One of the most important types of damage, however, may be what has been called diffuse axonal injury, resulting from shearing of neurons along the entire vertical axis of the brain, with more severe injury causing shearing further inferiorly into the brain stem.

A number of factors help predict the neuropsychiatric outcome of head injury. The patient's premorbid cognitive endowment, premorbid personality, psychiatric history, substance abuse history, and family psychiatric history must be investigated as with any neuropsychiatric disorder. Open brain injury (as opposed to closed head injury), deep initial coma, the presence of posttraumatic seizures (other than at impact), and long duration of the patient's posttraumatic amnesia (inability to learn new information because of confusional state) are all predictors of long-term neuropsychiatric compromise. The specific foci of brain damage will determine how severe the cognitive deficits will be and whether a specific organic personality syndrome will emerge. The psychiatrist must be aware of whether or not the injury was work-related and whether there is litigation pending, as these factors may influence the patient's presentation.

Apart from frontal-lobe personality syndromes, head injury may give rise to posttraumatic organic mood disorders, psychotic states, and seizure disorders, with their own neuropsychiatric morbidity. The ability of mild postconcussion syndromes to produce deterioration of work performance due to attentional deficits is often overlooked.

Interictal behavior syndrome of temporolimbic epilepsy

A cluster of personality traits has been described in some patients with temporolimbic epilepsy (Bear and Fedio 1977) (Table 12-8). This cluster has been referred to as the interictal behavior syndrome of temporolimbic epilepsy. Interictal (meaning "between seizures") is used to distinguish this syndrome from ictal behavior that occurs during the seizure itself according to the location of the seizure focus, and from postictal behavior commonly seen during the confusional state immediately following a seizure. The seemingly diverse interictal behaviors listed in Table 12-8 have two underlying themes in common: 1) the patient imbues all events—internal and external—with such importance that normal concepts of priorities are lost; and 2) in general, the patient's emotions become deepened and intensified (hyperemotionality).

The profound emotional experience of the patient with the interictal behavior syndrome of temporolimbic epilepsy can be contrasted with the shallow emotional world of the patient with frontal-

Table 12-8. Interictal traits associated with temporolimbic epilepsy (in order of decreasing discrimination from control subjects)

Humorlessness	Anger
Dependence	Religiosity
Circumstantiality	Hypermoralism
Sense of personal destiny	Paranoia
Obsessionalism	Sadness
Viscosity	Hypergraphia
Emotionality	Elation
Guilt	Aggression
Philosophical interest	Altered sexuality

Source. After Bear and Fedio 1977, with permission of the American Medical Association. Copyright 1977, AMA.

lobe behavior. When interictal rage occurs in the temporolimbic epileptic patient, it is likely to be planned, the patient may justify it by a perceived attack on deeply held values, and the patient may continue to feel very strongly about the incident. By contrast, a rage attack in a patient with frontal-lobe personality changes is likely to be an impulsive, unplanned episode that occurs in response to an immediate environmental precipitant. The rage of the frontal-lobe patient is short-lived. By the time the psychiatrist interviews the patient about a given incident, the patient is no longer concerned about it.

The interictal behavior syndrome should also be contrasted with the *Klüver-Bucy syndrome*, originally described in bilaterally temporal lobectomized rhesus monkeys. The Klüver-Bucy monkeys developed lasting behavioral changes, including visual agnosia (the inability to recognize familiar objects); tameness, with loss of normal anger and fear responses (hypoemotionality); hypermetamorphosis (constant manual exploration of the environment with mouthing of objects); hyperphagia (increased appetite, with diversified diet); and hypersexuality. In humans, the Klüver-Bucy syndrome includes apathy, prosopagnosia (the inability to distinguish among relatives, friends, and strangers), hypermetamorphosis, hyperphagia, and sexual disinhibition, and is usually associated with aphasia and amnesia. The syndrome occurs in conditions that cause bilateral temporal-lobe destruction, like herpes encephalitis, Pick's disease, Alzheimer's disease, and head trauma. Table 12-9 illustrates the contrast between the Klüver-Bucy syndrome of temporal-lobe destruction and the interictal behavior syndrome of temporolimbic epilepsy. The apathetic tameness (hypoemotionality) of the Klüver-Bucy syndrome is the opposite of the intense emotion of the interictal behavior syndrome. Whereas the Klüver-Bucy syndrome results in an increased tendency to explore the environment (hypermetamorphosis), patients with the interictal behavior syndrome have a great deal of trouble moving on to the next subject or task (hypometamorphosis). Finally,

Table 12-9. Klüver-Bucy syndrome compared to interictal behavior syndrome of temporolimbic epilepsy

Klüver-Bucy syndrome (bilateral temporolimbic destruction)	Interictal behavior syndrome (chronic temporolimbic seizure discharges)
Hypoemotionality	Hyperemotionality
Hypermetamorphosis	Hypometamorphosis
Hypersexuality	Hyposexuality

although several sexual alterations have been described in temporal-lobe epileptic patients, hyposexuality is the most common presentation, in contrast to the hypersexuality of the Klüver-Bucy syndrome.

Organic Psychotic Syndromes

The organic psychotic syndromes are characterized by isolated psychotic symptoms that occur in the setting of clear consciousness and are due to an organic factor. They are not diagnosed in primarily delirious or demented patients. Associated features of psychotic behavior, including disheveled appearance, incoherence, and agitation, do occur in these syndromes, but there is usually no history of schizoid development as in schizophrenia. In contrast to the flat affect seen in schizophrenia, the affect may be preserved in organic psychotic syndromes. For example, a 42-year-old businessman with no personal or family psychiatric history who suffers a closed head injury with bifrontal lesions and develops the persistent delusion that his wife has been replaced by an imposter, has an organic psychotic syndrome, specifically organic delusional syndrome. In organic delusional syndrome the principal symptom is delusion formation, while in organic hallucinosis, hallucinations are the most prominent feature. There have been numerous reported cases of organic delusional syndrome (see Table 12-10). Alcohol abuse is the most common cause of organic hallucinosis; hallucinations are usually auditory, but can be in any modality. Organic hallucinosis may also occur as a result of occipital or visual pathway pathology, seizures, or drug abuse.

Organic Amnestic Syndromes

Organic amnestic syndromes are memory disorders that occur in clear consciousness (i.e., without delirium) and that appear to be organically based. The most important amnestic syndrome is *Korsakoff's psychosis*, which occurs in cases of chronic thiamine deficiency. This is usually due to chronic alcohol abuse, but can be caused by malabsorption or dietary inadequacy. *Wernicke's encephalopathy*, which often repeatedly occurs prior to the development of Korsakoff's psychosis, is a combination of ataxia, eye movement abnormalities, and confusion that often improves with administration of thiamine.

Korsakoff's psychosis is a profound anterograde and retrograde amnesia that improves only little with abstinence from alcohol. The principal anatomic correlates of this syndrome are damage to the mammillary bodies of the hypothalamus and the dorsomedial nuclei of the thalamus. In patients with severe Korsakoff's psychosis, it is very difficult to demonstrate any short-term memory at all. Other causes of amnestic syn-

Table 12-10. Reported causes of organic delusional syndrome

Endocrinopathies
  Adrenal insufficiency
  Cushing's disease
  Hypothyroidism
  Hyperthyroidism
  Hypo- and hypercalcemia
  Panhypopituitarism
Deficiency states
  B$_{12}$
  Folate
  Niacin
Connective tissue disease
  Systematic lupus erythematosus
  Temporal arteritis
Drug medications
  Antiparkinson agents
  Antituberculosis agents
  Antimalarials, anticonvulsants
  Antidepressants
  Antihypertensives
  Hallucinogens
Miscellaneous
  Porphyria
  Huntington's chorea
  Amphetamines
  Corticosteroids
  Pentazocine
  Bromide
  Heavy metal toxicity
CNS disorders
  Multiple sclerosis
  Parkinson's disease
  Idiopathic basal ganglia calcification
  Spinocerebellar degeneration
  Temporal-lobe epilepsy
  Neoplasms
  Cerebrovascular disease

Source. Reprinted, with permission, from Stoudemire GA: Selected organic mental disorders, in *The American Psychiatric Press Textbook of Neuropsychiatry.* Edited by Hales RE, Yudofsky SC. Washington, DC, American Psychiatric Press, 1987, pp. 125–139. Copyright 1987, American Psychiatric Press.

dromes include head injury, herpes encephalitis, anoxic encephalopathy, and the transient amnestic syndrome associated with ECT that has decreased since unilateral ECT has become the common mode of treatment.

Organic Anxiety Syndrome

Organic anxiety syndrome refers to persistent or recurrent anxiety or panic etiologically related to an organic factor. The most common organic causes of anxiety are hyperthyroidism and stimulant abuse (caffeine, amphetamine, cocaine). Pheochromocytoma is a rarer cause of the syndrome.

Organic Mood Disorders

Mood disorders, too, can be caused by or precipitated by organic factors. You should suspect that a mood disorder is secondary to an organic disturbance when a person without personal or family history of mood disorder develops new onset of major depression or mania after age 45. Like other DSM-III-R diagnoses, the diagnosis is not made if the patient is primarily delirious or demented.

The reported causes of organic mood syndromes are legion. Among the more frequent causes of *organic mood syndrome, depressed type,* are medications such as alpha-methyldopa, propranolol, reserpine, steroids, and barbiturates; occult malignancy (especially pancreatic carcinoma); stroke; and endocrine disorders like Cushing's syndrome and hypothyroidism. Poststroke depression often follows anterior left-hemisphere strokes.

Organic mood syndrome, manic type, can also be caused by a number of medications, including antidepressants, stimulants, and steroids; by endocrine problems such as hyperthyroidism; and by focal brain lesions due to tumor, stroke, or infection. Studies of focal lesions causing secondary mania (organic mood syndrome, manic type) have shown that the lesions most likely to cause manic behavior are located in the right hemisphere, especially in the peridiencephalic area, the orbitofrontal cortex, and areas connected to them (and thus to the limbic system).

When examining a brain-damaged patient for the presence of a mood disorder, bear in mind that the patient may be incapable of producing some of the standard signs and symptoms associated with depression in neurologically normal individuals. An aphasic patient or a patient with a lesion that effectively disconnects the left-hemisphere language areas from the right hemisphere may not be able to produce the verbal complaints typically associated with depression. A patient with a right-hemisphere lesion may not be able to produce the affective changes in voice (emotional prosody), facial expression, or gestures, that help us recognize depression. Worse, these patients may completely deny their symptoms just as certain right-hemisphere stroke patients deny their deficits. The diagnosis of depression in this group requires questioning family members or ward staff as well as paying strict attention to neurovegetative signs. In some cases, for instance when there has been an unexplained increase in a preexisting neurological deficit, or an interruption in the progress of rehabilitation, the patient must be treated empirically for depression.

Congenital right-hemisphere syndrome, a specific learning disorder in which deficits are mostly in right-hemisphere functions, has been found to predispose some patients to recurrent depression. A combination of 1) visuospatial deficits; 2) impaired production of the affective components of language (emotional prosody), facial expression, and gesture; 3) a history of shyness; 4) poor eye contact; and 5) interpersonal difficulties, alert the clinician to the possibility of this disorder. The patient may recall having had difficulty adhering to the margins when learning to write, having been unable to copy drawings, or having poor directional abilities. Often there is a history of math difficulties as well as a positive family history of similar disorders on careful inquiry.

Psychomotility Disorders

A number of disorders exist that involve a combination of abnormal movements and psychiatric symptoms. This association has led some investigators to refer to these disorders as "psychomotility disorders" (Cummings 1985a) or disorders of motion and emotion. These disorders fall into two general categories: 1) extrapyramidal diseases associated with affective, psychotic, obsessive-compulsive, attentional, and dementia symptoms; and 2) psychiatric conditions associated with increased, decreased, or involuntary movements. Table 12-11 lists some of the more common of these conditions.

Psychiatric symptoms and movement disorders influence each other. For instance, it is well known that anxiety, emotional distress, suggestion, and environmental variables can exacerbate abnormal involuntary movements and that most of these movements disappear during sleep and decrease with relaxation. Many of the extrapyramidal diseases listed in Table 12-11 lead to the development of a primarily subcortical dementia. This type of dementia includes psychomotor retardation, forgetfulness (impaired memory retrieval as opposed to globally impaired new learning), decreased ability to manipulate acquired knowl-

Table 12-11. Psychomotility disorders: some examples

Extrapyramidal disorders	Psychiatric disorders
Encephalitis lethargica	Schizophrenia
Oculogyric crisis	Depression
Parkinson's disease	Mania
Huntington's disease	Anxiety
Wilson's disease	Obsessive-compulsive disorder
Idiopathic basal ganglia calcification (Fahr's disease)	Attention-deficit hyperactivity disorder
Tourette's syndrome	
Progressive supranuclear palsy	
Meige's syndrome	
Akathisia?	
Tardive dyskinesia?	

edge, mood disturbance, speech abnormalities such as dysarthria (as opposed to language abnormalities like aphasia in cortical dementia), and movement abnormalities. The dementias associated with Wilson's disease and Huntington's disease are good examples. Psychiatric symptoms are often the presenting complaints in extrapyramidal disorders. Even though abnormalities of movement are seldom the chief complaint in psychiatric disorders, movement plays an important role. The mannerisms and sterotypies of schizophrenia have long been known to clinicians. Psychomotor retardation and psychomotor agitation are key features of depression and mania, respectively.

There is some evidence that movement disorders and psychiatric disorders are genetically linked as well. Family members of patients with Tourette's syndrome have an increased incidence of tic disorder and obsessive-compulsive disorder. Patients with Tourette's syndrome have an increased tendency to develop obsessive-compulsive and attention deficit symptoms along with their tics.

The interplay between disorders of motion and emotion is so often a factor that one should not neglect to inquire about psychiatric symptoms in patients with extrapyramidal diseases, nor should observations of a patient's movement be omitted from the psychiatric evaluation.

TREATMENT

A thorough neuropsychiatric evaluation should lay the groundwork for individualized treatment or rehabilitation. Potentially reversible aspects of a patient's condition should be identified and appropriate interventions carried out. Commonly found reversible factors include superimposed anxiety, depression or psychosis, sensory deprivation, abnormal metabolic function, drug effects, nutritional problems, infections, environmental stressors, and effects of pathological family interactions.

The psychopharmacological treatment of anxiety disorders, mood disorders, and psychoses, when they are superimposed on brain damage, is similar to the treatment of these disorders in patients with uninjured brains. However, brain-damaged individuals are often sensitive to lower dosages of psychoactive medications and have lower thresholds for side effects as well as behavioral and cognitive toxicity. Antidepressants are often indicated in early dementia to treat superimposed depression that may look like cognitive deterioration. They are frequently used in posthead injury and poststroke patients when a failure to progress in rehabilitation appears related to superimposed depression. Recent studies have shown that the anticonvulsants carbamazepine and valproate may be useful in treating patients whose bipolar disorder is related to brain damage. In patients with *intermittent explosive disorder* or *organic personality syndrome, explosive type,* beta blockers have proven useful in controlling explosive outbursts.

When brain damage is present, insight-oriented psychotherapy is seldom possible. However, supportive therapy can be very helpful. The therapist may have to assume a more directive role than with nonbrain-damaged individuals. In the case of a patient who has suddenly declined from a higher level of functioning, the therapist may need to begin by helping the patient grieve the loss of function in order to enlist the patient as an active participant in rehabilitation. Some patients with organic personality syndromes may be treated most effectively in a group setting, where others can confront these patients with their maladaptive behaviors.

Rehabilitation following major brain injuries is best accomplished utilizing a mutlidisciplinary team that may include occupational, physical, vocational, and speech therapists, a social worker, a neuropsychologist, a neurologist, a physiatrist, and a neuropsychiatrist. Because brain-injured patients may be unable to report their own symptoms accurately or may even be unaware of their symptoms, the neuropsychiatrist often relies on input from other members of the treatment team for help in assessing a patient's symptoms or response to treatment. Other team members may be able to help devise objective methods for monitoring the patient's response to psychiatric treatment.

The neuropsychologist is often called on to perform a baseline assessment, with follow-up assessments at regular intervals to document the patient's deterioration or recovery and response to treatment. The neuropsychologist may work with the occupational therapist and the speech therapist to design a series of exercises aimed at teaching the patient compensatory strategies to circumvent cognitive deficits toward eventual return to gainful employment.

Family work is a critical part of neuropsychiatric treatment. The patient's deficits and how best to work around them must be carefully explained to family members to allow them to form appropriate expectations and learn to communicate with the patient. And if the neuropsychological testing or the bedside MSE reveal some cognitive strengths, these may be used to teach the family ways to attempt to work around the patient's deficits. The family must be given realistic prognostic information to allow them to plan appropriately for the future. Legal guardianship or conservatorship might become necessary if the patient's deficits render him or her incompetent to make certain decisions (e.g., consenting to medical procedures, managing money). In addition, the family should be warned of behaviors (e.g., outbursts, unusual seizure symptoms, confusional episodes) that may occur, and they should be told whom to call when they need help.

Neuropsychiatric findings should be carefully reviewed with the patient and the family. Understanding the origin of a problem behavior can help a family cope with the stresses of caring for their injured loved one. If the patient is capable of understanding his or her deficits, the neuropsychiatric explanation can help demystify the problem and foster a treatment alliance that will facilitate rehabilitation.

BIBLIOGRAPHY

Andreasen NC: Brain Imaging Applications in Psychiatry. Washington, DC, American Psychiatric Press, 1989

Bear D, Fedio P: Quantitative analysis of interictal behavior in temporal lobe epilepsy. Arch Neurol 34:454–467, 1977

Blumer D, Benson DF: Psychiatric manifestations of epilepsy, in Psychiatric Aspects of Neurologic Disease, Vol II. Edited by Benson DF, Blumer D. New York, Grune & Stratton, 1982, pp 25–48

Cummings JL: Clinical Neuropsychiatry. Orlando, FL, Grune & Stratton, 1985a

Cummings JL: Organic delusions: phenomenology, anatomical correlations, and review. Br J Psychiatry 146:184–197, 1985b

Hales RE, Yudofsky SC (eds): The American Psychiatric Press Textbook of Neuropsychiatry. Washington, DC, American Psychiatric Press, 1987

Lezak MD: Neuropsychological Assessment, 2nd Edition. New York, Oxford University Press, 1983

Lilly R, Cummings JC, Benson DF, et al: The human Klüver-Bucy syndrome. Neurology 33:1141–1145, 1983

Massion AO, Benjamin S: Manic behavior, in Outpatient Psychiatry. Edited by Lazare A. Baltimore, MD, Williams & Wilkins, 1989, pp 256–266

Roberts JKA: Differential Diagnosis in Neuropsychiatry. Chichester, UK, John Wiley, 1984

Ross ED, Rush J: Diagnosis and neuroanatomical correlates of depression in brain-damaged patients: implications for a neurology of depression. Arch Gen Psychiatry 38:1344–1354, 1981

Trimble MR: Biological Psychiatry. Chichester, UK, John Wiley, 1988

Weintraub S, Mesulam MM: Developmental learning disabilities of the right hemisphere: emotional, interpersonal and cognitive components. Arch Neurol 40:463–468, 1983

Part IV

Special Problems

13 Human Sexuality: Function and Dysfunction 383
14 Substance Abuse and Eating Disorders 413
15 Suicide 443
16 Violence 459

INTRODUCTION

The chapters included in this section cover subjects that every physician must understand. The clinical problems discussed in these chapters cross all diagnostic boundaries and often present as manifestations of other medical and psychiatric conditions.

Chapter 13 deals with sexual dysfunctions and deviations—concerns that are often overlooked in diagnostic evaluations. Eating disorders and substance abuse are discussed in Chapter 14. Problems of substance abuse have reached epidemic proportions in our society; but they, too, are missed in many medical and mental health assessments. Both of these chapters therefore emphasize diagnosis, with specific techniques for eliciting a history of problems with drugs or sexual functioning.

Suicide and violence are two of the most anxiety-provoking problems you will encounter in your clinical work. Chapters 15 and 16 focus on suicidal and violent patients, respectively, highlighting ways in which you can assess patients' potential for carrying out threats of harming themselves or others, and strategies for managing emergency situations.

13

Human Sexuality:

Function and Dysfunction

IN OUR SOCIETY, physicians are the professionals most often consulted about sexual problems. Ironically, although physicians are assumed by many to be experts in this field, they are frequently less knowledgeable about and less comfortable with various aspects of sexual behavior than some nonprofessionals. As a physician-in-training, you must gain some understanding of the broad range of human sexual behaviors, as well as an understanding of your own attitudes toward sex. Such awareness is essential to good clinical work in any specialty of medicine.

TAKING A SEXUAL HISTORY

To learn about the sexual aspects of your patients' lives, you must be comfortable in eliciting such information.

General medical workups and psychiatric histories should routinely include questions that will allow you to establish the patient's general attitude toward sex, his or her sexual functioning, and its bearing on important relationships. Sexual functioning should be explored in depth whenever the patient's complaints suggest possible sexual difficulties or concerns. Such common complaints as fatigue, headaches, dysmenorrhea, and depression should also alert you to the possibility of underlying sexual dissatisfaction.

When is it best to broach the subject during an interview? Obviously, if the patient's chief complaint is of a sexual nature, begin with a sexual history immediately. When this is not the case, it is usually best to wait until you and the patient have established some degree of rapport in the interview. A relaxed, matter-of-fact display of interest is most helpful. Ask questions as straightforwardly as possible.

The natural openings for discussion of sexuality are many. People usually talk about romantic relationships or marriages; use this as a point to introduce the topic with a general question, such as, "How has the relationship developed sexually?" or "Can you tell me about your sexual experience with this person?" When a patient talks about menstrual functioning, energy level, depression, or other general complaints, you can turn to the subject of sex with a question like, "How does this symptom affect your sexual relationships?" With some patients (e.g., adolescents or severely isolated individuals) who you suspect may have very limited sexual experience, you might begin with a general inquiry (e.g., "What have your sexual experiences been like?").

People are commonly concerned that some aspect of their sexuality is abnormal. It will be helpful to frame your questions so that you imply that many people have similar feelings and attitudes. For example, in inquiring about previous homosexual experiences, you might phrase your question as follows: "Many people have sexual experiences with members of the same sex at some point in their lives. Have you had any experiences with other men (women)?" Or concerning common practices that may be a source of embarrassment, you might word a question as follows, "How old were you when you began masturbating?" rather than "Have you ever masturbated?"

When inquiring about sexuality, take your language cues from the patient. This is particularly important in talking with gay and lesbian individuals. If you assume a heterosexual orientation (e.g., asking a man about girlfriends), you may make it more difficult for your patient to tell you about homosexual experiences. Thus, when talking about romantic relationships, use neutral terms such as "lover" until your patient offers specific names or pronouns that make sexual object choice clear.

Also, be sure to use your patient's terms whenever possible to describe sexual experiences and anatomy. Some patients use slang (e.g., "cock" for penis, "screwing" for intercourse), whereas others would find such terms offensive. Use your judgment, but remember that many words carry different connotations for different people. When in doubt, use the most neutral and widely accepted terms until you discover a common language with your patient.

Your Own Attitudes About Sex

Your comfort or discomfort in discussing sexual matters will undoubtedly be communicated to your patients. Many of us were raised in environments in which sex was never discussed, or only mentioned among intimates. It is no small task to learn to speak openly with patients about sexual functioning. You may find that you are embarrassed by or uncomfortable with some of what you encounter as a beginning clinician.

Unresolved conflicts about your own sexual life may hamper your ability to listen and evaluate sensitively. For example, an interviewer who is frightened by his or her own homosexual feelings may have difficulty in evaluating patients' homosexual concerns. Clinicians who believe that sex is "no one else's business" may be reacting to guilt feelings about their own unacknowledged sexual curiosity and may refrain from asking necessary questions. Or, such people may overcompensate, asking intrusive and overly detailed questions about matters irrelevant to the patient's complaints.

Those who are achievement oriented may tend to think of sex as a performance. Frequency of sexual intercourse, the number of orgasms attained, and the extent of the partner's visible satisfaction during lovemaking are all aspects of sexuality that can come to represent tests of competence. Such notions about sex can greatly distort not only your own sexual experiences but also your understanding of your patient's experiences.

Your job is to remain nonjudgmental and professional in your attitude toward your patient's sexual life. If you find yourself becoming anxious or imposing your personal values on a patient, you must stand back and (with the help of a colleague or supervisor) attempt to understand the source of the problem. Only then will you be able to be effective in helping patients to deal with sexual concerns.

Sample Interview Questions

Proceed from general questions to more specific ones in obtaining a sexual history. The following are suggestions for "openers":

- Tell me about your romantic life.
- How would you describe your sex life at this time?
- Is there anything troubling you about your sex life?
- Have you had any sexual thoughts that concern or disturb you?

The following questions on three more specific areas may help you to focus in on the particular concerns of your patient:

Orientation

- Are you primarily attracted to members of the opposite sex? Your own sex? Both men and women?

Current functioning

- How frequently do you have sexual contact? What does this involve? Are you (or your partner) concerned about the frequency with which you have sex?
- How often do you masturbate?
- What sort of sexual activities have been most (least) satisfying?
- Have you had any difficulties in reaching orgasm or in helping your partner to reach orgasm?
- Are you involved in any sexual activities that worry you or others, or that you must keep secret from others? (See the deviations described below.)

History

- What were your parents' attitudes toward sex?
- How would you describe your parents' sexual relationships?
- From whom did you learn about sex?
- Did you have any sexual experiences as a child with older people, e.g., parents, siblings? If so, what were the circumstances?
- Who prepared you for the onset of puberty/menstruation?
- When did you begin masturbating? (Ask about feelings and fantasies.)
- What was your sexual experience like as a teenager? As a young adult?
- How have you felt about yourself as a man/woman?
- Would you say that you are comfortable with yourself as a sexual person?

THE SEXUAL RESPONSE CYCLE

In evaluating your patients' sexual functioning, keep in mind the normal cycle of sexual response. Many texts (e.g., Masters and Johnson 1966) have excellent detailed discussions of this cycle. The brief discussion included here is only meant to provide an introductory overview.

Sexual stimulation produces characteristic responses in men and women that can be conceptualized as a four-phase cycle (see Table 13-1). These phases were described by Masters and Johnson in their research on human sexuality and have been useful to clinicians in understanding normal and disturbed sexual functioning.

Phase I: Excitement. Sexual excitement may be brought about by psychological stimulation (through fantasy or by the presence of a desired person), or it may be brought about by physical stimulation (e.g., kissing, caressing). Excitement is characterized by erection of the penis in the man and vaginal lubrication in the woman. Excitement may arise within 10 to 30 seconds after stimulation has begun, and it may last from several minutes to several hours. Another observable physical response in the excitement phase is nipple erection, more common in women than in men. Women also experience thickening of the labia minora and erection of the clitoris due to venous engorgement.

Phase II: Plateau. Continued sexual stimulation brings the individual to the threshold of orgasm, resulting in further physiological changes and increasing sexual tension in both men and women. In women, the vaginal barrel constricts along the outer third (the orgasmic platform), while the clitoris elevates and retracts behind the symphysis pubis (but may be stimulated indirectly through traction on the labia minora). Breast size increases, and the labia minora become bright or deep red because of venous engorgement. In males, the testes increase in size (up to 50%) and are brought up toward the body as the scrotal sac tightens and lifts. Two or three drops of mucoid fluid containing viable sperm are secreted from the penis at this stage as well, so that pregnancy can occur even if the man withdraws prior to orgasm. In both sexes, heart rate increases, respiration becomes more rapid, elevation of blood pressure is common, and there are voluntary contractions of large skeletal muscle groups. This preorgasmic phase is usually brief, lasting from 0.5 to 3 minutes.

Phase III: Orgasm. Increasing sexual tension generally culminates in orgasm, which is experienced as intensely pleasurable. In males, the

Table 13-1. The four phases of the sexual response cycle

Phase I—Excitement	Phase III—Orgasm
Phase II—Plateau	Phase IV—Resolution

testes, prostate, and seminal vesicles contract and expel sperm and seminal fluid into the entrance of the urethra. This is followed immediately by three to seven contractions of the urethra and muscles of the penis, ejecting the seminal fluid forcibly through the urethra and out of the penis. In females, orgasms consist of 3 to 15 involuntary contractions of the lower third of the vagina and strong, sustained contractions of the uterus. Both men and women also have involuntary contractions of the internal and external anal sphincters. In both sexes, muscular contractions during the height of orgasm occur at intervals of 0.8 seconds, and orgasm commonly lasts from 3 to 15 seconds. Other manifestations of orgasm include voluntary and involuntary movements of large muscle groups (e.g., extension of arms and legs), facial grimacing, and muscular spasm. Blood pressure rises by up to 80 mm systolic and 40 mm diastolic, while heart rate may increase to 180 beats per minute, and respirations, up to 40 per minute. Some people also experience a "sex flush," a blotching of the skin in variable patterns on the body that disappears within minutes after orgasm.

Phase IV: Resolution. After orgasm, the resolution phase brings the body back to its resting state by gradual disgorgement of blood from the genitals and a return of these organs to their resting size. If orgasm occurs, resolution is rapid and may take only 10 to 15 minutes. However, if orgasm does not occur, resolution may take 2 to 6 hours (in some cases even up to a day) and may be associated with pelvic discomfort. Resolution after orgasm is characterized by a subjective sense of well-being. For males, there is a refractory period after orgasm in which they cannot be stimulated to another orgasm. This may last from several minutes to several hours. There is no such refractory period in women; they are capable of multiple and successive orgasms.

Female Sexual Response

Most women have certain physical responses in addition to those mentioned above. The female vagina enlarges during sexual excitement and naturally accommodates to the size of the penis (or other object) inserted into it. Lubrication occurs internally, so lubrication of the outer labia must usually be accomplished by manual manipulation or through the thrusting of the penis.

At the moment of orgasm, the woman has a tendency to increase her pelvic thrusting, while the man tends to freeze his thrusting activity. Female orgasm seems to be triggered by stimulation of the clitoris, either directly—through masturbation—or indirectly—as when the thrusts of the penis cause traction on the labia minora, with resulting stimulation of the attached clitoris. Thus, female orgasm is triggered by clitoral stimulation and manifested by vaginal contractions.

Male Sexual Response

Men tend to show less variation in their sexual response cycles than women do, although there is some variation in the duration of each cycle phase. The man cannot generally have intercourse without first obtaining an erection that is sufficiently rigid to allow him to penetrate the vagina. Once erection occurs, it will normally wax and wane if the excitement phase is prolonged; this normal response should not be a cause for concerns about potency.

Men experience two stages of orgasm. The first is a moment of ejaculatory inevitability, when the testes, prostate, and seminal vesicles expel sperm and seminal fluid into the entrance of the urethra. The man "feels the ejaculation coming" and at this point can no longer interrupt the process voluntarily. The second stage is ejaculation, during which the semen is forcibly ejected out of the penis via the urethra. At the moment of orgasm, the man tends to stop his thrusting activity and hold the ejaculating penis in deep penetration.

Sex and Aging

Some of the most common misconceptions about human sexual response relate to the aging process. As the number of people over age 65 increases in this society, more attention is being focused on all aspects of geriatric life, including sexuality (see Chapter 9). People vary in their capacity for and interest in an active sexual life beyond middle age. Physical health is important, but, barring major physical illness, other factors seem to loom larger in determining sexual activity in later life—most obviously, the availability of a sexual partner. Also, people who have been sexually active in earlier years are more likely to remain so in later life, as are those who live in an environment that is accepting of their sexuality.

Changes in sexual responsiveness do occur with aging. In aging women, the vasocongestive response is diminished, and the elasticity and secretory capacities of the vagina decrease. However, women who continue to have intercourse regularly can minimize these changes and function effectively in spite of them. The aging man takes longer to have an erection, and erection may be less complete, although adequate to penetrate the vagina. The expulsive force of the ejaculation also diminishes, refractory time between orgasms is longer, and greater stimulation

is required to achieve erection in the first place. For men, erectile difficulty is the only sexual dysfunction that correlates with advancing age.
Some of this erectile failure is psychogenic in origin and can be treated
(see below); in other cases, impotence is due to neurological or vascular
disease.

Sexual interest and activity are the rule rather than the exception
among people in their fifties and sixties; some people continue to be
sexually active even in their eighties. One does not become "used up"
sexually; indeed, surveys suggest that a lifelong history of active sexual
functioning is a good predictor of sexual activity in old age—"If you use
it, you don't lose it."

SEXUAL DISORDERS: DEVIATION VERSUS DYSFUNCTION

Sexual deviations (also called "perversions") involve a disturbance of
sexual *aim*. Sexual dysfunction denotes a disturbance of sexual *function*.
The difference is thus that deviations are characterized by good and
pleasurable sexual functioning, whereas dysfunctions are not. The sexual deviant's choice of sexual object differs from the norm, and he or she
is aroused by stimuli that are not exciting to most people (e.g., a child, an
animal, a shoe). He or she may be excited by bondage or by receiving
punishment, by looking at or by exposing the genitals, or by inflicting
pain. But arousal and orgasm are physiologically normal and bring the
sexual deviant pleasure. Sexual deviations are treated with certain types
of behavior and insight-oriented therapy, as discussed below.

Sexual dysfunctions are psychophysiological disorders that make it
impossible for the person to enjoy sex or, in some cases, to have sex at all.
They involve inhibition of normal physiological responses—that is, venous engorgement of the sexual organs, and/or the orgasmic response
itself—that makes the experience of sexual activity in some way
unpleasurable. Sexual dysfunctions are quite common. Dysfunction that
results from medical illness may clear when the primary disorder is
treated, and those cases that are primarily psychological in origin respond to particular types of sex therapy and to a combination of sex
therapy and insight-oriented psychotherapy.

You will encounter patients with sexual dysfunctions in any setting
in which you practice, and you are likely to encounter sexual deviations
as well. Your receptivity to hearing about such issues, and your awareness of the possibilities for treating these disorders, can be crucial to
helping people who are often confused and embarrassed about problems
they do not understand.

Sexual Dysfunction

In evaluating people who come to you with sexual complaints, it is important to consider a variety of medical and psychological factors that can interfere with sexual pleasure and function. Your understanding of the etiology of the disorder will obviously determine how you decide to treat it, and treatment runs a wide gamut from hormone replacement for an endocrine deficiency to individual psychodynamic psychotherapy to couples behavior therapy.

Physical causes. While physical causes account for a small percentage (between 3% and 20%) of all cases, it is essential that these be considered. Many somatic causes of sexual dysfunction are treatable, and sexual dysfunction may be an early clue to occult medical illness. Therefore, every person who presents with a sexual complaint should have a routine physical examination and laboratory screening. Table 13-2 lists some of the most common medical causes of sexual dysfunction.

Psychological causes. The great majority of sexual dysfunctions are primarily psychogenic in origin. *Early sexual experiences* and *the attitudes of important figures* such as parents and siblings can have a profound effect on sexual functioning in adulthood. A history of sexual abuse (rape or incest), guilt about sexuality (e.g., the message from parents that sexuality is bad), and early homosexual experiences that arouse anxiety about one's sexual preference are among the more common factors thought to underlie sexual dysfunction. *Lack of information* about sex can result in ignorance about sexual techniques, perpetuation of myths about sex (e.g., "a real man is always potent and always interested in sex"), and unrealistic expectations of oneself and one's partner. Particular *life stresses* (e.g., death of a loved one, loss of a job, marital conflict) can precipitate problems in sexual fuctioning that may become self-perpetuating and require treatment. Couples who have trouble communicating often present with sexual problems, but *communication difficulties* may extend well beyond the sexual relationship.

Finally, a host of *intrapsychic problems* may precipitate difficulties in sexual functioning in one or both partners. The following are three of the most common intrapsychic factors underlying sexual dysfunction:

1. *Depression.* A depressive disorder (e.g., a major depressive episode or dysthymia) may be manifested by sexual dysfunction. It is often difficult to determine whether the sexual problem (e.g., impotence) is a symptom of an underlying depressive disorder, or whether the sexual problem has itself caused the individual to become depressed. You must be alert to the possibility of a treat-

Table 13-2. Medical causes of sexual dysfunction

Class of disorders	Specific examples	Effect on sexual functioning
Biochemical or physiological disorders	Cardiopulmonary, hepatic, renal, endocrine, and degenerative disorders; systemic infections, malignancies	Decreased libido, impaired arousal in women, decreased potency in men
Tumor infection	Mumps, tuberculosis, tumors of various origins	Invasion of specific structures (e.g., testes, ovaries); systemic symptoms that decrease libido or impair arousal
Anatomic or mechanical interference	Urethritis, prostatitis, endometritis, vaginitis, pelvic inflammatory disease, priapism, phimosis, clitoral adhesions, imperforate hymen	Pain, damage, irritation of the genitalia
Postsurgery with neurological or vascular damage	Prostatectomy, perineal resections, lumbar sympathectomies, abdominal aortic surgery, obstetrical trauma, complications of obstetrical procedures	Pain, obstructed vaginal introitus, erectile or ejaculatory disturbance, diminished or altered sensation
Neurological disorders	Temporal or frontal lobe damage (e.g., from trauma), amyotrophic lateral sclerosis, spina bifida, multiple sclerosis, spinal cord surgery or trauma, tertiary syphilis	Change in libido (from damage to higher centers of the brain); impaired erection, ejaculation, or female orgasm (from spinal cord injury)

Table 13-2. *Continued*

Class of disorders	Specific examples	Effect on sexual functioning
Vascular disorders	Interference with penile blood supply in males, due to thrombosis of penile veins or arteries, or to aortic thrombosis, leukemia, or sickle cell disease	Impaired penile erection
Endocrine disorders	Pituitary, adrenal, or gonadal diseases, which result in decreased androgen levels	Decreased libido or erectile responsiveness
Genetic or congenital disorders	*In males:* Klinefelter's syndrome (impotence), bladder exstrophy, hypospadias, undescended testicles *In females:* Imperforate hymen, congenital defects of internal and external genitalia	Impotence (Klinefelter's syndrome), decreased libido, pain or physical obstruction to sexual functioning
Drugs and medications	Numerous pharmacological agents alter sexual response. Among the most commonly implicated in sexual dysfunction are *CNS depressants* (alcohol, narcotics, sedatives); *anticholinergics; antiadrenergics*	Impotence and ejaculatory disturbance, decreased libido

able depressive disorder in anyone who comes to you complaining of sexual dysfunction.

2. *Control issues.* Sex involves a certain amount of loss of control as we abandon ourselves to erotic feelings. People who are concerned about losing control of their emotions may find sexuality threatening and may inhibit their sexual functioning.

3. *Low self-esteem.* People who suffer from low self-esteem, performance anxiety, and fear of failure may see sexual encounters as tests. They may become so anxious about "succeeding" at sex that they are unable to function.

Sexual dysfunction takes a variety of forms in females (see Table 13-3) and males (see Table 13-4). The most common problems are listed below.

Table 13-3. Types of female sexual dysfunction

Type	Definition
General sexual dysfunction	Inability to derive erotic pleasure from sexual stimulation
Orgastic dysfunction	Specific difficulty in reaching orgasm
Primary	Never experienced orgasm by any means of stimulation
Secondary	Experienced orgasm but subsequently developed this difficulty
Vaginismus	Impenetrability of the vagina because of involuntary spasm of the vaginal muscles
Dyspareunia	Pain on intercourse

Table 13-4. Types of male sexual dysfunction

Type	Impairment
Impotence (erectile dysfunction)	Impairment of penile erection that is recurrent and persistent
Primary	Never potent with a partner
Secondary	Potent in the past but subsequently developed erectile dysfunction
Premature ejaculation	Inability to exert voluntary control over the ejaculatory reflex
Retarded ejaculation	Inhibition of the ejaculatory reflex
Primary	Never ejaculated with a partner
Secondary	Ejaculated normally in the past but subsequently developed this difficulty

Female sexual dysfunction

General sexual dysfunction (frigidity). General sexual dysfunction is commonly called *frigidity*, but this is a nonspecific term that carries a pejorative connotation. General sexual dysfunction refers to an inability to derive erotic pleasure from sexual stimulation. Women with this disorder may show little or no physiological response to sexual stimulation (e.g., no vasocongestion or vaginal lubrication) and may experience themselves as essentially devoid of sexual feelings. Many of these women consider sexual activity an ordeal that they must endure to preserve a relationship, or sex may be so repugnant to them that any activity is impossible. Some women with this disorder are able to enjoy the nonerotic aspects of sexual contact (e.g., touching, physical closeness), despite their lack of sexual responsiveness. Among the psychological factors that seem to foster general sexual dysfunction are strict parental prohibitions against sexual expression in early life, overwhelming anxiety rooted in childhood conflicts or in current concerns, and hostility directed at, but not directly expressed to, the partner or men in general.

Orgastic dysfunction. Orgastic dysfunction is a more limited disorder that denotes a specific difficulty in reaching orgasm. Women who suffer from this disorder frequently have a strong sexual drive and may reach high levels of sexual arousal. The disorder is termed *primary orgastic dysfunction* if the woman has never experienced orgasm by any means of stimulation, and *secondary orgastic dysfunction* if she previously experienced orgasm and subsequently developed this difficulty. The difficulty in reaching orgasm may be present regardless of the setting, or it may depend on the situation. For example, some women can have orgasms with masturbation but not during coitus, while for others the situation is reversed. Some women rarely have orgasms with any partner and are surprised when they do, while others only experience difficulty with a particular partner. The diagnosis of a disorder is not always easy, since female response varies greatly. Failure to ever have an orgasm constitutes a disorder in almost all cases. However, not reaching orgasm during coitus (but being able to have orgasms during masturbation) is not necessarily a disorder but may be a normal variation of female functioning.

Women differ greatly in their thresholds for reaching orgasm and require varying amounts of clitoral stimulation, probably due to a combination of physiological and psychological factors. Coitus actually provides only mild clitoral stimulation (compared with masturbation and other more direct techniques), so only women who can be orgasmic with relatively mild stimulation will have orgasms in this way.

In this and other situation-specific cases, the diagnosis of a disorder depends to a large extent on whether the patient (and/or her partner) is disturbed by the problem and feels the need for treatment. If not, there is no reason to label the inability to reach orgasm during coitus "disordered." Many women are satisfied with other means of reaching orgasm and do not seek treatment.

Orgastic dysfunction is the most common complaint among women who do seek treatment for a sexual disorder. When a woman wants to have orgasms and cannot, the cause is often her involuntary inhibition of the response. She may unwittingly do this because the orgasm has acquired some symbolic meaning (e.g., losing control), because its intensity frightens her, because she is in conflict over her erotic feelings, or because she is uncertain about her commitment to her mate or even hostile toward her mate.

Vaginismus. Vaginismus refers to a very specific syndrome in which penetration of the vagina is impossible because of involuntary spasm of the muscles surrounding the vaginal entrance. Whenever penetration is attempted, the vaginal entrance literally snaps shut, so that coitus cannot take place. Even pelvic examinations must often be carried out under anesthesia. In addition to primary spasm of the sphincter vaginae and levator ani muscles, vaginismus may also involve a phobia of coitus and vaginal penetration that prompts avoidance of any situation in which coitus might occur. Some women with this disorder are quite sexually responsive as long as sexual contact does not lead to intercourse.

The diagnosis of vaginismus is made relatively rarely and can only be made definitely when involuntary spasm is noted on pelvic examination. Among the psychogenic factors that seem to be associated with this disorder are a history of sexual trauma, stern parental prohibitions against sexuality, confusion about choice of sexual object, and a partner's sexual dysfunction (particularly primary impotence).

Dyspareunia. Dyspareunia refers to pain in the genital area during coitus. While it occurs occasionally in men, it is more common in women. Obviously, there are numerous physical causes of pain upon intercourse (e.g., in various medical conditions and after surgical procedures), but *functional dyspareunia* refers to pain with no demonstrable physical cause. It is essentially a somatoform disorder (see Chapter 8) and is thought to be due to underlying fears of or conflicts over sexual activity.

Male sexual dysfunction

Impotence (erectile dysfunction). Because a great deal of male self-esteem is invested in the capacity for penile erection, there is probably no other physical condition that is as potentially frustrating or humiliating for a man. Impotence is simply an impairment of penile erection due to failure of the vascular reflex mechanism to pump a sufficient amount of blood into the cavernous sinuses of the penis to render it firm. Probably more than half of the male population have experienced occasional transient episodes of impotence, and these episodes are within the limits of normal sexual behavior.

The diagnosis of impotence is made when erectile dysfunction is recurrent and persistent. Men with primary impotence have never been potent with a partner, although they may have full erections when masturbating and may have spontaneous erections. Secondary impotence describes a condition in which a man has functioned well in the past but at some point developed erectile dysfunction. The impotent man may feel aroused and excited in a sexual situation and want to make love, and may even ejaculate, but his penis remains flaccid.

Psychological factors play a crucial role in an overwhelming majority of cases of impotence. Erectile function is impaired in most men when they become anxious. Thus, normal sexual functioning usually occurs only when the man does not feel threatened. There are great variations in the patterns of impotence among men with this complaint, because the precise aspect of the sexual act that arouses anxiety differs. Some men are impotent only upon entering the vagina. Some are impotent with one partner but not another, or are only impotent when they feel the expectation to perform. The source of anxiety may be in the man's current life, or the anxiety may stem from early childhood fears and experiences.

Why are some men more prone than others to become impotent when they are anxious? Some clinicians postulate that certain men have a physiological vulnerability to erectile dysfunction (perhaps because of a highly reactive vasocongestive system), while other men do not.

There are numerous medical conditions that cause impotence. Although these are much less common than psychological factors, they must not be overlooked. As noted above, any man who complains of impotence should have a medical and neurological workup in addition to a psychological evaluation. Among the most prevalent somatic causes of impotence are fatigue, early undiagnosed diabetes mellitus, low androgen levels, thyroid disease, kidney disease, liver disease, nonspecific debilitating illness, heart or respiratory illness, and abuse of narcotics, alcohol, or estrogenic and parasympatholytic medications. Neurological diseases that produce impotence include multiple sclerosis, lower spinal cord damage, and damage to the hypothalamic and temporal lobe regions of the brain.

Premature ejaculation. This is a condition in which the man is unable to exert voluntary control over his ejaculatory reflex, so that when he is sexually aroused, he reaches orgasm more quickly than he and/or his partner would like. Men who suffer from premature ejaculation cannot tolerate high levels of sexual tension and stimulation without ejaculating, and their partners are often left unsatisfied when orgasm occurs too soon and lovemaking ceases. The premature ejaculator may become anxious about reaching orgasm too soon and begin to avoid sexual activity so as not to face the difficulty.

When is ejaculation premature? The definition has been difficult, for no one criterion seems to suffice. The number of thrusts a man can tolerate before ejaculating, the number of seconds of coitus he can endure before ejaculation, and the satisfaction of his partner have all been put forward as criteria for the diagnosis, but all are relative and arbitrary. In fact, the crucial aspect seems to be the man's inability to voluntarily control his ejaculatory reflex, regardless of how many seconds have passed or how many thrusts he has made, and regardless of whether his partner has reached orgasm. The rapidity of orgasm is the primary complaint, but many premature ejaculators also have diminished perceptions of their erotic sensations as they become intensely aroused, and therefore are not aware when orgasm is imminent.

Many psychological theories have been put forward to explain the causes of premature ejaculation. Covert hostility toward women has been proposed by traditional psychoanalytic theorists, but it has become clear that the determinants of this disorder are more varied and complex. Many men with this disorder have otherwise good and satisfying relationships with wives or lovers. Other clinicians postulate that early hurried sexual experiences (e.g., with prostitutes or in the back seats of automobiles) play a role. However, many men with a history of such experiences do not go on to develop this disorder.

Clearly, anxiety plays a role in premature ejaculation, because it does not allow the man to perceive erotic sensations correctly. Also, marital difficulties and underlying psychiatric illness have been implicated in some, but not all, cases of premature ejaculation. Among the factors that do not seem to play a role are masturbatory practices and familial patterns.

Premature ejaculation is very rarely caused by physical factors. Among the physical conditions that may contribute to premature ejaculation are local disease of the posterior urethra (e.g., inflammation of the prostate), spinal cord injuries, multiple sclerosis, and other degenerative neurological disorders.

Retarded ejaculation. In this disorder (also called *ejaculatory incompetence*), the ejaculatory reflex is inhibited, although erection is usually not impaired. This may be primary, if the man has never ejaculated with a partner, or secondary, if the condition arose after an initial period of adequate functioning. The disorder may be so severe that the man cannot ejaculate when masturbating by himself, but in most cases extravaginal ejaculation is possible. This disorder may prompt the man to prolong intercourse for a very long period (e.g., more than an hour) or to fake orgasms with his partner and then either remain frustrated or achieve release only through masturbation following intercourse.

The causes of this disorder are rarely physical. Among the somatic illnesses that occasionally play a role are depressed androgen levels, undetected diabetes, spinal cord injuries, and drugs that impair the adrenergic mechanism of the sympathetic nervous system, which controls ejaculation (e.g., certain antihypertensive drugs). Thioridazine (Mellaril) can cause retrograde ejaculation, that is, ejaculation that forces semen up the urethra into the bladder rather than out of the penis. As this is painful, it is important to bear this side effect in mind when choosing an antipsychotic for males.

The most commonly reported psychological factors that seem to underlie ejaculatory incompetence include a strict religious upbringing that engenders sexual guilt, strongly suppressed anger, ambivalence toward a partner, fears of abandonment by a lover, and childhood fears of parental retaliation for sexual urges.

Treatment of sexual dysfunction

Whenever a patient presents with a sexual complaint, you should proceed with a thorough workup to determine which type of therapy is indicated. Some people present with complaints of sexual dysfunction but, in the course of giving you a psychiatric history, will reveal serious psychopathology (e.g., depression, psychosis) that requires treatment before sexual concerns can be addressed. In addition to a careful psychological evaluation, be sure that a thorough medical evaluation is carried out, including a medical history, physical examination, and, where indicated, a neurological, urological, or gynecological examination and appropriate laboratory studies.

Once you have ruled out organic pathology and serious psychopathology, you have a variety of treatment modalities from which to choose.

Dual-sex therapy (Masters and Johnson's techniques). The new sex therapy originated with the work of William H. Masters and Virginia E. Johnson. This type of therapy relies on behavioral techniques and makes the couple, rather than the dysfunctional individual, the focus of therapy. This is based on the premise that there is no such thing as a partner who is uninvolved in the sexual problem, nor is there one "sick half" in a couple. Both people are expected to participate fully in the therapy and to learn to focus on their own sexual feelings and desires, as well as to learn those of their partner and to improve communication within the dyad.

Treatment is based on the observation that performance anxiety and demands for sexual performance intensify and perpetuate sexual dysfunction. Using a man-woman team of cotherapists, sessions focus on correcting misinformation or ignorance about sexual functioning, providing support and reassurance, improving communication, and removing the demand to perform sexually.

After a thorough evaluation of the couple, sessions begin with "homework assignments"—exercises the couple carries out in private. All sexual activity, including intercourse, is prohibited until the therapists feel that the couple is ready. This enforced abstinence is the first step in removing the pressure for sexual performance. The first exercises are *sensate focus* exercises, designed to increase sensory awareness of oneself and one's partner. Each partner takes turns "pleasuring" the other, first touching all areas except breasts and genitals, and later including these areas.

Therapy sessions focus on the couple's experiences in carrying out the exercises; these provide crucial information to the therapists about where there is resistance to sexual activity (e.g., the man who is always too tired to do the exercises or the woman who develops a headache whenever exercises are initiated). Fears and misunderstandings can be clarified in the therapy sessions, and exercises repeated until they are pleasurable for both partners. Once this pleasuring is mastered, couples are usually communicating with each other more effectively than when they began treatment, and sessions move on to specific exercises directed at the particular dysfunction.

General sexual dysfunction is treated with sensate focus experiences to help the woman focus on erotic sensations, followed by genital stimulation by herself and with her partner. Intercourse is initiated when she chooses to do so and with no pressure to achieve orgasm. As she feels more secure in experiencing sexual feelings with her partner, the woman who suffers from this disorder is likely to be able to achieve considerable pleasure and even reach orgasm during sexual activity.

Organic dysfunction is treated with exercises that heighten the woman's arousal prior to coitus, to increase her awareness of and pleasure in her vaginal sensations and to maximize clitoral stimulation. This is done by using masturbatory techniques (and in some cases a vibrator), as well as teaching specific coital positions in which the partner can maximally stimulate the woman. All this is done in situations in which the pressure on the woman to reach orgasm is minimized.

Vaginismus is treated by teaching the woman and her partner to use fingers to gently dilate the vaginal opening, and to use mechnical dilators to accomplish the same purpose. Once vaginal dilation has been comfortably accomplished by these means, it is usually possible for the male to insert his penis into the vagina easily and without discomfort to his partner.

Premature ejaculation has been very successfully treated by using exercises that repeatedly stimulate the man to the point of near ejaculatory inevitability and then cease stimulation before inevitability occurs, thereby preventing ejaculation (the "stop-and-go" technique). This allows the man to experience intense sexual excitement repeatedly without ejaculating. This technique is accompanied by the forcible prevention when inevitability occurs by using the "squeeze" technique, which involves squeezing the head of the penis with the thumb and first and second fingers. The squeeze technique has had almost universal success in treating premature ejaculation.

Ejaculatory incompetence is dealt with in the opposite manner. Exercises are aimed at achieving intravaginal ejaculation, since in most cases ejaculation during masturbation is not impaired. The woman stimulates the man manually to orgasm in her presence, with the penis in gradually closer proximity to the vaginal opening. Eventually, she stimulates her partner to the point of ejaculatory inevitability and inserts the penis into her vagina without interrupting the ejaculation process. A single episode of intravaginal ejaculation often breaks the male's block against intravaginal ejaculation.

Impotence has been alleviated by creating nondemanding sexual situations in which the man can experience erections without the pressure to have intercourse. Exercises include masturbation, stimulation of the penis to erection by the partner, and gradual introduction of the penis into the vagina by the partner in the woman-on-top position. Even when the penis is inserted into the vagina, no thrusting is allowed at first, or only minimal movements to maintain the penis in a stimulated state. Thrusting is allowed in subsequent exercises, and orgasm naturally ensues. Relieved of the demand to perform, the man who can gradually achieve erections and achieve vaginal penetration usually proceeds at his own pace to have effective coitus.

Masters and Johnson have reported high rates of success for these treatment approaches, with an overall rate of 80% success for all dysfunctions combined. They report the greatest success with premature ejaculation (97%) and the most limited success with primary impotence

(59%). Although some critics argue that results are temporary, these behavioral techniques have proved valuable in the treatment of sexual dysfunction.

Psychodynamically oriented sex therapy. Combining psychodynamic psychotherapy and sex therapy enables clinicians to treat people whose sexual complaints are associated with other mental disorders. This therapy may continue for longer than the usual 10 to 15 sessions involved in sex therapy alone, and it may involve individual work with each partner as well as work with the couple. This approach is particularly useful for couples who have difficulties in their relationship that clearly extend beyond the realm of sex. Couples are given "homework assignments" as described above, but sessions also focus more intensively on the psychological conflicts and distortions that hamper the relationship—often problems that originated for each partner in early childhood relationships.

When one partner is more obviously in need of psychological support and help than the other, individual sessions can be tailored to that person's needs and carried out in addition to the couple's therapy sessions. For example, if a woman who complains of general sexual dysfunction discovers in couple therapy that she harbors deeply rooted hostility toward men, she may want to work with the therapist individually to understand more about the origins of this anger, while continuing in joint meetings to explore the ways in which she unwittingly distances her husband.

The combination of psychodynamic and sex therapy is commonly used in general mental health facilities, while sex therapy alone is often used in those clinics and facilities that limit their work to the treatment of sexual dysfunctions.

Hypnotherapy. Some clinicians have found hypnotic suggestions useful in alleviating anxiety (e.g., in a man with secondary impotence) and in removing psychological impediments to vaginal lubrication, erections, and orgasm. This is not a couple's approach, and is aimed at specific symptoms rather than at an individual's general ability to experience and communicate his or her sexual feelings in a relationship.

Behavior therapy. This therapy was initially developed to treat phobias, but the technique of systematic desensitization has also been applied to sexual situations that arouse anxiety (see Chapter 17). The patient identifies situations that arouse anxiety and foster symptoms (e.g., when vaginal penetration results in impotence), and the therapist gradually desensitizes the patient to these anxiety-provoking situations. Like hypnotherapy, this approach is generally for individuals rather than couples.

Group therapy. Groups have been useful in treating people with sexual dysfunction, because they can impart sexual information, provide reassurance, and offer mutual support to people who suffer from similar difficulties. Some groups consist of people of one sex who have the same disorder; others are composed of couples. Groups are particularly useful for people who need to explore interpersonal difficulties, as well as specific sexual problems.

Individual psychotherapy. Classical psychodynamic theory holds that sexual dysfunctions have their roots in early childhood experiences and conflicts that therapy can help to elucidate. When irrational fears and fantasies are brought to light and understood, the symptoms of sexual dysfunction often lessen. However, the psychodynamic approach is less effective than the behavioral approach of Masters and Johnson in rapidly removing specific sexual symptoms. Individual psychotherapy is most useful for people whose sexual dysfunction is part of a larger constellation of psychological difficulties and who have other symptoms for which psychotherapy is indicated.

Sexual Deviations

Sexual deviations (also called *perversions* and *paraphilias*) are disorders that involve unusual sexual-object choices or sexual acts (see Table 13-5). The person who suffers from a perversion generally requires these specific acts or objects or images in order to be sexually aroused and to achieve orgasm. He or she must repeatedly recreate the needed situation or fantasy. Perversions most often involve one of the following: the use of a nonhuman object for sexual arousal (excluding vibrators and other objects designed for that purpose), the experience of suffering on the part of the individual or of his or her partner, or sexual activity with a nonconsenting partner.

Many people with perversions do not regard themselves as ill and only come to mental health facilities for help when their behavior has brought them into conflict with society (e.g., with their families or with the law). People with sexual perversions are grossly impaired in their ability to participate in mutually gratifying sexual relations with consenting adults, and marital difficulties are common.

Perversions are much more common in men than in women, but the reasons for this are not clear. Environmental factors (particularly early childhood experiences) appear to play a major role in the genesis of sexual perversions, and sons often develop the specific perversions of their fathers. Because these disorders are relatively uncommon, they will be discussed only briefly.

Table 13-5. Types of sexual deviations

Type	Definition
Transsexualism	Persistent sense of discomfort about one's anatomic sex and strong desire to change one's genitals and secondary sex characteristics
Transvestitism	Dressing in clothes appropriate to the opposite sex for purposes of arousal
Fetishism	Use of a nonhuman object as the preferred method of achieving sexual excitement
Zoophilia	Repeated sexual arousal through contact with an animal
Pedophilia	Sexual contact with prepubertal children as the preferred means to sexual excitement
Exhibitionism	Exposure of the genitals in public to unsuspecting strangers to achieve sexual excitement
Voyeurism	Repeatedly looking at unsuspecting people who are disrobing or engaging in sexual activity
Sexual masochism	Obtaining sexual gratification through mental suffering or bodily pain
Sexual sadism	Inflicting physical or psychological pain on another to achieve sexual excitement

Transsexualism. This disorder involves a persistent sense of discomfort and inappropriateness about one's anatomic sex and a wish to change one's genitals and secondary sex characteristics in order to live as a member of the opposite sex. Transsexualism must be distinguished from transvestitism and homosexuality (see below), neither of which necessarily involves a desire to change one's sexual anatomy. Cross-dressing and homosexual behavior are common among transsexuals, but the eventual goal for these people is often surgical and hormonal treatment leading to reassignment of gender. Surgical procedures to change external anatomy from male to female are more common than the reverse procedure.

Transsexualism is often associated with moderate to severe personality disturbance. Surgical correction does not bring about a satisfactory sexual adjustment for some transsexual individuals, and depression and suicide attempts are frequent complications of this disorder. Thus, careful and detailed psychiatric evaluation must be a prerequisite to surgical procedures for anyone wishing to change his or her sex.

Transvestitism. Transvestitism involves dressing in clothing appropriate to members of the opposite sex for purposes of arousal and as an adjunct to masturbation or coitus. This generally occurs among *het-*

erosexual males and may range from occasional cross-dressing to intense involvement in an elaborate transvestite subculture. When not cross-dressed, the transvestite usually appears and acts masculine. Homosexual experiences are reported in this population, but sexual preference is generally for members of the opposite sex. Cross-dressing often begins in adolescence, but may start earlier, and is often used to alleviate anxiety in addition to providing erotic stimulation. Transvestitism must be distinguished from cross-dressing by homosexuals, which is often carried out in order to attract homosexual partners; and from transsexualism, which involves a conscious desire to change one's anatomy in order to become a member of the opposite sex.

Fetishism. Fetishism involves the use of a nonhuman object as the preferred (or only) method of achieving sexual excitement. These objects tend to be shoes, corsets, gloves, or other items of apparel closely associated with the human body. Fetishes may also involve body parts (e.g., feet, hair) rather than inanimate objects. The object may be the sole focus of sexual activity (e.g., masturbation into a shoe) or may be integrated into sexual activity with a partner (e.g., the demand that the partner wear high-heeled shoes).

The fetish differs from simple experimentation to achieve sexual arousal, because people with true fetishes require the presence of a specific object (at least in fantasy) for arousal to occur, and the object is preferred over human beings. The desired object is usually linked to someone important from the individual's childhood and serves to help maintain some special relationship in fantasy with that person.

Zoophilia. Zoophilia involves repeated sexual arousal through contact with an animal. Sexual contact with animals (masturbation or coitus) is not uncommon among adolescents, particularly those raised in rural settings. However, true zoophilia involves preference for sexual contact with an animal even when other sexual outlets are possible.

Pedophilia. Pedophilia involves sexual contact with prepubertal children as the preferred or only means of achieving sexual excitement. Pedophiles tend to fall into two distinct groups: those who choose children of the opposite sex (heterosexual pedophiles) and those who choose children of the same sex (homosexual pedophiles). Virtually all pedophiles who come to the attention of mental health professionals are men.

Heterosexual pedophiles tend to be socially maladjusted men, often alcoholic individuals with troubled marriages. The incidence of heterosexual pedophilia peaks among late adolescent boys and among men in their forties and sixties. They generally prefer to engage in sexual activity with 8- to 10-year-old girls.

Homosexual pedophiles tend to be men who have never married, and they tend to prefer prepubertal or pubescent boys as the objects of sexual activity. Many of these men were themselves sexually abused by older men when they were children.

There are few reliable statistics on the relative incidences of homosexual and heterosexual pedophilia, but a great majority (some estimates are as high as 90%) of incidents are perpetrated by heterosexual men. Especially common is sexual activity between fathers (or stepfathers) and their preadolescent or early adolescent daughters. Thus, contrary to popular myth, homosexual men do not pose the most significant sexual threat to children in our society.

Exhibitionism. Exhibitionism involves exposure of the genitals in public to unsuspecting strangers as a means of achieving sexual excitement, with no attempt at further sexual activity with these strangers. The exhibitionistic person is usually aware of the desire to shock observers. Exhibitionistic individuals are exclusively men, and they generally expose themselves to women and girls. They may begin this practice at any time after the onset of puberty, but the disorder most commonly begins in the mid-20s. These men are frequently arrested for their behavior, but they generally do not constitute a danger to those to whom they expose themselves.

Voyeurism. Voyeurism involves repeatedly looking at unsuspecting people (usually strangers) who are disrobing or engaging in sexual activity. This activity is the voyeur's preferred means of achieving sexual excitement. No sexual activity with the person is sought, but the voyeur often reaches orgasm through masturbation during the voyeuristic activity or afterward, while recalling the activity. Such people (mostly men) are usually isolated, withdrawn individuals who prowl neighborhoods looking for opportunities to "peep." This behavior often gets the voyeur into minor legal difficulties.

Voyeurism differs from sexual excitement achieved by watching a partner undress, or by viewing pornography, in that sexual partners and pornographic entertainers are willing participants and are aware of being watched.

Sexual masochism. Masochism consists of sexual gratification obtained through mental suffering or bodily pain. The individual prefers to be excited or can only be excited by being bound, beaten, humiliated, or tortured. The diagnosis is made on the basis of one or more episodes in which an individual achieves excitement through suffering. Masochistic sexual behavior occurs among heterosexuals and homosexuals. It may begin at any time, but most commonly begins in early adulthood. It may be quite dangerous, particularly if the individual must engage in increasingly harmful activities in order to be aroused. Permanent bodily injury, castration, and even death may result from such activity. Masochistic individuals often engage in sadistic sexual practices as well. Sexual masochism is distinct from masochistic personality disorder in that masochistic personality traits are not associated with conscious sexual excitement.

Sexual sadism. Sexual sadism involves inflicting physical or psychological pain on another person as a means of achieving sexual excitement. The partner may be consenting or nonconsenting, and this mode of sexual arousal is both repeated and preferred over others. Sexual sadism occurs among both heterosexuals and homosexuals, and most commonly begins in early adulthood. The harm inflicted on a partner may be mild and may not escalate over time, or harm may be quite severe and result in death or permanent disability or disfigurement of the victim. Severe sadistic practices can result in legal action and imprisonment. Sexual sadists sometimes engage in masochistic activities as well. Sexual sadism differs from sadistic personality disorder in that the latter does not involve conscious sexual excitement through the infliction of pain on others.

Treatment of sexual deviations

Sexual deviations are thought to be psychologically based and rooted in early childhood experiences. Thus, many clinicians have used psychodynamic psychotherapy in treating these disorders, albeit with limited success. Psychoanalysis attempts to elicit and resolve early childhood conflicts that are responsible for the perversion, but many disturbed people (e.g., those with severe personality disorders or psychoses) cannot tolerate such intense treatment. Individual psychotherapy aims at helping patients identify the feelings and fantasies that prompt deviant sexual behavior, find more acceptable means of obtaining sexual gratification, and diminish the extent to which perverse behaviors interfere with other aspects of their lives.

Antiandrogen agents such as medroxyprogesterone (Depo-Provera) have been used in men with sexually hyperactive perversions (e.g., in those who are involved in compulsive sexual assaults) to decrease sexual activity and thereby decrease dangerousness to self and others. Psychotropic medications (e.g., antipsychotics, lithium, anticonvulsants) have also been used to decrease paraphilic arousal, but to date there have been no controlled studies of their effectiveness.

Behavior therapies have been used to treat paraphilias. *Aversive conditioning* couples an unpleasant stimulus (electric shock, nausea) with paraphilic arousal in an attempt to negatively reinforce deviant behavior. *Covert sensitization* is a similar technique, in which the patient learns to pair his paraphilic sexual fantasies with unpleasant, anxiety-provoking mental images. *Satiation* is a technique that involves the patient going over his paraphilic fantasies repeatedly after orgasm to make the fantasies and behavior boring.

No treatment has yet proved dramatically effective with these disorders. Sexual deviations remain troubling and difficult to treat.

Homosexuality

Imagine a textbook discussion of heterosexuality as a clinical entity. Most of us take heterosexuality for granted in our dealings with other people; it is considered the norm. Yet a large portion of the population consists of men and women who prefer same-sex partners for sexual activity. You undoubtedly have encountered and will continue to encounter gay people in your personal and professional life. Whether your gay friends, colleagues, and patients feel they can tell you about their sexual orientation will depend in large part on your sensitivity and receptivity to nonheterosexual orientation and life styles.

It has been said that gay people have as much in common as coffee drinkers. There is tremendous diversity in personality traits, life-styles, and sexual practices among people whose primary orientation is homosexual. It is difficult even to define the gay population. How would one classify the many people who are heterosexual in practice and homosexual in fantasy, or those who are sexually active with both men and women, or others who make abrupt midlife changes in their sexual-object choices?

Prevalence. Homosexual behavior occurs in virtually all societies. The prevalence of homosexuality is difficult to determine, in part because of problems in defining what constitutes homosexuality and in part because much homosexuality goes unreported because of societal prejudices and pressures against open disclosure of a homosexual orientation. The best data probably remain those of Kinsey and his coworkers, who in their 1948 and 1953 studies of sexual behavior in men and women interviewed more than 11,000 men and nearly 8,000 women. Kinsey found that 4% of men were exclusively homosexual throughout their adult lives, while another 13% were predominantly homosexual for at least 3 years between the ages of 16 and 55. Most surprising to the American public was the disclosure that 37% of the men in Kinsey's sample reported at least one sexual experience with another man leading to orgasm during their postpubertal years. His findings showed the prevalence of homosexuality among women to be roughly one-third that found among men. About 28% of the women in his sample reported some homosexual experience or arousal at some time from the onset of puberty, with 13% experiencing associated orgasm. He estimated the prevalence of exclusive homosexuality among women in his sample to be between one-half and one-third of that among men.

Causes. Why do some people grow up with a heterosexual orientation and others with a homosexual one? There are no clear-cut answers. In attempting to elucidate the causes of homosexuality, researchers have explored a variety of psychological and biological hypotheses.

Traditional psychoanalytic theory views homosexuality as an arrest of psychosexual development. For men, the disturbance is thought to result from early childhood experiences with a close-binding, intimate mother and a passive, hostile, or absent father. For women, no such clear-cut family pattern has been hypothesized, but traditional theorists believe that female homosexuality involves unresolved developmental difficulties. These psychoanalytic hypotheses have not been consistently validated in clinical studies of gay men and women. And this research is significantly flawed, for most of it has been conducted by using populations of gays who have consulted a psychiatrist for emotional difficulties, thus biasing the sample toward those individuals who are psychologically troubled.

Genetic theories of the origins of homosexuality have been supported by twin studies that show a substantially higher rate of concordance for homosexuality among monozygotic (identical) than among dizygotic (fraternal) pairs of twins. However, cases of discordance among identical twins have been reported, and studies of twins reared together versus those reared apart (which would better separate genetic from environmental factors) have yet to be carried out. Thus far, it has been impossible to prove or disprove that genetic factors play a role in homosexual orientation.

Neuroendocrine studies of possible causes of homosexuality have focused on the hypothalamus and the pituitary gland. Studies of serum testosterone levels have not consistently shown differences between homosexual and heterosexual populations. However, new research is focused on the hypothesis that variations in sex hormone levels in the uterus may program the developing fetus for a heterosexual or homosexual orientation. To date, no conclusive data have emerged from this research.

In summary, the numerous theories about psychological and biological causes of homosexuality remain unproven. It is likely that both developmental and biological factors play a role in the genesis of homosexuality, as they do in the genesis of heterosexuality.

Life-style. Much publicity has been given to the gay life-style, which stereotypically involves frequent anonymous sexual contacts and little sustained emotional attachment. The subculture of gay bars and baths that facilitates such impersonal contacts has come increasingly into the public eye in recent years as the sexual transmission of AIDS has aroused concern about sexual practices. To be sure, such stereotypes do hold for some gay people, more commonly for men than for women. However, the pattern of frequent anonymous sexual contacts is typical of only one subset of the gay population; those who are involved in stable, intimate relationships are often less visible.

Some clinicians cite fleeting relationships as evidence that gay men in particular cannot sustain intimate emotional ties; others argue that our society provides no social supports that encourage gay people to form lasting relationships in the way that the institution of marriage is socially sanctioned. It is also true that as the divorce rate climbs to nearly 50% and singles bars become a more prominent part of heterosexual culture, heterosexuals and homosexuals come to look increasingly similar with respect to the frequency with which they sustain intimate relationships. In dealing with either heterosexual or homosexual patients, you must never make assumptions about life-style or sexual behavior; wait until your patient shares that information with you.

Psychopathology. There continues to be considerable controversy within our society and within the mental health profession about whether homosexuality per se is a mental disorder. Although Freud did not believe it to be so, many later psychiatrists have adhered to the notion that homosexuality is pathological. Recent studies of large nonpatient populations of heterosexuals and homosexuals do not support the thesis that homosexuality is associated with pathological personality traits or increased emotional distress or social dysfunction. Thus, the American Psychiatric Association has removed homosexuality from its *Diagnostic and Statistical Manual of Mental Disorders* as of the third edition (DSM-III 1980).

Obviously, the range of psychopathology found among homosexuals is as broad as that found among heterosexuals. But homosexuality per se is only cited as a disorder in DSM-III-R ("Sexual Disorder Not Otherwise Specified") when it is ego-dystonic, that is, when an individual strongly desires to change his or her homosexual orientation to a heterosexual one in order to lead a heterosexual life-style.

Treatment. Whether mental health professionals should be involved in helping people try to change their sexual orientation is a matter of controversy. Many different treatments have been employed to help people who want to change their homosexual orientation. Psychotherapy, psychoanalysis, and behavior therapy have been the modalities most commonly employed, and all have met with very limited success. Some clinicians estimate that one-third of gay men who enter treatment with this goal in mind achieve a heterosexual orientation through therapy. However, others are more pessimistic about the possibility of achieving a

lasting reorientation of sexual preference through any form of treatment. For men, factors reported to weigh in favor of achieving a heterosexual reorientation include youthfulness (under 35), some experience of
heterosexual arousal, and high motivation. Few data are available for
homosexual women.

Many experienced clinicians advocate that treatment for people
who are distressed by a homosexual orientation should not aim to
change sexual preference. Instead, psychotherapy should be directed
toward helping the person to be more comfortable with a gay life-style—
decreasing the shame, guilt, and anxiety that are too often associated
with homosexuality.

At the time of this writing, acquired immune deficiency syndrome
(AIDS) continues to be an epidemic of major proportions. The populations in the United States most at risk of infection are homosexual males
and intravenous drug users. Many gay men seek psychiatric treatment
with a variety of symptoms both directly and indirectly related to the
AIDS epidemic. Direct central nervous system involvement of the AIDS
virus can result in dementia. Indirectly, fear of AIDS and the loss of
friends and loved ones to the disease can result in depression and anxiety
that become disabling and require therapeutic intervention.

Advice to the clinician. Unfortunately, many health care professionals are either insensitive or openly hostile to the concerns of those
with a bisexual or homosexual orientation. You can do a great service to
all of your patients by paying attention to some simple interviewing
techniques:

- Do not assume that you know your patient's sexual orientation
  until you are told.
- Do not assume that you understand your patient's sexual practices or life-style until he or she tells you.
- Do not assume that a patient who is homosexual is troubled by his
  or her sexual orientation.
- When you are taking a sexual history, use neutral terms like
  "lover" and "relationship" until your patient tells you whether
  sexual relationships have been with men or women, or both.
- Use your patient's words for his or her sexual behavior—some
  people call themselves "homosexual," but for others this term
  carries negative connotations and "gay" is more comfortable.

BIBLIOGRAPHY

American Psychiatric Association: Diagnostic and Statistical Manual of Mental Disorders, 3rd Edition. Washington, DC, American Psychiatric Association, 1980

Faulstich ME: Psychiatric aspects of AIDS. Am J Psychiatry 144:551–556, 1987

Group for the Advancement of Psychiatry: Assessment of Sexual Function: A Guide to Interviewing. GAP Publications, Vol 8, Report No 88. New York, Group for the Advancement of Psychiatry, 1973

Hetrick ES, Stein TS (eds): Innovations in Psychotherapy With Homosexuals. Washington, DC, American Psychiatric Press, 1984

Kaplan HS: The New Sex Therapy. New York, Brunner/Mazel, 1974

Kaplan HS: Disorders of Sexual Desire and Other New Concepts and Techniques in Sex Therapy. New York, Brunner/Mazel, 1979

Kinsey AC, Pomeroy WB, Martin CE: Sexual Behavior in the Human Male. Philadelphia, PA, WB Saunders, 1948

Kinsey AC, Pomeroy WB, Martin CE, et al: Sexual Behavior in the Human Female. Philadelphia, PA, WB Saunders, 1953

Masters WH, Johnson VE: Human Sexual Response. Boston, MA, Little, Brown, 1966

Meyer JK: Paraphilias, in Comprehensive Textbook of Psychiatry, 4th Edition. Edited by Kaplan HI, Sadock BJ. Baltimore, MD, Williams & Wilkins, 1985, pp 1065–1077

Nadelson CC: Problems in sexual functioning, in Treatment Interventions in Human Sexuality. Edited by Nadelson CC, Marcotte D. New York, Plenum, 1983, pp 11–35

Sadock VA (ed): The psychiatric aspects of sexuality (Section 1), in Psychiatry Update: The American Psychiatric Association Annual Review. Edited by Grinspoon L. Washington, DC, American Psychiatric Press, 1982, pp 7–73

Stein T, Cohen C (eds): Contemporary Perspectives on Psychotherapy with Lesbians and Gay Men. New York, Plenum, 1986

Stoller RJ, Herdt G: Theories of origins of homosexuality. Arch Gen Psychiatry 42:399–404, 1985

14

Substance Abuse and Eating Disorders

ALCOHOL AND DRUG ABUSE

Drug abuse and drug dependence are major social problems in our culture, yet it is difficult to define exactly what sort of behavior constitutes abuse. The use of mind-altering substances is sanctioned in almost every group in Western society. Which substances, then, are not permissible? And among sanctioned substances, how much is too much? It may be useful to begin with some definitions.

Psychoactive substance abuse is defined in DSM-III-R (p. 169) as a maladaptive pattern of substance use, present for at least 1 month, and evidenced by 1) continued use of the substance even when the person knows that it has adverse social, psychological, occupational, or physiological consequences; and 2) recurrent use in situations where it is physicially hazardous, such as driving while intoxicated. Some drug abuse results in *tolerance*, which is an altered physiological state caused by continuous use of a drug, resulting in a diminished response to the same dose of the drug over time, so that progressively larger doses are required to produce the same drug effect.

Psychoactive substance dependence, as defined in DSM-III-R (pp. 166–168), refers to a cluster of behavioral, psychological, and physical symptoms which indicate that the person has inadequate control over the use of the substance and continues to use it despite adverse consequences. To qualify for a diagnosis of psychoactive substance dependence, the person must demonstrate at least three of the following nine features:

1. The substance is taken in larger amounts or over a longer period than the person intended.
2. The person has repeatedly desired to control substance use or has made at least one unsuccessful attempt to do so.
3. The person spends a great deal of time trying to procure the substance, taking it, or recovering from its effects.
4. The person frequently suffers from intoxication or withdrawal symptoms while fulfilling obligations at school, at home (e.g., child care), or at work; or uses the substance when it is physically hazardous (e.g., drunk driving).
5. The person gives up or reduces important social, occupational, or recreational activities because of substance use.
6. The person continues to use the substance even though he or she is aware that it causes or exacerbates a social, psychological, or physical problem.
7. The person experiences marked tolerance, needing at least a 50% increase in the amount of the substance taken to achieve the desired effect, or experiencing a diminished effect with the original amount used.
8. The person experiences characteristic withdrawal symptoms.
9. The person uses the substance to avoid or relieve withdrawal symptoms.

As you can see, this list is long, and the combinations of traits that qualify for the diagnosis of dependence are varied. One need not have physical symptoms of dependence (e.g., withdrawal symptoms) to warrant this diagnosis—psychological and behavioral problems are sufficient. The disturbance must be present for at least 1 month or must have occurred repeatedly over a long period of time. Table 14-1 lists some of the more commonly abused substances and their effects.

Obviously, not all substance abuse results in dependence, nor does every instance of abuse imply the presence of an illness. When does the use of mind-altering substances constitute a disorder that requires treatment? *Drug use is pathological when it in any way impairs an individual's family and social relationships, health, job efficiency, or ability to avoid legal difficulties.* This definition, like the DSM-III-R definition, is deliberately broad in order to include the almost infinite variety of ways in which drugs can hamper people's lives.

Table 14-1. Effects of some commonly abused substances

Drug	Tolerance	Psychic dependence	Physical dependence
Alcohol	+	++	++
Amphetamines	++	++	O?
Barbiturates	++	++	++
Caffeine	+	+	+
Chlordiazepoxide	++	++	++
Cocaine	+	++	+
LSD	++	+	O
Marijuana	+	+	−+
Nicotine	++	++	+
Opiates	++	++	++

Note. O = no effect, + = mild effect, ++ = marked effect.
Source. Reprinted, with permission, from Vaillant GE: The alcohol-dependent and drug-dependent person, in *The New Harvard Guide to Psychiatry*. Edited by Nicholi Jr AM. Cambridge, MA, Harvard University Press, 1988, pp. 700–713. Copyright 1988, President and Fellows of Harvard College.

Alcoholic individuals and polydrug abusers

What sorts of people use particular drugs? Although drug abusers are often classified by clinicians according to the substances they abuse, such categorization actually tells us very little about the people involved. One common myth is that alcoholic individuals tend to remain "faithful" to alcohol and do not generally go on to abuse other substances, while those who abuse opioids, barbiturates, or hallucinogens are likely to abuse other drugs, including alcohol, during the course of their lives. In fact, many people—whether primarily categorized as alcoholic or as polydrug abusing—use whatever substances are available to alter their psychic state.

What causes people to abuse drugs and alcohol?

Obviously, there is no single factor that accounts for why some people develop these disorders and others do not. The following variables seem to be important in determining patterns of drug abuse.

Availability of drugs. People who live and work in situations where drugs are readily accessible are more prone to abuse them (e.g., bartenders). While availability is a necessary condition for drug abuse, it does not, in and of itself, cause people to abuse drugs.

Onset of action of the drug. Drugs that act quickly (e.g., alcohol, fast-acting benzodiazepines) are more prone to be abused than those that exert their effects more slowly.

Development of tolerance and physical dependence. Withdrawal symptoms are unpleasant and may be life-threatening. The avoidance of these symptoms is a powerful factor in the continued use of drugs that create physiological dependence (e.g., alcohol, heroin).

Genetic background. The child of an alcoholic person, adopted at birth into a nonalcoholic family, is at a greater risk of developing alcoholism than the child of a nonalcoholic person who is adopted into a nonalcoholic family. The incidence of alcoholism is four times higher in the male offspring of alcoholic fathers than in the male offspring of nonalcoholic fathers, whether these children are raised by their biological parents or by others. There thus appears to be some genetic predisposition to alcoholism, although the importance of this factor has yet to be fully elucidated. Moreover, it is not clear exactly what is inherited that predisposes one to alcoholism. Among the most prominent hypotheses currently under study are 1) that susceptible individuals have an inherited deficiency of serotonin or prostaglandins, which is altered by alcohol ingestion; 2) that these individuals have more pronounced alterations in endorphin activity in response to alcohol; 3) that there is an increased relaxation response to alcohol among susceptible individuals; and 4) that these individuals are more prone to tolerance than are those without genetic susceptibility.

With the identification of endogenous opioids and opioid receptors in recent years, there is increasing interest in a possible genetic predisposition to opioid addiction based on inborn variations in the relationship among receptors, endogenous endorphins, neurotransmitters, and other substances such as adrenocorticotropic hormone (ACTH). However, studies of possible genetic determinants of opioid addiction and other substance abuse disorders are lacking.

Childhood environment. In addition to the genetic factors mentioned above, alcoholic individuals (particularly men) are more likely than nonalcoholic individuals to have alcoholic parents and siblings. The process by which drinking habits are "handed down" from one generation to another is thought to be based on the mechanism of *identification*, whereby children unconsciously adopt characteristics of important caregivers and others who are role models as they grow up. No general statements can be made with certainty about the childhood experiences of polydrug abusers. Some writers claim that polydrug abusers tend to come from noncohesive home environments where one or both parents were neglectful of or abusive toward the children, but this hypothesis has yet to be well substantiated empirically.

Culture. Drug abuse is less likely where drug use is prohibited on religious grounds or where there are clear guidelines for nonabusive drug use. Thus, rates of alcoholism are very low among Moslem and Mormon communities, where alcohol is prohibited, and among Italians and Jews, who allow children to drink in socially sanctioned ways but frown upon drunkenness.

Socioeconomic status. Drug abusers often fail to conform to popular stereotypes. To be sure, there are sociopathic addicts who live on the street and steal to finance a heroin habit. But other "hard-core" addicts and alcoholic individuals include physicians, teachers, housewives, and students—people from all backgrounds and socioeconomic groups.

Mental illness. Many people who abuse drugs and alcohol suffer from mental disorders. It is often difficult to distinguish between psychiatric symptoms that result from substance abuse and those that prompt it. However, it is clear that many patients begin to abuse drugs to "medicate" preexisting emotional disorders such as depression, anxiety, and psychosis (e.g., the depressed student who becomes addicted to cocaine). Disorders that commonly coexist with drug abuse include affective disorders, anxiety disorders, somatoform disorders, and personality disorders (e.g., borderline, narcissistic, and antisocial personality disorders). No one personality type has been found among substance abusers. People who become alcoholic have often been stereotyped as passive, dependent, and depressed; polydrug abusers are thought to be primarily sociopathic. But these generalizations are not valid. Alcoholic individuals and polydrug abusers vary greatly with respect to personality type and underlying psychopathology.

Mental health professionals are often consulted for treatment of emotional problems by people who minimize the extent to which their drug use affects their mental health. It is virtually impossible to get an accurate picture of a substance abuser's baseline state of mental health while he or she continues to use drugs. Thus, accurate assessment and effective treatment of mental illness are not possible until substance abuse has ceased.

Alcoholism

It is estimated that 5% to 10% of the adult population in the United States is afflicted with alcoholism, and that the lifetime prevalence of the disorder is 13.6% of the general population. It is more prevalent among men than women, but the incidence among women is increasing. Not surprisingly, it is also more prevalent among the poor and less educated, although it cuts across all class, ethnic, and geographical lines. Alcoholism is responsible for an estimated 200,000 deaths per year. It increases one's risk of suicide by 10- to 20-fold, and alcohol is strongly associated with violent crime and traffic fatalities. The yearly cost of alcohol-related problems in the United States is estimated in billions of dollars.

A public health problem of major proportions, alcoholism is also significantly underdiagnosed—perhaps as many as half of the alcoholic individuals seen by health care professionals go entirely undiagnosed. This occurs in part because alcoholic individuals tend to strongly deny that they have a problem; in many cases, only family and friends can supply accurate information about drinking habits and resulting impairment of functioning. The alcoholic person is likely to rationalize job difficulties and interpersonal problems as the *causes* rather than the *results* of drinking. And clinicians do not generally suspect alcohol abuse among people who do not conform to the stereotype of the skid-row bum.

Alcoholic individuals commonly do not seek treatment until they are forced to by others. This often involves some sort of confrontation or coercion. For example, an exasperated spouse may threaten to leave if the alcoholic person does not stop drinking. Or an irate employer may give the alcoholic person one last chance to sober up or be fired. Unless the alcoholic individual's way of life seems significantly threatened, he or she is not likely to view drinking as a problem that requires treatment.

You will most often deal with alcoholic patients who want to hide the severity of their drinking problem from you, from friends and family, and from themselves. They will tend to minimize the extent to which they abuse alcohol, and see their current physical or psychological symptoms as unrelated to drinking. Alcoholic individuals tend to hide their alcoholism best from those outside the home, so that problems at work tend to develop late in the illness. The people affected earliest and most severely by someone's drinking are family members, so it is important to interview the family in addition to the patient when you suspect a drinking problem.

You will not diagnose alcoholism if you do not look for it. A drug and alcohol history is part of every psychiatric evaluation. You must be particularly diligent about pursuing any clues or intuitions you have about the presence of alcohol abuse, or else you may miss a problem that is primary to your patient's complaints.

Diagnosis

Ask every patient about the amount and frequency of alcohol use. *Assume* alcohol use and begin with such questions as, "How much do you drink? In what situations? How often do you take a drink?"

Give patients who are vague about amounts and frequency some suggestions that are more likely to *overestimate* drinking than to underestimate it (e.g., "Do you have several drinks each day?"). When you suspect a problem, the following questions may help you clarify the situation. They are grouped roughly according to the severity of the symptoms they are designed to elicit.

- Do you sometimes feel a little guilty about your drinking?
- Do you often find that you want to continue drinking after your friends say they have had enough?
- Are you irritated when your family or friends comment on your drinking?
- Have you ever argued with someone close to you about your drinking?
- When drinking with others, do you try to have a few extra drinks when others will not know it?
- Did you ever wake up "the morning after" and discover that you could not remember part of the evening before, even though your friends tell you that you did not pass out?
- When you are sober, do you ever regret things you have done or said while drinking?
- Do you try to avoid family or close friends when you are drinking?
- Are you having more financial or work problems lately?
- Do you eat little or irregularly when you are drinking?
- Have you ever been in a car accident after you have been drinking, or have you ever been arrested for drunk driving?
- Do you sometimes have "the shakes" in the morning and find that it helps to have a little drink?
- Do you sometimes drink steadily for several days at a time?
- After periods of drinking, do you sometimes see or hear things that aren't really there?

Positive answers to any of the questions at the beginning of this list should make you think seriously about alcoholism and explore the matter further. If you suspect that your patient is denying the seriousness of the problem, ask to speak with family members, and do so with the patient in the room. This should help you assess the extent to which alcohol has impaired work, home life, or health, and whether it constitutes an illness requiring treatment. In particular, be alert to a history of withdrawal symptoms ("the shakes," delirium tremens) or "blackouts" (memory loss while intoxicated), for these are clear signals that the problem is significant and may result in serious withdrawal reactions in the future.

Treatment

Once you have diagnosed alcohol abuse, you must decide what forms of treatment are indicated and assess your patient's motivation for treatment. Obviously, emergency situations must be treated first. Anyone presenting with severe intoxication that threatens to compromise respiratory functioning, or with severe withdrawal symptoms such as delirium tremens or seizures, should be admitted immediately to a medical ward or intensive care unit. For information on the management of these situations, consult a general medical textbook.

Patients who present for mental health evaluation are generally those for whom there is no medical emergency, but they may nevertheless require careful medical and psychiatric treatment in order to avert consequences of alcohol abuse or withdrawal.

Detoxification. Detoxification is the first step in the treatment of those who are addicted to alcohol and have experienced significant withdrawal symptoms when they have stopped drinking in the past. Detoxification is generally carried out on a medical or psychiatric inpatient unit, in order to allow careful monitoring of physical status and to prevent potentially lethal withdrawal reactions. Inpatient treatment also allows the alcoholic individual to begin other types of therapy (discussed below), which can be continued on an outpatient basis.

Physiological withdrawal from alcohol usually begins 6 to 24 hours after the person has stopped a period of heavy drinking, and may begin as late as 36 hours after the alcoholic patient's last drink. The early signs and symptoms of alcohol withdrawal are shown in Table 14-2.

The later complications of alcohol withdrawal typically include the following:

Table 14-2. Early manifestations of alcohol withdrawal

Signs	Symptoms
Tachycardia (increasing pulse rate)	Irritability
Elevation of systolic blood pressure	Agitation
Sweating	Difficulty concentrating
Fever	Insomnia
Hyperventilation	Abdominal pain
Hyperreflexia	Nausea, vomiting
Diarrhea	Tremulousness ("shakes")

- *Worsening of early symptoms* (see Table 14-2), *especially rapid pulse, sweating, agitation, and tremor.*
- *Seizures.* These are most likely to occur in the first 24 to 48 hours after the last drink. They are usually nonfocal and generalized, as well as self-limiting, and generally precede agitation, delirium, and hallucinations.
- *Alcoholic hallucinosis.* This condition most commonly occurs in the first 24 to 48 hours after the last drink. It may involve visual or auditory hallucinations, or both.
- *Delirium tremens* (DTs). These usually occur 50 to 100 hours after the last drink and may last up to 2 weeks. DTs are characterized by hallucinations and delusions, and a hypermetabolic state, including elevated body temperature, dehydration, and blood chemistry imbalance. The mortality rate is as high as 15%.

Major withdrawal syndromes can usually be prevented by treating earlier manifestations before they become severe. The key is early and aggressive treatment, for it is much more difficult to "catch up" once withdrawal has progressed beyond the preliminary stages.

Treatment of early signs of alcohol withdrawal. Chlordiazepoxide (Librium) is an effective pharmacological substitute for alcohol that has a wide margin of safety, little respiratory depression, low addiction potential, anticonvulsant effects, and a long half-life (24 to 30 hours). It both alleviates the signs and symptoms of early withdrawal and prevents progression to more severe syndromes (DTs, seizures).

Treatment, as outlined below, should be begun as soon as patients show any of the early signs of withdrawal: evaluated pulse rate (over 100 beats per minute), elevated systolic blood pressure, sweating, or elevated temperature. These signs are more reliable indicators than subjective symptoms such as anxiety and agitation, which may be present for many reasons other than withdrawal.

1. Give 25 to 100 mg of chlordiazepoxide orally at the first signs of withdrawal. (The dose will depend on the person's physical size and extent of recent alcohol abuse.) For persistent symptoms, the dose may be repeated in an hour.
2. Patients experiencing withdrawal can then be put on an ongoing regimen of 25 to 100 mg of chlordiazepoxide orally every 4 to 6 hours as needed to keep vital signs stable during the first day. The average person will require 300 to 400 mg/day on the first day; the total daily dosage should not exceed 600 mg.
3. Further doses should be given as needed for agitation, high blood

pressure, or rapid pulse. A useful guideline is to medicate so as to keep the pulse rate below 100, provided the person is alert.

4. After the first 24 hours, if symptoms are controlled, the dosage of chlordiazepoxide may be cut by 20% each day until it is tapered off within 5 to 7 days.

Once withdrawal symptoms have been controlled, other forms of treatment may be initiated.

You may be surprised by the onset of alcohol withdrawal among people who are admitted to the hospital for seemingly unrelated medical or psychiatric reasons but who have a history of recent heavy drinking. These people may only admit to the full extent of their alcohol abuse when, in a setting where alcohol is suddenly unavailable, withdrawal symptoms set in. You must therefore consider the possibility of alcohol withdrawal whenever you see a hospitalized patient who has a history of alcohol abuse.

Wernicke's encephalopathy and Korsakoff's syndrome (alcohol amnestic disorder). The medical consequences of alcohol addiction, such as hepatic cirrhosis and polyneuropathy, are well outlined in general medical texts. One neuropsychiatric syndrome, Korsakoff's syndrome, deserves special mention here because it is characterized by dramatic psychological symptoms. Chronic alcoholic individuals develop the syndrome, presumably because of a prolonged inadequate diet that results in thiamine deficiency.

Wernicke's encephalopathy is an acute, life-threatening condition characterized by clouding of consciousness, ophthalmoplegia (weakness of the muscles controlling movement of the eyes), and ataxia (a wide-based gait, falling, or inability to walk or stand).

At autopsy, people who develop this condition are found to have brain-stem hemorrhages, particularly in the area of the mammillary bodies. The condition comes on rapidly and requires emergency treatment with thiamine to prevent death and minimize residual brain damage. *Anyone* with a history of chronic alcohol abuse who manifests acute psychiatric or neurological symptoms should be given 100 mg of thiamine intramuscularly. Symptoms often respond dramatically to treatment, but residual impairment is common.

Korsakoff's syndrome, also known as *alcohol amnestic disorder*, is a chronic condition that remains when Wernicke's encephalopathy is treated. It may also occur after one or more episodes of DTs. The most prominent feature of Korsakoff's syndrome is *recent memory impairment*, although peripheral neuropathy, ataxia, and oculomotor difficulties may also be present. Classically, these people have been described as using confabulation—that is, fabricating answers to questions in an attempt to fill in details they do not recall. However, confabulation is actually infrequent and is not necessary to establish the diagnosis. The most common memory impairment involves difficulty in learning new information (e.g., your name). Korsakoff's syndrome improves in about 75% of people who stop alcohol abuse and are maintained on an adequate diet for 6 months to 2 years, but only about 25% of those with this syndrome achieve full recovery. The only prevention against Wernicke's encephalopathy–Korsakoff's syndrome is an adequate diet, and, after emergency treatment with thiamine, diet is the only necessary treatment for those recovering from the syndrome.

Long-term treatment of alcoholism. Most clinicians consider alcoholism a disease rather than a moral failing. This viewpoint is useful in helping to alleviate the heavy burden of guilt carried by many alcoholic individuals. However, the disease concept does not absolve alcoholic individuals from responsibility for their drinking, nor does it imply that other people can bail them out of their difficulties. The treatment of alcoholism is long and difficult for the patients, families, and treaters alike. Alcoholic patients are asked to give up forever a substance they truly (if ambivalently) love.

Effective treatment involves giving patients a nonchemical substitute for the lost addiction; reminding them continuously that even one drink can lead to relapse; repairing the social and medical damage that has occurred; and restoring their self-esteem. A variety of treatment modalities have been employed to achieve these goals, the most effective of which are listed below.

Alcoholics Anonymous (AA). This is the most effective treatment known for alcoholic individuals. It provides continuously available group support by individuals who have themselves suffered from alcoholism. Meetings are held in many cities and towns at every hour of the day and night, so that support is available as frequently as the alcoholic individual wishes it. These meetings involve peer support and gentle confrontation of the ways in which alcoholic individuals deny their illness. AA techniques also help the alcoholic person understand the conditioned and impulsive aspects of drinking. AA replaces drinking companions with a new group of peers with whom the alcoholic person can identify. It allows members not only to receive help from other alcoholic individuals but also to give help to others, thereby enhancing self-esteem.

Many alcoholic patients are initially reluctant to participate in AA. In recommending this treatment, you should be consistently supportive and, if possible, find a way for other AA members to personally introduce the patient to these meetings.

Because alcoholism often takes a devastating toll on the families of alcoholic patients, you may want to refer them to *Al-Anon*, a self-help group that helps spouses deal with their own emotional difficulties, as well as teaching them about alcoholism and how to avoid interfering with the alcoholic patient's recovery. *Alateen* is a similar organization that offers support to adolescents who are coping with alcoholic parents. In recent years, groups for *adult children of alcoholics* (ACOA) have become widespread, helping people who grew up with an alcoholic parent to understand the effects of the alcoholic parent's inconsistent availability and emotionally depriving behavior on the family. It also helps these people understand ways in which they may serve as "co-dependents"—that is, facilitators of a loved one's addictive behavior. Children of alcoholic individuals often feel forced into a parental role, develop mistrust of people in caregiving roles, and have difficulty establishing and maintaining intimate relationships. Peer support and education can help such people understand and change these maladaptive patterns.

Psychotherapy. Individual psychotherapy is not the primary treatment of choice for alcoholism, for it cannot provide the continuous support that is often required. However, when used adjunctively with other modalities like AA, it can be extremely useful, for example, in helping to uncover family problems that perpetuate the patient's drinking and in helping the patient to see ways in which drinking provides him or her with certain benefits (*secondary gains*). In most cases, psychotherapy cannot be effective until the patient stops drinking, for only then can the therapy address the uncomfortable feelings and symptoms the alcoholic individual habitually "medicates" away with ethanol. Thus, when psychotherapy is undertaken with a person who is actively drinking, the need to stop drinking is the first agenda.

Disulfiram (Antabuse). This medication blocks the normal oxidation of alcohol so that acetaldehyde accumulates in the bloodstream and causes unpleasant symptoms such as tachycardia and vomiting. Obviously, the use of this medication is voluntary (usually in orally administered doses of 125 or 250 mg/day), and patients must be made aware of its adverse interactions with alcohol. Although disulfiram provides a deterrent to drinking, it does not help with such factors as low self-esteem and the loss of the addicting substance. By itself, therefore, it is of limited use in the treatment of alcoholism. However, many clinicians use it in conjunction with AA or psychotherapy.

Behavior modification. Hypnosis, desensitization, relaxation training, and aversion therapy (coupling alcohol use with noxious stimuli such as shocks or nausea) have been somewhat successful in treating alcoholism. In particular, aversion therapy that couples alcoholism with vomiting has shown some promise.

Adjunctive services. Halfway houses, vocational rehabilitation programs, and other social institutions that give alcoholic individuals support and help them recover lost skills have been useful as part of a treatment plan that includes other modalities like AA.

Opioids

Opium is an ancient drug around which entire cultures and economies have revolved. Today, many opium-related compounds are used illegally in this country. In addition to the natural alkaloids of opium—morphine and codeine—there are important synthetic derivatives such as heroin, hydromorphone hydrochloride (Dilaudid), oxycodone (Percocet), and oxymorphone hydrochloride (Numorphan); as well as purely synthetic opioids such as meperidine (Demerol), methadone (Dolophine), pentazocine (Talwin), and dextropropoxyphene hydrochloride (Darvon).

All of these drugs are sedating; more importantly, they are the strongest painkillers known. Thus, they are highly useful for medical purposes. However, they have strong potential for the development of tolerance, as well as psychological and physiological dependence.

In 1980, there were nearly 500,000 opioid addicts in the United States. Although the majority of narcotic addicts live in the slums of large cities and obtain drugs on the street, addiction cuts across all class and social lines. Some health care professionals who have ready access to narcotics become addicted to them. Men outnumber women by three to one among narcotic addicts, and addiction is most prevalent among people between the ages of 18 and 25. Few addicts manage to break the habit, and recidivism is estimated to be as high as 90%.

Among the most serious complications of opioid addiction include infection, suicide, and homicide. In recent years, spread of the AIDS virus through shared needles has made heroin addiction a major risk factor for contracting the virus. The death rate from all causes among young addicts is more than 20 times that of their age-matched cohort in the general population.

Many addicts seek treatment for their addiction in outpatient settings, but you may also encounter them in hospital emergency rooms where they are experiencing acute symptoms of overdose or withdrawal.

Overdose

Overdose with narcotics often occurs because the user is unaware of the strength of the illicit supply he or she has purchased. Also, one's tolerance to a given dose of narcotic varies according to how much one has used recently; addicts may overdose even on their usual "fix" if their tolerance has been lowered by short supply of the drug.

The signs of acute overdose are the following: constricted pupils, diminished pulse rate, diminished respiratory rate, pulmonary edema, and stupor or coma. Acute overdose requires emergency treatment. First, the person's vital functions must be supported, and glucose must be administered intravenously. Then, an *opioid antagonist* must be given to block the effects of the drug. Although there are several drugs that block the action of opioids, naloxone hydrochloride (Narcan) is the drug of choice, because it has no physical effects in the absence of opioids and therefore will not complicate the situation if the diagnosis of opioid overdose is incorrect. The usual initial adult dose of naloxone hydrochloride is 0.4 mg intravenously administered, although up to 1.2 mg may be required to reverse coma and respiratory depression. Comatose patients should be put into physical restraints before this agent is given, because they may be combative as they emerge rapidly from coma. Naloxone hydrochloride will reverse the signs of acute overdose within minutes, but its effect may wear off within 30 to 120 minutes, at which time the narcotic will again produce symptoms of overdose. Thus, people who emerge from coma must not be allowed to leave the hospital but must be monitored carefully for up to 48 hours, repeating the administration of naloxone hydrochloride as needed.

Withdrawal

Withdrawal from opioids has been given much publicity in films and on television, and the abstinence syndrome associated with narcotics is very unpleasant. However, abrupt withdrawal is *not* life-threatening in otherwise healthy people, as it may be from severe alcohol or barbiturate addiction. In fact, in terms of discomfort and medical danger, opioid withdrawal has been compared to a 1-week bout with influenza. The symptoms are listed in Table 14-3.

Table 14-3. Symptoms of opiate withdrawal

Early (12–36 hours after last dose)	Late (48–72 hours after last dose)
Yawning	Abdominal cramps
Sweating	Diarrhea
Gooseflesh (piloerection)	Vomiting
Insomnia	Elevated blood pressure
Dilated pupils	Increased respiratory rate
Anorexia	Increased heart rate
Muscle cramps	Fever
Tremor	

Treatment

Treatment strategies are many, but divide into those that employ some long-term chemical substitute for the abused opioid and those that aim for abstinence.

Methadone substitution. Methadone is a synthetic opioid that has proved effective in treating withdrawal from narcotics because it is long-acting and produces less euphoria than some other opiate drugs. (Even so, it is commonly abused by addicts.) It is used for withdrawal primarily on an inpatient basis and in certain specialized outpatient clinics. It is given orally, beginning with 10 mg every 4 to 6 hours as needed for signs of withdrawal, and generally no more than 40 mg in a 24-hour period. The dose is adjusted to the minimum level that will suppress symptoms and is then decreased by 5 mg (or 20%) every day until it is discontinued. It is important to use objective signs (blood pressure, temperature, heart rate) to assess the person's condition, rather than relying on subjective complaints.

Outpatient methadone maintenance. This is a treatment designed to provide addicts with methadone as a long-term substitute for street drugs in order to reduce the craving for these drugs. Methadone is given in doses of up to 120 mg orally per day, and addicts are monitored carefully with urinalyses and other control measures. However, abuse of methadone and its illicit sale on the street have been complications of such programs. Methadone maintenance must be carried out in conjunction with other support services (e.g., group therapy, vocational rehabilitation) that address the psychosocial aspects of addiction.

Two relatively new long-acting opioid agonists may be preferable to methadone for maintenance therapy. A-L-Acetylmethadol (LAAM) has a longer half-life than methadone and can therefore be given three times per week rather than daily, obviating the need to send outpatients home with supplies of the drug. It is less prone to abuse than methadone. Buprenorphine hydrochloride (Buprenex) is a mixed agonist-antagonist that may have lower abuse and overdose potential than methadone, but has yet to be fully tested in clinical settings.

Clonidine. Recent studies have demonstrated that clonidine is effective in alleviating the autonomic signs of withdrawal from opioids, presumably by suppressing the activity of the locus coeruleus that appears to mediate the withdrawal process. Clonidine is a nonopioid, is nonaddicting, and produces no euphoria, so it is not likely to be abused. At the time of this writing, clonidine is not approved by the FDA for opioid detoxification. Follow-up studies suggest that detoxification with clonidine and with methadone are no different with respect to relapse rate.

Naltrexone. Naltrexone is an opioid antagonist that blocks opioid receptors and therefore is effective in blocking the "high" achieved from opioid intoxication. This has been used as a maintenance treatment to extinguish drug-seeking behavior by making drug use ungratifying. However, this treatment has been refused by the vast majority of addicts in urban outpatient populations. It remains a useful treatment for highly motivated addicts, particularly those who have extensive social and family supports.

Psychosocial treatments. *Therapeutic communities* have been used to remove addicts from the drug environment and to confront them with their own responsibility for their addiction in the context of intensive peer group support. Patients must be highly motivated to stay in treatment, however, and drop-out rates are high. *Narcotics Anonymous*, like Alcoholics Anonymous, is a program of group support that has proved effective for some addicts. Again, however, many addicts refuse to engage in this form of treatment. *Psychotherapy* alone is not a sufficient treatment for opioid addiction, but in conjunction with other modalities it has been shown to improve the long-term outcome for the many addicts with underlying concurrent psychiatric illnesses (e.g., personality disorders).

Central Nervous System Stimulants

Cocaine

Cocaine use has increased dramatically in the United States in recent years. Less than two decades ago it enjoyed a special status as the recreational drug of the affluent. However, the recent availability of less expensive and highly addictive derivatives of cocaine, such as the freebase form known as "crack," have made it ubiquitous in all socioeconomic groups. The National Institute of Drug Abuse (NIDA) estimated that 5.4 million Americans had tried cocaine by 1974, and by 1986 that estimate more than quadrupled. Once thought to be rare, addiction to cocaine is now commonplace, and cocaine-related deaths have increased more than fourfold in the last 15 years. The drug is commonly absorbed via the nasal lining after "snorting," through the lungs after smoking, or directly via intravenous use. The rise in intravenous use of cocaine has introduced the many complications common among intravenous heroin users—most notably, the spread of AIDS.

Cocaine intoxication results in an initial stimulation of the central nervous system (CNS) like that seen in amphetamine use, followed by CNS depression. Stimulation includes euphoria, hyperalertness, disinhibition, enhanced sense of mastery, and improved self-esteem. Prolonged use and high doses may cause psychomotor agitation, hypervigilance, and a transient delusional psychosis resembling paranoid schizophrenia. Because intoxication is highly reinforcing, cocaine use may escalate into binges that end in overdose. Overdose may result in tachycardia, respiratory acidosis, grand mal seizures, and respiratory and cardiac arrest.

The abstinence syndrome following cocaine use involves an acute "crash," or post-use dysphoria, which is characterized by depression, anxiety, insomnia, irritability, and intense cocaine craving. This state lasts from several hours to three days. Over several subsequent days, the person may experience milder craving for cocaine, along with mild irritability and anxiety. At any time during this period, a subsequent dose of cocaine will temporarily relieve abstinence symptoms, creating a cycle of repeated use to avoid withdrawal.

Many cocaine abusers have concurrent psychiatric disorders. The most common are affective disorders, personality disorders (particularly borderline, narcissistic, and antisocial disorders), other substance-use disorders, and attention deficit disorder. No single personality type has been related empirically to cocaine use, but clinical lore holds that narcissistic personalities are particularly drawn to the drug, given its power to create euphoria and inflated self-esteem.

Treatment. Psychosocial treatments have been the mainstay of therapy for cocaine dependence. Some patients require initial *hospitalization*, particularly when heavy and prolonged use results in psychosis or severe abstinence symptoms. Hospitalization is often necessary when patients are dependent on other drugs in addition to cocaine (e.g., benzodiazepines), when they lack social and family supports, when they have serious medical complications, and when outpatient treatment has failed.

Rehabilitation of the cocaine addict relies on the same techniques used in other forms of addiction: 12-step programs such as Narcotics Anonymous or Cocaine Anonymous, therapeutic communities or halfway houses, and group and individual psychotherapy. Patients in therapy must be confronted with their denial about their illness. They must be educated about the illness, and they must begin to identify the psychological and social factors that stimulate their cravings for cocaine. Most of these patients need help making plans to reconstruct their damaged lives, and building the supports needed to avoid further use.

Medications. Some investigators have found that tricyclic antidepressants are of use in treating the anhedonia that is part of the cocaine "crash." Desipramine and imipramine have been studied as possibly being effective in diminishing the craving for cocaine and diminishing the euphoria caused by intoxication. However, the use of antidepressants, either during the acute "crash" or as prophylaxis against further abuse, remains experimental and controversial.

Amphetamines

Amphetamines are prone to abuse by a wide variety of people, including students who want to be able to stay up for many hours preparing for examinations or writing papers. However, amphetamine use in large doses can produce acute delirium and psychosis. Overdose is potentially lethal. The symptoms of amphetamine intoxication and overdose are listed in Table 14-4.

Treatment of acute intoxication involves decreasing CNS irritability and controlling psychotic symptoms. Toward this end, support and reassurance in a quiet setting may suffice in mild intoxication. In more severe cases, 25 to 50 mg of chlorpromazine (Thorazine) administered orally every 6 hours will ease agitation and diminish psychosis.

Amphetamine psychosis occurs in a more chronic form after prolonged use of the drug. The psychotic symptoms can be difficult to distinguish from schizophrenia. Symptoms include talkativeness, hyperactivity, stereotyped or repetitive behavior, bruxism (grinding the teeth), picking movements, suspiciousness, and (in more severe cases) persecutory delusions, hallucinations, ideas of reference, and hypersexuality. Management of amphetamine psychosis is also carried out with antipsychotic medication (e.g., chlorpromazine in the doses noted above) to decrease agitation and diminish psychotic symptoms.

Although physical addiction to amphetamines does not develop, a sudden withdrawal of the stimulant after prolonged use or administration of high doses results in a marked decrease in CNS activity, known as

Table 14-4. Symptoms of amphetamine intoxication and overdose

Mild	Severe
Restlessness	Confusion
Irritability	Delirium
Weakness	Hallucinations
Confusion	Paranoia
Talkativeness	
Anxiety	
Tremor	
Hyperreflexia	
Insomnia	
Euphoria, with lability of mood	

"crashing," which is characterized by drowsiness, fatigue, apathy, and severe depression that may lead to suicidal ideation. People who "crash" need sleep, as well as physical and emotional support, until CNS activity returns to normal.

Central Nervous System Depressants

Sedatives, hypnotics, and antianxiety agents all depress the CNS. They are often referred to as *downers*. Most are prescription drugs that are either obtained illegally or obtained legally from physicians but misused. The pharmacological properties of these drugs are described in Chapter 18. Downers are commonly abused along with alcohol and opioids, and both abuse and overdose frequently involve combinations of drugs. Individuals who use barbiturates and other sedative-hypnotics are very prone to develop psychological dependence, followed by increasing tolerance and physical dependence.

Benzodiazepines are now widely used in medical practice, and barbiturates are less often prescribed than they were three decades ago. Accordingly, clinicians have seen more benzodiazepine abuse and dependence in recent years and a decline in barbiturate abuse. Although benzodiazepines produce less euphoria than other CNS depressants, and are therefore less prone to abuse, they can nevertheless produce tolerance even at low doses. Long-term use (months to years) of even 10 to 40 mg of diazepam (Valium) per day can result in physical dependence, as can the use of high doses over a period of weeks. This fact is important because you will see many patients who use benzodiazepines chronically and who are at risk for withdrawal.

Overdose

The symptoms of intoxication and overdose resemble those of drunkenness—drowsiness (coma in severe overdoses), slurred speech, lack of coordination, memory impairment, confusion, nystagmus, tremor, decreased muscle tone, agitation, paranoia, and inappropriate affect. Intoxication and overdose with benzodiazepines occur at much higher doses than with barbiturates, but small amounts of alcohol or other CNS depressants may interact with benzodiazepines to precipitate overdose.

Management of overdose. If the person is *awake*, induce vomiting or perform gastric lavage to clear the stomach of any unabsorbed substance. Send blood and urine samples and gastric contents for toxicological analysis. Monitor and support respiratory and cardiac functions for at least 24 hours.

If the person is *comatose* or *semicomatose*, attempt gastric lavage if the drug was taken less than 12 hours before. Alkalinize the urine to increase excretion. Support basic life functions through intubation, administration of oxygen, plasma expanders, and vasopressors.

Obviously, severe overdose with CNS depressants requires immediate medical attention and necessitates admission to a facility where intensive care can be provided.

Withdrawal

Withdrawal from CNS depressants can be quite dangerous if it occurs abruptly. In particular, withdrawal can result in seizures and cardiovascular collapse, and it carries a significant risk of death. The possibility of withdrawal must be considered for every person who presents with a history of abuse of or dependence on CNS depressants. The withdrawal symptoms for all types of CNS depressants are similar and are listed in Table 14-5.

Treatment of withdrawal. Treatment of acute withdrawal is generally conducted on an inpatient basis and relies on substitution of a barbiturate or long-acting benzodiazepine (e.g., diazepam) for the abused CNS depressant, with subsequent gradual tapering. Treatment begins with a pentobarbital tolerance test on day 1, to determine how much sedative must be given initially to prevent severe withdrawal.

Pentobarbital tolerance test. First, a 200-mg test dose of pentobarbital is given orally. If intoxication results (with nystagmus and/or ataxia), then tolerance is not presumed to be great, and the person is maintained on 150 to 200 mg of pentobarbital orally every 6 hours for the first day of treatment.

If no intoxication results from the 200-mg test dose, 100 mg is given

Table 14-5. Symptoms of withdrawal from CNS depressants

Mild	Severe
Agitation	Seizures
Anxiety	Delirium
Anorexia	Hypothermia
Vomiting	Cardiovascular collapse
Increased heart rate	
Postural hypotension	
Hyperreflexia	
Tremor	

orally every 2 hours until intoxication develops. The total dose required to produce intoxication is then given every 6 hours for the first 24 hours of treatment. That is, if intoxication develops after 400 mg has been given, the dose for day 1 is 400 mg orally every 6 hours.

After the first 24 hours, the dose of sedative is reduced by 10% each day and withdrawn gradually over a period of about 3 weeks. Subjects are monitored carefully for signs of intoxication or withdrawal, with subsequent adjustments in dosage.

Some clinicians use phenobarbital instead of pentobarbital in the treatment of withdrawal because there is less fluctuation in blood levels of phenobarbital and because it has antiseizure activity. In this procedure, 30 mg of phenobarbital is substituted for each 100 mg of pentobarbital, in three divided doses, and the dose is decreased 30 mg/day.

If someone is dependent on both opioids and barbiturates, barbiturate withdrawal is carried out first.

Patients who have not demonstrated signs of tolerance or withdrawal, but who have histories of longstanding benzodiazepine use, must be tapered off the medication slowly. It may take several weeks to discontinue a benzodiazepine, with careful monitoring by the physician to avoid precipitating withdrawal.

Hallucinogens

Hallucinogens include a wide variety of substances grouped together somewhat arbitrarily based on their ability to induce altered states of awareness that resemble those of natural psychoses. Some hallucinogens, like psilocybin (mushroom) and mescaline (peyote cactus), come from natural sources, whereas drugs like D-lysergic acid diethylamide (LSD) and dimethyltryptamine (DMT) are synthetic.

Signs and symptoms of hallucinogen intoxication include alteration of mood (often euphoria), vividness of real or fantasied sensory illusions and hallucinations, synesthesia ("overflow" from one sensory modality to another), and confusion. Many other psychological manifestations may be present, including a sense of time slowing, a loss of body boundaries, and feelings of grandiosity or omnipotence.

Although each hallucinogen has slightly different characteristics and produces somewhat different signs and symptoms, they all produce adverse reactions in some people. These reactions include acute panic attacks, psychosis, flashbacks, and precipitation of underlying psychosis (e.g., in people with latent schizophrenia). Whether a person has an adverse reaction to a hallucinogen (a "bad trip") depends on such factors as the dose of the drug, the setting in which it is used, and the personality characteristics of the user. LSD intoxication is particularly common and is manifested by such physical signs as dilation of pupils, increased deep tendon reflexes, muscle weakness, hypertension, tachycardia, and fever.

Treatment of hallucinogen intoxication generally involves support, reassurance, and diminishing stimulation around the person until the drug wears off. In many cases, putting the person in a quiet, dimly lit room and talking to help him or her distinguish psychotic symptoms from reality will suffice to weather the crisis. However, severe panic may be treated effectively with orally administered diazepam. Unless psychosis is unusually severe and prolonged, it is best to avoid using antipsychotic medication because of possible adverse anticholinergic reactions resulting from the combination of a hallucinogen and an antipsychotic.

Phencyclidine

Phencyclidine (PCP) is unique in action compared with other psychedelic drugs, and it is not a true hallucinogen. A synthetic drug initially developed as a possible anesthetic agent for humans, it is now licensed only for use as an immobilizing agent for nonhuman primates. Often called "angel dust," it is a common drug of abuse. Its psychological effects include changes in body image (e.g., "My head is growing larger"), depersonalization, anxiety, disorganization of thought, depression, and hostility. PCP abusers sometimes behave with great violence under the influence of the drug. Physical signs of intoxication include elevated blood pressure, tachypnea, and neurological signs such as nystagmus, muscle spasm and rigidity, and ataxia. PCP intoxication can result in coma and death.

Treatment of mild to moderate intoxication is different from that for hallucinogens in that "talking people down" is not usually helpful and may even increase the person's anxiety. Instead, placing the subject in a quiet, dimly lit room with a minimum of stimulation is successful in most cases. Diazepam is used intravenously if severe muscle spasm or seizures result. Antipsychotics are not generally helpful. Most cases of intoxication resolve after several hours of reduced stimulation (e.g., in a secluded room in an emergency ward), but some cases result in prolonged and severe behavioral disturbances, exaggeration of any preexisting thought disorders, and serious medical complications that require hospital admission.

Cannabinoids

Cannabinoids, such as marijuana and hashish, are mild euphoriants with some sedative effects. Many people use these drugs as others use alcohol socially. It is estimated that as many as 30 million Americans have had some experience with marijuana, but only a fraction of that number use the drug heavily on a continuous basis. Signs and symptoms of acute intoxication include disconnected speech, recent memory impairment, emotional lability, depersonalization, and confusion, as well as increased heart rate, conjunctival injection (redness of the eyes), and decreased body temperature. While adverse reactions such as panic, psychosis, and depression do occur as a result of cannabis intoxication, these reactions are rare.

The effects of chronic use of cannabinoids are the subject of some debate. Chronic psychotic states secondary to cannabis use have been reported in Eastern cultures where doses are presumably much higher, but such reactions have been rare in the West. Some clinicians have identified an *amotivational syndrome* of low drive, poor judgment, introversion, loss of insight, poor communication skills, and depersonalization. This syndrome occurs in people who use marijuana heavily on a regular basis for many months or years. At this time, however, it is not clear whether heavy cannabis use causes or results from this condition of low motivation, and adverse effects of intermittent cannabis use have not been identified.

Treatment of Polydrug Abuse

Your first task in dealing with people who abuse drugs is to avoid stereotyping them. As was noted above, polydrug abusers come from all backgrounds, including highly educated professionals and "sweet little old ladies." If you only look for people who come in covered with tattoos and needle marks, you will fail to notice the many cases in which substance abuse is a major problem.

Your second task is to take a nonjudgmental approach to the evaluation and treatment of drug abusers. Clinicians often see addicts as hopeless cases. Your first impulse in dealing with such people may be to try to usher them out of your office as quickly as possible. *Every drug abuser you see deserves a thorough medical and mental health evaluation, with particular attention to possible accompanying mental illness (e.g., affective illness, anxiety disorders, personality disorders).* You should either do the evaluation yourself with supervision or refer the patient to a clinician who is experienced in the treatment of drug abuse, or to a drug treatment center.

Treatment of drug abuse is difficult. Detoxification and crisis management are only the beginning of a long and difficult course to recovery. Like alcoholism, polydrug abuse involves substituting a substance for human contact. Many addicts' lives revolve around the process of obtaining drugs, and this provides a daily structure and a set of personal contacts that must be replaced even after physical addiction is eliminated. Also, polydrug abusers often "medicate" unpleasant feelings (anxiety, depression) that are likely to persist or worsen when the drug is taken away.

Recovering drug abusers who come from lower socioeconomic groups often find little support among peers who are likely to be antisocial and to encourage drug abuse. Thus, an important part of treatment for many people consists of helping them to establish new support systems. This may take the form of self-help groups like *Narcotics Anonymous* (similar to Alcoholics Anonymous), vocational rehabilitation programs, day care centers, or drug-free residential communities (e.g., Phoenix House).

Psychotherapy cannot, in and of itself, provide the continuous support and peer group encouragement many recovering substance abusers require. However, as an adjunct to other treatment programs, psychotherapy can help some drug abusers to cope more effectively with feelings and problems that may have promoted drug use in the first place. Family therapy can also be useful in pointing out the family's pathological patterns of coping with stress. Group therapy can be especially useful in providing support, as well as in confronting drug abusers with the consequences of their self-destructive and antisocial behaviors, especially when other group members are themselves recovering or recovered drug abusers. No one treatment modality is as useful as a combination that provides the patient with support, daily structure, and vocational skills that help to increase self-esteem.

EATING DISORDERS

Eating disorders have become the focus of much interest among mental health professionals in recent years. An increasing number of people (predominantly women) report gross disturbances in their eating behavior. The eating disorders are grouped here with alcohol and drug abuse because they share common addictive features. Like substance abuse, eating disorders involve compulsive misuse of a substance—food—to achieve some desired psychological equilibrium. Unlike alcohol and drugs, food is essential to human life. Therefore, abstinence is not a solution, and proper use of food is a central element of recovery.

The two most prevalent syndromes are *anorexia nervosa* and *bulimia* (see Table 14-6). Although these eating disorders are described as primary—that is, as not resulting from some medical illness—a great many patients with anorexia nervosa and bulimia also suffer from other diagnosable mental disorders. In fact, eating disorders occur in people

Table 14-6. Major categories of eating disorders

Anorexia nervosa

    Intense fear of becoming obese and a disturbance of body image that leads to willful restriction of food intake, significant weight loss, and refusal to maintain a minimal normal body weight

Bulimia

    Recurrent episodes of binge eating accompanied by a fear of not being able to stop eating, and followed by depressed mood and self-deprecating thoughts

Bulimarexia

    Features of both bulimia and anorexia nervosa—particularly binge eating and refusal to maintain a minimal normal body weight

who span the entire range of psychopathology, from psychosis to anxiety disorders and neurosis. In particular, many people with severe disturbances in their eating behavior suffer from personality disorders.

Thus, when you see people who report eating problems such as binge eating and vomiting, or who engage in self-starvation, you should look carefully for underlying psychosis, affective disturbances, and personality disorders before assuming that the eating disorder is an isolated problem.

Anorexia Nervosa

Anorexia nervosa is a syndrome of self-starvation in which the individual willfully restricts food intake and overexercises in an effort to ease the intense fear of becoming obese. Anorexic individuals report feeling fat when they are at normal body weight and even when they are emaciated, because weight loss does not decrease their fear of obesity. They suffer from a distorted perception of their bodies and have difficulty identifying bodily sensations, including the feeling of hunger. However, anorexia nervosa is not primarily a disturbance in appetite. Rather, it is related to disturbances in the sense of self, identity, and autonomy. The anorexic individual struggles desperately to control appetite and weight, often to combat an underlying and global sense of helplessness.

Anorexic individuals are almost exclusively female (95%)—most commonly adolescent girls and young adults. Estimates are that as many as 1% of high school students suffer from anorexia nervosa. The syndrome often begins unnoticed by others, as the anorexic person goes on a diet "to slim down." But as weight loss progresses and food intake decreases, family and friends gradually become alarmed, while the anorexic individual remains adamant in her desire to lose weight because she is fat. Many anorexic teenagers give histories of being overly compliant "model children," who become angry and negativistic as the syndrome develops and they begin to struggle with their families over eating practices. Besides using diet and exercise to accomplish their starvation, anorexic individuals may use self-induced vomiting, laxatives, and diuretics. Weight loss, by definition, proceeds to at least 15% of the anorexic person's original body weight (or projected normal body weight in growing teenagers) and may go well beyond this mark toward a state of total emaciation.

Anorexic individuals typically deny that they have a problem, and do not want treatment. Anorexic adolescents often manifest delayed sexual development, and adults with this disorder show little interest in sex. Amenorrhea, or loss of menstrual periods, is often one of the earliest results of the anorexic person's stringent dieting, and the diagnosis of anorexia nervosa is made only after a female has missed three expected menstrual periods. Many psychological theorists postulate that a fear of sexuality contributes to the anorexic individual's drive to become emaciated.

The etiology of anorexia nervosa remains a matter of controversy. Psychological theories of eating disorders are numerous. Cognitive theories emphasize the distortions of body image so prominent among anorexic individuals. Psychodynamic theorists postulate that the anorexic person's rigid perfectionism and insistence on control may stem from experiences of chronic helplessness in early family life—for example, when faced with the demands of a self-absorbed parent who cannot help the child learn to attend to her own bodily and emotional needs. Family systems theorists emphasize the anorexic individual's central role in maintaining some equilibrium in a dysfunctional family. For example, the child's illness might be seen as the "glue" that keeps an unhappy marriage together, thus making separation and growing up dangerous.

Biological factors are difficult to elucidate, as starvation itself brings about abnormalities in neuroendocrine and metabolic functioning. Dopamine, serotonin, and norepinephrine all influence appetite, and some indirect evidence suggests possible dysregulation of these three neurotransmitters in anorexia nervosa. Familial occurrence of the disorder (e.g., higher rates of concordance among monozygotic twins) suggests some genetic component to the etiology of the illness, but studies in this area are preliminary.

The relationship between eating disorders and affective disorders is controversial. As many as one-quarter to one-half of patients with eating disorders meet criteria for a major depressive episode. Many investigators have suggested that anorexia nervosa and bulimia are variants of affective disorder. However, this hypothesis has not been substantiated by recent research. While studies have reported an increased incidence of affective disorders and alcoholism among the first- and second-degree relatives of patients with eating disorders, the reverse has not been demonstrated. Certainly a subgroup of anorexic patients has concurrent depression.

Fortunately, most anorexic patients experience a single episode of the eating disorder and then recover completely without recurrence. Factors associated with a good prognosis include onset of the problem before age 15 and weight gain within 2 years after treatment is begun. Among this group, more than half remain maladjusted in family relationships and demonstrate unusual eating behaviors despite return to normal weight.

Some people have recurrent periods of anorexia nervosa, and a sizable proportion take an unremitting course, with progressive starvation. Factors associated with poor prognosis include later age of onset, previous psychiatric hospitalizations, premorbid personality difficulties, and greater disturbance of the patient's relationships with his or her family members.

If weight loss becomes profound, physical signs ensue, including hypothermia, pedal edema, bradycardia, hypotension, and lanugo (fine, soft body hair). Medical complications include electrolyte imbalances (particularly hypokalemic alkalosis), fatty liver degeneration, and leukopenia. Electrolyte imbalances commonly cause cardiac arrest. **The morbidity and mortality for anorexia nervosa are among the highest for any psychiatric disorder.** Studies estimate mortality at from 5% to 20% in long-term follow-up of anorexic patients. Hospitalization and forced feeding are often necessary to prevent starvation, and forced feeding procedures often come to be the focus of the severely anorexic person's angry struggles to maintain rigid control over her body.

Treatment of anorexia nervosa is extremely difficult. The first goal must be improvement of the person's nutritional status, both to stabilize her medical condition and to reverse the psychological disturbances (such as difficulty in assimilating new information) that specifically result from starvation. Only when the worst malnutrition is reversed can you get an accurate picture of the person's baseline psychological condition (e.g., the presence of a thought disorder or severe personality disturbance). Hospitalization is often necessary in the beginning of treatment, especially for patients who are emaciated (e.g., have lost 30% or more of body weight), who suffer from medical complications such as electrolyte imbalance, or who are in the midst of a suicidal or family crisis.

Clinicians have reported some success in treating anorexia nervosa with a combination of behavior therapy aimed at maintaining weight at an adequate level and cognitive psychotherapy aimed at elucidating and correcting anorexic patients' inner confusion and misconceptions about their own feelings and needs, their self-worth, and their ability to control their lives. An important (some would say essential) adjunct to this treatment is family therapy aimed at decreasing the family's characteristic overinvolvement with the anorexic patient and helping the family to allow the patient more autonomy. Individual psychodynamic therapy can also be useful in addressing long-standing personality problems and difficulties in interpersonal functioning.

Bulimia

Bulimia is a disorder characterized by recurrent episodes of binge eating that are associated with self-induced vomiting, strict dieting, vigorous exercise, and/or diuretic or laxative abuse to prevent weight gain. DSM-III-R criteria require a minimum of two binges per week for at least 3 months to make the diagnosis.

Binge eating involves rapidly consuming large amounts of food in a short period of time. In contrast to people with anorexia nervosa, bulimic individuals are generally aware that their eating patterns are abnormal, and they feel they cannot stop eating voluntarily. Bulimic individuals often become depressed after binges and frequently berate themselves for their behavior.

Binges commonly consist of high-calorie foods, many of which are sweet and can be eaten quickly. Eating is usually done secretively, and the binge eater often stops only when abdominal pain becomes severe, sleep intervenes, or social circumstances make it impossible to continue gorging. Bulimic individuals frequently vomit after binges to relieve abdominal pain, reduce guilt, and control their weight. Their weight may fluctuate widely, because of alternating periods of binge eating and fasting, or it may remain stable. When it is severe, binge eating may disrupt bulimic individuals' social and occupational lives, because they may spend hours secretly procuring food, gorging themselves, and rushing to a bathroom to induce vomiting after each binge.

Bulimia typically begins in adolescence or early adulthood. It is much more common in women than in men (a ratio of 8 or 9 to 1). Bulimia is much more prevalent in the higher socioeconomic classes, although the reasons for this are not known. It is estimated that between 4% and 9% of high school and college students have bulimia at any given time. Bulimia generally follows a chronic course, occurring intermittently over many years, and episodes of binge eating are often precipitated by life stresses. Most bulimic individuals have problems in interpersonal relationships and poor self-esteem. Many are impulsive in other ways in addition to eating; drug abuse and stealing are common in this group of patients.

Medical complications are usually the result of chronic vomiting, purging, and diuretic abuse. Hypokalemic alkalosis may develop in severe cases. Vomiting can cause erosion of teeth and parotid gland enlargement with elevated serum amylase. In fact, it is possible to "screen" for continued vomiting episodes by monitoring serum amylase levels.

The etiology of bulimia is not known, but, in many cases, the eating disorder is related to more global psychopathology (e.g., an underlying personality disorder). Some have argued that bulimia is a variant of affective disorder, but, to date, empirical evidence suggests that the two disorders are distinct entities. Psychodynamic theorists have looked at bulimia as evidence of a failure to develop the ability to evoke soothing images of mother in times of separation from her (lack of object constancy). They describe many bulimic patients who use food as a substitute for maternal comfort.

A variety of treatment modalities have been used with bulimic patients, including behavior modification techniques, insight-oriented psychotherapy, and cognitive therapy—all with limited success (see Chapter 17). Group psychotherapy using cognitive and behavioral techniques has been reported to be particularly effective, in that it can provide support and education as well as structured techniques for managing eating problems. However, no well-designed empirical studies have yet been done to test the relative efficacy of this modality. Psychodynamic therapy is commonly used to focus on personality problems and interpersonal difficulties that accompany the eating disorder.

Antidepressant medication has been used effectively in a subgroup of bulimic patients. It is possible that those who respond to antidepressant medication have a concurrent atypical depression. Studies have also shown that two anticonvulsants, phenytoin and carbamazepine, are somewhat effective in reducing episodes of binge eating. To date, however, pharmacotherapy appears to be effective in only a minority of bulimic patients.

Bulimarexia

This term is used to describe a disorder that includes features of both bulimia and anorexia nervosa—that is, binge eating, vomiting, and self-starvation with severe weight loss. The overlap between the two syndromes is significant; it is estimated that between 40% and 50% of people with primary anorexia nervosa exhibit bulimic behavior.

BIBLIOGRAPHY

Bruch H: Eating Disorders: Obesity, Anorexia Nervosa, and the Person Within. New York, Basic Books, 1973

Bruch H: Anorexia nervosa: therapy and theory. Am J Psychiatry 139:1531–1538, 1982

Dackis CA, Gold MS: Psychopharmacology of cocaine. Psychiatric Annals 18:528–530, 1988

Herzog DB, Copeland PM: Eating disorders. N Engl J Med 313:295–303, 1985

Herzog DB, Keller MB, Lavori PW: Outcome in anorexia nervosa and bulimia nervosa: a review of the literature. J Nerv Ment Dis 176:131–143, 1988

Levy AB, Dixon KN, Stern SL: How are depression and bulimia related? Am J Psychiatry 146:162–169, 1989

Millman RB: Evaluation and clinical management of cocaine abusers. J Clin Psychiatry 49 (No 2, suppl):27–33, 1988

Scaturo DJ: Toward an adult developmental conceptualization of alcohol abuse: a review of the literature. Br J Addict 82:857–870, 1987

Searles JS: The role of genetics in the pathogenesis of alcoholism. J Abnorm Psychol 97:153–167, 1988

Treece C, Khantzian EJ: Psychodynamic factors in the development of drug dependence. Psychiatr Clin North Am 9:399–412, 1986

Vaillant GE: The Natural History of Alcoholism. Cambridge, MA, Harvard University Press, 1983

Vaillant GE: The alcohol-dependent and drug-dependent person, in The New Harvard Guide to Psychiatry. Edited by Nicholi AM Jr. Cambridge, MA, Harvard University Press, 1988, pp 700–713

Weiss RD, Mirin SM: Cocaine. Washington, DC, American Psychiatric Press, 1987

Woody GE, McLellan AT, Luborsky L, et al: Psychotherapy for substance abuse. Psychiatr Clin North Am 9:547–562, 1986

15

Suicide

THE INTENTIONAL DESTRUCTION of one's own life is an act of enormous power. Suicidal intent and suicidal behavior constitute one of the most emotionally charged of medical emergencies—for patients, for their families, and for clinicians.

The majority of those who commit suicide consult a physician within 6 months before their death. Each year, the average physician encounters half a dozen patients who are seriously contemplating suicide. Suicide is ubiquitous, confronting practitioners in every branch of medicine.

The pathways to suicide are many, but virtually all suicidal people have reached a state of intolerable psychological pain. The rage, defiance, despair, and helplessness that you will encounter in such people are often frightening and confusing.

Suicidal people invariably arouse intense emotions in those close to them. Families and friends may react to suicide threats with sympathy, anxiety, or hostility. They may feel impotent and overwhelmed; they often blame themselves for the crisis; and they usually feel responsible for its outcome.

You, too, are likely to find your equanimity challenged by the suicidal patient. As a physician-in-training, you are charged with helping people to improve the quality of life. Yet people who are intent on killing themselves often go to great lengths to thwart those aims. They may reject every offer of aid, thereby making you feel what they feel—helpless and angry. Or they may attribute to you unrealistic powers over life and death, and make you believe that you alone will be responsible if they carry out their self-destructive plans. Suicidal patients force you to confront the limitations of how much responsibility you or anyone else can take for another's life. If you are to deliver effective care in such situations, you must learn to tolerate your own fear, anger, and frustration without retaliating against the patient.

Often, in the midst of emotional turmoil, you will be called on to make a considered judgment about the lethality of the patient's intentions and actions. You must use that judgment to intervene in a quick and decisive manner. There are no fool-proof formulas for the prediction of suicide risk, and estimation of intent and lethality remains a matter of clinical judgment. But the study of suicide has yielded valuable guidelines for emergency assessment, and these guidelines, along with a heightened sensitivity to your own reactions, can make the care of the suicidal patient safer and more efficient.

MYTHS ABOUT SUICIDE

A great many misconceptions about suicide have flourished, even among mental health professionals, and these can hinder clinical work:

1. *Suicidal people are fully intent on self-destruction and have the right to die.* Nearly all suicidal people are ambivalent about dying: they want to die and at the same time wish to be saved from death. For many, the fact that they have reached your office is evidence of these mixed feelings.
2. *Once decided upon, suicide is inevitable.* Strong suicidal intent usually represents an acute condition, and intent generally falls sharply when the immediate circumstances compelling the event are survived.
3. *People who talk about killing themselves are not the ones who actually do it.* In the majority of cases, people who succeed at suicide have given definite warnings of their intent to die.
4. *Improvement following a suicidal crisis means that the period of risk is over.* Most completed suicides occur within 3 months after an acute crisis, when "improvement" affords the suicidal person more energy with which to put his or her intentions into effect.
5. *Discussing suicidal thoughts and plans with the patient will fix ideas of suicide more firmly in his or her mind.* In fact, the

careful eliciting of such thoughts and plans can be enormously relieving to people who have been unable to share their feelings of desperation. Sensitive and open discussion may well ease the crisis and will rarely if ever exacerbate it.

EPIDEMIOLOGY OF SUICIDE

Suicide is the eighth leading cause of death in the United States:

- Roughly 10 out of every 100,000 people kill themselves each year in the United States (in 1984, 11.8 per 100,000 population).
- Estimates of the total number of suicides in the United States each year range from 25,000 to 55,000. (Many suspected suicides are never proved.) In 1987, 29,453 suicides were recorded in the United States.
- One out of every 10 people in the general population have at some time had suicidal feelings that *they* would label "serious."
- For every completed suicide, there are between 10 and 40 attempts. (Many attempts are never reported.)

RISK FACTORS

Suicidologists have long searched for "suicide profiles." They have looked at everything from the phases of the moon to birth order in the family in an effort to solve the mystery of why certain people resort to suicide. The following are the risk factors most consistently identified in recent studies:

Age. The risk of suicide among white males increases with age, and peaks in the ninth decade. For white females, the risk steadily increases to age 50 and then declines somewhat in later years. Suicide risk is greatest for nonwhite males in their 20s and early 30s, and rises again in the eighth decade. Nonwhite females have the highest suicide rate in young adulthood to age 40, with a decline thereafter. In the last 25 years there has been a more than threefold increase in the rate of suicide among adolescents and young adults.

Sex. Men commit suicide three times more frequently than women. However, women *attempt* suicide two to three times as often as men. Men tend to use knives, firearms, and other violent methods of suicide, while women show a preference for self-poisoning.

Race. The suicide rate is higher for whites than for nonwhites.

However, the rate among young black adults in ghetto areas has recently increased sharply.

Marital status. Suicide rates are lowest for married people and higher for those who are separated, divorced, or widowed.

Living situation. People who live alone are at a higher risk of suicide than people who live with others.

Employment status. People who are unemployed are at higher risk of suicide than those who are working in or out of the home. Professionals (especially male physicians) are also at a disproportionately high risk.

Physical health. Physical illness, or the perception that one is ill, is more frequent among those who commit suicide. In particular, there is a high correlation between completed suicide and visits to a physician for medical complaints during the preceding 6 months. The risk of suicide is significantly increased among people suffering from cancer and from acquired immune deficiency syndrome (AIDS).

Mental health. Among the mental illnesses that have been correlated with a high risk of suicide are depression, manic-depressive illness (bipolar disorder), and schizophrenia. Nonfatal attempts are more prevalent among people with personality disorders, and adjustment disorders. In general, the presence of major mental illness should alert the clinician to the possibility of suicide. More than 90% of adults who commit suicide have an associated psychiatric illness.

Alcohol abuse or addiction. Alcoholism markedly increases the risk of suicide.

Previous suicide attempts. A history of suicide attempts has been estimated to increase the risk of completed suicide by as much as 64 times that of the general population. At least 10% of suicide attempters eventually kill themselves.

The following factors, while less easily quantifiable, have also been associated with completed suicides:

Hopelessness. Several studies have concluded that the specific symptom of hopelessness about one's life situation is more highly correlated with suicide than is the more general category of depression.

Interpersonal loss. There is a high correlation between interpersonal loss and suicide. *Loss* is defined as the separation from, divorce from, or death of a significant other, and may include relatives, friends, lovers, and therapists. The risk of suicide is particularly high among alcoholic individuals who have suffered interpersonal losses within the previous 6 weeks.

Life stresses. A high frequency of major life events in the previous 6 months has been found among those who commit suicide. Such events include job changes, moves, births, graduations, financial reversals, marriage, retirement, and menopause. Such changes are important to identify in assessing both the precipitants of a suicidal crisis and the possibilities for therapeutic intervention.

Interpersonal conflict. Long-standing intense interpersonal conflict with family members or other important people is associated with a high risk of suicide and has led some observers to characterize suicide as a fundamentally dyadic event. Such conflict, if unremitting, may continue to jeopardize the life of the patient after a particular crisis has passed.

BIOLOGICAL FACTORS IN SUICIDE

It has long been known that a family history of suicide is a significant risk factor for suicide. How suicidal behavior is transmitted from one generation to another is not clear and is likely to be multidetermined. Relatives of people who commit suicide (especially children) may come to see suicide as a means of coping with seemingly intolerable life situations. According to this explanation, transmission occurs via the psychological process of *identification* (see Chapter 2).

In recent years, investigators have begun to look for *genetic factors* that might predispose an individual to suicidal behavior. There is a high concordance rate for suicide in identical twins. Moreover, a large Danish study of people adopted at birth who subsequently killed themselves found that the incidence of suicide was six times greater among the biological relatives of those adoptees than was found among their adoptive relatives.

Recent biochemical studies have shown that suicide victims and violent suicide attempters have low levels of 5-hydroxyindoleacetic acid (5-HIAA), a major metabolite of serotonin, in their cerebrospinal fluid (CSF). This supports the hypothesis that a central nervous system (CNS) serotonin deficiency may be related to suicidality. However, low levels of CSF 5-HIAA are also found in people who behave violently, suggesting that this may be a biological marker for impulsive aggressivity in general, rather than a more specific marker of self-directed aggression. Other studies have shown increased serotonin receptor sites and decreased binding of imipramine in the frontal cortex of suicide victims. These studies do not, however, differentiate between suicidal behavior and depression.

No conclusions can yet be drawn about neuroanatomic or neurochemical correlates of suicidal behavior. Nevertheless, these lines of research hold promise for helping clinicians identify people who are at risk for suicide and develop effective pharmacological treatment interventions for these people.

ASSESSING THE SUICIDAL PATIENT

When to Assess

Like many other potentially lethal conditions, suicidal intent can present itself to the clinician in a variety of subtle and obscure ways. Many suicidal people express their desperation covertly, and the danger to their lives may go unnoticed.

You must ask about suicide *whenever* it crosses your mind, and with each new patient who presents with an emotional complaint. Even this will not be sufficient unless you are attuned to the types of verbal and nonverbal clues that desperate people often give.

Verbal clues. Direct statements about suicide are easy to identify, but people may couch these in an offhand or joking manner. *Statements about killing oneself are to be taken seriously until proven otherwise.* Suicidal people will often speak indirectly about their desire to die. They commonly express frustration with particular aspects of their lives ("My job is too much—I can't handle it any more") or they describe a general state of unhappiness ("I can't take it—nothing is going right"). Hopelessness is particularly evident among people who are suicidal. Statements such as "I might as well give up because I can't make things better for myself," or "I don't expect to get what I want," may allude to a patient's deep-rooted sense that the future is intolerable. Such declarations often sound like everyday "garden variety" complaints, but it is at these times that careful inquiry often elicits profoundly self-destructive ideas and plans.

Behavioral clues. People who are unable to verbalize their wish to die may act it out in a number of ways. The patient who abruptly decides to make a will, buy a casket, or give away prized possessions may be putting affairs in order prior to suicide. Nonlethal experimentation with potentially lethal agents (drugs, weapons) may be a prelude to a serious attempt. A new interest in life insurance policies, cemetery plots, or gravestones may seem like prudent planning and may only in retrospect appear to reflect suicidal intent. Accidents and accident-proneness are very common among suicidal people, who may be genuinely unaware of the ways in which they put themselves in danger so as not to have to acknowledge the existence of suicidal impulses. All of these behaviors should alert you to the possibility of suicide and should prompt the sort of examination described below.

How to Assess

People on the verge of suicide are desperate. Their usual methods of coping with life have failed, and they may feel very ashamed of their condition. A nonjudgmental, objective concern on the part of the clinician may do much to alleviate these patients' burdens of humiliation, enabling them to be more open about their feelings and plans.

Whenever possible, the suicidal patient should be interviewed in a quiet and relatively private setting. When the patient has made a suicide attempt, it is essential that the interview be conducted only *after* the patient has had a full medical evaluation and is medically stable. Initially, you will usually want to speak with the patient alone, and at some later point speak with friends or family in person or by telephone. You should make it clear to everyone involved how the evaluation will proceed. A calm and organized approach will help to ease the extreme tension that suicide threats inevitably generate in patients and family members or friends. Avoid premature reassurance, for the patient may interpret this to mean that you do not understand the seriousness of the situation.

Obviously, this sort of assessment requires time and thoughtful attention to emotional nuances, and both of these factors are usually in short supply in such places as a busy emergency room. Nevertheless, you must take care to establish a setting in which you can gather the data you need.

What to Assess

Assessment of suicide risk must focus on suicidal intentions, suicide attempts (if any have been made), general psychiatric condition, and potential resources for correcting the situation. An outline is provided in Table 15-1.

Suicidal ideation

You must entertain the possibility of suicide with every new patient you see in a psychiatric setting and with every nonpsychiatric patient who appears depressed. In such cases, you need to ask about suicidal ideation even when no attempts have been made and the patient has not spoken of feeling suicidal.

The exploration of suicidal thoughts can usually be done most

Table 15-1. Outline for suicide assessment

Assessing suicidal ideation
    Pervasiveness of suicidal thoughts
    Extent to which plans have been formulated
    Lethality and availability of proposed method
    Likelihood of rescue from proposed attempt

Assessing a suicide attempt
    Damage done
        Agent used
        Impairment of consciousness
        Extent of physical harm
        Reversibility of physical harm (recovery time)
        Treatment required

    Likelihood of rescue
        Location of attempt
        Person who acted as rescuer
        Probability of rescue
        Patient's participation in rescue
        Delay until discovery

General psychiatric evaluation
    Social situation—important relationships and recent changes in these
    Occupation—change in status or performance
    Psychiatric history—previous suicide attempts, depression, psychosis,
        current treatment
    Drug and alcohol history
    Medical history—recent change in physical health
    Mental status examination
    Availability of community resources (family, friends, etc.)

tactfully and yield the most useful information when the interviewer begins with general questions and proceeds to specifics. A sequence of inquiries might go as follows:

> How is your life going?
> How are you feeling in general?
> How bad does it get?
> Do you sometimes feel like giving up?
> Do you ever think you would be better off dead?
> Have you thought of ending your life?
> Do you ever feel close to harming yourself?
> How would you do it?

Where would you get the means to do it?
At what time and in what place would you do it?
How close have you come to killing yourself?
Do you feel that you will kill yourself in the near future?
What has kept you from killing yourself until now?
Does anyone else know of these feelings?

Each question narrows the focus of the discussion. In some cases, you will find that your patient's responses to general inquiries do not point toward suicidal thoughts; more detailed questioning about suicide plans will then be unnecessary. In other cases, the patient will gradually divulge carefully worked-out schemes for self-destruction.

In discussing suicide plans, the *key factors* are the *lethality* of the method, the *availability* of the method, and the *likelihood of rescue*. Tactful questioning does not increase a patient's desire or ability to plan for suicide.

Direct denials of suicidal intent are usually truthful. People often admit to seriously considering suicide, but insist that they would not actually harm themselves, citing children, spouses, jobs, or other factors in their lives that keep them from killing themselves. Such reassurances are usually reliable, at least temporarily. Of course, one can be misled; you must be especially wary of patients who act self-destructively and at the same time deny any suicidal intent. In such cases, judge patients by their actions rather than their words.

Attempted suicide

Physicians are often called upon to treat people who have survived a suicide attempt. In such a situation, you must make a judgment about the risk of another attempt in the immediate future. This involves a careful evaluation of the suicide attempt itself, because the lethality of an attempt has considerable prognostic significance for later self-destructive behavior. *No one* who has made a suicide attempt should be sent home from a treatment facility without a psychiatric evaluation.

Below are a number of questions you can ask to quickly estimate the lethality of a particular self-destructive act. These questions evaluate the damage caused by the attempt, and the degree to which rescue from this attempt was likely. The possible answers are listed in order of increasing dangerousness.

Physical harm done in the suicide attempt. The following questions can help you evaluate the physical damage done in an unsuccessful suicide attempt. Because superficial wrist scratches will inspire less alarm than a gunshot wound, the management of two such cases would differ greatly.

1. What agent was used?
   a. Least lethal: ingestion, cutting, stabbing
   b. Intermediate: drowning, asphyxiation, strangulation
   c. Most lethal: jumping (e.g., off a bridge), shooting
2. Was consciousness impaired?
   a. Alert
   b. Semicomatose, confusion
   c. Coma
3. How much physical harm did the person do?
   a. Mild: superficial, self-limited (e.g., scratching without significant blood loss)
   b. Moderate: requires a physician's attention, but not life-threatening (e.g., wound that requires sutures, fractures of small bones, damage to small arteries)
   c. Severe: penetration of vital organs or large blood vessels, skull or large bone fractures, neurological changes
4. How quickly can the patient recover from the physical effects of the attempt?
   a. Within 24 hours
   b. Within 1 to 6 days
   c. Questionable, possible residual damage
5. What medical treatment is required?
   a. First aid
   b. Hospital admission
   c. Intensive care

The likelihood of rescue from the suicide attempt. A person who has attempted but not completed suicide has obviously been rescued, and it is useful to determine how likely that rescue was. For example, taking an overdose at home in the living room with others nearby is quite different from taking the same dose while alone in a hotel room in a strange city. The likelihood of rescue provides one measure of the lethality of any given suicide attempt, as well as data for judgment about continued suicide risk.

The following five questions will give you some idea about how far the patient went to conceal or publicize the attempt:

1. What was the setting in which the attempt was made?
   a. Familiar: where the subject would be recognized (e.g., home, office, school)

b. Nonfamiliar but not remote: where the subject would not be recognized, but where he or she could be observed to be in trouble by a passerby (e.g., bridges, subways, public buildings)

c. Remote: where discovery could not be counted on (e.g., deserted areas, alleys, rural roads)

2. Who initiated the rescue?

a. Key person: someone who knows the subject (friend, relative, therapist)

b. Professional: someone whose job is such that he or she would initiate rescue (e.g., physician, police officer, taxi driver, telephone operator)

c. Passerby: someone with no obligation to initiate rescue, who happened on the scene by chance (e.g., hotel maid, pedestrian, washroom attendant)

3. What was the probability that someone would rescue the patient?

a. High, almost certain: rescuers were nearby or were faced with the attempt immediately (e.g., spouse was expected home)

b. Moderate, uncertain: for example, a rescuer was nearby but would not know of the attempt

c. Low, accidental: rescue was by chance (e.g., subject took precautions to avoid discovery)

4. To what extent did the patient participate in the rescue?

a. Asked for help

b. Left clues (e.g., staggered, left notes or empty bottles in conspicuous places)

c. Did not ask for help

5. How much time elapsed before the attempt was discovered?

a. Less than 1 hour

b. One to four hours

c. More than 4 hours

General psychiatric evaluation

Suicidal ideation and attempts only make sense in the larger context of a person's life. A careful general history will help you to identify risk factors for suicide, as well as problems that might be amenable to change. One question to keep in mind is "Why now?"—what prompted this person to choose suicide at this particular point in life? Another question to ponder as you hear about the patient's current life is "What would this suicide accomplish for the patient?" Explore the following areas:

1. *Social situation.* Current living situation, family, recent changes in or losses of love relationships or important friendships.
2. *Occupation.* Job, home responsibilities, school; recent changes in status or performance.
3. *Psychiatric history.* Previous suicide attempts (method, severity), manic and/or depressive episodes (depressed or elated mood, sleep or appetite disturbance, diurnal variation in mood), psychotic symptoms (hallucinations, delusions), psychotropic medications used (if any), psychiatric hospitalizations, current therapy.
4. *Drug and alcohol history.* Patterns of use or abuse; consider psychosis or depression secondary to drug use or drug withdrawal.
5. *Medical history.* Ongoing conditions and treatment; recent changes in physical health.
6. *Mental status examination.* Focus on presence or absence of depression, psychosis, and homicidal ideation. The wish to kill others is commonly associated with the wish to kill oneself. Also, hallucinations or delusional beliefs may dictate suicide (e.g., a voice commands the person to leap from a window), and the patient is at serious risk as long as this form of psychosis persists.

Availability of resources

You must listen to the patient's story with an ear for possible interventions. Hospitalization is indicated for many who are at risk of suicide, but others can be treated as outpatients if they have adequate resources in the community.

Family and friends. The attitudes of those closest to the patient provide important information about treatment possibilities. Significant others who are concerned but not panicked, and who recognize both the seriousness of the situation and the need for treatment, are likely to promote the patient's safety and recovery. Such people, if available to stay with the patient, can be instrumental in helping the patient to weather the suicidal crisis. At the other end of the spectrum, a person who has no one to whom he or she is close would leave the emergency room facing the prospect of returning to an impoverished world.

Often, those closest to the patient are overwhelmed with panic and confusion, or with anger. They may be incapable of assisting in follow-up care. It is even more lethal if friends and family are indifferent to the crisis. They may minimize the dangerousness of the situation and discourage the patient from seeking professional help.

Most lethal is the setting in which significant others covertly encourage the patient to commit suicide. The husband who ignores his depressed wife's suicide threats, or who leaves a bottle of tranquilizers lying about, may consciously or unconsciously wish for his wife's death. If the history demonstrates such collusion, you must arrange to get the patient out of this environment until some intervention can be made.

Other resources. "Significant others" whose help can be enlisted in follow-up care include psychotherapists, family physicians, and clergy. Important people in the patient's life should be identified and considered as possible resources, particularly if you contemplate outpatient treatment. As a rule, any ongoing caregivers (e.g., physicians, therapists) should be contacted while the evaluation is taking place.

TREATING THE SUICIDAL PATIENT

Use your judgment about continued risk and available resources to arrive at a plan of action. Do this with the help of the patient, the family, friends, and any ongoing caregivers who are available to collaborate in the process. The options are essentially the following three:

Send the patient home. The patient who has not made a suicide attempt and who expresses vague ideas but denies any clear self-destructive plan or intent is probably a candidate for outpatient treatment, consisting of follow-up by you, the family physician, or a clinician at a mental health facility. The choice will depend on the patient's preferences and the cooperation of those to whom the referral is made. A definite appointment within the following day should always be confirmed before the patient is allowed to leave.

For the person who *has* attempted suicide, hospital admission is often the treatment of choice. However, if the patient denies further suicidal intent, if the attempt itself indicates low risk, if the patient is not locked into a hopeless or frightened position by depression or psychosis, and if concerned relatives or friends can stay with the patient, you may consider sending the patient home. Follow-up care by a mental health professional should take place *the next day*. This may be through a community mental health center or other local facility, or with a private therapist. It is essential that a definite follow-up plan be formulated, that the relevant agencies be contacted, and that the patient have an appointed time and place for follow-up care before he or she is allowed to go home.

Outpatient treatment will be based on the patient's needs and diagnosis, and may range from a few sessions of crisis intervention work to long-term psychotherapy and pharmacotherapy. Possibilities include individual treatment, couples or family therapy, and group therapy. For a description of various treatment modalities, see Chapters 17 and 18.

Voluntary admission to a hospital. Many people who have definite plans for suicide, and most who have actually made serious attempts, will need hospital admission. Hospitalization affords a safe place in which to weather the crisis, as well as the chance for intensive evaluation and prompt initiation of treatment. Desperate suicidal people will often agree to hospitalization, especially if family or friends support such a move. If you suspect that the patient may attempt suicide again, even in the hospital, arrange admission to a locked psychiatric unit where the patient will be under careful observation.

Forced hospitalization. Unlike most other conditions, suicidal intent carries with it a legal mandate for involuntary hospitalization. A person whom you judge to be at immediate risk of suffering serious bodily harm can be hospitalizad against his or her will, according to the law in most states. The patient who is bent on self-destruction and refuses voluntary admission should be committed to a psychiatric unit. Commitment is generally done by a licensed physician, who must explain this course of action clearly and decisively and, if necessary, use ancillary personnel to detain the patient against his or her will. Because suicidal people often have enormous conflicts about their wishes, present your plan of treatment as clearly and firmly as possible. Decisions about suicide risk should be clearly documented in the patient's chart.

Hazards in Treating the Suicidal Patient

The mirage of health. A patient may look healthiest immediately *after* a suicide attempt, if the attempt has mobilized support from family, friends, and caregivers. People who give perfectly rational explanations for their attempts (eliciting sympathy, getting attention) may convince you that they are out of danger. Do not discharge such a person (from a medical ward or emergency room) after medical treatment without a psychiatric evaluation or follow-up. The probability of a subsequent, more serious attempt is extremely high if the patient's condition and life circumstances remain unchanged.

Debating the wisdom of suicide. You may find yourself drawn into an argument over the pros and cons of suicide. Remember that almost all suicidal people are ambivalent about dying, and may well opt to live once the crisis has passed. Impromptu existential debates are rarely helpful.

Monitoring your own reactions. You may be quite disturbed by a suicidal patient's despair or by what you see as the patient's manipulativeness. Some treaters find themselves furious or frightened by talk of suicide. Other clinicians find their patients to be "kindred spirits" and may unwittingly ignore distress signals in an effort to see patients as healthier than they really are.

You must be attuned to your own reactions to suicide so that your blind spots and personal prejudices do not obscure the nature and severity of the illness. When you sense that your feelings are in some way interfering in your work with a suicidal patient, do not hesitate to seek help from a colleague or supervisor. No one needs to manage a difficult crisis alone, and knowing when to ask for support is an essential aspect of good clinical care.

BIBLIOGRAPHY

Blumenthal SJ: Suicide: a guide to risk factors, assessment, and treatment of suicidal patients. Med Clin North Am 72:937–971, 1988

Havens LL: The anatomy of suicide. N Engl J Med 272:401–406, 1965

Jacobs D, Brown HN (eds): Suicide: Understanding and Responding. Madison, CT, International Universities Press, 1989

Klerman GL: Clinical epidemiology of suicide. J Clin Psychiatry 48 (No 12, suppl):33–38, 1987

Maltsberger JT: Suicide: The Formulation of Clinical Judgment. New York, New York University Press, 1986

Mann JJ: Psychobiologic predictors of suicide. J Clin Psychiatry 48 (No 12, suppl):39–43, 1987

Paykel ES, Myers JK, Lindenthal JJ, et al: Suicidal feelings in the general population: a prevalence study. Br J Psychiatry 124:460–469, 1974

Pfeffer CR: The Suicidal Child. New York, Guilford, 1986

Robins LN, Kulbok PA: Epidemiological studies in suicide. Psychiatric Annals 18:619–627, 1988

Shneidman ES: Definition of Suicide. New York, John Wiley, 1985

Sletten IW, Barton JL: Suicidal patients in the emergency room: a guide for evaluation and disposition. Hosp Community Psychiatry 30:407–411, 1979

Tefft BM, Pederson AM, Babigian HM: Patterns of death among suicide attempters, a psychiatric population, and a general population. Arch Gen Psychiatry 34:1155–1161, 1977

Weisman AD, Worden JW: Risk-rescue rating in suicide assessment. Arch Gen Psychiatry 26:553–560, 1972

16

Violence

THREATENED AND ACTUAL VIOLENCE are ever more pervasive in our culture. Mental health professionals have long been prominent among those who work with "dangerous" individuals, but the issue of which violent acts to attribute to mental illness continues to cause heated debate in both courtrooms and emergency rooms.

Popular wisdom holds that insane people are dangerous people. Yet this notion does not hold up under scrutiny. Although some investigators report slightly higher rates of violent crime committed by released psychiatric inpatients than by the general population, this difference can be accounted for by patients who have a record of criminal activity prior to hospitalization. Psychiatric patients who do not have prior criminal records are, if anything, less prone to violent behavior than the general populace. The President's Commission on Mental Health addressed this issue in its 1978 report (p. 56):

> The sporadic violence of so-called "mentally ill killers" as depicted in stories and drama is more a device of fiction than a fact of life. Patients with serious psychological disorders are more likely to be withdrawn, apathetic, and fearful. We do not deny that some mentally ill people are violent, but the image of the mentally ill person as essentially a violent person is erroneous.

Our understanding of violence is sadly limited. The literature abounds with studies that show psychiatrists' poor record in the prediction of dangerousness. Yet psychiatrists continue to be called upon for expertise in evaluating violent individuals and forecasting their future behavior. Psychiatric assessment of dangerousness remains central to the decision to commit a potentially violent person to a psychiatric hospital against his or her will. Such opinions are often influential in distinguishing "patients" from "prisoners" and in determining whether a violent person is to be treated or punished. Although the complex relationship between mental illness and criminal justice is beyond the scope of this discussion, it is of critical importance in modern psychiatry.

This chapter deals with violence on a personal level: how it affects you in your clinical work. Although most mentally ill people are not violent, threatening behavior does occur in mental health settings—and indeed in all health care facilities—for we regularly deal with people who are under severe emotional stress. You may be faced with violence where you least expect it (e.g., from an enraged father who cannot accept the death of his hospitalized child), so it is essential that you become familiar with some basic principles of management. As an informed clinician, you can make critical interventions that prevent injury, diminish fear, and deliver much-needed care to people who are on the verge of losing control or who have already lost it.

SOME BASIC PRINCIPLES

Violence generally denotes an assault on objects or people. When people are involved, it implies an intrusion that threatens another person's sense of safety or well-being. We often speak of verbal violence as well as physical violence, but "violence" will be used here to denote physical harm done by one human being to another.

Violence is a behavior, not a diagnosis. Violent behavior cuts across all diagnostic categories, and it is common among people who have no diagnosable mental disorder. It is not an illness, but in some cases it is a symptom of an underlying illness.

Violence or the threat of violence preempts all efforts at treatment. It demands immediate management, for you cannot care for someone competently when you feel that you are in danger. Much like a cardiac arrest, the violent act in a medical setting is an emergency that must be responded to and effectively controlled before you can step back and think about underlying causes and possible remedies.

Minimizing or denying your own fear is the most dangerous thing you can do in dealing with people who may act violently. It is also the most common error made by inexperienced clinicians. Your own reaction to a patient constitutes important data about how safe you are and how close the patient is to losing control. It may be your only clue to an imminent attack. If you do not pay attention to your own responses, you put yourself, your patient, and other people in real danger of being harmed, even killed. If this sounds overly dramatic, remember that health care professionals are at times the unfortunate victims of those they treat.

Why are we so prone to deny our fears in working with potentially violent people? As professionals, many of us harbor the unrealistic belief that we should be able to cope with any problem under any and all circumstances. Admitting that we are afraid, or that we need help, is not consonant with that belief. You are not omnipotent if you summon security guards, or end an interview and leave the room after acknowledging to your patient that you are concerned about his or her threatening behavior. You may be accustomed to putting your personal feelings aside until a crisis is over. But in fact, failing to attend to your own fears as you sit with a threatening patient is like failing to monitor someone's pulse and blood pressure during a cardiac arrest—you ignore critical data and thereby risk making the situation worse.

CLUES TO VIOLENCE

Potential violence may be easy to ignore, and it often goes unrecognized. Physicians who are hurried, emotionally withdrawn, or overly sympathetic may screen out clues to dangerousness and allow their patients' warnings to go unnoticed. You must be attentive to a variety of verbal and behavioral clues if you are to help people who cannot keep their violent impulses in check.

Threats. Roughly 5% of homicidal threats culminate in murder. Even when made in an offhand manner, threats of harm to others must be taken seriously and actively explored. A patient may make casual threats to test your receptivity to the problem, and a concerned response allows the patient to make a more explicit request for help.

Body space. The individual who remains constantly vigilant may be ready to lash out violently in self-defense. Such people reveal their inner terror in a variety of ways:

- Shrinking from physical contact (such as when approached for a handshake)

- Feeling crowded (paranoid people require roughly four times as much space as others do to maintain comfortable conversational distance)
- Retreating when approached suddenly
- Protecting the rear (a fear of being approached from behind and surprised by an assailant)

Physical findings. Unusual numbers of scars, lacerations, bruises, old fractures, head injuries, and missing teeth may indicate that a patient is habitually involved in violent activities.

Your gut response to the patient. This is often the only clue to dangerousness. It is better to be overcautious and to overestimate possible danger than to underestimate it and be sorry.

EMERGENCY MANAGEMENT OF THE VIOLENT PATIENT

When people become violent or threaten violence in mental health care facilities, your first priority is to *ensure safety*—the patient's, the staff's, and your own. No effective treatment can begin until treaters and patient feel that the threat of danger has been removed.

Your second task is to *quiet the patient and develop an alliance.* Many violent people assume a hostile and aggressive posture to defend themselves against intense feelings of helplessness and fragility. They are often fearful of losing control over their violent impulses. The following measures will help maintain a safe environment in which some collaboration between you and the patient can take place (see Table 16-1).

When a Patient Is Potentially Violent but Danger Is Not Imminent

If you are interviewing someone who has a history of violent behavior, or who you sense might become agitated and lose control, you must structure your interview so as to maximize everyone's safety.

Show available force. Before you begin, or at any point when you sense danger, bring security guards and other personnel into the interview room, or station them outside the room within the patient's view. People who fear losing control of their impulses will find outside controls reassuring, and you will feel more comfortable with help nearby.

Establish a nonthreatening setting for the interview. Remain at least at arm's length from the patient. Leave the patient and yourself

Table 16-1. General guidelines for managing a violent patient

When there is a possibility of violence	When violence is present or imminent
Show available force.	Summon help.
Establish a nonthreatening setting for the interview.	One staff member should assume leadership.
Establish a collaborative tone in the interview.	Remove all weapons from the patient.
Set verbal limits on threatening behavior.	Seclude the patient.
Monitor your own reactions.	Set physical limits on violent behavior when verbal limits do not suffice.
Know when to stop the interview.	Administer medication (antipsychotics, benzodiazepines) if needed to ease agitation and combativeness.

clear access to an exit so that either one of you has the freedom to leave at any time (e.g., do not sit between your patient and the door). The door to the interviewing room should remain open at all times. *Never approach the patient from behind.*

Establish a collaborative tone in the interview. The most helpful interviewing style is a straightforward and respectful manner that honors the patient's reasonable requests. You should show empathetic concern, but avoid appearing too warm or too friendly at the outset—this may frighten a paranoid patient. Openly inquire about any veiled threats made against you or others, and encourage the paranoid patient to see you as an ally against perceived enemies.

Set verbal limits on threatening behavior. When dealing with someone who is obviously agitated, try to help him or her *verbalize* feelings rather than acting on them. You may want to reassure the patient that you will not allow anyone to be harmed—neither the patient nor others. (Many paranoid people lash out because they are frightened that they will be attacked.)

Monitor your own reactions. Your gut responses to the patient throughout the evaluation and treatment process may be your only clue to the patient's level of hostility and degree of self-control. If you begin to feel unsafe, address this openly with the patient and then remedy it; otherwise, the patient will sense your uneasiness, and his or her own fears of losing control may intensify. You could, for example, ask security personnel stationed outside the interviewing room to come in, so that both you and the patient feel safer to proceed.

Know when to stop. If you have taken precautions as noted above, but the patient continues to be agitated and threatening, do not continue the interview. Instead, let the patient know that you sense his or her difficulty in maintaining self-control and that you are going to continue the interview at another time, when both of you can feel safer. Remember, you have nothing to lose by stopping an interview when you sense danger, and everything to lose by continuing.

When a Patient Behaves Violently or Is on the Verge of Losing Control

Summon help. Call for help at the first sign that a patient may become violent (or before a violent person arrives, if advance warning is given). This help may include security guards, police (where necessary), or anyone capable of helping to restrain an assaultive individual.

Assume leadership. Both staff and patient must feel that you can take charge and direct a team effort. Give your directions clearly and tell the patient what to expect at each step.

No surprises. Keep your distance from the patient and do not block the doorway.

Remove all weapons. No treatment can be delivered to an armed patient. This includes pills and alcoholic beverages as well as knives, guns, and other instruments of force. Do not take a weapon directly from the patient, but ask that it be placed on a table; then remove it. Explain that it will be held for safekeeping. Police help must be enlisted if an armed patient refuses to cooperate with staff, and the patient may need to be searched for weapons.

Seclude the patient. Take the patient away from large, populated areas (e.g., a waiting room) to a more secluded setting. This will limit the potential targets of any violent outbursts and quiet the patient, especially when hostility and hypervigilance are due to fear of others. Seclusion is a common technique for decreasing agitation, because a seclusion room diminishes sights, sounds, and voices when the patient's normal ability to screen out such environmental stimuli is impaired.

Set physical limits on violent behavior when verbal limits do not suffice. Remember that severe agitation is very frightening for the patient as well as for others, and physical and/or mechanical restraint is often relieving. *Physical restraint* refers to another person or persons holding the patient to prevent violent or self-destructive behavior. *Mechanical restraint* refers to the use of belts, straps, or other devices to restrict the patient's movements, often by strapping the person's arms and legs to a bedframe as he or she lies on a mattress. Physical and mechanical restraints provide concrete external controls when the patient has lost his or her internal controls. Wrist and ankle restraints must not be used punitively, but only when physical harm to self or others appears imminent.

The primary clinician should generally not take part in restraining the patient for two reasons: 1) others are usually more skilled in this procedure, and 2) physical struggles between therapist and patient may make later work impossible.

One person should generally be assigned to restrain each of the person's extremities; this should be done with a minimum of struggling and as humanely as possible. The use of restraints does not replace personal contact. Do not attempt physical restraint alone, and be sure that someone involved in the restraint is experienced in this procedure.

Medication. The use of medication against the patient's will as a *chemical restraint* is warranted only when there is immediate danger of injury to the patient or to others. However, patients who are acutely anxious will often willingly accept medication if the reasons for treatment and the effects of the medicine are carefully discussed in advance, and the plan of treatment is presented in a firm and confident manner.

Antipsychotics may be given orally or intramuscularly to control agitation and combative behavior. They are particularly effective in acute psychosis secondary to mania and schizophrenia. They should be given with caution (or not at all) to delirious or intoxicated patients, and a toxic screen is indicated.

You may, for example, prescribe 2 to 10 mg of haloperidol (Haldol) orally or intramuscularly every 30 minutes or every 4 hours (depending on the rapidity with which tranquilizing effects are needed) until agitation subsides. This is the drug of choice in many cases, because it does not cause the rapid drop in blood pressure that commonly results from using other major tranquilizers. Another likely choice would be chlorpromazine (Thorazine), with 25 to 75 mg given intramuscularly or 50 to 100 mg given orally every 4 hours until agitation subsides. Chlorpromazine is more likely than the higher-potency neuroleptics (e.g., haloperidol) to cause hypotensive reactions (sudden drops in blood pressure) and must therefore be used intramuscularly with caution.

Benzodiazepines (minor tranquilizers) are particularly useful for those who are agitated but not actively violent and for the elderly, who are more sensitive to hypotensive reactions. A physician might call for 5 to 20 mg of diazepam (Valium) to be administered orally every 4 to 6 hours, or 50 to 100 mg of chlordiazepoxide (Librium) every 6 to 8 hours.

For severe alcohol withdrawal, a physician might prescribe 10 to 30 cc of paraldehyde orally every 4 hours.

Amobarbital sodium (sodium Amytal) is another powerful sedative, which may be used in oral doses of 100 to 200 mg as needed to produce sedation.

PROFILES IN VIOLENCE

There is enormous diversity among those who resort to violence, but certain personal characteristics are common. If you are alert to these correlates of violence, you can use them to put your patient's threats or behavior into perspective and to judge his or her potential to act violently in the future.

Previous violent behavior. Previous violent behavior is the most valid predictor of violent behavior in the future. The probability of future violence increases with each violent act. This includes a history of arrests, assaults on people or property, and a history of accidental or intentional involvement in another person's death.

Age. Violent behavior peaks among teenagers and those in their early 20s. Juvenile violence is increasing at nearly twice the rate of violence among adults. The earlier that one is violent, the greater the likelihood that one will continue to be violent.

Sex. Ninety percent of those arrested for violent crimes are male. But much domestic violence (e.g., child abuse) perpetrated by women goes unreported.

Race. Blacks account for 12% of the population but 48% of all arrests for violent crime in the United States each year. The rate of violence is also higher among Hispanics than in the general population. The reasons for this disproportionate representation of nonwhites among violent criminals are not entirely clear. Social injustice and economic discrimination are obvious contributing factors and appear to be more important than the influence of so-called "violent subcultures" in the genesis of violent behavior.

Drug and alcohol abuse. Substance abuse is highly correlated with violent behavior and predisposes one to violence through a variety of mechanisms (see below).

Socioeconomic status and employment stability. Violence is markedly increased among members of lower socioeconomic groups and among those with a history of unemployment or irregular employment. Two of the prime determinants of homicidal behavior appear to be absolute poverty and marital disruption.

Self-destructive behavior. This factor is often overlooked. Self-mutilation and suicide are disproportionately common among people who act violently toward others.

Other factors that correlate with violent behavior include increased residential mobility ("absent roots"), being single, lower IQ, and lower level of educational attainment.

Childhood Correlates of Violence in Adults

Which children grow up to be violent? We do not know, but the following factors have been found to be particularly prevalent in the childhood experiences of people who behave violently as adults:

- *Parental deprivation and abuse.* Violent people frequently give histories of parental neglect or abandonment, as well as parental abuse (verbal and/or physical). It is estimated that roughly one in three people who were victims of violence as children commonly become victimizers as adults.
- *Early exposure to violence.* Parental and sibling brutality witnessed in the home provides a model for conflict resolution through violence.
- *Frequent disruptions in family life.* This includes parental separation or divorce, frequent moves, and school changes.
- *Temper tantrums and frequent fights.*
- *Authority problems.* These include truancy, school problems, and difficulties in the military.

ETIOLOGIES OF VIOLENCE

In evaluating a patient who has acted violently, you must consider the possible causes of this behavior. Many mental disorders underlie violence; some of the most important ones are listed below. But because most violence is perpetrated by people who do not suffer from a major mental disorder, your first task is to determine whether the problem is psychiatric.

You may find it helpful to try to fit your patient's behavior into a broader conceptual scheme of the etiology of violence. Most of us keep our violent impulses in check most of the time. What, then, has prompted this person to act on his or her violent impulses in this setting at this time?

Does the person suffer from an impaired ability to test reality? People who are hallucinating may hear voices commanding them to act violently—for example, a man may hear his dead mother's voice commanding him to kill his father. Someone who is having visual hallucinations might see you as a vampire who is about to attack.

Paranoid thinking plays a prominent role in many acts of violence. People who resort to the use of violence frequently believe that they are being persecuted, harassed, or unfairly treated; they view the world as hostile and threatening, and they often lash out in "self-defense." Paranoid ideas generally begin with the misinterpretation of real events. The paranoid person who acts violently often does so because of a distorted view of his or her situation.

Does the patient suffer from an impaired ability to control his or her impulses? We all have violent impulses. On a daily basis, we hear ourselves and others make such statements as "I wanted to wring his neck!" Yet we control these urges, sometimes so rigidly that we push them out of our awareness entirely. We do not attack others whenever we feel like it. People who do not control themselves may not have developed a normal capacity for self-control as children because of poor parental control, neurological impairment, a severely disturbed home environment, or other factors we have yet to elucidate. Such people often give histories of impulsivity in many areas of their lives, including sexual behavior, employment, drug abuse, and reckless driving. Other people lose the ability to control their impulses only temporarily—for example, under the influence of disinhibiting substances such as opiates or alcohol.

Does the patient show impaired judgment? Judgment is a complex mental function involving a variety of cognitive skills. Obviously, psychosis or drug use can impair one's ability to judge how to behave in a given situation. Other factors that may impair judgment include anxiety, depression, and neurological impairment (e.g., as a result of head trauma).

Does the patient use violence explicitly to manipulate others? Many people suffer from no impairment in mental functioning, but simply use physical force deliberately and in a calculated fashion to intimidate or to achieve what they want at others' expense. Such people do not require mental health care, but disciplinary action.

Mental Disorders and Violence

Some of the more common mental disorders may foster violent behavior. They are listed in Table 16-2 and described briefly below.

Psychotic illnesses

Schizophrenia. Delusional beliefs and hallucinations become the "motives" for violence.

Mania. Delusions and hallucinations, coupled with uncontrolled rage and hyperactivity, predispose the patient to violence.

Psychotic depression. The hopeless person may kill family members or a lover in the delusional belief that this "spares them grief," and

Table 16-2. Some disorders that may underlie violent behavior

Psychotic illnesses	Drug intoxication or withdrawal
Schizophrenia	Alcohol
Mania	Opiates
Psychotic depression	Amphetamines
Brief reactive psychosis	Barbiturates
(postpartum depression)	Cannabis
	Cocaine
Personality disorders, especially:	LSD
Paranoid personality disorder	Phencyclidine (PCP)
Borderline personality disorder	
Obsessive-compulsive personality	**Organic conditions**
disorder	
Antisocial personality disorder	Temporal lobe epilepsy
	Brain damage
Sexual disorders	Dementia
	Adult minimal brain dysfunction
Sexual dysfunction	Altered androgen levels?
Homosexual panic	Delirium

may go on to commit suicide. Elderly people with agitated depression can be surprisingly combative.

Postpartum depression. This is a special category of depression. Typically, the mother becomes anxious prior to delivery, develops the delusion that her husband is unfaithful, and becomes depressed after delivery. She is at risk of harming her newborn child.

Personality disorders

Any of the personality disorders may be accompanied by violence, particularly those listed below.

Paranoid personality disorder. Constant, pervasive paranoia may erupt into violence when the paranoid person feels that he or she is under attack.

Borderline personality disorder. Poor impulse control and persistent anger may prompt borderline individuals to behave violently toward those who are important to them, but anger turned against the self is more common.

Obsessive-compulsive personality disorder. The highly controlled, obsessional individual may "explode" under severe stress.

Antisocial personality disorder. This disorder is characterized by failure to accept social norms, recklessness, impulsivity, and unstable relationships. Often labeled "sociopaths," people who have this disorder characteristically feel no remorse for antisocial behavior.

Sexual disorders

Sexual dysfunction. Threats to sexual identity, particularly impotence from any cause, may prompt a show of force to demonstrate virility.

Homosexual panic. Men whose unconscious homosexual strivings come to the surface (e.g., in the military or other situations of forced intimacy) may become acutely anxious and paranoid. In the midst of such panic, the individual in homosexual panic believes others are accusing him of "forbidden" homosexual wishes and practices, and he may pick fights to prove his manhood. Such men frequently brawl in barrooms with "drinking buddies."

Drug-related violence

Drugs may precipitate violence in three basic ways:

1. *Substances with disinhibiting effects* can take away an individual's self-control, particularly when that control was tenuous in the first place.
2. *Intoxication may result in delirium or toxic psychosis*, in which confusion, delusions, and hallucinations prompt violent behavior.
3. *Drug withdrawal syndromes* may include agitation, confusion, and psychosis.

Some drugs commonly implicated in acts of violence are alcohol and opiates (nearly half of all violent crimes are committed by people who are under the influence of one of these classes of substances), amphetamines, barbiturates, cannabis (marijuana, hashish, synthetic tetrahydrocannabinol), LSD, and phencyclidine (PCP). Cocaine use is increasingly associated with violence in our society, both because of criminal behavior around the sale and distribution of the drug and because of the paranoia that results from severe intoxication.

Less common causes of violent behavior, but sometimes encountered among medical and psychiatric patients, are L-dopa, benzodiazepines, and tricyclic antidepressants.

Organic conditions

Some organic conditions may produce violent behavior.

Temporal-lobe epilepsy. People who experience psychomotor seizures are at risk for developing impulsive and irritable behavior patterns, characterized by angry outbursts. These outbursts do not occur at random but are often provoked. They do not occur during seizures, they do not commonly result in serious injuries, and they alternate with prolonged periods of "good behavior." Families often note that the person seems to have undergone a gradual personality change. Recent studies suggest that violence among patients with temporal-lobe epilepsy is relatively uncommon and may be no more prevalent in this population than among those without epilepsy.

Brain damage. Traumatic lesions most often associated with violence are those involving the frontal or temporal lobes, particularly the limbic system and the area of the amygdala and hippocampus. Brain damage that prompts subsequent violent behavior may occur at birth, or later in life as the result of falls, motor vehicle accidents, etc.

Dementia. Alzheimer's disease and senile dementia diminish integrative capacity and produce confusion, which often results in combative states, even among seemingly frail elderly people.

Adult minimal brain dysfunction. This syndrome of aggressiveness, impulsivity, and mood disorder is often found in people with a history of minimal brain dysfunction in childhood.

Delirium. Delirium may result from a variety of causes, including metabolic encephalopathies (see Chapter 9).

Factors that *have not* been proven to be associated with violence include:

Neurotransmitter abnormalities. While low levels of 5-hydroxyindoleacetic acid (5-HIAA) have been found in the cerebrospinal fluid (CSF) of people with histories of aggressive behavior, they have also been found among people with histories of suicidal behavior. Low CSF 5-HIAA levels may be a marker of impulsivity rather than a specific marker for violent behavior.

Altered androgen levels. Once thought to be elevated among violent men, androgen levels have not been correlated with violence in recent empirical studies.

Sex chromosome abnormalities. XYY and XXY chromosomal abnormalities have been thought to be related to increased aggressive behavior, but research has failed to support this hypothesis.

ASSESSMENT

Clinical evaluation of people who behave violently must include a detailed exploration of violent acts and impulses, along with thorough psychiatric and medical histories. People rarely exhibit random violence, but become dangerous to others only under specific circumstances. You must therefore pay close attention to the particular social, biological, and psychological stressors that trigger violent impulses in each person.

Only by constructing individual "profiles" of violence can you tailor treatment to individual patients' needs. Also, if you can identify specific settings, events, and other factors that trigger violence in your patient, you will improve your ability to predict when he or she may act violently in the future.

Evaluating Violence

The following questions may help you assess a patient's current status after a recent episode of violent behavior or violent threats:

Current Crisis

- What happened?
- Who decided that you needed help? (You? A relative? A friend?)
- Do you think your behavior is a problem? Do others think so? If so, in what way?
- What prompted this crisis? (Fears of others? Threats from others?)
- Where did it happen? (In a bar? At home? At work?)
- Who was involved? (Spouse? Policeman? Passerby?)
- In as much detail as possible, reconstruct exactly what was said, what was done, and who was involved. Also note whether alcohol or drugs were involved. What were the patient's thoughts and feelings throughout the episode?

Potential Victims

- Who do you feel angry at now?
- Is there anyone you would like to hurt or kill?
- Is there anyone you feel wants to hurt you?
- Are you likely to see these people soon?

Available Weapons

- How would you carry out your threat or protect yourself?
- Do you have a gun, knife, etc.?

History of Violent Behavior

- How far back does your trouble with violence (getting into fights) go?
- What is the most violent thing you have ever done?
- How badly have you hurt someone in the past?
- What is the closest you have come to killing someone?
- Do you get into fights (with X) more or less often than you used to?
- Are the fights getting worse?
- Have you ever been arrested? (Document dates.)
- Have you been convicted of any crimes? (Document crimes and sentences.)
- Have you ever been hospitalized because of your violent behavior?
- What weapons have you used in the past? Against whom?
- Do you ever hit your spouse or your child?
- Where do fights usually occur? With whom? What do you usually fight about?

Try to get a detailed picture of previous situations in which the patient has acted violently—for example, when intoxicated, upon ending a relationship, when fired from a job, when manic.

Environment

Assess the family situation and peer pressure:

- Has anything recently changed at home or with friends? (Is an important relationship suddenly threatened?) Note that 75% of all emergency commitments occur when family members are attacked or threatened. Half of all homicides are committed by family members or lovers.
- Are you the only one at home/at work/among your friends who gets into fights?
- Have you had trouble at work lately?

Judgment

Determine whether the patient can accurately appraise situations and anticipate the consequences of his or her actions:

- Do you think you will need to behave violently again?
- What do you think will happen to you if you do what you have in mind?

Psychiatric Evaluation

A general psychiatric evaluation is part of every assessment of the violent patient. Special attention should be paid to the following areas:

- History of drug and alcohol use
- Childhood history (abuse or neglect, violence in the home, tantrums, frequent fights, school difficulty, delinquency problems with authority)
- Sexual concerns
- The mental status examination, particularly delusions (e.g., thought control, thought broadcasting), hallucinations (commands or threats from imaginary beings), depersonalization, paranoia, suicidal ideation, and impulsivity

TREATMENT

When a patient comes to you in an outpatient clinic or emergency room with a history of recent violent or threatening behavior, you must judge whether it is safe to allow that person to return to the community. Obviously, your decision will be based on many factors, including the patient's mental status, the presence of underlying medical or psychiatric illness, and your assessment of the likelihood that the patient will harm someone if released.

If you are concerned that a patient will be violent if allowed to go home, it is safest to hospitalize him or her so that you have more time to thoroughly evaluate the situation. Again, it is better to be safe than sorry.

Hospitalization

Indications for hospitalization include 1) specific homicidal intent with a definite, workable plan and the availability of weapons and intended victims; 2) lack of internal controls—impulsivity, poor judgment, faulty reality testing; 3) lack of social supports—family and friends are unavailable or are themselves in danger; 4) acute psychosis; and 5) toxic states that do not clear rapidly.

People who fear their own violent impulses may willingly agree to hospitalization. Involuntary commitment is justified in most states only when there is a substantial risk of physical harm to others or evidence that the patient has placed others in a reasonable fear of harm.

When involuntary commitment is indicated. Involuntary commitment must be presented to the patient in a firm and nonpunitive manner. Staff must remain with the patient at all times to prevent escape, and transportation must be carried out by ambulance and/or by security forces. Hospitalization should not mean rejection; whenever possible, if you do the initial assessment, you should make a follow-up visit once the patient is admitted to the hospital.

When involuntary commitment is not indicated. You face a dilemma when the patient does not fit the criteria for commitment and refuses voluntary hospitalization, but there is concern that a specific intended victim might be harmed. Recent court rulings (e.g., *Tarasoff v. Regents of University of California*) have upheld the idea that clinicians are obligated to warn intended victims when patients express homicidal intentions toward specific people. Because it constitutes a breach of confidentiality in the therapist-patient relationship, this concept is under heated debate. Also, given mental health professionals' demonstrated inability to reliably predict their patients' future violent behavior, many feel that the profession has become legally bound to perform a task of which it is incapable. Nevertheless, the clinician must contact and warn intended victims if patients are sent home with persistent thoughts of violence focused on particular individuals. A useful therapeutic stance, at the start of treatment or when the patient's potential for violence becomes clear, is to inform the patient that the rules of confidentiality do not hold in cases where the patient's or someone else's life is in danger.

When you make judgments about a patient's dangerousness, it is essential that the basis for these judgments and subsequent interventions be carefully documented in the patient's record.

Outpatient Treatment

Patients who reveal no clear violent intention or plan, and who have no history of violence, may be followed up in outpatient treatment if they appear capable of allying themselves with you and seeking help before they act on violent impulses. Before the patient is sent home, it is essential that precise arrangements for follow-up be made, ideally involving you if you performed the initial assessment.

Psychotherapy

Psychotherapy can be helpful to patients who want and can use an ongoing relationship. The therapist should assume an interested but nonintrusive attitude, avoiding all physical contact and initially avoiding the use of humor, which may be misunderstood by a suspicious patient. The focus of work is on helping the patient recognize violent urges and behavior patterns and on finding verbal or other means of ventilating these urges without acting them out. Patients must learn to predict the times and situations when they are likely to act violently, and to develop means of preventing such acts.

Some clinicians have used specific techniques of behavior therapy with violent individuals. Therapist and patient identify behaviors such as hitting, pushing, and hair pulling, which they then target to be extinguished. They then construct a behavioral program that reinforces the patient with concrete rewards when he or she refrains from these behaviors. The program may actively discourage the patient from exhibiting violent behaviors by establishing adverse consequences when they occur.

Clinicians disagree about the best treatment regimen for violent patients in psychotherapy. Some consider regular outpatient appointments with one therapist the treatment of choice. Others recommend treatment on an "as needed" basis at one facility by a variety of treaters, in order to dilute the intense and potentially overwhelming feelings that might develop in a therapy relationship and that could actually promote violence toward the therapist. Most clinicians agree that violent people need access to one institution on an ongoing basis for crisis intervention.

Pharmacological treatment

There are no specific medications for the long-term management of violent behavior. Medication should be used only when it is likely to alleviate an underlying mental disorder, and only after a thorough discussion with the patient (see Table 16-3).

In rare cases of intractable violence, psychosurgery has been effective. In violence associated with sexual activity, antiandrogen therapy with drugs that reduce blood levels of male sex hormones—for example, medroxyprogesterone (Depo-Provera)—has proved useful. However, both treatments raise particular ethical problems for the clinician.

Table 16-3. Some medications that may be indicated in the management of violent behavior

Medication	Indication
Antipsychotics	Psychosis and overwhelming anxiety
Lithium	Affective disorders and disorders of impulse control (e.g., episodic dyscontrol)
Antidepressants	Depression
Benzodiazepines	Anxiety
Anticonvulsants	Underlying seizure disorders, including psychomotor seizures
Disulfiram (Antabuse)	Alcohol addiction

YOUR REACTIONS TO VIOLENCE

Anxiety in dealing with violent people is real and must be used as data rather than ignored. In the struggle to remain in control of the situation, you may defend against your own uneasiness in a variety of unproductive ways:

Denial. You may overlook important evidence of the patient's dangerousness (e.g., not hearing veiled threats, forgetting to ask about weapons) and see only the patient's nonthreatening qualities.

Reaction formation. "I'm afraid of you" may become "I'm not afraid of you," and your fear may be transformed into an overly warm and solicitous manner that can raise a paranoid patient's level of anxiety.

Withdrawal. If you feel helpless in treating a violent individual, you may avoid or openly reject the patient without being aware of your own emotional withdrawal.

Retaliation. Anger at the patient can be expressed through punitive treatment (e.g., the unnecessary use of restraints). You may find yourself enraged at someone who threatens you, and you may actually find pleasure in the "revenge" involved in restraining a violent person with medication or by physical force. If this happens, simply step back from the situation and allow others to take over for you. Anger and fear are normal reactions to violence—you need not be ashamed of them. However, you are obliged as a professional to remove yourself (at least temporarily) from the treatment situation if such feelings begin to influence your clinical decisions.

Treatment for the Treaters

Working with people who resort to violence is extremely stressful. Witnessing violent behavior and fearing for your own safety are experiences that arouse some of our most primitive emotions. You must have support in doing such work, including the following:

1. *Group support.* Staff members who have been involved in a crisis with a violent patient commonly meet when the crisis has passed to "decompress" and discuss their reactions to what has happened.
2. *Supervision.* Supervisors who have experience in working with violent people can help you understand your reactions to threatening patients and improve your therapeutic skills.
3. *Review of security procedures in the facility where you work.* This may allay some anxiety and will improve your future efficiency in managing crises with violent patients. Review in detail plans for summoning help and procedures for carrying out physical restraint.
4. *Visit a maximum security psychiatric facility.* This is likely to broaden your perspective on how violent behavior can be controlled and treatment facilitated.
5. *Peer support.* The most helpful support usually comes from your colleagues, who best understand your reactions as a trainee in a stressful situation.

Violence, perhaps more than any other clinical situation, highlights the fact that you cannot care effectively for others if you do not take care of yourself.

BIBLIOGRAPHY

"Drugs that cause psychiatric symptoms." The Medical Letter Vol 23, Feb 6, 1981, pp 9–12

Eichelman B: Toward a rational pharmacotherapy for aggressive and violent behavior. Hosp Community Psychiatry 39:31–39, 1988

Kaufman J, Zigler E: Do abused children become abusive parents? Am J Orthopsychiatry 57:186–192, 1987

Lion JR: Evaluation and Management of the Violent Patient. Springfield, IL, Charles C Thomas, 1972

Monahan J: The clinical prediction of violent behavior (DHHS Publ No ADM-81-921). Washington, DC, U.S. Government Printing Office, 1981

President's Commission on Mental Health: Report to the President. Washington, DC, President's Commission on Mental Health, 1978, p 56

Rada RT: The violent patient: rapid assessment and management. Psychosomatics 22:101–109, 1981

Rockwell DA: Can you spot potential violence in a patient? Hospital Physician 10:52–56, 1972

Tardiff KJ: Violence, in The American Psychiatric Press Textbook of Psychiatry. Edited by Talbott JA, Hales RE, Yudofsky SC. Washington, DC, American Psychiatric Press, 1988, pp 1037–1057

Weiger WA, Bear DM: An approach to the neurology of aggression. J Psychiatr Res 22:85–98, 1988

Part IV   Treatment

17 Psychotherapies 483
18 Somatic Therapies 515
    Psychotropic Medications 515
      Antipsychotic Medications 527
      Antidepressants 541
      Lithium 556
      Anticonvulsants 561
      Antianxiety Agents 563
    Electroconvulsive Therapy 569

INTRODUCTION

The two major forms of treatment in modern psychiatry are the psychotherapies and the somatic therapies. Chapter 17 is a discussion of several different types of psychotherapy. The array of psychosocial treatments now used in mental health care is vast. This chapter could not begin to teach you about all of them, and no attempt is made to do so. Instead, the chapter includes an extensive discussion of traditional psychodynamic psychotherapy and briefer descriptions of some of the most important nonpsychodynamic modalities.

Why the emphasis on psychodynamics? First, as a medical practitioner, you will need to have more than a superficial understanding of this approach to mental illness, since psychodynamic principles such as transference and resistance are important in *all* encounters between doctor and patient, regardless of the medical problems being addressed. Second, Freudian psychodynamic theory is the foundation upon which

481

many subsequent theories of the mind were constructed, and it is the school of thought against which many psychological theorists have reacted. Your understanding of the "basics" will greatly enhance your ability to think critically about the many ways in which these principles have been modified in later efforts to understand and treat psychiatric disorders.

Chapter 18 covers the somatic therapies, beginning with a general discussion of the principles of using psychotropic medications. You may want to read this section in its entirety. The subsequent sections on specific classes of medication are there for you to refer to as questions about particular medications arise in the course of your clinical work. Electroconvulsive therapy is discussed at the end of the chapter.

17

Psychotherapies

CONTACT WITH OTHER HUMAN BEINGS can relieve distress, change behavior patterns, and alter our views of ourselves and the world. All psychological therapies rely on this fundamental premise. From the infinitely complex ways in which people interact, psychosocial theorists attempt to tease out the factors that promote emotional well-being and those that foster ill health. These studies have yielded a variety of schemes for understanding emotional life and treating psychological impairment.

The term *psychotherapy* includes those means by which a therapist attempts to provide new interpersonal experiences for another human being. These experiences are designed to enhance one's ability to manage subjective distress and to participate in loving relationships and satisfying work.

To be sure, these are ambitious goals. They are, in essence, no different from the goals any physician brings to work with patients, for the aim of all therapeutics is to improve the quality of life. Most medical practitioners rely heavily on the use of concrete aids in their therapeutic interventions—medications, surgical procedures, and an ever-increasing array of tools and machines. Psychosocial therapists, by contrast, rely on themselves as the primary agents of treatment. Yet the medical and psychosocial models of therapy are much closer than they at first appear to be. Regardless of their specialty, experienced medical practitioners invariably attest to the therapeutic power inherent in the doctor-patient relationship.

HOW CAN A HUMAN RELATIONSHIP BE THERAPEUTIC?

Each type of therapy discussed in this text emphasizes a particular view of mental illness and particular treatment techniques. Yet all therapeutic situations share certain important factors that promote recovery.

The patient brings to therapy an expectation that help is possible. Psychotherapy prescribes that the therapist and the patient work together in specific ways that they both believe will be a means of restoring health. The therapist offers a sincere, interested, attentive, and reliable presence; the patient generally comes to view the therapist as a benign and powerful force. Most patients come to treatment with the hope that the therapist has benevolent powers. This hope underlies the majority of doctor-patient relationships in all areas of medicine.

Where does this hope come from? Human beings spend many years in a dependent relationship with their parents and other caregivers. As children, we learn that needs can be satisfied, fears allayed, and pains eased by the care and attention of adults. This learned expectation of help becomes activated in many situations in our adult lives, as when we consult health care professionals.

These hopes serve as the cornerstone for successful treatment. In psychoanalytic terms, this phenomenon is referred to as *positive transference*, because we transfer positive expectations we had for early caregivers to people who we expect to play similar roles in our adult lives. As a rule, people who have not learned to trust in this manner were deprived of care during early infancy. Such people may bring to therapy ingrained attitudes of suspicion and hatred that take months or even years to overcome, or their mistrust may be so pervasive that it is impossible to establish a therapeutic relationship.

Psychotherapy gives the patient a conceptual scheme for making sense of bewildering mental phenomena. Each type of psychotherapy provides a set of concepts that people can use to label and explain confusing subjective states and seemingly inexplicable behaviors. This enhances the person's sense of control over problems. (This also occurs in other forms of medical treatment.)

The therapist offers the expectation that the patient can make positive life changes. Although this may appear obvious, many people come to therapy believing that they are incapable of self-improvement. Relatives and friends may share this pessimism, and everyone in the patient's life may be quite comfortable with the view that the patient is "disturbed" or "a mental case," or that he or she is "the one with problems." In such situations, the therapist offers a different perspective and an unwillingness to share these stereotyped views.

The patient adopts certain of the therapist's positive attitudes. This happens through *identification*, a process that occurs in all of us from early childhood onward, as we consciously and unconsciously take on the characteristics of important others (e.g., parents, teachers) whom we want to be like. The patient in psychotherapy identifies with the therapist's attitude that problems can be faced squarely and that seemingly unbearable thoughts and feelings can be tolerated and managed. For example, a patient who is brutally self-critical can identify with the therapist's more tolerant and realistic view, thus gaining the ability to be more flexible and less demanding of perfection.

Therapy offers a safe place for taking risks. The patient learns that it is possible to discuss "forbidden" feelings, attitudes, and experiences with another person without being judged or reprimanded. Developing a trusting, confiding, emotional relationship with the therapist is, in and of itself, a considerable achievement for many isolated and inhibited people and serves as a model for developing more satisfying relations with others. The patient can also use therapy to experiment with new behaviors in a situation that carries no real threat of punishment.

The safety of therapy lies in its structure: the sessions have clear boundaries of time and space, the therapist is restrained and professional, and the activities that go on between patient and therapist are strictly limited. These limitations are at times frustrating, but also reassuring. For example, a patient who is frightened by sexual impulses can learn that it is possible to talk about such feelings without having to act on them.

Therapy expands one's horizons and increases one's options. This occurs in innumerable ways. Many forms of therapy help the patient arrive at a fuller awareness of self, particularly those aspects of the self that were previously disavowed or distorted. Therapy also helps patients see the ways in which they repeatedly distort their perceptions of others. This opens up the possibility of dealing with people in more productive and satisfying ways. Some therapists explicitly teach new behaviors; others attempt to teach new cognitive styles. All therapies offer new possibilities for viewing oneself and dealing with the world—that is, they reopen the future by facilitating growth.

Psychotherapy cannot alter the problems of the world in which the patient lives. It cannot, for example, eliminate stress or poverty. But therapy can enhance self-acceptance and help the patient cope more effectively with the environment.

MODELS OF PSYCHOTHERAPY

There are many models of psychotherapy. This discussion could not begin to describe all of them, but will instead focus on two very different models at some length. Psychodynamic therapy and behavior therapy may be seen as two ends of a broad spectrum of psychological treatments. The former emphasizes self-exploration and self-understanding, while the latter is more directive and task-oriented, aiming at the acquisition of new, more adaptive behaviors and elimination of maladaptive ones.

Psychodynamic therapies are based on the idea that people can achieve greater understanding of the psychological forces that motivate their actions, and that insight achieved through psychological exploration opens up possibilities for change in personality and behavior. The classic insight-oriented therapy is psychoanalysis, which will serve as a prototype for our discussion of psychodynamic change.

Behavior therapies do not aim to develop insight or bring about personality change, but instead use directive techniques to remove specific symptoms. Persuasion and learning theories provide the theoretical bases for these therapies.

In reality, most therapists do not adhere rigidly to one theoretical model when they conduct psychotherapy. Rather, they use a mix of supportive-directive and insight-oriented techniques, based on their own personal styles and the needs of the individual patient. We will look at psychodynamic therapy and behavior therapy in "pure" form to orient you to each type, and, in addition, this chapter will cover cognitive therapy and hypnosis, two widely-used methods of treatment.

PSYCHODYNAMIC THERAPIES

The Psychodynamic Model of Change

Psychodynamic therapy encompasses a vast array of treatment modalities, including individual, group, couples, and family therapy. Sigmund Freud (1856–1939) is generally acknowledged to be the major figure in the genesis of this approach, for he was the first person to systematize a method of understanding seemingly unintelligible behavior in adult life by relating such behavior to childhood experiences.

All psychodynamic therapies share the assumption that the present is shaped and governed by the past—that is, that our present attitudes and styles of reacting to the world are, to some extent, carryovers from our attitudes and reactions to people and events earlier in life. Psychodynamic theorists focus on childhood—particularly on early childhood experience—in attempting to understand mental health and mental illness. This is not to say that childhood trauma is invariably the cause of psychological difficulties in adult life. Indeed, human behavior cannot be reduced to simple causal explanations. Nonetheless, how children experience pleasure and pain, punishment and reward, in the context of family and social life prompts the gradual development of personality traits, ideas about oneself, and expectations of others.

Each of us develops along different lines. We have different caregivers as children and different family constellations; we play different roles within those constellations; and we bring different inborn characteristics to our dealings with the world. Each person's "take" on the world is unique, and the psychological traits and forces that develop early in our lives are highly individual, like fingerprints. These forces are modified as life proceeds, but the extent to which early roles and attitudes persist into adulthood and rule our adult lives is considerable.

Many of these psychological forces operate without our being aware of them. They are *unconscious*. The unconscious consists of fantasies, feelings, expectations, memories, attitudes–virtually all types of mental phenomena (see Chapter 2).

Why do some things that were once known to us lie outside our awareness? According to psychodynamic theory, material is pushed into the unconscious because it reflects experiences that are unacceptable at the time and in the circumstances in which they first occur. For example, a small boy may be totally unaware that he is angry at his abusive mother. The child *represses* his anger—that is, banishes it from his consciousness—because he cannot resolve the conflict between his anger at his mother and his very real need for his mother's care and protection.

Conflicts and deficits

The idea of *conflict* is central to the psychodynamic model of mental illness. Conflict refers to the opposition between seemingly irreconcilable forces. Examples include a wish to excel and a wish not to defeat others, a wish to please someone that can only be achieved by doing something that is considered wrong, and a wish to both grow up and remain a child.

Many of those who seek psychiatric treatment are enmeshed in conflict and are in some way hampered by it. Battles between opposing psychological forces can consume a tremendous amount of energy and leave the individual exhausted and incapable of effective functioning, as in the following example:

> A young man who had unconsciously adopted his parents' strong prohibitions against sexuality found himself caught in a desperate struggle between his own sexual longings and the dictates of a stern conscience. Sexually frustrated and incapable of forming a satisfying sexual relationship, he sought gratification in other, less intimate activities. He turned to auto racing, which, although objectively more dangerous, was emotionally safe. Despite his considerable success in this endeavor, he remained unsatisfied with his life and preoccupied. Moreover, he began to have difficulty completing projects at work and was increasingly unable to concentrate on even the simplest of tasks.

In many cases, such as this one, people who are caught between conflicting intrapsychic demands or desires find themselves unable to derive satisfaction from work or play. They may feel anxious or depressed, or develop discrete symptoms such as phobias; but because the conflict is unconscious, they are not aware of the cause of their distress.

Psychoanalytic theory holds that conflict fosters the development of symptoms in three stages:

1. The presence of an unresolvable conflict
2. An attempt to repress the conflict
3. The return of the repressed conflict to conscious life in a disguised form: as a symptom (e.g., anxiety) or as a pathological character trait (e.g., passive-aggressive characteristics)

Life events and the process of growing up can ease internal conflicts, and many people find their way out of such dilemmas without psychotherapeutic intervention. However, some people become "stuck" and cannot find satisfactory solutions on their own.

The notion of conflict provides a framework for understanding some of the symptoms of mental illness. However, many people—particularly those who are more severely impaired—seem to have an absence of important emotional and cognitive capacities that are normally acquired in the process of growing up. They are thought to have psychological *deficits* that make them incapable of certain activities most of us take for granted. Examples of psychological deficits include a lack of the capacity to control violent or sexual impulses, the inability to anticipate the consequences of one's acts, the inability to delay gratification, and the inability to understand the difference between one's own and another person's feelings.

How do such deficits arise in the course of personality development? Psychodynamic theory emphasizes the importance of early experiences with caregivers in explaining the origins of developmental deficits as well as developmental gains. For example, the capacity to channel a violent impulse into more socially acceptable behavior is commonly learned from parents, both in how they explicitly instruct the child and in how they themselves act. Children can *internalize* this capacity—that is, incorporate it into their personalities—if parents have modeled it. However, children who grow up without such models, and with models of violent impulsive behavior, are themselves more likely to have difficulty with impulse control.

Deficits in development may be repaired by life experiences. For example, a young man with poor impulse control may learn this capacity in adolescence through identification with an admired high school football coach, or through experiences in the military. But some people come for psychiatric treatment because developmental defects persist in adult life and hamper their ability to maintain satisfying relationships and to work productively.

In pursuing the nature of mental illness, psychodynamic theorists and clinicians continue to debate whether certain symptoms and character traits result from conflicts or from deficits. This controversy has important implications for treatment.

Sources of data in psychotherapy

People come to psychotherapy because they have problems and need help. Their presenting complaints usually involve immediate life events and specific symptoms, but they are generally unaware of the deeper issues that underlie their complaints, as in the following case:

> A 23-year-old woman sought therapy after breaking up with her 45-year-old boyfriend. She reported that she became inexplicably anxious and had to flee the relationship as it became more intimate. She was aware that other relationships, also with older men, had ended in a similar fashion, but she did not understand why. In the treatment that followed, the patient and her therapist explored the origins of her need to flee from intimacy, particularly when it involved older men. Eventually she recalled a childhood experience in which an uncle's physical affection had frightened and excited her. She was also able to recall the shame she felt not only because her uncle had caressed her body but also because from time to time she wished that he would do it again. In her adult life she found herself pursuing older men, but, at the same time, she unconsciously equated sexual intimacy with her fear of sexual exploitation and with her forbidden interest.

As a therapist, how would you work with a patient to understand the presenting problem? The therapist has several sources of data about how patients' minds work. First, patients offer information about their past experiences: their relationships with important people and how they felt and behaved in a variety of situations. Second, as sessions proceed, patients generally bring up information about their current lives and relationships. Third, the patient forms a relationship with the therapist. This relationship is a powerful tool, because patients bring into therapy the same set of unconscious conflicts and styles of relating that they bring to their dealings with other people in their lives. Thus, they are bound to recreate in therapy many of the pathological patterns that brought them into treatment in the first place. The therapist can then help the patient step back from the relationship and attempt to understand its unsatisfying and destructive aspects.

This brings us to two of the most important concepts that psychoanalytic theory has contributed to our understanding of the human mind: transference and resistance.

Transference

We are not born knowing how to relate to other people. From the first moment of life, the infant begins to form relationships and, in doing so, learns patterns of dealing with others that are not arbitrary but are determined both by the infant's inherent temperament and by the environment into which he or she is born. The way we learn to form relationships is strongly influenced by the particular people who are important to us early in life—most often, parents or other primary caregivers, and siblings. We carry our feelings for these people with us into adult life, and they serve as templates on which we form later relationships.

Thus, our reactions to new people in our lives are not only based on how we experience them in reality. We also tend to displace onto new people the feelings and attitudes we had toward early significant figures (parents, siblings, etc.), *transferring* feelings from old relationships to new ones. This happens with particular intensity when someone in the present resembles someone important from the past. The resemblance may be in very particular details (appearance or tone of voice), or it may simply be in the nature of the relationship itself (for example, an authority figure). An individual may thus stir up intense feelings of worship or hatred, longing or fear, that are totally inappropriate to one's real knowledge or experience of that person. This is transference, and it is, for the most part, unconscious.

Transference feelings are present to some extent in all of our relationships, and they help determine our choices of friends, lovers, and colleagues. But transference reactions are likely to occur with particular intensity toward people who perform functions such as teaching, caregiving, and disciplining that were originally carried out by parents. Thus, we are likely to have strong transference reactions to teachers, lovers, bosses, and, of course, therapists.

Patients instinctively reenact their earliest interpersonal patterns and conflicts in the relationship with the psychotherapist. They do this by attempting to coerce the therapist into being something other than a therapist—for example, a lover, a protector, or a competitor, as the following case example illustrates:

> A patient complained that throughout his adult life he had always established highly idealized relationships with women, but the women he went out with always fell short of his expectations. Similarly, in the therapeutic situation, his therapist (who happened to be a woman) always disappointed him in that she "never quite understood what I was driving at," sometimes had to change his appointment time, and occasionally had the temerity to go on a family vacation. Eventually the patient began to realize that what he really wanted in a relationship was the nurturance he believed his mother had provided. Further exploration, however, revealed that in fact his mother had been somewhat cold and ungiving. Thus, what he expected from other people (especially women) was the perfect "idealized" mother of his fantasy life. Anger at others for continually disappointing him and anger at himself for feeling so dependent colored all his relationships and eventually caused others to become angry at him and to leave, proving to him that they were in fact as undependable as his mother had been.

Because psychotherapy sessions are unstructured and the therapist remains a relatively neutral, nondisclosing figure, the psychotherapeutic situation encourages transference feelings to blossom. When these feelings become sufficiently intense, the therapist can help patients discover their distortions of the doctor-patient relationship and thereby to discover how they misperceive and misjudge other relationships in their lives. Such revelations can have major therapeutic impact because they are based on patients' actual experiences in the therapy sessions.

Countertransference

Countertransference is, in essence, the therapist's transference to the patient. Like transference, countertransference feelings are inappropriate to the therapy situation because they belong to a relationship in the therapist's past. For example, a male psychiatry resident may find in talking with an older female patient that he is reluctant to explore the sexual concerns for which the patient has come to him for help. At the root of the difficulty is that fact that the patient reminds him of his mother, and he reacts to her in subtle ways as if she *were* his mother. He is embarrassed and feels that it is forbidden for him to be curious about her sexual functioning. In this case, the resident must recognize his distortions (e.g., with the help of a supervisor) in order to be of assistance to his patient. Countertransference is, for the most part, unconscious. Thus, it is imperative that therapists-in-training have supervision so that they become well enough acquainted with their countertransference responses to be able to deliver effective treatment without imposing their own distortions onto therapeutic relationships.

Resistance

People come to therapy for help and usually express a desire to cooperate in the hope of getting better. Toward this end, they try to form an alliance with the therapist. Paradoxically, they also try to keep the therapist and themselves at a distance from the sources of their emotional pain. Indeed, people in emotional distress have often spent much time and psychic energy warding off pain, and many have achieved a tenuous, if unsatisfactory, emotional balance. The therapeutic relationship offers the prospect of psychological insight and change, and any change threatens to upset this hard-won emotional balance.

Even patients who suffer distressing symptoms will feel safer holding on to familiar ways of coping with the world than venturing into unknown territory. And they may have "good" reasons for not getting better: increased attention from others, decreased responsibility, a desire to make others feel guilty for their suffering, or a need to punish themselves. Thus, patients may be aware of wanting to get better, but largely unaware of their fears about change. They are also likely to be unaware of how they attempt to keep themselves and others away from their real feelings and concerns. This distancing process is known as *resistance*.

Resistance can assume innumerable forms, and examples are easy to find in daily clinical work. Patients may arrive late for appointments, leaving less time to do the work, or, once in the therapist's office, they may find that they have nothing to say. Others discover that they are suddenly well after one visit and need no more help ("flight into health"). Some deliberately withhold information, while others "forget" important data because of unconscious conflict over whether to disclose it. Any means of distracting attention from the task of therapy can be seen as resistance—for example, when the patient is seductive or amusing, when the patient tries to divert the discussion to talk about the therapist's private life, or when the patient rejects the therapist's efforts to engage in conversation. The use of psychiatric jargon is also a resistance when it is used to ward off genuine understanding.

Resistance may be so strong as to completely undermine the therapy, but such sabotage can often be avoided if the therapist addresses the problem, along with the feelings that prompt resistances. However, resistance is more than just an obstacle that needs to be overcome. Like everything else in therapy, resistance constitutes important data about how the patient's mind works. The ways in which patients keep their true feelings out of the interviews are likely to be the ways in which they avoid them in other areas of their lives. In therapy, people can learn to recognize these defensive maneuvers and understand how they get in the way of forming satisfying relationships.

To facilitate the clear emergence of transference distortions and resistances in the therapy hours, particular therapeutic techniques—free association and dream analysis—are especially helpful. They are used most often in psychoanalysis but also, to a lesser extent, in other types of dynamic therapy.

Free association is a process by which patients say whatever comes to mind as they talk with the therapist. They are instructed not to change the sequence of undirected thoughts, and not to withhold feelings or thoughts that seem irrelevant, illogical, or distressing. This sort of uncensored, uninhibited verbalization is most often the ideal rather than the reality, for true freedom to say whatever comes to mind is not easy to achieve. The flow of thoughts is repeatedly interrupted by the patient's various resistances to the work of therapy. Over time, patterns of resistance can be understood and clarified as they emerge to obstruct the free flow of material.

Dream analysis is another means of discovering unconscious material. Dreams differ from most mental content in that they lack some of the careful censorship the mind exerts over unconscious ideas during waking life. Thus, dreams often reveal underlying motives and yearnings more clearly than do consciously directed thoughts.

Psychoanalytic theory holds that dreams reveal our childhood wishes in symbolic form. Recent theories have emphasized the role of dreams in our efforts to solve problems from waking life as we sleep. Dreams also provide evidence of the patient's feelings for his or her therapist.

It should be noted that the interpretation of dreams and their usefulness for understanding hidden motivations or conflicts is a subject of debate. Indeed, there are some who view dreams as simply random neuronal discharges that have little relevance for understanding human behavior. Others suggest that, although dream content itself may be of limited value, the patient's associations to (i.e., thoughts about) the content reveal a great deal about what he or she finds emotionally significant.

The Process of Psychodynamic Change

Lifting repression

One of the fundamental assumptions of classical psychodynamic theory is that we handicap ourselves by banishing certain anxiety-arousing thoughts and feelings from our awareness and relegating them to the realm of the unconscious. This process of *repression* fosters the development of a great many psychological symptoms and irrational behaviors. A primary aim of psychodynamic treatment is to undo the repression that has taken place over many years, in order to give people access to material buried in the unconscious. When unconscious material is made conscious, decisions become more rational, and we cease to feel like the victims of feelings, thoughts, and behaviors that seem beyond our comprehension and control.

The lifting of repression in treatment occurs gradually. As it happens, patients remember matters that were previously inaccessible to them. Repressed wishes—often the unrealistic pleasure-seeking demands we had as small children—and repressed traumatic experiences can be examined by our adult minds. By bringing adult reason and logic to bear, patients can lessen some of the anxiety, distortions, and guilt connected with them. People can also abandon their ways of defending themselves against the recognition of these early childhood experiences, freeing up energy to deal with the adult world more creatively and more effectively.

Interpretation and working through

Life events (past and present), dreams, associations, and the patient's mode of relating to the therapist are all invaluable sources of data about how the patient's mind works. It is the therapist's job not only to elicit this information but to help the patient find meaning in it. The therapist perceives connections between various aspects of the patient's mental life and can offer tentative interpretations, the validity of which the therapist and patient can then test out together. Through interpretation, the patient gains some insight into the dynamic motivations that lead to persistent symptoms. Interpretation connects thoughts, feelings, and behaviors in the patient's current life with those in the unconscious, and it clarifies the defensive maneuvers the patient uses to keep from recognizing unconscious material.

Interpretations make the unthinkable thinkable. They are therefore bound to stir up anxiety and must be timed so that the patient is more or less receptive to them. This usually involves waiting until the patient has worked on a problem long enough that unconscious material is very close to awareness. Interpretation may also be necessary when the patient's level of frustration is so great that it becomes difficult to continue the work of therapy unless the source of the frustration is clarified.

Ideally, a single interpretation of the origin of a symptom or behavior would bring about change and cure. However, this is rarely the case. Intellectual understanding is not equivalent to emotional understanding and real integration of new knowledge. Any new awareness that comes from an interpretation must be relearned and tested in different situations and in association with other experiences—it must be integrated more fully into the patient's self-concept. This process, known as *working through*, involves amassing evidence from memories, current life situations, and the therapy relationship itself to confirm the truth of a new piece of information. It is one of the rate-limiting steps in psychotherapy and a major reason that insight-oriented psychodynamic therapy takes longer than many people think it should.

Corrective experiences

As originally formulated by Freud, the task of psychodynamic therapy was to make the unconscious conscious using interpretation. However, it is clear that much more is accomplished in dynamic psychotherapy than the integration of well-timed interpretive comments. One of the most important aspects of all psychotherapies involves providing patients with experiences they have not previously had (e.g., the experience of confiding a shameful secret to a nonjudgmental person). Experiential learning is an important element in psychodynamic therapy. As they come to feel that therapy is a safe place, patients can try out new ways of relating to the therapist and new "risky" behaviors (e.g., asking directly for what one wants) without fear that the therapist will criticize or abandon or retaliate against them.

Experiential learning is particularly important for people with the sorts of psychological deficits discussed above. While a conflict—for example, between unconscious hatred and conscious love for a parent—can be interpreted verbally, deficits such as poor impulse control and low anxiety tolerance are thought to be ameliorated by interpersonal experiences. How might this happen in psychotherapy? Therapists serve as role models with whom patients can identify, as is illustrated in the following case example:

> A young woman found it difficult to tolerate the anxiety that she felt when there was uncertainty in an important relationship. Whenever a boyfriend began to express doubts or criticism about her, she became so afraid of his

leaving her that she immediately broke off the romance. She made similarly impulsive moves from one job to another in response to minor criticism from bosses. The patient felt that her life was a "roller coaster" and despaired of ever settling down. Over time in psychotherapy, she found that her therapist dealt with anxiety and uncertainty differently. When the patient criticized the therapist for being too passive and not understanding the patient's problems, the therapist did not break off the relationship, but instead wanted to understand all she could about her patient's discontent. When the patient talked about moving to another city and terminating her psychotherapy, the therapist did not take any action or insist that the patient make up her mind, but instead explored with her all of the pros and cons of the proposed move. Gradually, the patient began to appreciate the stability in her relationship with the therapist and to identify with the therapist's ability to tolerate anxiety and to delay action. She began to have more stable relationships with friends and lovers and to work more steadily at one job.

The repair of deficits, and the development of new psychological capacities, can occur through experiential learning with any patient. But this kind of learning is thought to be most important for people who are more disturbed—for example, people with severe personality disorders. Whether and to what extent experiential learning is an essential factor in psychodynamic psychotherapy is a subject of debate among clinicians.

Varieties of Psychodynamic Psychotherapy

Psychodynamic principles can be used to help you make sense of any doctor-patient encounter, and they can be applied with greater or lesser "purity" in any type of psychotherapy. Treatment that is predominantly psychodynamic in orientation usually falls into one of three categories, as described below.

Psychoanalysis

Psychoanalysis was the original mode of treatment developed by Freud and his followers. It aims at a reorganization of character structure, with an emphasis on self-understanding and the correction of developmental lags. Symptom relief usually occurs as a result of this understanding but is not the immediate objective of the treatment. The patient lies on a couch, while the analyst is seated behind the patient and out of view. Free association, dream analysis, and the development and working through of transference distortions in the relationship with the analyst are the most salient features. Sessions are usually held four or five times a week, and a completed analysis generally takes 3 to 5 years, but length of treatment varies considerably with the nature of the problems being treated.

People in psychoanalysis must be able to tolerate a fair degree of frustration and ambiguity because of the lack of structure in the analytic situation. Analysis is therefore suitable for people at the healthier end of the spectrum of psychological disorders—people with neurotic conflicts and personality disorders of lesser severity. The usefulness of psychoanalysis in the treatment of severe personality disorders is questionable, and its use in treatment of schizophrenia and other psychotic illness is generally contraindicated. Psychoanalysis is practiced by clinicians who have undergone specialized training in this area after residency training. This treatment modality is less widely used than exploratory and supportive treatments.

Exploratory psychotherapy

Like psychoanalysis, exploratory psychotherapy aims at understanding motivations and unconscious forces that hamper daily living. However, exploratory psychotherapy focuses less on the analysis of infantile experiences and more on current life situations and dynamic patterns of dealing with others in the here and now. Analysis of transference remains a central feature, but transference reactions are often less intense than in analysis, where the therapist's relative inactivity allows such reactions to flower. The sort of temporary regression that is fostered in psychoanalysis is usually avoided in psychotherapy.

The patient does not lie on a couch but sits in a chair, promoting a more "real," face-to-face interaction with the therapist. Sessions are usually held one to three times a week (occasionally more frequently), depending on the patient's motivation and capacity to tolerate the intense feelings that are more likely to be stirred up when sessions are frequent. Treatment may last for several sessions, or several years, depending on the nature of the problem and the extent of the patient's motivation. Medication may be used in combination with exploratory therapy if the patient's symptoms warrant pharmacotherapy.

Exploratory psychotherapy is employed in the treatment of a wide range of psychiatric illnesses, including many psychotic conditions, depression, personality disorders, anxiety disorders, and neuroses. Patients must be motivated to understand their inner life and its manifestations in their dealings with the world. The major contraindication to exploratory psychotherapy is the inability to tolerate the exploration of feelings without having to act on them in destructive ways (e.g., suicidal behavior or violent acts toward others). The therapist must be alert to such adverse reactions in therapy, adjusting the frequency and intensity of sessions according to what the patient can tolerate.

Supportive psychotherapy

Although all forms of psychodynamic therapy involve some measure of support, supportive therapy is distinct from exploratory work and psychoanalysis because its goal is not the development of insight, but the lessening of anxiety. The therapist does this through reassurance, advice, modification of social factors where possible, and the bolstering of the patient's personal strengths and more adaptive defenses (see Chapter 2). The therapist is generally more active and more directive than in the other modalities.

One potential danger in doing supportive therapy is that it may foster a dependency relationship that is harmful and infantilizing rather than helpful. But some patients who have little interest in or capacity for achieving psychological insight can function much better in the world when "maintained" by a supportive relationship with a therapist. Supportive therapy generally occurs once a week or less, but at times it is carried out more frequently. Supportive treatment is indicated for those in need of temporary emotional support during a crisis, for those who are resistant to or too severely disturbed to respond to insight-oriented treatment, and for those who are not interested in changing their lives but simply in returning to a previous level of adjustment.

Short-term psychotherapy

While any psychotherapy may be long or short, psychodynamic therapy has traditionally been an open-ended enterprise. In recent years, a time-limited form of psychodynamic treatment was developed as an alternative to more prolonged and more costly treatments. The aim of short-term psychotherapy (also called time-limited therapy or "brief therapy") is to help the patient understand the roots of and achieve some resolution of a particular emotional problem that is a source of acute distress. The focus is on current life situations, and dependence and regression are discouraged. Brief therapy may focus on the patient's transference to the therapist or it may leave this area largely unaddressed.

The key element that distinguishes brief therapy from other psychodynamic therapies is that the number of sessions is agreed upon at the outset of treatment (from 8 to 20 or more). There is an emphasis on personal autonomy and independent functioning throughout the course of therapy. The therapist is active in maintaining the focus of the sessions on a central issue that is identified by therapist and patient at the beginning of treatment. This often keeps the patient's anxiety level relatively high throughout treatment. The sense of limited time also keeps the patient's motivation high.

Short-term therapy may be more desirable than prolonged work for people who are in an acute crisis that has an easily identified focal issue, and who are interested in crisis resolution rather than a thorough exploration of themselves with the potential for a deeper restructuring of character.

Common Misconceptions about Psychodynamic Therapy

Among the most frequently voiced erroneous ideas about psychodynamic treatment—particularly psychoanalysis—are the following three:

Myth: Treatment uncovers original childhood traumas that are the causes of symptoms in adult life. In fact, there are rarely single original traumatic events underlying psychological problems. People learn to behave as they do over many years by being treated in certain ways over and over again, and by repeating behaviors in similar situations. The goal of treatment is to examine the patient's current experiences in life and in the relationship with the therapist, and to demonstrate how old patterns of thinking, feeling, and behaving are still active in the patient's current relationship to the world. Memories of the past simply confirm the continuity between present and past attitudes. Human behavior cannot be reduced to simple causal explanations. So rather than playing detective and looking for the single childhood trauma that "caused" an adult symptom, the therapist looks for evidence of recurrent trauma and for ways in which the patient has repeatedly dealt with stressful experiences in maladaptive ways. We can almost never answer the question of why someone developed a symptom, any more than we can know why someone else with similar childhood experiences remains symptom-free and well-adjusted in adult life.

Myth: The psychodynamic therapist must be a "blank screen" and not a real person in the therapy. Psychodynamic therapy involves very different degrees of self-disclosure on the part of the therapist, depending on the needs of the patient. But all therapies rely to a considerable degree on the reactions of the therapist as a real person. The patient needs this aspect of the doctor-patient relationship to highlight the ways he or she distorts this (and other) relationships.

Myth: Psychodynamic therapy makes the patient unnecessarily dependent on the therapist. Doctor-patient encounters usually stir up our deepest longings to be cared for by an all-powerful parent. In an intensive psychodynamic therapy, a patient may come to feel at times as though he or she were a child and may behave in childlike ways toward the therapist. However, this is only a temporary phase of treatment that helps the patient see how new relationships become distorted by feelings from the past. In fact, psychodynamic therapy aims to give patients the skills to continue to understand their own mental life long after treatment has ended—that is, to become more autonomous rather than less so.

The Goals of Psychodynamic Treatment

People seek psychotherapy for a wide variety of problems. The specific therapeutic modalities and the intensity of their application are determined only after careful assessment of the patient's needs. Each of the dynamic therapies seeks to increase the person's sense of self-acceptance and well-being, while improving his or her ability to obtain satisfaction in work and at play.

Two general categories of beneficial effect can be discerned in people who have undergone psychodynamic psychotherapy. The uncovering of unconscious sources of conflict acts to free people from the burden of irrational fears and inhibitions carried over from early life experiences. Further, it enables them to handle the stresses and conflicts of everyday life more effectively. The second benefit is a gradual shift in the patient's view of self and others. The therapeutic relationship provides a unique opportunity for self-exposure and intimacy in a protected setting. At the same time, heightened awareness of the complexity and ambiguity of human interaction gradually replaces the "tunnel vision" and automatic behavior that often characterize people who seek this form of treatment. The result is a richer and deeper recognition of life's inherent difficulties and limitations, and the development of a more flexible repertoire of responses to these limitations.

BEHAVIOR THERAPY

Behavior modification, or behavior therapy, is an approach to the treatment of specific behavioral symptoms such as phobias, compulsions, anxiety, and speech disorders. Behavior therapy focuses on observable actions rather than inferred mental states, and it aims at eliminating maladaptive behaviors by means of techniques that are based largely on learning theory.

The phenomenon of *classical conditioning*, discovered by the Russian physiologist Ivan Pavlov (1849–1936), is one of the central principles of behaviorism. Pavlov discovered that a neutral stimulus, when repeatedly paired with a nonneutral stimulus (one that routinely elicits an emotional or physiological response), eventually loses its neutrality and can, by itself, bring about the same response. For example, a man who suffers a series of spontaneous panic attacks (see Chapter 8) while away from home may come to associate being out of the house with the feeling of panic. He may refuse to leave home thereafter, even though he had no negative feelings about being away from home prior to the onset of his panic attacks. In this case, he arrives at an end state of agoraphobia via classical conditioning.

A second fundamental paradigm of behaviorism is *operant conditioning*. This paradigm rests on the observation that much of our learning occurs via a gradual process of trial and error. When an individual is stimulated in a given situation and responds, if the response is followed by positive consequences, the response will tend to be repeated. If the response is followed by negative consequences, it will tend not to be repeated. So, for example, a child who throws tantrums at bedtime may find that when he does so, his mother allows him to stay up later. The tantrums are reinforced by mother's positive response, and the child is likely to throw tantrums every night to get what he wants. However, if mother consistently puts the child to bed despite these tantrums, the behavior will not be reinforced and will be likely to cease. Desired responses can be reinforced and undesirable ones extinguished by a variety of techniques, some of which are described below.

Behavior therapy begins with an analysis of the responses that cause the patient distress or diminish his or her satisfaction and productivity. This analysis outlines the types of situations and reinforcing factors that have elicited and maintained the problematic behavior (e.g., stuttering). The next step consists of developing a detailed schedule of exercises for eliminating these behaviors and replacing them with more desirable ones. Among the most important forms of behavior therapy currently in use are systematic desensitization, flooding, positive reinforcement, extinction, and aversive conditioning (Table 17-1).

Systematic Desensitization

Systematic desensitization is widely used in modern mental health care. It is based on the premise that people can master anxiety-provoking situations by approaching them gradually and in a relaxed state that inhibits anxiety. Patients are essentially "counterconditioned"—that is, conditioned anxiety responses to feared situations (e.g., flying) are blocked by the patient's self-induced state of relaxation. Patients are first taught the technique of progressive relaxation, which consists of tensing major muscle groups and then relaxing them in a fixed order (often

Table 17-1. Models of behavior therapy

Systematic densensitization
   Mastering anxiety-provoking situations by approaching them gradually and
      in a relaxed state that inhibits anxiety
Flooding
   Confronting the feared stimulus for prolonged periods until it is no longer
      frightening
Positive reinforcement
   Strengthening behavior and causing it to occur more frequently by
      rewarding it
Negative reinforcement
   Causing a behavior to occur more frequently by removing a noxious
      stimulus when the desired behavior occurs
Extinction
   Causing a behavior to diminish by not responding to it
Punishment
   Causing a behavior to occur less frequently by applying a noxious stimulus

beginning at the top of the head and working down). In the next step, the patient and therapist determine which situations produce anxiety and construct a hierarchy of feared situations.

For example, in the case of a man who is afraid to fly in an airplane, the hierarchy would involve 10 to 12 scenes that might include buying a ticket, walking to the gate, entering the plane, taking off, and landing. These scenes are ordered according to how much anxiety they produce. The patient then puts himself into a relaxed state, using progressive relaxation, and he is asked to vividly imagine the first scene while in his deeply relaxed state. He repeats the exercise for the first scene until he experiences only minimal anxiety, at which time he can move on to the next scene. The goal is to be able to imagine the most anxiety-provoking scene (e.g., the plane landing) while remaining calm. This inhibition of anxiety carries over into corresponding real-life situations. It is often helpful for the patient to practice entering actual feared situations between treatment sessions, once the fears have been overcome in therapy.

Systematic densensitization is commonly used with great efficacy in treating phobias. It is also helpful to some people with compulsive behaviors and sexual dysfunctions (e.g., secondary impotence). Densensitization is less useful for more diffuse anxiety that is not specific to particular situations.

Flooding

Flooding is another approach to treating situation-specific anxiety. In flooding, patients confront the feared object or situation (e.g., a spider) at full intensity for prolonged periods of time until it is no longer frightening. The confrontation may be done by having the patient imagine the frightening scene (a technique called *implosion*), but results are better when the exposure is to a real-life situation. This technique is less widely used than systematic desensitization, in part because it involves such a high degree of anxiety that many people do not tolerate it well.

Positive Reinforcement, Negative Reinforcement, Extinction, and Punishment

The basic premise of *positive reinforcement* is that behavior will be strengthened and will occur more frequently if it is rewarded—for example, with praise, increased attention from others, or the avoidance of pain. *Negative reinforcement* involves strengthening a desired behavior by withdrawing a negative stimulus when the behavior occurs. So, for example, the baby who stops crying when the mother picks him up is negatively reinforcing mother's behavior. The theory behind *extinction* holds that a specific behavior will diminish if it is not responded to at all. *Punishment* applies a noxious stimulus to an undesirable behavior in an effort to diminish its frequency.

You may see these principles put into use in constructing treatment programs for severely disturbed patients on hospital wards or in day-care facilities. You may, for example, work on an inpatient unit that has a *token economy*—a system in which patients earn tokens for adaptive, socially sanctioned behaviors and are fined for maladaptive ones. Patients may earn tokens for such activities as grooming themselves properly, cleaning rooms, or helping in group activities. They can then use the tokens to buy snacks, watch television, or take a trip off the hospital grounds to go to a movie. They are fined tokens for such behavior as disrupting meetings, becoming physically abusive, or remaining isolated and uncommunicative. Such a system can be individually tailored to each patient's needs, to help him or her acquire the skills and behaviors that will promote better functioning and more autonomy. Such systems have also been useful in other communities, for example, in treatment facilities for juvenile delinquents or the mentally retarded.

Aversive conditioning involves applying negative stimuli to well-established behaviors. A maladaptive behavior is coupled with a noxious stimulus, so that the person experiences a motivational conflict between the desired behavior and the unpleasant consequences that go with it. For example, aversive conditioning has been used to treat alcoholism, by giving ethanol along with an emetic that produces severe nausea and vomiting. Repeated administration of this treatment suppresses many people's desire to drink. Critics argue that this approach provides only a temporary solution to what is usually a chronic problem.

Aversive conditioning has also been used to treat people who want to change a homosexual orientation to a heterosexual one. Patients are shown erotic homosexual scenes on film, and concurrently receive either emetics that produce nausea and vomiting or mild electric shocks. The patients are then shown erotic heterosexual films, without concurrent noxious stimuli. This form of treatment has also been used for sexual perversions (see Chapter 13). Its use in changing the choice of sexual object from homosexual to heterosexual is quite controversial, and it has not been clearly demonstrated to be effective in achieving this goal.

In general, behavior therapy is very useful in treating relatively specific symptoms. It is less effective in addressing deeper and more global psychological problems, such as those encountered among people with neurotic conflicts or personality disorders. It is not the primary mode of treatment in any of the psychotic illnesses, but may be a useful adjunctive treatment.

Every clinician should know about behavioral treatments and ideally should be able to practice some simple techniques.

HYPNOSIS

Hypnosis is neither a form of sleep nor a form of therapy. Rather, it is a particular type of concentration that is attentive, receptive, and focused. It is accompanied by diminished awareness of peripheral stimuli. You have undoubtedly experienced hypnotic or trance-like states—for example, when you get so absorbed in a novel that you ignore what is going on around you and must reorient yourself to the environment when you stop reading.

In a treatment situation that employs hypnosis, the patient cooperates with the therapist to develop this form of intense concentration in a way that facilitates and accelerates the achievement of particular psychotherapeutic goals. Hypnosis is most often used for the relief of specific symptoms such as anxiety, insomnia, phobias, conversion reactions, and pain. It is also used to control habits—particularly smoking and overeating, among others.

Treatment involves teaching people self-hypnosis techniques so that they can put themselves into a trancelike state and then use hypnotic suggestions that "restructure" their thinking about the problem being treated. For example, people who want to quit smoking are taught to put themselves into a trancelike state every few hours and at any time they crave a cigarette. In this state, they run through several points that are designed to reorient their thinking—for example, "Smoking damages my body. I need to take care of myself. I will not harm myself in this way." Similar suggestions for use under self-hypnosis can be designed by therapists and patients to ease anxiety, curb overeating, help overcome phobias, and lessen the psychological components of chronic pain.

Hypnosis has significant limitations as a therapeutic technique. It cannot, for example, treat more global difficulties, such as neurotic conflicts, psychotic illnesses, or personality disorders. Its usefulness even for the isolated symptoms mentioned above is questioned by some clinicians, who argue that symptom relief resulting from hypnotherapy is only temporary in many cases. Nevertheless, hypnosis continues to be a valuable tool in modern clinical practice when applied judiciously.

COGNITIVE THERAPY

Cognitive therapy is a relatively new mode of short-term psychotherapy. Specifically developed for the treatment of depression and anxiety, it is now more widely applied to a wide range of mental disorders. It is based on the premise that our moods and feelings are influenced by our thoughts and that psychological disturbances are frequently caused by habitual errors in thinking. By correcting these distorted ways of thinking, the cognitive therapist restructures patients' views of themselves, the world, and the future—substituting more realistic thoughts that reduce such painful feelings as anxiety, guilt, and hopelessness, and improve patients' abilities to function in the world. Behavior modification is combined with verbal therapy to help patients test the reality of distorted cognitions. In fact, this form of therapy is commonly called *cognitive-behavior therapy*, reflecting the use of behavioral techniques as a common element of treatment.

Cognitive therapy is based on the idea that the way people cognitively structure a situation influences how they feel and behave. When people are stressed, they tend to lose some of their normal cognitive abilities and develop selective and egocentric conceptualizations of their situation. They typically distort some aspects of the situation and ignore others. These conceptualizations commonly have to do with themes of danger, loss, or self-enhancement. Stressors are different for different people. So, for example, one person might tend to significantly distort conversations with people in authority ("My boss thinks I'm worthless"), while another might be stressed by dating ("Women can see I'm anxious and inadequate"). These kinds of stressful, distorted interactions "snowball" and become mutually reinforcing. For example, Mr. A. fears that women will find him anxious and inadequate, and he is so worried about himself that he approaches each date with great trepidation. Because he is so anxious, he finds himself tongue-tied with women even though he is normally a good conversationalist. He has thus created a self-fulfilling prophecy. Mr. A.'s dates do indeed find him stiff and anxious, and their lack of enthusiasm reinforces his worst fears about himself. Dating then becomes even more highly charged with anxiety.

Cognitive therapists help to guide the patient in discovering distorted ways of thinking that lead to uncomfortable feelings and maladaptive behavior. In addition, the cognitive therapist plays an active role in proposing and rehearsing with the patient specific cognitive and behavioral techniques that will promote corrective experiences outside therapy. In this respect, the cognitive therapist is more active in making suggestions, giving advice, and structuring sessions than is the psychodynamic therapist. Like psychodynamic therapy, cognitive therapy pays attention to patients' negative reactions to the therapist and resistances to progress in treatment. The cognitive therapist uses these negative reactions to demonstrate that the same dysfunctional beliefs cause patients to distort the therapy relationship as they do other relationships in their lives.

Because cognitive therapy is usually time-limited (often 10 to 15 weekly sessions), both therapist and patient feel pressure to use the time efficiently. Patients are asked to carry out homework assignments that help them identify cognitive distortions and master the cognitive and behavioral skills that they learn during sessions.

Certain cognitive distortions are typical among people who are depressed, anxious, and who suffer from low self-esteem. Among the most common are the following:

Arbitrary inference. This distortion involves drawing conclusions without supporting evidence. Mr A., who fears dating, may infer that any woman he is attracted to would never want to go out with him.

Selective abstraction. This distortion refers to taking one detail out of context and basing one's whole assessment of a situation on it, while ignoring other more salient details. For example, Mr. A. noticed that an attractive woman did not say hello to him at work one morning, and decided that she was repelled by him. He ignored the fact that she was rushing to catch the elevator, and that the day before she had gone out of her way to sit with him in the employee cafeteria.

Overgeneralization. Overgeneralization involves drawing a general conclusion across all situations based on a single incident. Mr. A. found that one woman in college did find him too anxious and at the end of their first date said she did not want to see him again. On the basis of this incident, he concluded that all women would react to him in this way.

Magnification. This distortion refers to blowing things out of proportion. In Mr. A.'s case, he assumed that having sweaty palms when he shook hands with a woman was an obvious sign of his anxiety that would disgust her.

Minimization. Minimization involves shrinking relevant details to relative unimportance. Mr. A. dismissed his colleague's sitting with him in the cafeteria as insignificant.

Personalization. This distortion occurs when one relates external events to oneself without any basis for the connection. (This is a nonpsychotic, milder form of ideas of reference, described in Chapter 4.) For example, Mr. A. assumed that when a woman friend did not return his phone call within the hour, it was because she did not want to talk to him. He neglected to consider the many other possible explanations for her behavior.

Dichotomous thinking. This type of thinking refers to categorizing events and situations in black-and-white, all-or-nothing terms. This is the basis for perfectionism, for example, "I am worthless if I cannot do things perfectly."

The so-called "silent assumptions" that people make on the basis of the cognitive distortions described above are usually outside of the person's awareness. An initial goal of cognitive therapy is to help the patient become aware of these assumptions. In this respect, it is akin to the psychodynamic goal of making the unconscious conscious.

Patients in cognitive therapy are asked to identify and write down negative thoughts—at first with the help of the therapist, and subsequently on their own. The therapist can then help the patient identify the distortions in these thoughts and substitute more rational responses. The therapist also helps the patient recognize self-defeating silent assumptions and exchange them for more realistic ones.

Patients in cognitive therapy are encouraged to test out their assumptions in real-life situations. Mr. A. might be assigned the task of making casual conversation with a woman in his office one week, then asking her on a date. He would be encouraged to monitor his thoughts and feelings as he carried out these homework assignments, and they would be the focus of discussion in subsequent therapy sessions. The therapist might use relaxation training to help Mr. A. block anxiety when he is out on dates. In a more relaxed state, Mr. A. would be better able to perceive stressful situations more accurately, and he would probably both have more fun and *be* more fun as a result. This would ideally start a positive cycle that might replace the negative one in which he was stuck when therapy began.

Cognitive therapy has been used increasingly in recent years with considerable success. Critics of this approach have argued that negative thoughts do not cause painful feelings, but result from them, and that changing one's thinking is not sufficient to bring about a lasting change of mood. However, in outcome studies, cognitive therapy has compared favorably with antidepressant treatment for depression. Its short-term structure makes it particularly useful in busy mental health centers where resources are limited and more open-ended psychotherapies are less available. Further research is needed to determine the relative efficacy of cognitive therapy in the treatment of different mental disorders.

MODALITIES OF PSYCHOTHERAPY

All of the treatment strategies described above, and the many more not covered in this chapter, can be applied in different settings with different combinations of therapists and patients over different time courses. The most frequently used modalities are individual psychotherapy, group therapy, couples therapy, and family therapy (Table 17-2). With respect to time frame, some therapies are open-ended, whereas others involve making contracts for a specified number of sessions from the outset of treatment.

What follow are brief descriptions of group, couples, and family therapies—each of which differs in important ways from the model of one therapist treating one patient.

Group Psychotherapy

Group psychotherapy is a powerful treatment modality. Both because of its therapeutic effects and because it is less costly than individual therapy, group therapy has been widely employed in many mental health care settings.

Groups vary greatly in structure and in the way meetings are run.

Table 17-2. Modalities of psychotherapy

Individual therapy	Couples therapy
Group therapy	Family therapy

Group membership may range from 2 or 3 to more than 15, but most groups have 6 to 10 members. Groups of this size are large enough for a sense of group identity to develop and for clear patterns of group interaction to emerge, but not large enough to lose sight of each individual's issues and needs. There is usually one leader, but co-leaders are not uncommon. Groups generally meet once a week for 1 to 2 hours, but sessions may vary in length and frequency.

The goals of group therapy vary as do those of individual therapy. Self-understanding and self-acceptance may be the goals of a psychodynamic group, while social skills training might be the focus of an inpatient group, and control of binge eating the focus of a cognitive-behavior therapy group for bulimic individuals. The tools used in group therapy include the entire range of therapeutic techniques discussed in this chapter, from transference interpretation to cognitive restructuring to relaxation training.

Group therapy has some distinct advantages over individual work. The very fact that several people with emotional difficulties come together with therapists in one room to discuss their lives opens up the possibility for a wider range of interactions than can take place between one patient and one therapist. Patients can provide each other with mutual validation of experiences, so that individuals feel less isolated by what they think are unique and unacceptable emotional difficulties. They also give one another advice, which may be helpful in its content and in its demonstration of concern and caring. People who have felt like burdens to family and friends are able to experience being helpful to other group members as they offer support, insight, and reassurance in group meetings.

Groups are effective in recapitulating family situations. Patients interact with group leaders and other group members as they once interacted with parents and siblings. In groups with a psychodynamic orientation, therapists interpret patients' transference reactions so that patients can see the ways in which they distort relationships in the group based on past experience.

Group members can also learn such skills from one another as how to resolve conflicts, how to be more responsive to others, and how to be less judgmental of others' behaviors. As members come to be more comfortable with one another, they can take risks and try out new behaviors that are too threatening to test out elsewhere (e.g., a patient may begin to experiment with increased assertiveness). The group becomes a microcosm of larger social groups, and patients can relate their behavior in therapy to how they operate in group situations outside therapy (e.g., at work).

Group therapy has been used for virtually all types of mental illness.

It is particularly useful for people with personality disorders, whose character problems are obvious to others but not to themselves. Such people can often tolerate being confronted by their peers with evidence of their maladaptive behaviors better than they can tolerate confrontation by an authority figure like the group leader. Sociopathic, drug-addicted, and alcoholic individuals are among those who have benefited from such treatment. Group treatment is also used for people who are psychotic (e.g., schizophrenic patients). Group meetings with psychotic people are usually fairly structured and actively guided by the therapist, often focusing on specific tasks such as the improvement of social skills.

Group therapy may be used alone or in conjunction with other forms of treatment (e.g., medication). People may be in group therapy for months or years, depending on their motivation and the type of treatment used. Groups may contain members with many different types of problems, or may be limited to people with one particular illness (e.g., alcoholism, obsessive-compulsive disorder). Groups may also be organized around a particular life experience that is not in itself an illness—as in groups for adult children of alcoholic individuals and victims of sexual abuse. Groups are used for both outpatient therapy and inpatient work, and they are useful in such diverse settings as prisons and college health services.

Couples Therapy

Couples therapy deals with a partnership between two people and the problems that arise within this relationship. Sometimes called "marital therapy," it is useful not only for married couples but also for heterosexual and homosexual couples who are living together or committed to each other in some fashion other than marriage.

Psychodynamic couples therapy focuses on the intrapsychic conflicts and dynamics of each member of the dyad, but only insofar as these issues affect the relationship. Therapy is aimed at facilitating communication within the couple, clarifying individual goals, and resolving conflicts. Psychodynamically oriented therapy looks at each member's distortions of the relationship based on earlier life experiences with parents, siblings, and other important people. Such therapy is not necessarily aimed at keeping the couple together, but at helping the couple to understand how the relationship works and does not work, and whether problems can be resolved.

Couples therapy with a cognitive or behavioral orientation is often used to solve specific problems such as discrepancies between verbal and nonverbal communication, and problems in sexual functioning (see Chapter 13). In fact, the Masters and Johnson behavioral techniques for sex therapy are now the standard treatments for couples with sexual dysfunction.

Sessions are usually held weekly, but may be more or less frequent. Couples therapy may be done in combination with individual therapy (for one or both partners) or may be used as the only treatment modality. Although treatment by a single therapist is common, couples treatment is also effectively carried out by two therapists of different sexes, since this may enable each member of the couple to feel that he or she has a same-sex "ally" to identify with in therapy. Sessions are usually carried out with both partners present, but there may be individual sessions at the outset and at various times during the course of therapy as issues arise that need one-on-one attention.

Contraindications to couples treatment are few, but include acute psychosis in one or both partners, obvious psychopathology in one or both partners that requires individual therapy before couples work can proceed, and the harboring of an "unexposable" secret by one partner.

Family Treatment

Family relationships have always been of intense interest to psychotherapists, but the actual direct treatment of entire family units is a relatively new development in mental health care.

Dynamically oriented family therapy explores how family members interact during sessions with one or more therapists. The therapists observe patterns in styles of communication among family members, family patterns of becoming organized or disorganized in response to specific challenges, and alliances adopted by various members. Families generally do not notice these patterns because they are caught up in perpetuating them in order to maintain some equilibrium within the family unit. Family therapists not only observe behaviors that create disharmony and dysfunction in the family but also ask the family to step back and look at themselves as they have been unable to do in the past. Family therapy provides a setting in which the members often become more aware of how other members feel. As family members come to understand more about the consequences of their pathological behavior patterns, they have the possibility of changing behaviors and exploring more satisfying ways of dealing with one another.

Structural family therapy is a treatment approach based on systems theory. This approach assumes that the family system itself is more influential than the individual personality traits of its members. It assumes that the way the family is structured is an important determinant of how individuals within the family behave. So the therapist observes the family and develops a "structural family map" that characterizes the different roles that members play and the way they interact. The therapist looks at such variables as who in the family has power, who gets blamed for various problems, and whether boundaries between parents and children are rigid or flexible. The therapist then works with the family to alter aspects of the family structure that may be contributing to problems.

Like group therapy, family therapy generally requires more activity by the therapist than does individual therapy. It may also require directive techniques aimed at realigning alliances, proposing alternative means of managing problems, and insisting upon the rights or needs of particular family members to be heard. Behavioral techniques have been used with some success to help family members decrease hostility and improve communication in their dealings with one another.

Family therapy is often carried out in conjunction with couples therapy and/or individual therapy for one or more family members. Sessions are generally held weekly. As in couples work, many family therapists work in pairs, both to model interactions between the therapists and to check with one another on their perceptions of the family's style of behaving.

FUTURE DIRECTIONS: INTEGRATING THE PSYCHOTHERAPIES

There are over 400 different "schools" of psychotherapy, each claiming a distinct theoretical base and a distinct set of treatment techniques. Psychodynamic therapies and cognitive-behavior therapies represent the most widely used and best articulated of these systems.

In the past decade, there has been a growing movement of psychotherapists who propose to break down the barriers that have traditionally separated these different schools of therapy, and to define what they have in common and what is therapeutically effective in each of them. Many therapists use a mixture of techniques in their work. One of the best examples is the new sex therapy (see Chapter 13), which combines behavioral techniques with psychodynamic couples therapy to treat sexual dysfunction.

No single theory of therapy has proved adequate to treat all types of mental illness. In addition, psychotherapy outcome studies have failed to show that any one approach is clearly superior to others in terms of the quality of results it can achieve. Studies suggest that the particular characteristics of patients and therapists are more important than therapeutic technique in determining the outcome of psychotherapy.

Given these realities, many psychotherapists are searching for "active ingredients" that promote healing in many different types of therapy. They hope to develop a common language to describe the techniques and goals of psychotherapy. And they hope to be able to tailor therapy more explicitly to the needs of the individual patient.

BIBLIOGRAPHY

Beck AT: Cognitive Therapy and the Emotional Disorders. New York, International Universities Press, 1976

Beck AT, Rush AJ, Shaw B, et al: Cognitive Therapy of Depression. New York, Guilford Press, 1979

Beitman BD, Goldfried MR, Norcross JC: The movement toward integrating the psychotherapies: an overview. Am J Psychiatry 146:138–147, 1989

Frank JD: General psychotherapy: the restoration of morale, in American Handbook of Psychiatry, Vol 5. Edited by Arieti S. New York, Basic Books, 1974, pp 117–132

Frankel FH: Hypnosis: Trance as a Coping Mechanism. New York, Plenum, 1976

Fromm-Reichman F: Principles of Intensive Psychotherapy. Chicago, IL, University of Chicago Press, 1950

Greenson RR: The Technique and Practice of Psychoanalysis, Vol 1. New York, International Universities Press, 1967

Gustafson JP: The Complex Secret of Brief Psychotherapy. New York, WW Norton, 1986

Marks IM: Review of behavioral psychotherapy, I: obsessive-compulsive disorders. Am J Psychiatry 138:584–592, 1981

Marks IM: Review of behavioral psychotherapy, II: sexual disorders. Am J Psychiatry 138:750–756, 1981

Minuchin SA: Families and Family Therapy. Cambridge, MA, Harvard University Press, 1976

Roth S: Psychotherapy: The Art of Wooing Nature. Northvale, NJ, Jason Aronson, 1987

Strachey J: The nature of the therapeutic action of psychoanalysis. Int J Psychoanalysis 15:127–159, 1934

Yalom ID: The Theory and Practice of Group Psychotherapy, 3rd Edition. New York, Basic Books, 1985

18

Somatic Therapies

THE SOMATIC THERAPIES used in modern psychiatry consist of psychotropic medications and electroconvulsive therapy (ECT). This chapter covers general principles of the pharmacological treatment of mental disorders and the use of specific classes of psychotropic drugs. ECT is discussed briefly at the end of the chapter.

PSYCHOTROPIC MEDICATIONS

Psychotropic medications are chemical agents that have an effect on the mind. Many mind-altering substances are abused in our society for "recreational" purposes. Several types of psychotropic agents are useful in the treatment of mental disorders.

Why Are Psychotropic Medications Used in Psychiatry?

The question is not an idle one. The media and popular literature have, at times, painted a rather gloomy picture of mental institutions in which patients are kept "spaced out" on large doses of drugs. The mention of major tranquilizers conjures up images of mind control and the repression of individual freedom.

Yet, the advent of modern psychopharmacology in the last four decades has revolutionized the treatment of mental illness, giving millions of people relief from symptoms that are both frightening and crippling. Prior to the 1950s, there were few methods available for treating severely disturbed people. Seclusion behind locked doors and barred windows and the use of physical restraints were more common and more necessary than they are today. Treatment included "hydrotherapy," insulin shock, neurosurgery, and sedation with narcotics, barbiturates, and bromides. These treatments have virtually disappeared from psychiatry, and for good reason. Mania, florid hallucinations, severe agitation, and life-threatening depression have all proved responsive to modern psychopharmacological agents. Fewer people require long-term treatment behind locked doors, and it has been possible to return many chronically mentally ill persons and many treatment facilities to the community.

The number of patients hospitalized in psychiatric facilities has been drastically reduced over the last 20 years. To be sure, this is due in part to society's increased awareness of the detrimental effects of chronic institutionalization on human behavior, as well as to economic and political considerations. Also, new applications of group therapy techniques in day-care programs and outpatient clinics have proved effective in helping people live outside a structured inpatient setting. But much of the credit for this shift from inpatient to outpatient treatment must go to the use of psychotropic medications. They have not only proved effective in relieving acute psychotic symptoms but have also been useful in preventing recurrences and stabilizing functioning over long periods of time.

We must temper this praise, however, with some perspective on the limitations of the psychotropic medications. In fact, these medications only alleviate symptoms—*they do not cure.* Also, many people do not respond to these medications, even when classic symptoms would predict a good response. The medications carry side effects and toxicity that range in severity from uncomfortable to lethal. Finally, they are generally slow to work in at least one crucial respect: the antipsychotic effect of the neuroleptic agents may take days or weeks to become optimal, and the antidepressant effects of the tricyclics often appear more than a week after the medication is begun.

What Do Psychotropic Medications Do?

It is useful to think of these medications as falling into discrete groups (see Table 18-1), with each group of psychotropics alleviating a particular set of symptoms.

The major groups of psychotropics—antipsychotic agents, antide-

Table 18-1. The types of psychotropic medications

The major groups—act against specific symptoms
    Antipsychotic agents
    Antidepressants
    Antimanic agents
    Anticonvulsants
Other classes—produce particular effects without regard to presence or
   absence of illness
    Antianxiety agents
    Psychomotor stimulants
    Sedative-hypnotics

---

pressants, antimanic agents, and anticonvulsants–have actions that are directed against specific symptoms of mental illness. Unlike "uppers" or "downers," these medications do not work through simple arousal or sedation, but through more specific effects. Normal subjects do not experience euphoria when they take antidepressants or depression when they take antimanic medications, and they do not find their thought processes altered by the antipsychotics. If anything, the major psychotropic medications produce little more than sedation or other side effects in normal subjects, but they produce specific therapeutic effects in those who are ill.

The other classes of psychotropic medications are less specific in their actions. Antianxiety agents, psychomotor stimulants, and sedative-hypnotics produce similar effects in most people who use them, whether a mental illness is present or not. These medications are of little value in treating psychosis and mood disorders. It is because of their nonspecific effects that these classes of psychotropic medications are much more commonly abused than the major psychotropics.

A word about terminology is in order. The term *tranquilizer* is frequently used incorrectly to describe any sedating medication. There are two very different types of medications to which the term is correctly applied. *Major tranquilizers* are also called antipsychotic agents; their effects are both antipsychotic and sedating. This group includes such medications as chlorpromazine (Thorazine), trifluoperazine (Stelazine), and haloperidol (Haldol). *Minor tranquilizers* are the antianxiety agents, such as diazepam (Valium) and chlordiazepoxide (Librium). Other sedating medications (e.g., the barbiturates) are more commonly labeled *sedative-hypnotics*.

Included in Appendix E is a table listing commonly used psychotropic medications by trade names, with their corresponding generic names and medication type. When you hear a medication referred to by its brand name, you can use this table to quickly find its chemical name and major use in clinical practice.

Principles of Prescribing Psychotropic Medications

For every patient you see, you must make a judgment as to whether pharmacotherapy is both warranted and prudent. This requires facts.

Clinical evaluation

First, your clinical evaluation must be thorough. You must arrive at a tentative diagnosis based on the following factors.

History. You should enlist the help of family members in getting a history if the patient's reliability is questionable. In particular, a delineation of symptoms, previous treatments and responses, history of drug or alcohol abuse, family psychiatric history, medical history, and current medications are important.

Physical examination. You, or another clinician, must assess the patient's physical health and rule out underlying medical disorders that might mimic psychiatric illness. For outpatients, a routine examination done by the family physician in the previous 6 months will suffice if no medical problems are suspected.

Laboratory tests. These tests should include routine studies to rule out organic causes of psychiatric symptoms (e.g., hypothyroidism as the basis for depression). The routine laboratory workup for each type of medication is discussed below.

Period of observation. When there is no acute problem (such as severe agitation or life-threatening behavior) that requires immediate use of medication, it is helpful to observe the patient in a drug-free state for several days to see how symptoms appear over time. This is particularly useful if there is some question about whether medication is likely to be helpful, or when there is confusion about the diagnosis. You can then make an assessment, including differential diagnosis and treatment recommendations, with the understanding that you may need to change course as you learn more about the patient's illness and as you have more data about how the patient responds to your initial interventions.

Course of the illness

You must know the expected course of the illness you have diagnosed. Some psychiatric conditions are self-limiting (e.g., drug-induced psychosis). When it is safe to do so, it is preferable to treat such cases with medical support and without psychotropic medication until the illness runs its course. However, a major depressive episode is not likely to remit quickly without pharmacological intervention, and support alone would be insufficient treatment.

Risks of treatment

You must weigh the risks of not treating your patient against the risks of the various forms of therapy available. Tricyclic antidepressants, for example, are potentially lethal when taken in acute overdose; with suicidal people, this possible hazard must be weighed against the patient's need for relief from a life-threatening illness. Major tranquilizers produce potentially long-lasting *tardive dyskinesia* (discussed below) in a minority of people. Pharmacotherapy should never be undertaken lightly.

Choosing a medication

Once you decide to prescribe psychotropic medication, you must determine which class of medication to use. This will depend on the diagnosis and the patient's symptoms. But once you have decided to use an antidepressant, an antipsychotic, or an anxiolytic, there is a wide assortment of specific medications from which to choose. Within the groups of medications mentioned above, individual agents differ little in their ability to affect particular constellations of symptoms. Thus, the choice of which particular antipsychotic or anxiolytic to use will often be based on factors other than the symptoms you are trying to alleviate. These might include the following:

Previous treatment response. The patient's previous treatment response can be a useful indicator of what to try and what not to try. If something worked once, it is likely to work again. The converse may also be true. Thus, if a patient tells you that haloperidol was of no help in relieving his psychotic symptoms 10 years ago, it would be wise to avoid it now. If, however, he tells you that loxapine was the only medication that took away his auditory hallucinations, and he suffers from the same symptom at present, loxapine is likely to be your best bet. This is, perhaps, stating the obvious. Yet, too often we forget that we are frequently dealing with chronic conditions, that many patients have considerable prior experience with medication, and that they often know what has worked for them in the past. *Do not forget to ask.*

Medication histories of biological relatives. These can be valuable in helping with this decision. Treatment response and side effects may be determined, at least in part, by genetic factors. So, for example, if a depressed patient reports that her father was depressed and got better on imipramine, then imipramine would be a good first medication to use with her.

History of side effects. The patient's history of side effects is equally important. No one is likely to take a medication that produces unbearable side effects. When you are dealing with someone who has been given a variety of antipsychotics in the past, find out which of those medications were least unpleasant for the patient to take.

Your familiarity with particular medications. Familiarity with a particular medication is very important, including detailed knowledge of a medication's effects, side effects, and toxicity. When using a medication with which you are unfamiliar, it is important to get consultation from a more experienced colleague and to read the relevant literature in order to expand your therapeutic capabilities responsibly.

Cost. Cost of the medication may be a factor, particularly if long-term treatment is required. Medication prices vary greatly according to the availability of generic forms and the extent of competition in the market. As a rule, newer medications are more expensive.

Determining medication dosages

Unlike many other medications used in medical practice, there are no precise dosages prescribed for most of the psychotropic medications. Rather, there is a dosage range within which the physician must determine the amount that best meets the patient's needs. And dosage requirements are highly individual. One person may require two, three, or even four times the amount of medication needed by another person of similar body weight in order to achieve similar therapeutic effects. Prescribing thus involves a process of fine tuning the therapy according to the symptoms and responses of the individual.

There is a high correlation between the severity of the target symptoms at which treatment is aimed and the minimum dose that produces a favorable response. Severe symptoms will generally require higher doses of medicine, while mild symptoms may respond to dosages at the lower end of the therapeutic range. The most important considerations in determining medication dosages are *safety* and *therapeutic efficacy*.

Several of the antidepressants have a therapeutic window—range of blood levels within which a therapeutic response is to be expected. Levels that are outside the therapeutic window (i.e., too high or too low) are likely to be less than optimally effective or even to have adverse effects on the patient. New research is showing that the antipsychotics also have such windows, although neuroleptic plasma levels are less widely used in clinical practice at the time of this writing.

Administering psychotropic medications

The two major routes of administration are oral and intramuscular. Intravenous administration of psychotropics is sometimes used, particularly in well-controlled inpatient settings.

Doses administered by injection are roughly two to four times as potent as the same doses taken by mouth. This is largely because the liver, which does the bulk of the body's work in metabolizing psychotropics, is bypassed by intravenous injection on the first pass through the circulation, so that more unmetabolized medication reaches the central nervous system.

Although the minor tranquilizers and some other sedating medications are at times given by injection, the medications most often given intramuscularly are the antipsychotics. Injection is used for the following reasons:

- To produce rapid relief of severe agitation and other symptoms that might pose a danger to the patient or to others
- If the patient is unable or unwilling to take medication orally
- When oral absorption of the medication is thought to be poor (a relatively rare indication)

The disadvantages of giving these medicines intramuscularly are the following:

- Some of them are painful (e.g., chlorpromazine) and may cause irritation at the site of injection.
- Intramuscular injection may be seen by some severely disturbed people as an assault, and it may disrupt an already tenuous therapeutic alliance.

In addition to controlling severe agitation on inpatient units, the most common situations in which intramuscular administration of medication is used are 1) in emergency rooms, where people present in crisis and need rapid relief, and 2) in outpatient programs when people who cannot comply with daily oral regimens are given *depot* forms of antipsychotic medication by injection every 2 to 4 weeks. (A depot medication is in a chemical form that is absorbed very slowly into the bloodstream from the muscle into which it has been injected. Because this occurs over days, or weeks, it eliminates the need for frequent doses of medication.)

Advising your patients about medication

As with any form of treatment, the way in which you present the treatment plan to your patient can make a great difference in the amount of cooperation you receive. Not only is compliance important, but, in most cases, the patient must tell you whether or not the treatment is working. There are no laboratory measures of medication response with the psychotropics, so you and your patient must agree on specific target symptoms that you are trying to alleviate, and then together you must evaluate whether, in fact, those symptoms have been affected by the medication.

When the patient is confused, unreliable, or otherwise unable to comply with the regimen on his or her own, a responsible friend or relative should be included in the discussion of how the medicine is to be taken. Assure the patient that you are available to talk about the medication when questions arise.

Especially at the beginning of medication treatment, it is important that you and/or other staff members be available by telephone or in person so that the patient is not left alone with distressing side effects or other unexpected adverse reactions. In explaining the treatment plan to the patient, be sure that the following information is included:

What you are trying to treat (target symptoms). People will expect medication to help all their psychiatric symptoms, and this is almost never the case. Your patient must know which specific symptoms the medication treatment is aimed at and which symptoms the medication cannot be expected to alleviate.

For example, if an antidepressant is prescribed for a recently widowed woman with severe melancholic depression, she should be told that the medication could help her sleep better and perhaps increase her appetite, but that she will continue to feel sad about her husband's death and may mourn his loss for some time to come. If a patient is receiving another form of treatment (e.g., psychotherapy) in addition to medication, be sure the patient knows what each treatment is meant to accomplish. Too often, people assume that medications are panaceas, that the problem is all "chemical," and that there is no need to cooperate in other forms of therapy. Such assumptions set the stage for disillusionment when the medication fails to cure everything that ails the person. (The same is true for the converse assumption that one's problems are entirely "psychological.")

Side effects that might occur. You want your patients to have some idea of what to expect when they take medication, but they could be frightened by a long list of serious but remote possibilities. Here, judgment is critical. It is generally useful to describe common side effects and to explain how the patient can handle them if they occur. When dry mouth is a potential side effect, you might note this and explain that chewing gum or hard candy can help keep the mouth moist. If drowsiness or dizziness is a common side effect, then the patient must be cautioned about driving a car. If the effects of alcohol are enhanced by the medication, then caution the patient about even social drinking. The patient must be alerted to the warning signs and symptoms of medication toxicity (e.g., symptoms of lithium toxicity, such as nausea, vomiting, diarrhea, and stupor).

Above all, let the patient know that you are available and that it is important to share questions or problems with you as they arise. If patients feel that they ought not to bother you with their concerns about medication, they may suffer distressing side effects (e.g., impotence) without reporting these, or they are likely to discontinue the medication without discussing their concerns with you first.

Managing side effects

Virtually all psychotropic medications have side effects, but we cannot predict which people will be particularly sensitive to which effects. The management of side effects is crucial to the successful pharmacotherapy of mental illness, because treatment is commonly necessary for months or years. Compliance depends upon the patient's willingness and ability to tolerate the medication. People often discontinue their medication without consulting a physician, most commonly because they believe that the medication is not helpful or that they no longer require it, because they cannot bear unpleasant side effects, or because they believe their discomfort is due to side effects when it is in fact due to the symptoms of their illness.

Side effects can be difficult to recognize. Psychotic individuals may report bizarre symptoms that are actually manifestations of their illness, or they may be uncommunicative and incapable of reporting side effects at all. In dealing with people who are in emotional distress and who have impaired cognition, the therapeutic alliance is particularly important. The following are some effective ways that you can work to minimize or eliminate side effects:

1. Monitor the patient's mental and physical status regularly, including frequent meetings with the patient. When the patient

cannot reliably report on his or her condition, include a family member or close friend.

2. Pay attention to all the patient's complaints, even when they seem trivial.

3. Work as a team with other people involved in the patient's care—nurses, mental health workers, social workers, psychologists, and physicians. Professionals who see the patient in other settings may be able to give you much needed information about your patient's reactions to medication.

4. The patient should be taking the lowest dosage that produces the desired effect. Many side effects are related to dosage.

5. Advise and reassure the patient. Many patients are capable of tolerating a significant amount of discomfort and inconvenience, provided they know that it is in their interest to do so and that you are concerned and supportive.

6. Use of adjunctive medication. Particularly in the case of antipsychotics, side effects can be effectively relieved by antiparkinsonian medications (discussed below).

7. Discontinue the medication and try another medication if side effects become intolerable.

8. Frequently reevaluate the patient's need for the medication. If medication regimens are not reevaluated, medication maintenance may be prolonged unnecessarily.

9. Avoid polypharmacy—the prescribing of several medications concurrently for a patient in the hope that something will work. Each medication should be carefully chosen and its effects frequently evaluated.

Combining psychotropic medications

As a rule, combining two or more medications of the same basic type (i.e., two antipsychotics or two antianxiety agents) is not desirable. Rather than enhancing the desired therapeutic effect, such combinations generally result in an increased risk of toxicity, increased side effects, and little or no therapeutic advantage.

However, combinations of *different* types of medications are often useful. Antipsychotics, anticonvulsants, antidepressants, lithium, and antianxiety agents are used frequently in combination. Ideally, medication combinations are prescribed as a result of—and not instead of—a careful diagnostic evaluation. When medications are added to a regimen with no rationale and no target symptoms in mind, the result is usually a muddled and sometimes dangerous treatment.

A cardinal rule in medical treatment: Whenever possible, do one thing at a time. Too often, the clinician tries unsuccessfully to make several changes in the treatment regimen at the same time. The results can be confusing. For example, if you lower the dose of a patient's antipsychotic medication and simultaneously increase the dose of an antidepressant, the patient may take a turn for the better or worse, but you will be unable to assess which change made the difference.

By making one change in a treatment regimen at a time, you will have a much better chance of understanding the effects of your interventions. This is true not only for medications but for other elements in a patient's treatment. For example, if you decide to lower the dosage of your patient's antipsychotic medication just as the patient is about to begin weekly psychotherapy, you may not know whether an increase in psychotic symptoms during the first weeks of therapy is due to the lowered dosage of the medication or to the stresses of forming a new relationship.

Failure of pharmacotherapy

The four most likely possibilities if medication treatment does not seem to work are as follows (in approximate order of frequency):

- You have not obtained your patient's cooperation in taking the medication reliably.
- You selected the correct medication, but the wrong dosage.
- You selected the wrong type of medication.
- You selected the correct medication and dosage, but the patient has not yet been taking the medication long enough to produce a therapeutic effect.

When pharmacotherapy appears to fail, do not give up. Consider the points noted above and try to determine whether any of these factors is responsible for the treatment failure. Also remember that individuals respond idiosyncratically to psychotropic medications: a patient who does not benefit from one medication may respond to a different medication in the same class.

Gather all the information you can from the patient, from family members, and from other members of the treatment team, and then determine what changes you can make—one at a time and systematically—to try to achieve the therapeutic effect you seek. If it is feasible, get a consultation.

The treatment team

Often you will be treating patients in collaboration with others. While you prescribe medication, other professionals may be involved with the patient in psychotherapy, behavior therapy, group therapy, rehabilitation, and a host of other treatment modalities. You must talk with other members of the treatment team and enlist their cooperation in the psychopharmacological intervention, preferably *before* any new medication is prescribed.

There are several reasons for this emphasis on communication within the treatment team. First, it makes for good patient care. Those who do not prescribe medication must nevertheless know what to expect when such a treatment is introduced. They must know what side effects to watch for, and they must know the goals of the somatic treatment in order to help the patient understand and comply with the plan. Second, the patient must have the sense that members of the treatment team are coordinating their efforts—that the right hand knows what the left hand is doing. If you prescribe a potentially lethal medication for a suicidal patient, everyone involved in the treatment *must* know the risks and benefits involved in this plan, so that the patient's use of the medication and suicidal impulses can be carefully monitored.

Finally, you should include other clinicians in your efforts as a matter of professional courtesy. When members of a treatment team do not feel that you value their input, it is easy for treatment goals to be subtly sabotaged. This may happen out of anger or out of ignorance of what you are trying to accomplish.

The following are some basic points to remember about your role as a member of a treatment team:

1. Keep yourself informed of what other clinicians are doing. Ask questions. Remember: no question (e.g., about a treatment strategy) is too elementary.
2. Keep other clinicians informed about your own work with a patient, and share your observations about the patient's responses to various interventions (e.g., apparent reactions to a change in medication).
3. Consult with other clinicians before you make major changes in a patient's treatment regimen, and expect that other treaters will do the same.
4. If you are part of a treatment team in which this sort of communication is not occurring, meet with all concerned to discuss and remedy the problem. Otherwise, it is your patient who will suffer. As a rule, the physician must act as the coordinator of the

treatment team, and it is up to you to maintain contact with all other clinicians involved in a patient's care.

The basic guidelines above for the use of psychotropic medications apply to each of the specific classes of medications discussed in the following sections.

Antipsychotic Medications

Antipsychotic (neuroleptic) agents are useful primarily in the treatment of thought disorders and, more acutely, to relieve severe agitation.

How do they work?

The mechanism of action of the antipsychotics is not completely understood. The areas of the brain most affected by these medications are the reticular formation, basal ganglia, hypothalamus, and limbic system. At the cellular level, the medications inhibit the transmission of nerve impulses in the central nervous system (CNS) by blocking the action of dopamine, a neurotransmitter, at postsynaptic receptor sites. These medications also have delayed actions on presynaptic dopamine activity. It is not known whether this dopamine-blocking activity is the mechanism by which psychosis is ameliorated, but it probably contributes to the extrapyramidal side effects of these agents (discussed below).

The mechanisms of action of the antipsychotics probably go beyond simple dopamine blockade, and this is currently an area of active research. In large-scale studies, these medications have been shown to be effective in ameliorating acute psychosis and reducing relapse or exacerbation rates in chronic schizophrenic patients.

What are the indications for using an antipsychotic?

Several illnesses usually call for the use of an antipsychotic, as follows.

Schizophrenia. This is the major condition for which antipsychotics are indicated. They are used in the following ways:

- By intramuscular injection to control acute, severe psychotic agitation or excitement (usually short-term use)
- Orally in daily doses to control acute episodes of illness (e.g., to suppress auditory hallucinations)
- As maintenance therapy to prevent recurrent exacerbations, in daily oral doses, or in intramuscular doses of a depot agent such as

the decanoate ester of fluphenazine or haloperidol every 2 to 4 weeks

Bipolar disorders (manic-depressive illness). Manic excitement often is rapidly alleviated by antipsychotics, which are commonly used in combination with lithium in cases of acute mania and then discontinued when mania abates. The efficacy of long-term maintenance therapy of manic-depressive illness with antipsychotics is unproved (see Chapter 6).

Amphetamine psychosis. Antipsychotics are the medications of choice. They are used until the psychosis remits, and then discontinued (see Chapter 14).

Drug-induced psychosis. If the drug cannot be identified, it is better in most cases to talk the person down rather than use medication. However, if agitation is life-threatening, antipsychotics can be of great benefit. (Antipsychotics are not used to treat psychosis caused by anticholinergic medications or phencyclidine [PCP].)

Agitated or psychotic depression. Antipsychotics are effective, particularly in combination with an antidepressant or ECT. The efficacy of antipsychotics in retarded or bipolar depression is less clear.

Chronic brain syndromes. Dementia and other chronic neurological syndromes that involve psychotic symptoms may be treated symptomatically with antipsychotics.

Anxiety. Antipsychotics are not appropriate medications for anxiety and can even worsen anxiety symptoms by causing akathisia (see below).

Gilles de la Tourette syndrome. Antipsychotics may be used to control the symptoms of Tourette syndrome (see Chapter 12). Haloperidol and pimozide are the medications most frequently used in treating this disorder.

Personality disorders. Recent research suggests that antipsychotics in low doses may be helpful on a short-term basis in treating anxiety, depression, somatization, and psychotic ideation in patients with borderline and schizotypal personality disorders. However, the effects of these medications in personality disorders are modest, and this is an area of pharmacotherapy that needs further study before any firm treatment recommendations can be made.

If one of the above-mentioned illnesses has been diagnosed, you must still determine which features of the illness are likely to respond to an antipsychotic (Table 18-2). The symptoms that are most likely to respond are combativeness, hyperactivity, tension, hostility, hallucinations, sleeplessness, poor hygiene and self-care, acute delusions (of recent onset), and social isolation. Symptoms less likely to respond are lack of

Table 18-2. Responsiveness of symptoms to antipsychotic medications

Most likely to respond	Less likely to respond
Combativeness	Lack of insight
Hyperactivity	Poor judgment
Tension	Impaired memory
Hostility	Disorientation
Hallucinations	Chronic delusions
Sleeplessness	
Poor hygiene and self-care	
Acute delusions (of recent onset)	
Social isolation	

insight, poor judgment, impaired memory, disorientation, and chronic delusions.

Before treating someone with an antipsychotic, the following basic workup is indicated:

- History and physical examination
- Blood pressure, both standing and reclining, to note baseline postural changes
- Laboratory studies—complete blood count (including white blood cell count with differential), liver function tests, urinalysis, thyroid function tests (T_3, T_4, thyroid-stimulating hormone [TSH])
- A baseline electrocardiogram (EKG) for people with any history of cardiac problems and for anyone over 40

Types of antipsychotic medications

There are several pharmacologically distinct classes of antipsychotics, but all have similar therapeutic actions and are similarly effective. There is no need to describe here in detail the different pharmacological properties of these classes. Excellent discussions of the pharmacology of the antipsychotics can be found in the references at the end of this chapter. Clinically, there are three important differences among the groups of antipsychotics:

Potency. Because the antipsychotics are of such different potencies, medication doses vary by a factor of up to 1,000. Thus, for example, if it takes 300 to 400 mg of chlorpromazine (Thorazine) to relieve a patient's psychotic symptoms, it would take roughly 6 to 8 mg of haloperidol

(Haldol) to achieve the same effect, as the potency of haloperidol is about 50 times that of chlorpromazine, although they are equally effective agents.

Side effects. The side effects, discussed below, vary greatly from one type of medication to another.

Patient's idiosyncratic responses. Some people who do not respond well to a medication of one class may respond satisfactorily to a medication that is chemically distinct.

Table 18-3 presents the most commonly used antipsychotic agents. They are listed according to their pharmacological group. The potencies of these agents are given relative to the potency of chlorpromazine.

Table 18-3. Equivalent doses of commonly used antipsychotic agents by chemical type (chlorpromazine = 100)

Generic name	Trade name	Potency relative to chlorpromazine
Phenothiazines		
Aliphatic		
Chlorpromazine	Thorazine	100
Piperidine		
Mesoridazine	Serentil	50
Piperacetazine	Quide	12
Thioridazine	Mellaril	100
Piperazine		
Acetophenazine	Tindal	20
Fluphenazine	Prolixin	2
Perphenazine	Trilafon	10
Trifluoperazine	Stelazine	5
Thioxanthenes		
Aliphatic		
Chlorprothixene	Taractan	65
Piperazine		
Thiothixene	Navane	5
Dibenzazepines		
Loxapine	Loxitane, Daxolin	15
Butyrophenones		
Haloperidol	Haldol	2
Indolones		
Molindone	Moban	10
Rauwolfia alkaloids		
Reserpine	Serpasil, etc. (generic)	1–2

This table can serve as a guide to determining proper doses of the antipsychotics. Essentially, the table helps you think of the dosage of any antipsychotic in terms of chlorpromazine equivalents—that is, the strength of the dosage relative to an equivalent dosage of a standard agent, chlorpromazine.

Suppose, for example, that you want to treat an acutely psychotic young man with trifluoperazine (Stelazine). It has been determined that the minimum dosage of chlorpromazine that is likely to be effective in treating acute psychosis in a young adult is about 300 to 500 mg orally per day. How much trifluoperazine is the daily equivalent of 400 mg of chlorpromazine (CPZ)?

The arithmetic, as shown in Figure 18-1, is simple. For example, 400 mg of CPZ equals 20 mg of trifluoperazine. Thus, you would want to give your patient about 20 mg/day of trifluoperazine to adequately treat his condition.

$$\frac{\text{Potency of drug X}}{\text{Potency of CPZ}} \times \frac{\text{Desired dose in}}{\text{CPZ equivalents}} = \frac{\text{Desired dose}}{\text{of drug X}}$$

$$\frac{5}{100} \times 400 \text{ mg} = 20 \text{ mg}$$

If this psychotic man showed no improvement on trifluoperazine, even at increased doses, you would probably try another antipsychotic of a chemically different class, going back to the table to choose a medication like haloperidol. You would then determine the dosage of the new medication on the basis of its potency relative to chlorpromazine. However, the new medication should be begun at a lower-than-optimal dose and increased slowly to prevent unwanted side effects (e.g., dystonia—see below).

Side effects

All antipsychotics carry side effects (see Table 18-4). You can expect to see side effects in most people treated with these medications.

Sedation. Sedation occurs in a majority of cases. This may be a desired effect (for insomniac patients), or it may be a problem (e.g., for students or for those who feel drowsy when driving an automobile). To treat sedation, try lowering the dosage, giving the entire daily dose at bedtime, or using a less sedating, more potent medication.

Table 18-4. Side effects of antipsychotic medications

Sedation	Postural hypotension
Extrapyramidal side effects (EPS)	Allergic or toxic side effects
Dystonia	Agranulocytosis
Parkinsonism	Dermatitis
Akathisia	Allergic hepatitis
Akinesia	Metabolic or endocrine side effects
Tardive dyskinesia	Toxic retinopathy
Lowered seizure threshold	EKG changes
Anticholinergic side effects	Retrograde ejaculation
Dry mouth	
Blurred vision	
Constipation	
Urinary retention	

Extrapyramidal side effects. "Extrapyramidal" side effects refer to disturbances in functioning of the extrapyramidal motor system of the brain. These side effects occur in the vast majority of cases. There are several types:

Acute dystonia (a state of abnormal muscle tension) occurs early in treatment, often within the first two days. Manifestations include spasms of the eyes, eyelids, face, neck, and back muscles, which can produce bodily contortions that are dramatic and frightening. In rare instances, spasm of the larynx and pharynx can cause asphyxia. Dystonia is most commonly experienced as simple muscle stiffness. Acute dystonic reactions are easily and rapidly treated as described below. For recurrent dystonias, lower the dose, switch to a less potent antipsychotic, or use antiparkinsonian medications prophylactically in conjunction with the antipsychotic.

Parkinsonism—a cluster of symptoms like those seen in Parkinson's disease—arises generally over 1 to 4 weeks after treatment is begun. Symptoms include bradykinesia, shuffling gait, decreased energy, masklike facial expression, and variable tremor. Parkinsonism (see below) is treatable by the same means as are dystonias.

Akinesia or bradykinesia (severe parkinsonism) is relatively uncommon, but its insidious onset makes this problem easy to miss. It involves markedly decreased or absent body activity that can be mistaken for a symptom of psychosis or depression and wrongly treated by raising the dosage of the antipsychotic or adding an antidepressant.

Proper treatment involves lowering the dosage, switching to another medication, or using antiparkinsonian medication.

Neuroleptic malignant syndrome (NMS) is rare among patients treated with antipsychotics, but it is life-threatening. Patients become rigid, catatonic, and stuporous. Symptoms include fever, elevated white blood cell count, tachycardia, blood pressure fluctuations, tachypnea, and sweating. Creatine phosphokinase (CPK) is elevated because of muscle breakdown, which can lead to myoglobinuria and acute renal failure. Treatment involves immediately discontinuing all medications and providing intensive medical support, which may be required for several days. Specific treatments have not yet proven to be of value in NMS, but among those under investigation are dantrolene, bromocriptine, amantadine, benzodiazepines, and anticholinergic medications.

Akathisia is very common, occurs within 1 to 6 weeks after treatment has begun, and can be severely distressing and long-lasting. It involves restlessness, pacing, rocking, and an inability to sit still. It is often experienced as "jumpy legs." Akathisia is treatable with benzodiazepines (e.g., lorazepam) or propranolol (in doses up to 120 mg/day), but it is easy to mistake for psychotic agitation; *do not mistreat it by raising the dosage of the antipsychotic!*

Tardive dyskinesia is the most ominous of the side effects of the antipsychotics. This syndrome develops late in treatment (after 6 months to 20 years of maintenance therapy); it is estimated to occur in about 20% of chronic schizophrenic patients. It involves involuntary movement, including lip smacking and sucking, jaw movements, "flycatcher" tongue movements, writhing movements of the extremities, and occasional difficulty swallowing. Although rare cases are irreversible, most remit partially or completely (often very slowly) when antipsychotic medication is discontinued or the dose is lowered. Antiparkinsonian medications are of no help in treatment and may increase the severity of the movements. The best (and probably the only) treatment for tardive dyskinesia is prevention, by using antipsychotics only when indicated and in the lowest effective doses, and by monitoring patients on antipsychotics frequently with trials off medication to assess their ongoing need for the medication. Obviously, the discomfort and impairment caused by these involuntary movements (they are often mild and not noticed by the patient) must be weighed against the patient's psychotic illness in determining whether antipsychotic medication is warranted even when symptoms of tardive dyskinesia develop. All patients taking antipsychotic medication must be monitored for tardive dyskinesia by examining them for abnormal movements every 3 to 6 months. Patients and families must be apprised of the risk of tardive dyskinesia before therapy with an antipsychotic is begun.

Lowered seizure threshold. All antipsychotics increase the likelihood of seizures in people who have preexisting seizure disorders. Among the antipsychotics, molindone and fluphenazine have the least potential for lowering seizure threshold. Therapy with antipsychotics must be undertaken with caution (but is not contraindicated) with patients who are prone to seizures.

Autonomic side effects. These are very common, usually mild, but somewhat annoying. Peripheral anticholinergic effects include dry mouth, blurred vision, rapid heartbeat, nasal congestion, and constipation. Occasionally, peripheral side effects are severe, such as ileus or urinary retention. Patients must be carefully screened for preexisting narrow-angle glaucoma, because antipsychotics can precipitate acute exacerbations of this condition, which may eventually result in loss of eyesight. Central anticholinergic effects include impairment in concentration, memory, and attention, as well as anorgasmia and ejaculatory incompetence.

Toxicity results in *anticholinergic delirium*, which includes dry mucous membranes, hot dry skin, dilated pupils, absent bowel sounds, distended bladder, and sinus tachycardia. This delirium tends to be worse among the elderly and among people taking low-potency antipsychotics. This is a medical emergency that is treatable with physostigmine, 1 to 2 mg, intramuscularly or via slow intravenous infusion.

Postural hypotension. This is particularly common in the elderly and must be monitored closely to prevent falling and possible head trauma or hip fractures. As a general rule it is best to avoid using low-potency antipsychotics in those over age 65.

Toxic and allergic effects. Although toxicity is not common, you must be alert to possible adverse effects:

Agranulocytosis occurs in the first 3 to 8 weeks of treatment in roughly 1 in 10,000 to 20,000 people taking chlorpromazine, and somewhat less commonly with other medications in this class. Clozapine is an exception, with agranulocytosis occurring in as many as 0.2% to 0.5% of patients. Early manifestations are fever and sore throat that usually precede a falling white blood cell count. It can be treated by stopping all medication and working to prevent infection.

Dermatitis, or skin rash, is common—not only an allergic reaction to the medication, but also as a result of medication-induced sensitivity to sunlight. People taking phenothiazines must be forewarned to use sun blockers, or they can be badly and dangerously sunburned.

Allergic hepatitis occurs chiefly with use of chlorpromazine (about 1 in 500 people) during the first 4 weeks of treatment. It is manifested by jaundice and is a benign condition that remits when the medication is stopped.

Metabolic or endocrine side effects. These uncommon effects include weight gain, menstrual irregularity, abnormal production of breast milk and breast enlargement (in both sexes), hyperglycemia, and hyper- or hypothermia.

Toxic retinopathy. This rare condition has been associated with use of thioridazine (Mellaril) in doses above 800 mg per day.

EKG changes. Arrhythmias, T-wave inversions, and prolongation of EKG intervals are relatively trivial, but they are more common with thioridazine use than with use of other antipsychotics.

Retrograde ejaculation. Ejaculation of semen up into the urinary bladder instead of out of the penis is a painful condition that is primarily caused by use of thioridazine, so other antipsychotic agents are recommended in treating men for whom this might be a problem.

Treatment of extrapyramidal side effects

Dystonias, parkinsonism, and akinesia are all responsive to antiparkinsonian medications. The most commonly used medications in the treatment of extrapyramidal side effects are the following:

Diphenhydramine (Benadryl). This agent is an anticholinergic antihistamine that is safe, not prone to being abused, and especially useful in acute dystonias because parenteral administration brings relief within minutes. It can be given orally, intravenously, or intramuscularly. Sedation and pronounced anticholinergic effects make this medication less desirable for treating extrapyramidal side effects on a long-term basis. The dosage is 25 to 50 mg intramuscularly or intravenously for acute dystonia, and 25 to 50 mg orally every 4 to 6 hours to prevent recurrent dystonic episodes.

Benztropine mesylate (Cogentin). This is an antiparkinsonian medication that is very effective for acute and long-term treatment of extrapyramidal side effects. Administer 1 to 2 mg orally one to three times a day as needed to control and prevent these side effects. It may be used on a long-term basis and is also available in intramuscular and intravenous forms (in doses of 0.5 to 2 mg) for treatment of acute reactions.

Trihexyphenidyl hydrochloride (Artane). This agent, another antiparkinsonian medication, is quite similar to benztropine mesylate. Many people find it less sedating than either benztropine mesylate or diphenhydramine, and therefore more suitable for long-term treatment. The usual dosage is 2 mg orally (and sometimes higher) one to three times a day.

If the patient requires an antiparkinsonian medication for side effects, continue the medication for 1 to 3 months, and then taper it off to determine whether it is still required. A majority of people will no longer require the antiparkinsonian medication for dystonia. However, a significant number of patients require antiparkinsonism therapy for symptoms of parkinsonism as long as they take the antipsychotic.

Note that some people experience a high from benztropine mesylate and trihexyphenidyl hydrochloride and will abuse these drugs when the side effects are no longer present.

Medication interactions

Some medications that interact with the antipsychotics include the following:

1. The efficacy of *oral anticoagulants* is decreased by phenothiazines.
2. *Antacids* may decrease the absorption of antipsychotic medications.
3. The phenothiazines potentiate (i.e., exaggerate) the effects of *antihistamines, antihypertensives, CNS depressants* (e.g., alcohol), *oral hypoglycemics,* and *succinylcholine.*
4. *Anticonvulsants* lower blood levels of antipsychotic medications, and when the two are used concurrently, antipsychotic dosages must be adjusted upward.
5. *Scopolamine* overdose (e.g., Compoz, Sominex) or *diuretics* in combination with the phenothiazines can cause a hypotensive crisis (a precipitous drop in blood pressure).

Choosing an antipsychotic

Since antipsychotics are almost all of similar efficacy, how do you decide which one to use for a particular patient?

Rely on the patient's history. If your patient has had antipsychotic medication in the past, find out which medications worked and which did not.

Consider compliance. If you work with an outpatient who does not take daily oral medication reliably, you can consider giving fluphenazine decanoate or haloperidol decanoate by intramuscular injection every 2 to 4 weeks.

Decide which side effects are least likely to be troublesome to the patient. Because all antipsychotics produce side effects, you must weigh one set against another. In most cases, you are choosing between low-potency medications, which have primarily autonomic and sedating effects, and high-potency medications, which are less sedating but more likely to cause extrapyramidal reactions (dystonias, parkinsonism, and akathisia). For a severely agitated individual who cannot sleep well, you might deliberately choose a more sedating (low-potency) medication like chlorpromazine (Thorazine) because sedation would be desirable. Paranoid patients might be particularly frightened by muscle spasm (dystonia), so a high-potency medication might be avoided, or given along with prophylactic antiparkinsonian medication. For a college student who is studying for examinations, a low-potency antipsychotic might cause too much drowsiness and blurred vision, whereas a high-potency medication like haloperidol (Haldol) would be less likely to compromise his or her studying capacity because of sedation (but might cause akathisia).

Table 18-5 lists some of the most commonly used antipsychotics, showing their relative potencies and the degree to which they cause sedation and/or extrapyramidal side effects.

Prescribing the antipsychotics

Once an antipsychotic is chosen, how is it prescribed?

Emergencies. Severely combative, aggressive, and destructive psychotic people can be rapidly and effectively treated with repeated intramuscular injections of an antipsychotic to decrease excitement and to protect the patient and others from harm. Before such a treatment is used with a patient who is unknown to you (e.g., in a hospital emergency room), the following conditions that might be obscured or worsened by the administration of an antipsychotic must be ruled out:

- Head injuries
- Space-occupying intracranial lesions (e.g., a subdural hematoma, or blood clot, pressing on the brain)
- Epilepsy
- Severe hypotension or hypertension
- Intoxication with drugs that have anticholinergic effects
- Imbalance of serum electrolytes (sodium, potassium)

Table 18-5. Commonly used antipsychotics, their relative potencies, and their sedating and extrapyramidal effects (EPS)

Generic name	Trade name	Relative potency	Sedation hypotension	EPS
Phenothiazines				
Aliphatic				
Chlorpromazine	Thorazine	100	+++	++
Piperidine				
Thioridazine	Mellaril	100	+++/++	+
Piperazine				
Fluphenazine	Prolixin	2	+	+++
Perphenazine	Trilafon	10	+	+++
Trifluoperazine	Stelazine	5	+	+++
Thioxanthenes				
Aliphatic				
Chlorprothixene	Taractan	65	++	++
Piperazine				
Thiothixene	Navane	5	+	+++
Dibenzazepines				
Loxapine	Loxitane	15	++	+++
Butyrophenones				
Haloperidol	Haldol	2	+	+++
Indolones				
Molindone	Moban	10	+	++

If none of these is present, any one of the antipsychotics listed below may be used via intramuscular injection (initial doses are suggested, along with an acceptable dosage range):

- Haloperidol (Haldol) 2 mg—range 1–10 mg
- Perphenazine (Trilafon) 10 mg—range 4–12 mg
- Fluphenazine (Prolixin) 2.5 mg—range 1–10 mg
- Trifluoperazine (Stelazine) 5 mg—range 1–10 mg
- Thiothixene (Navane) 5 mg—range 4–15 mg

The end point of this initial treatment is a decrease in excitement, and the process is commonly continued until the person falls asleep. To achieve this, the dose may be repeated every hour (even every 30 minutes if excitement is severe), to the maximum of the above dose ranges within the first 12 hours. Intramuscular doses can be safely repeated as long as there is no significant drop in blood pressure. Frequent monitoring of blood pressure is essential during this treatment. Additional treatment can be given orally, and doses can be limited if antipsychotic treatment is supplemented by potent benzodiazepine sedatives such as lorazepam or clonazepam.

Acute psychosis. For patients who are acutely psychotic but who do not exhibit severe agitation, parenteral antipsychotic therapy may not be necessary. Instead, begin with oral doses of the medication. Start at a moderate dose (e.g., 5 mg of haloperidol or fluphenazine) and increase it gradually to a maximum of perhaps 15 to 20 mg per day until the desired effect is achieved or until side effects become intolerable and the dose must be lowered. The phases of acute treatment, when effective, are likely to be as follows:

- *1 to 5 days*: Excitement and hyperactivity disappear, and the patient becomes more cooperative.
- *2 days to 4–6 weeks*: The patient's thought disorder persists, but he or she functions better in daily living.
- *1 to 6 weeks (or more)*: Amelioration of the patient's thought disorder.

Many cases of acute psychosis respond to a minimum of 300 to 400 mg per day of chlorpromazine (or the equivalent dose of another medication). The average dosages required for the acutely psychotic individual range from 300 to 750 mg a day orally. How quickly this dosage is reached will depend on the person's size (larger people often require higher dosages), age (the elderly generally require or respond to lower dosages), and history (tolerance of high dosages in the past permits rapid increase in the dosage). For young, healthy individuals who have had no prior experience with antipsychotics, it is best to start with 100 to 150 mg chlorpromazine-equivalent per day (in bid or tid doses) and increase the dosage by 50 to 100 mg every other day or more slowly as tolerated.

How high is too high? The dosage of an antipsychotic can be increased to fairly high levels to achieve the desired result if the side effects are tolerable, but daily dosages above 500 to 750 mg orally do not usually result in faster or additional improvement.

The antipsychotics have elimination half-lives of at least 20 hours—that is, they are eliminated from the body slowly and are relatively long-acting. Thus, provided that side effects are tolerable, the entire daily dosage may be given at one time to achieve continuous antipsychotic effects, if the patient can comply more easily with a once-a-day regimen.

Maintenance therapy

Once the patient has been stabilized on an antipsychotic, how long does treatment continue? The answer is not clear. Prolonged therapy with an antipsychotic given more often than every other day carries significant risks, particularly the risk of tardive dyskinesia. Thus, maintenance therapy should only be used if there is a clear indication that the patient requires such treatment.

Acute drug-induced psychoses generally remit rapidly; prolonged antipsychotic treatment is not necessary. Mania is treated acutely with antipsychotics, but most bipolar (manic-depressive) patients are not continued on antipsychotics once the acute psychosis has cleared and they are stabilized on lithium.

A patient who suffers a first psychotic episode of unknown etiology (particularly an adolescent) should be tapered off the medication after several months of successful medication treatment so that the ongoing need for medication can be assessed. Such a person may never have a subsequent psychotic break and should not be medicated indefinitely.

Maintenance therapy is required for conditions in which psychosis recurs within weeks or months after treatment is stopped. Most people who fall into this category are chronic schizophrenic or schizoaffective patients, and those bipolar patients who do not remain symptom-free on lithium alone. (However, the efficacy of antipsychotics in long-term treatment of bipolar disorders has not been proven.) About 40% to 60% of people who are diagnosed as chronic "schizophrenics" have relapses within 6 months after antipsychotic treatment is stopped, and 60% to 90% relapse within 1 year. For these people, long-term maintenance has been shown to decrease their rates of relapse and rehospitalization by at least three times.

Even the most chronically or recurrently ill people should be given occasional closely supervised trials off medication to be sure that treatment is not being prolonged unnecessarily.

Long-term maintenance dosages of antipsychotics can usually be lowered to 20% to 50% of the dosage required during the acute psychotic episode. There is no standard maintenance dosage, so it must be arrived at by monitoring symptoms carefully and determining the lowest dosage at which target symptoms are kept in abeyance. Some patients may be maintained on as little as 50 mg chlorpromazine-equivalent per day.

If treatment seems ineffective, consider whether the dosage is adequate and whether the patient is taking the medication. *Plasma levels* of antipsychotics are now available, but standard therapeutic plasma levels for the antipsychotics have not been established. While blood levels are not particularly helpful in determining dosage, they can be used qualitatively to determine whether a patient is taking the medication.

If the patient shows no response or little response to an apparently adequate dosage of medication after 6 to 8 weeks of treatment, it is useful to try another medication. Lack of response to one antipsychotic does not always mean that the person will fail to respond to another.

Other antipsychotic agents

Lithium carbonate. Studies have shown that between one-third and one-half of schizophrenic patients show a positive response to treatment with lithium carbonate. It is not clear whether lithium is effective in schizophrenia, or whether this group consists primarily of patients who have undiagnosed affective illness. Lithium is not as effective as standard antipsychotics, but may be useful in patients who do not respond adequately to these standard treatments. A more complete discussion of lithium is included later in this chapter.

Anticonvulsants. These agents, especially valproate, have been shown to be effective antipsychotic medications. The uses of anticonvulsants in psychiatric practice are discussed later in this chapter.

New medications. New medications, such as benzamides and clozapine, are being investigated as treatments for schizophrenia. It is hoped that they will be effective against psychotic symptoms but have fewer extrapyramidal effects, including tardive dyskinesia. Clozapine is scheduled for release in 1990. The benzamides are still used only experimentally.

Antidepressants

Medications that alleviate and prevent depression have proved invaluable in the treatment of mood disorders. These medications fall into two major classes—the tricyclic antidepressants (TCAs) and the monoamine oxidase inhibitors (MAOIs). These medications, along with ECT, are the most effective somatic therapies now available for the treatment of severe (major) depression. Stimulants such as amphetamine and methylphenidate were once widely used to attempt to elevate the depressed person's mood, but since the advent of these more effective and more specific antidepressant agents, mood elevators are rarely used for this purpose.

As was mentioned in Chapter 6, symptoms and clinical courses of various depressive syndromes are quite varied. No one treatment is uniformly effective for all types of depression, and the efficacy of the antidepressants is imperfect. Nevertheless, a majority of people with severe depression respond favorably to antidepressants, and many who do not respond to one medication will respond to another or to ECT.

Psychotherapy or medication?

This choice is not an either-or proposition. Medications and psychotherapy work in complementary ways for many depressed patients: the medication alleviates many of the physiological symptoms of the illness, while psychotherapy helps to ease emotional pain and promote more effective functioning in the world. Empirical studies of depressed patients have shown the combination of psychotherapy and pharmacotherapy to be more effective than either treatment alone, and contemporary studies show especially good results of cognitive and interpersonal forms of psychotherapy in milder cases of major depression.

Which depressed people are most likely to benefit from an antidepressant? Two factors should be considered in answering this question: the symptoms and the syndromes (as shown in Table 18-6).

The depressive *symptoms most likely to be alleviated by antidepressant medication* are the *vegetative signs:* appetite disturbance and weight loss, sleep disturbance (especially early morning awakening), decreased energy, decreased sexual drive, psychomotor agitation or retardation, and diurnal mood variation (depression worse in the morning).

The *symptoms less likely to respond to antidepressants* are those that are the more *subjective* and *psychological signs:* demoralization, low self-esteem, hopelessness, and helplessness. Such feelings are more responsive to psychotherapeutic interventions, at least in depression of mild to moderate severity.

The depressive *syndromes most likely to respond to antidepressants* include vegetative signs and discrete episodes of illness that seem to have a life of their own. Discrete episodes of depression have a clear time

Table 18-6. Responsiveness of symptoms and syndromes to antidepressant medications

Most likely to respond	Less likely to respond
Symptoms	
Appetite disturbance and weight loss	Demoralization
Sleep disturbance	Low self-esteem
Decreased energy	Hopelessness
Decreased libido	Helplessness
Psychomotor agitation or retardation	
Diurnal mood variation	
Syndromes	
Major depressive episodes	Dysthymic disorder
Agitated depression	Personality disorder

of onset, as opposed to more chronic depression, which the patient regards as having always been present. *Major depressive episodes* (endogenous depression) are not greatly influenced by changes in the person's environment or by specific social or therapeutic interactions; they generally include vegetative signs. *Agitated depression* (including involutional melancholia) is common in people over 45 and is characterized by pacing, hand-wringing, hair-pulling, and vocal expressions of psychic pain. Antipsychotics and ECT are also particularly useful in these cases. *Delusional depression* is poorly responsive to treatment with antidepressants alone, but responds well to the combination of an antidepressant and an antipsychotic or ECT.

The *syndromes less likely to respond to antidepressants* are those that have no clear onset or discrete episodes, but have a clear relationship to environmental events (e.g., the patient's wife has left him) and minimal vegetative disturbance. These syndromes include *dysthymia* (chronic, low-grade depression) that has been present for at least 2 years in adults and is characterized by long-standing feelings of hopelessness, inadequacy, and low self-esteem without severe physiological disturbance; and *personality disorders* in which depression is a concomitant of long-standing interpersonal difficulties and chronically impaired functioning. For example, people with borderline personality disorder often complain of depression, and may even report sleep and appetite disturbance, but these symptoms are often the direct result of the underlying personality disorder and current life events. Such difficulties are not resolved by pharmacotherapy.

Syndromes that are self-limiting do not require antidepressant therapy. *Reactive depression* due to severe environmental stress includes, for example, grief reactions after the death or loss of a loved one. Support, psychotherapy, and brief symptomatic treatment (e.g., with antianxiety agents) usually suffice. *Drug-induced depression* (e.g., depression caused by the antihypertensive reserpine) is usually resolved when the offending drug is discontinued. *Depression secondary to physical illness* often resolves when the underlying physical condition improves (e.g., anemia, hypothyroidism); but, especially in cases where the underlying illness is incurable, antidepressant therapy may be helpful.

Syndromes that are sometimes responsive to antidepressant treatment include *bipolar disorders* (manic-depressive illness) and *schizoaffective disorders*. Although lithium treatment is more common and generally more effective on a long-term basis, antidepressants can be useful in treating the acute depressive phases of bipolar disorders. A word of caution, however. Because antidepressants can precipitate mania, they must be used cautiously with people who are prone to manic episodes, and in such cases are best used briefly in moderate doses in combination with lithium. For schizoaffective disorders, antipsychotics and antidepressants are often used in combination when people manifest both prominent affective symptoms and psychosis. Again, antidepressants must be used with caution, because they exacerbate psychosis in some cases.

Other psychiatric syndromes for which antidepressants are believed to be useful, but for which these agents have not been approved by the Food and Drug Administration, include panic disorder, obsessive-compulsive disorder, and bulimia. Nevertheless, empirical data support their use in these disorders.

Antidepressants must be used with caution in patients with recurrent affective episodes. Antidepressants have been shown to decrease the intervals of time between affective episodes in some unipolar patients, and to produce more rapid cycling in and out of manic and depressive episodes in bipolar patients. Thus, it is important to keep track of the intervals between depressive episodes, and if they appear to be decreasing, to consider the use of lithium instead of an antidepressant to prevent relapses.

In cases of depression that are not clear-cut, when symptomatology is not clearly vegetative, the decision to medicate or not to medicate remains a matter of clinical judgment. Most clinicians agree that it is best to try antidepressants when there is a reasonable possibility that medication could be of benefit to the patient and when a trial of the medication can be carried out safely.

Dexamethasone suppression test

As the discussion above suggests, there is some disagreement over which people are likely to respond to antidepressants. In the past decade, much publicity has been given to the dexamethasone suppression test (DST), which promised to be a definitive biochemical test for depression that would enable clinicians to reliably sort out those depressed people who would respond to antidepressant therapy from those who would not. Because you may encounter the DST in your work, a brief discussion of this laboratory-based method of assessment is provided here.

The development of the DST began with the observation that many depressed people had elevated serum cortisol levels and poor regulation of adrenocorticotropin (ACTH) production. In normal people who are given a small dose of dexamethasone (a synthetic steroid), the body's production of cortisol is suppressed over the next 24 hours. However, in some depressed people given the same oral dose of dexamethasone, cortisol production is only partly suppressed or recovers too early, suggesting an abnormality in the regulation of hormone production somewhere in the body's regulatory system (i.e., in the hypothalamus, the pituitary, or the adrenal gland).

The DST is given as follows: 1 mg of dexamethasone is given orally at 11 P.M., and venous blood is drawn for cortisol assays, usually at 8 A.M., 4 P.M., and 11 P.M. the following day. (In outpatients, the test is usually limited to a 4 P.M. sample.) The DST is considered abnormal if any of the samples show a plasma cortisol level above 5.0 micrograms/deciliter.

Investigators have reported that 40% to 60% of people who have melancholic or endogenous depression have an abnormal (positive) DST—a low rate of sensitivity for this test. Ideally, the DST could help clinicians establish or rule out the presence of endogenous depression if the clinical findings were equivocal. However, the test is neither highly sensitive nor specific, for only about 50% of people who are diagnosed clinically as suffering from major depression have abnormal DST responses; the rest are not identified by this screening measure, or rapidly correct to normal DST even before clinical recovery.

To complicate matters, many medical conditions other than depressive illness can give positive DSTs—including Cushing's disease, liver disease, pregnancy, and drug use (e.g., alcohol, phenytoin, carbamazepine, or sedatives). New research suggests that the DST may not specifically identify people who are endogenously depressed, but may also be positive in some cases of mania, acute psychosis, chronic schizophrenia, stroke, and dementia. The DST is consistently positive in eating disorders.

The DST has not been shown to be superior to clinical findings in predicting whether someone will respond to antidepressant therapy, nor has it proved helpful to clinicians in choosing particular medications for treating depression. Some psychiatrists use serial DSTs to follow an individual's response to treatment, but it has not been shown that this technique for monitoring improvement is more reliable than clinical judgment. Therefore, the clinical examination continues to be the most accurate and sensitive method available for the diagnosis and treatment of depression responsive to somatic therapy, and the DST remains of more research interest than clinical utility.

Clinical evaluation

Before you begin a patient on an antidepressant, it is important to collect certain data that might influence the choice of treatment (Table 18-7).

History. When taking a history, pay particular attention to the following:

Current medications. Medications like reserpine, methyldopa, cocaine or other stimulants, oral contraceptives, alcohol, marijuana, and other drugs of abuse can cause depression.

Family history. A family history of depressive episodes that were responsive to medication or ECT is a good predictor of response. Note which medications alleviated depression in relatives, because medication responsiveness, like depression itself, may have genetic determinants, and what worked for grandfather may work for grandchild as well. If there is a family history of mania, proceed with caution in using antidepressants, because they can precipitate mania in those who have an underlying bipolar illness.

Current medical conditions. Cardiac problems are particularly important to elucidate, given the side effects of the antidepressants (discussed below). Question the patient carefully about a history of congestive heart failure, heart attacks, arrhythmias, and postural hypotension. Other problems to screen out include prostatic enlargement (antidepressants can cause obstruction of the urinary tract and urinary retention) and narrow-angle glaucoma (antidepressants can precipitate acute exacerbations and result in loss of eyesight).

Suicidal ideation. This is a tricky problem, because many depressed people are prone to suicidal ideation and attempts. Tricyclic antidepressants (e.g., imipramine, amitriptyline) are potentially lethal in overdose; the lethal dose is only 10 to 20 times the typical daily therapeutic dosage. MAOIs can interact with certain tyramine-containing foods (discussed below) to cause severe hypertension, resulting in stroke and death. They can also cause a catastrophic toxic interaction with certain medications (e.g., TCAs, meperidine hydrochloride). For suicidal people, prescribing

---

Table 18-7. Medical workup for antidepressant therapy

Medical history
   Current medical conditions
   Current medications
   Family history

Physical examination

Baseline laboratory studies
   Complete blood count with differential
   Routine blood chemistry–SMA-12
   Thyroid function tests (T_3, T_4, TSH)
   Urinalysis

EKG (if patient over 40 or any history of cardiac symptoms)

---

medications must be done with care. Antidepressants for suicidal outpatients can be dispensed weekly or even every few days if necessary as a sign to the patient of your concern and attention. Severely suicidal people can be treated in the hospital to prevent overdose in the initial phases of treatment, or given ECT.

Physical examination. A careful examination should be performed by the psychiatrist, family physician, or internist. If a depressed outpatient has had an examination within the previous 6 months and is in stable health, this will suffice in most cases.

Baseline laboratory studies. The following laboratory studies are useful in ruling out an underlying medical illness that causes depression:

- Complete blood count (CBC) with differential
- Routine blood chemistries (serum sodium and potassium, blood sugar, blood urea nitrogen, etc.)
- Thyroid function tests (T_3, T_4, and thyroid-stimulating hormone)
- Urinalysis
- EKG (if patient is over 40 or has any history of cardiac symptoms)

Tricyclic antidepressants

The tricyclic and the tricyclic-like compounds form a class of medications with similar therapeutic properties and side effect profiles. As a group they are referred to as *tricyclic antidepressants* (TCAs), to distinguish them from the other major class of antidepressants, the MAOIs, and from certain newer atypical agents (notably trazodone, fluoxetine, and bupropion). TCAs are the medical treatment of choice for most cases of major depression. Except in a limited number of cases for which ECT is more clearly indicated, the TCAs should be the first treatment you consider when you think about somatic therapy for depressed people.

Despite considerable research, we do not know how these medications alleviate depression. However, we do know that the TCAs affect the concentration of serotonin and norepinephrine at nerve synapses in the central nervous system (CNS) by blocking their reuptake by presynaptic neurons, thus increasing their availability at the junctions between neurons. In addition to this effect, many of the TCAs decrease the sensitivity of β-adrenergic receptors and increase neuronal responsiveness to serotonergic and α-adrenergic stimulation when administered for more than several days or weeks, paralleling the time course of clinical improvement in medication-responsive patients. It has been hypothesized that these neurotransmitter effects are the mechanisms by which the TCAs alleviate depression, but this theory has yet to be proven empirically.

Clinically, it is useful to know which TCAs increase CNS levels of serotonin and which increase levels of norepinephrine, because a patient whose depressive symptoms do not respond to one medication may respond to a medication of the other type (see Table 18-8 for the characteristics of the commonly used antidepressants).

The tricyclic antidepressants. *Imipramine* (Tofranil, etc.) and *amitriptyline* (Elavil, etc.) are the oldest and best studied of the tricylic antidepressants. They are still widely prescribed, but newer medications with fewer side effects are beginning to be used extensively in clinical practice. Amitriptyline is quite sedating and has some prominent serotonergic effects; it is useful in treating people who have insomnia. Imipramine is less sedating and has prominent noradrenergic effects.

Doxepin (Sinequan) is another tertiary amine that has two major disadvantages: severe anticholinergic side effects and profound effects on the heart at therapeutic doses. It is contraindicated in geriatric patients.

Desipramine (Norpramin, etc.) is a demethylated metabolite of imipramine; it is purer in its noradrenergic effect. It has lesser anticholinergic side effects (dry mouth, blurred vision, constipation) than do imipramine and amitriptyline. *Nortriptyline* (Aventyl, etc.) is a demethylated metabolite of amitriptyline with lesser anticholinergic side effects. *Protriptyline* (Vivactil) has little in the way of sedative properties and is therefore useful for patients who would find sedation unpleasant.

Heterocyclic compounds. Other antidepressant agents that are related to the tricyclics have recently come onto the market or are under investigation.

Amoxapine (Asendin) is related both to the tricyclics and to the dibenzazepine group of antipsychotics. It has both antidepressant and sedating properties, and its onset of action is more rapid than that of the tricyclics (often as little as 4 to 7 days). Amoxapine carries a risk of extrapyramidal side effects, perhaps including tardive dyskinesia, because of its chemical similarities to the antipsychotics.

Maprotiline (Ludiomil) is a tetracyclic antidepressant that has mild anticholinergic and sedating side effects, but a high risk of inducing seizures at doses of greater than 200 mg per day.

Trazodone (Desyrel) is chemically distinct from all other available antidepressants. It has proved fairly effective in relieving mild depressive symptoms and anxiety. It has limited anticholinergic and cardiovascular side effects, and suicide by trazodone overdose has been relatively uncommon. Priapism has been reported in a small number of men treated with trazodone. This effect is potentially hazardous enough to warrant prescribing trazodone for men only when other antidepressant treatments have failed.

Table 18-8. The most commonly used tricyclic and related antidepressants and their characteristics

Generic name	Trade name	Chemical group	Noradrenergic or serotonergic	Daily dosage range (mg)	Comments
Dibenzocycloheptadienes					
Amitriptyline	Elavil and others	Tricyclic	Mostly serotonergic	75–300	Sedating
Nortriptyline	Aventyl	Tricyclic	Both	40–100	Demethylated metabolite of amitriptyline
Protriptyline	Vivactyl	Tricyclic	Both	15–60	Least sedating tricyclic
Dibenzazepines					
Imipramine	Tofranil and others	Tricyclic	Mostly noradrenergic	75–300	Oldest, most widely studied
Desipramine	Norpramin, Pertofrane	Tricyclic	Noradrenergic	75–300	Demethylated metabolite of imipramine; least anticholinergic
Dibenzoxepines					
Doxepin	Sinequan, Adapin	Tricyclic	Both	75–300	Very sedating; least cardiotoxic
Dibenzoxazepines					
Amoxapine	Asendin	Tricyclic	Both	200–200	Rapid onset of action
Dibenzo-bicyclo-octadienes					
Maprotiline	Ludiomil	Tetracyclic	Noradrenergic	150–250	May have more rapid onset of action
Triazolopyridines					
Trazodone	Desyrel	Triazole	Serotonergic	200–300	Little cardiotoxicity, some antianxiety effects
Serotonin uptake inhibitors					
Fluoxetine	Prozac	Noncyclic	Serotonergic	20–80	Little anticholinergic effect, long half-life

Fluoxetine (Prozac) has now been approved by the FDA for clinical use. It is a potent and selective serotonergic reuptake blocker with very little anticholinergic effect and little postural hypotension or cardiac depressive effect. It may cause restlessness, irritability, and insomnia, as well as gastrointestinal distress, but has been well tolerated by many patients and is less likely to be lethal in overdose than the tricyclics. It is very long-acting and can increase the blood levels of other medications (including TCAs).

Bupropion (Wellbutrin) is a new medication that is chemically unrelated to other known antidepressant agents. Preliminary studies have shown it to be an effective treatment for major depression. However, it carries an increased risk of inducing seizures (relative to other antidepressants) and is contraindicated in patients with seizure disorders and eating disorders.

Side effects. *Autonomic effects.* Mild anticholinergic effects are quite common and are to be expected in most people. They include dry mouth, blurred vision, and constipation—all of which resolve spontaneously or with symptomatic treatment. Sweating may also occur. Less common anticholinergic effects include urinary retention, paralytic ileus, and the acute exacerbation of narrow-angle glaucoma.

Central nervous system effects. CNS effects include agitation, fine tremor, irritability, mania, and psychosis. Some people report sudden falls and balance problems. Sedation is a property of many TCAs. TCA-induced drowsiness may be unpleasant or welcome, depending on the patient's symptoms.

Cardiovascular effects. Postural hypotension is a potentially hazardous effect of the antidepressants, as it may result in falls that cause hip fracture or subdural hematoma. To avoid sudden drops in pressure, patients may need to make slow changes in posture or wear elastic stockings. TCAs in therapeutic doses can exacerbate preexisting heart block by prolonging the P-R, QRS, and Q-T intervals. Thus, they must be used with great caution in people who have conduction defects, have recent myocardial infarction, or are being treated with other cardiac depressants such as quinidine. A thorough cardiac evaluation, including physical examination and EKG, is essential for people who have cardiac symptoms or a history of cardiac illness. In overdose, the TCAs may cause life-threatening ventricular arrhythmias and severe hypotension, so their use in people who are suicidal must be closely monitored.

Sexual side effects. Sexual dysfunctions reported by patients treated with TCAs include impotence, ejaculatory dysfunction, and decreased libido. Because depressed patients commonly suffer from low self-esteem and sexual dysfunction, such disturbances in sexual functioning can be particularly devastating.

Weight gain. This is a side effect of some TCAs.

Medication interactions. Medication interactions of most TCAs include potentiation of the effects of quinidine and antagonism of the antihypertensive effects of guanethidine. TCAs can also cause severe toxic reactions when added to the treatment of a patient already on an MAOI. In shifting a patient from an MAOI to a TCA, it is safest to wait 1 to 2 weeks after the MAOI is discontinued before beginning the TCA, and then to administer it cautiously in gradually increasing doses.

Overdose. An acute overdose of most TCAs results in severe cerebral intoxication, convulsions, increased deep tendon reflexes, confusion, coma, severe EKG disturbances, and death. The lethal dose of most TCAs is about 10 to 20 times the typical daily therapeutic dose. As a rule, trazodone and fluoxetine (two of the nontricyclics) are significantly less dangerous than the TCAs in overdose.

Prescribing regimen. The following is the recommended prescribing regimen for the TCAs and related compounds:

- Begin with a low dose.
- Raise the dosage slowly (over 1 to 2 weeks) to within the recommended effective dosage range or until side effects prohibit further dosage increases. A typical daily dosage for someone starting on imipramine would be as follows:

Day 1	50 mg
Days 2–4	75 mg
Days 5–7	100 mg
Days 8–10	150 mg

    Similar regimens are suitable for most of the other TCAs. Doses may be divided (two or three times per day) to lessen side effects. Once the patient's dosage has been stabilized, single daily doses (especially if less than or equal to 150 mg/day) are acceptable and may make compliance easier.

- If the patient has not responded adequately to 150 mg/day (or its equivalent), increase the dose to 200 to 300 mg per day as tolerated.
- Obtain a *plasma antidepressant level* when your patient has not responded to an adequate trial of the usual therapeutic dosage (up to 200–300 mg/day) of imipramine, nortriptyline, or desipramine. While a majority of patients will respond to usual dosages, the rates at which patients metabolize these agents vary, and many patients will have plasma levels that are above or below the therapeutic range. The plasma levels shown in Table 18-9 have been

Table 18-9. Plasma levels associated with maximal therapeutic response to tricyclic antidepressants

Drug	Plasma level (ng/ml)
Nortriptyline	50–100
Imipramine (+ desipramine)	200–300
Desipramine	100–250
Amitriptyline (+ nortriptyline)	200–300
Doxepin (+ desmethyldoxepin)	probably >100

associated with maximum therapeutic response. Plasma levels should be drawn 5 to 7 days after the patient has been at a given dosage (i.e., six times the half life of the medication), and 10 to 14 hours after the last dose has been ingested. For medications whose therapeutic levels have not been established, you may need to raise the dosage to the upper limits of the recommended therapeutic range or beyond, as long as no intolerable side effects develop.

- Wait at least 2 weeks after the patient is receiving an adequate dosage to evaluate therapeutic effects. If no therapeutic response occurs during this time, raise the dosage of the TCA unless side effects become intolerable. Six weeks at a therapeutic dosage constitutes an adequate trial of an antidepressant. If partial response occurs in this time period, add lithium carbonate, which may result in further improvement in symptoms. If no response occurs, switch to a dissimilar TCA or to an MAOI, or consider ECT (see below). Thyroid hormone (triiodothyronine) has also been used to potentiate antidepressant effects in people with refractory depression, particularly those whose thyroid function tests reveal subclinical hypothyroidism.

A summary for the treatment strategy for pharmacology of depressed patients is given in Figure 18-1.

Continuing therapy. Once the initial depressive symptoms have remitted, how long should you continue antidepressant therapy? Studies have demonstrated that medication should not be withdrawn until the patient has been symptom-free for 4 to 5 months after an acute depressive episode. Medication should then be tapered off slowly (e.g., imipramine might be decreased by 25 mg per week). This will help to avoid withdrawal symptoms—including insomnia, anxiety, malaise, and depressed mood—which may be mistaken for a recurrence of the depressive symptomatology. You can differentiate withdrawal from recurrent

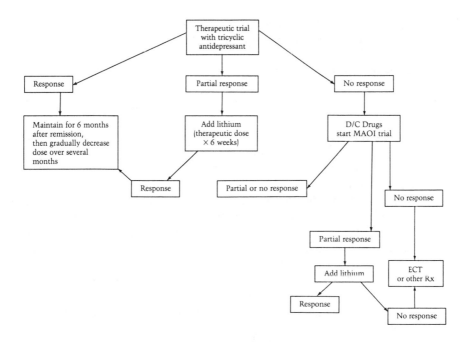

Figure 18-1. Summary of strategy for the pharmacological treatment of depressed patients. Reprinted, with permission, from Silver JM, Yudofsky SC: Psychopharmacology and electroconvulsive therapy, in *The American Psychiatric Press Textbook of Psychiatry*. Edited by Talbott JA, Hales RE, Yudofsky SC. Washington, DC, American Psychiatric Press, 1988, pp. 767–853. Copyright 1988, American Psychiatric Press.

depression by the time course: withdrawal symptoms occur immediately upon discontinuation of medication, whereas a recurrence of depression is more likely to take weeks or even months to appear. If medication is tapered slowly and depressive symptoms recur, the medication should be reinstated.

Maintenance therapy. Which people need long-term maintenance on an antidepressant? This is not an easy question to answer. Some people have one episode of depression and never experience a recurrence. For them, maintenance therapy is unnecessary. Other people have recurrent depressive episodes, but so infrequently (e.g., every 10 years) that maintenance therapy is not warranted. On the basis of large follow-up studies, it appears that people who have two depressive episodes within 5 years are likely to experience recurrences. For such people, preventive treatment of depressive episodes is recommended.

Recurrence of major depressive episodes may be as high as 85% within the first 3 years after an initial episode.

Monoamine oxidase inhibitors

The MAOIs block the action of the enzyme monoamine oxidase (MAO), which inactivates biogenic amines such as norepinephrine, serotonin, dopamine, and tyramine. By inhibiting the action of MAO, the MAOIs increase the tissue concentration of these transmitters and may potentiate their activity. This effect is believed to be related to their antidepressant action.

MAOIs have traditionally been second-line medications in treating depression because their side effects can be particularly dangerous, and patients who use them must comply with a diet that restricts foods rich in tyramine, drugs with sympathomimetic effects, and certain analgesics (e.g., meperidine). As a rule, MAOIs should be used when other treatments such as TCAs have failed or are contraindicated. The available MAOIs are shown in Table 18-10.

Some clinicians report that MAOIs are more effective than TCAs in "atypical" depressions—that is, for depression characterized by oversleeping, overeating, labile mood, and prominent anxiety. However, the TCAs remain the medications of first choice for treatment of most forms of depression.

Prescribing a monoamine oxidase inhibitor. As with TCAs, MAOIs are begun only after a thorough history, a physical examination, and the indicated laboratory studies (see above section on clinical evaluation for TCA use) to rule out underlying physical illness. Begin the medication slowly: for example, give an initial dose of 15 to 45 mg of phenelzine once or twice daily, and increase it by 15 mg every other day

Table 18-10. Available MAOIs and their average dosages

Generic name	Trade name	Average daily dosage (mg)
Hydrazides		
Isocarboxazid	Marplan	10–30
Phenelzine	Nardil	45–75
Nonhydrazide		
Tranylcypromine	Parnate	20–40
Pargyline	Eutonyl	40–100

until a dosage of 45 to 60 mg per day is reached, going to a maximum as needed of up to 75–90 mg per day. The same principles of dosage adjustment, monitoring of response, and considerations for maintenance therapy apply to the use of MAOIs as they do to the use of TCAs.

Side effects. *Orthostatic hypotension.* This is the most common cardiovascular side effect of the MAOIs and can be particularly problematic in the elderly and in those with congestive heart failure. Dose reduction sometimes remedies the problem, but substitution of another form of therapy (a TCA or ECT) may be the only way to manage this side effect in some patients. MAOIs do not affect cardiac conduction or rhythm.

Sexual dysfunction. Among patients taking MAOIs (particularly high doses of phenelzine), impotence and anorgasmia are relatively common. As noted above, it is important to ask patients about these side effects, as many will be too embarrassed or ashamed to bring up the subject themselves. Dose reduction or switching to a different medication will usually resolve the problem.

Weight gain. This is another side effect that can be troubling to patients.

Adverse effects. *Hypertensive crisis.* Hypertensive crisis (a sudden, dramatic increase in blood pressure) is perhaps the most widely known side effect of the MAOIs. It occurs primarily when the patient on an MAOI eats foods that contain tyramine. Because tyramine is not inactivated by MAO, it will result in the release of increased amounts of norepinephrine at synapses and can cause massive α-adrenergic vascular stimulation. The foods to be avoided are numerous and include certain types of cheese, wine, beer, pickled herring, chicken livers, cream, chocolate, and yogurt. Hypertensive crisis may be mild, with headache, flushing, and nausea; or it may be severe, resulting in intracranial hemorrhage and death. A patient taking an MAOI must be able to comply with a diet that involves the strict avoidance of many foods.

Drug interactions. The drugs with which MAOIs interact are too numerous to list here, but the major ones include cold and sinus remedies, pain killers, amphetamines, alcohol, narcotics (particularly meperidine), diuretics, antihypertensives, and hypoglycemics. The combination of these drugs with an MAOI can cause severe hypertension, hypotension, or CNS depression. Patients taking MAOIs should be told to discuss all medications (including over-the-counter remedies) with you or another physician prior to using any other drug. Local anesthesia for dental work must be given without vasoconstrictors such as epinephrine. You should routinely give patients lists of foods and medications to be avoided when you prescribe MAOIs.

Interaction with tricyclic antidepressants. As a rule, these medications are not used in combination with TCAs, except in special cases under the close supervision of a psychopharmacologist. It is particularly hazardous to add a TCA when a patient is already being treated with an MAOI.

Overdose. The lethal dose of an MAOI is relatively low—6 to 10 times the average daily dosage. Thus, the potential for injury or suicide by overdose or by the abuse of tyramine-containing foods is high.

Precipitation of mania. Like TCAs, MAOIs may precipitate mania in bipolar patients. These medications must therefore be used with caution in anyone with a history of manic or hypomanic episodes, or with a family history of bipolar disorder.

Lithium

As early as 1871, the antimanic properties of the lithium ion were described in the literature. By 1970, lithium carbonate was approved for clinical use in the United States. It has been a mainstay in the treatment of manic-depressive illness ever since. Lithium has been shown to be effective against the symptoms of acute mania, as well as in preventing recurrent episodes of major affective illness during long-term maintenance.

We do not know how lithium works. Its physical, chemical, and biological properties are similar to those of sodium and potassium. However, it crosses cell membranes slowly, and a therapeutic response is not generally achieved until 5 to 10 days after treatment is begun.

Uses

Acute manic episodes. Lithium has been shown to be effective in controlling acute mania in roughly 80% of people within 1 to 2 weeks after treatment is begun. During the lag period between the start of treatment and the beginning of the therapeutic effect of the medication, clinicians usually treat patients with antipsychotic and sedative agents to control agitation and diminish psychosis.

Bipolar disorder (maintenance therapy). Lithium has proved effective in preventing severe relapses of both manic and depressive episodes in bipolar disorder. It appears to be more effective in preventing mania than depression. Lithium diminishes both the severity of the episodes and the frequency of recurrence.

Recurrent unipolar depression (maintenance therapy). Although the TCAs are currently the treatment of choice for prevention of depressive episodes, increasing attention is being paid to the benefits of lithium for this purpose. Lithium has also been used to potentiate the effects of antidepressants in refractory unipolar depression.

Schizoaffective disorder. Lithium is of limited use in treating this illness, because the affective features are atypical and mixed with symptoms of psychosis. Antipsychotics are probably the treatment of choice in schizoaffective disorder, but lithium is often added to the regimen when an antipsychotic alone does not sufficiently ameliorate the symptoms or prevent recurrent exacerbations.

Other uses. Much research is being done on other psychiatric conditions that may be responsive to lithium. Various cyclic mood disturbances are under consideration, along with impulse disorders, other aggressive states, and unstable personality disorders. It appears that a family history of affective illness and/or a favorable response to lithium in some family member favor a therapeutic response in people with a variety of atypical mood disorders.

Effects

Although lithium takes away the subjective experience of being high and ameliorates manic psychosis and excitement, it has almost no effect on normal people. There is little or no sedation, and no appreciable effect on thinking or motor activities in the nonmanic person. Nevertheless, people who have bipolar disorder (manic-depressive illness) often dislike the medication because it takes away the euphoria that can be a subjectively pleasant aspect of mania.

Lithium is given orally and is rapidly absorbed into the bloodstream. It reaches peak levels in 1 to 3 hours after ingestion. Lithium is distributed throughout the body and is eliminated by the kidneys. Kidney functioning must be monitored throughout treatment. The rate of lithium excretion by the kidney may vary as a result of several factors. Most notably, as sodium intake decreases, lithium retention by the kidney increases. Thus, such variables as diet and the use of diuretics can significantly affect blood levels of lithium and even result in lithium toxicity.

Side effects

The *early side effects* of lithium treatment, which are very common and usually subside within a few days, include the following:

- Gastrointestinal distress, including nausea, vomiting, diarrhea (especially with the slow-release form of lithium carbonate), and stomach pain

- Muscle weakness and the subjective experience of being dazed or tired
- Hand tremor (a fine tremor, in contrast to the more coarse tremor of parkinsonism)
- Increased thirst and frequency of urination

The *later side effects* include the following:

- Persistent hand tremor
- Increased thirst and frequency of urination that may be severe and persistent, and that can be treated by stopping the medication or by carefully adding concurrent treatment with a thiazide diuretic (paradoxical effect)
- Weight gain and/or edema (retention of fluid by the body)
- Precipitation of hypothyroidism or goiter
- Leukocytosis (greater than 12,000/m³), which is common and relatively benign
- EKG changes (common), including T-wave depression and widened QRS complexes
- Kidney abnormalities

Concerning kidney abnormalities, a small proportion (less than 10%) of people develop interstitial nephritis that may be associated with diabetes insipidus: increased thirst, frequent urination, and difficulty in concentrating urine, resulting in loss of large quantities of body water. To prevent this condition, it is wise to monitor people on lithium maintenance by measuring their serum creatinine levels at 3-month intervals; any severe increase in the frequency of urination should be carefully evaluated.

Lithium poisoning

Lithium toxicity is common. It occurs when the amount of lithium in the bloodstream is as little as 50% above therapeutic levels. Mild lithium toxicity can be reversed simply by omitting several doses and then beginning again at a lower dosage when the serum lithium level has fallen to within a nontoxic range and toxic symptoms have remitted. Severe toxicity must be managed in the hospital, usually by osmotic diuresis.
Common causes of an elevated serum lithium level include:

- Overdose
- Sodium or fluid loss (e.g., vomiting, diarrhea, diuretic use)
- Concurrent medical illnesses

A patient who contracts even a minor illness (especially with fever and gastrointestinal symptoms) should let you know immediately and refrain from taking lithium if he or she experiences vomiting or diarrhea. The level of lithium in the blood should be measured at such times to reassess the dosage.

It is important that both you and your patient be aware of the signs of lithium toxicity (see Table 18-11).

Clinical evaluation

Before a patient is started on lithium, the following evaluations must be completed.

Medical history and physical examination. Elicit any history of kidney, cardiovascular, or thyroid disease. Contraindications to treatment with lithium include pregnancy, chronic diarrhea, organic brain syndromes, and old age or severe debilitation. A low-salt diet and the use of diuretics require decreased dosage and closer monitoring of lithium blood levels. Any of the above-mentioned conditions require caution in prescribing lithium.

Baseline laboratory tests. Baseline laboratory tests should include the following:

- Blood urea nitrogen (BUN), creatinine, and urinalysis to assess kidney function
- Complete blood count with differential, since leukocytosis is common in the course of therapy
- Thyroid function tests (T_3, T_4, and TSH). Decreased thyroid functioning can occur during treatment

Table 18-11. The signs of lithium toxicity

Early signs	Late signs
Slurred speech	Impaired consciousness—
Drowsiness	somnolence, confusion, stupor
Muscle weakness	Hypertonic muscles and
Coarse tremor and muscle twitching	fasciculations
Anorexia	Increased deep tendon reflexes
Vomiting and diarrhea	Hyperextension of arms and legs
Ataxia	Seizures
Confusion	Coma
	Death

- Electrolytes, especially sodium, potassium, and calcium. This test is typically most useful if you suspect that your patient may be dehydrated.
- EKG—for people with cardiac symptoms and for those over age 40
- Liver function tests and serum glucose characterization—for people who may have liver disease or who have a history of alcoholism or hypoglycemia

Follow-up laboratory studies for lithium maintenance. During maintenance therapy with lithium, the following studies should be performed periodically as indicated:

- Lithium level every 1 to 2 months
- Serum creatinine every 3 months
- White blood cell count (WBC), T_3, T_4, TSH, and urinalysis every 3 to 6 months

Administration

Lithium comes in three oral forms: regular lithium carbonate, a slow-release form of lithium carbonate, and a liquid form of lithium citrate. Lithium carbonate is the most commonly used preparation in the United States and comes in 300-mg tablets and capsules. Lithium is commonly given in divided doses, generally two or three times daily (the slow-release form can be given twice a day). Dosages are individually determined for each person according to his or her serum level of lithium. Therapeutic blood levels are generally 1.0 to 1.25 meq/l in acute mania, and 0.6 to 1.0 meq/l for long-term maintenance. Note that samples for determining blood levels are drawn approximately 12 hours after the last dose of medication (and usually before the first dose in the morning); blood levels are higher and change rapidly in the hours immediately following ingestion.

Acute mania. Treatment usually begins with a dose of 300 to 600 mg of lithium carbonate per day (less in small or elderly people). Measure serum levels every 2 to 3 days, raising the dosage until serum levels reach 1.25 meq/l or until signs of toxicity develop. Some people require as little as 300 mg per day to reach a therapeutic level, while others require as much as 3,600 mg per day. After 1 to 2 weeks, when mania subsides, it is usually necessary to lower the dosage, since the patient will no longer require as much medication and may become toxic. A level of 0.6 to 1.0 meq/l will usually suffice for maintenance beyond the acute manic phase.

Maintenance

Research data indicate that lithium is somewhat more effective in the prevention of manic episodes than depressive episodes. Lithium has been clearly demonstrated to decrease both the severity and the frequency with which mania and depression recur in bipolar patients. It has also been shown to prevent depressive episodes in some apparently unipolar patients.

Who is a candidate for lithium maintenance? Only those people who have a history of *recurrent* manic and depressive episodes. Those who have suffered a first episode may be taken off lithium and observed, because subsequent attacks may never occur or may not recur for many years.

Lithium maintenance involves careful monitoring of blood levels (monthly, or at least bimonthly) to prevent toxicity. Toxic blood levels range from mild toxicity at 1.5 to 2.0 meq/l, to a potentially lethal condition at 4.0 meq/l or greater. *Remember: Lithium treatment should be discontinued and blood levels checked immediately whenever the dosage is adjusted, when any signs of toxicity develop, when hypomanic or depressive symptoms occur, and when any but the most trivial illness develops.*

Anticonvulsants

Although anticonvulsants have been the mainstays of pharmacological treatment of epileptic disorders for many years, their use in the treatment of psychiatric disorders is relatively new. At this time, anticonvulsants are used as second-line or adjunctive treatments in a variety of mental illnesses, particularly mania.

Carbamazepine

Carbamazepine (Tegretol) has been found to be effective in the treatment of acute mania and may also prevent recurrent manic episodes. It is especially useful for patients who do not respond to treatment with lithium, or for whom the side effects of lithium are intolerable. Some investigators report that bipolar patients who are "rapid cyclers" (that is, who have four or more episodes of mania or depression per year) or who have frequent recurrent episodes of mania respond better to carbamazepine than to lithium. Carbamazepine also has been shown to be effective as an adjunct to lithium in manic patients who respond only partially to lithium. Carbamazepine probably is less effective in the treatment and prevention of depression, but reports indicate that a minority of depressed patients may respond favorably to this treatment. It has not been demonstrated to be as effective in treating schizoaffective disorder or atypical psychosis. Recently, a controlled study of patients with borderline personality disorder showed that carbamazepine was associated with limited improvement in impulsivity and behavioral dyscontrol. However, further work in this area is needed to substantiate these findings.

Treatment usually begins with 200 mg orally twice daily. The dosage can be increased by 200 mg per day every 5 to 7 days until a plasma level of 6 to 12 micrograms/ml is obtained. The maximum dosage recommended is 1,200 mg per day, but some clinicians have used higher doses guided by blood level assays with good effect. Because carbamazepine can induce its own metabolism, plasma levels may decline slowly over the first weeks to months of treatment, and the dosage may need to be readjusted.

Carbamazepine has potentially serious hematological and hepatic toxicity, so patients on this medication must be carefully monitored to prevent life-threatening complications. Patients rarely (less than 1 in 50,000) develop aplastic anemia, but 10% develop reversible leukopenia. Thrombocytopenia and persistent leukopenia develop in 2% of the patients. Hepatotoxicity usually involves a hypersensitivity hepatitis that occurs several weeks into treatment and is manifested by elevated serum glutamic-oxaloacetic transaminase (SGOT), serum glutamic-pyruvic transaminase (SGPT), and lactate dehydrogenase (LDH). This is generally reversible once the medication is discontinued, but if carbamazepine is reintroduced in hypersensitive patients, as many as 25% may die. Patients should be monitored with CBC and platelet counts every 2 weeks for the first 3 months, and every 3 months thereafter. In addition, SGOT, SGPT, LDH, and alkaline phosphatase should be monitored every month for the first 2 months and every 3 months thereafter.

Minor autonomic side effects of carbamazepine include blurred vision, constipation, and dry mouth. Some patients also report drowsiness, ataxia, and dizziness.

Valproate

The use of valproic acid (Depakene) and sodium valproate (Depakote) in psychiatric disorders has been largely experimental to date, and most of the studies on these medications are uncontrolled. However, valproate has been reported to be effective in treating manic episodes in bipolar and schizoaffective patients. It is less effective in depression and schizophrenia. Some clinicians report that it may potentiate the effects of lithium, antidepressants, and antipsychotics when used in combination with these medications.

Clonazepam

Clonazepam (Klonopin) is a very potent long-acting benzodiazepine (see above) with antiepileptic properties. It has been used experimentally in treating patients with panic disorder and mania. It appears to be about as effective as alprazolam in the treatment of panic disorder. Clonazepam has a much longer half-life than alprazolam, thus reducing the likelihood of withdrawal symptoms. In this respect, clonazepam may be superior to alprazolam. Clonazepam also may be a safe adjunct to neuroleptic treatment of acute mania and lithium maintenance of manic patients, given the risk of tardive dyskinesia inherent in high-dose and long-term use of neuroleptics.

Antianxiety Agents

Anxiety is a symptom we have all experienced. In many cases, it is adaptive to the situations in which we find ourselves. However, anxiety can become overwhelming and incapacitating, and leave people unable to carry on with their daily lives. This has prompted an age-old search for medications that alleviate anxiety.

Virtually any sedating drug will diminish the effects of acute anxiety, but many sedatives (e.g., the barbiturates) significantly impair one's ability to think, to perceive and react to stimuli rapidly, and to exercise normal motor skills. Most sedatives are also highly addictive; many are widely abused and have such low lethal doses that suicide with these agents is common.

The antianxiety agents are among the most frequently prescribed medications in medicine, primarily because the demand for relief from anxiety is great and because antianxiety agents are safer than sedative-hypnotics. The former cause less impairment of cognitive and motor functioning, dependence is relatively uncommon, and they are much less lethal when taken in overdose.

The major class of antianxiety agents used in clinical settings is the *benzodiazepines*. A new antianxiety agent, *buspirone*, is chemically unrelated to all other anxiolytics, and in preliminary studies it appears to have fewer side effects and adverse effects than the benzodiazepines.

Antianxiety agents do not cure anxiety, they only alleviate it. Thus, these agents are not the treatment of choice for long-term treatment of psychiatric disorders. They are most clearly indicated for *short-term* treatment of transient forms of anxiety. Because most people tolerate anxiety without becoming dysfunctional, antianxiety agents are indicated only when the patient becomes in some way disabled by his or her distress.

Why the emphasis on short-term treatment, and only when the

anxiety is disabling? First, because the medications are not without hazards, especially when given for long periods of time. Some people become tolerant to the antianxiety, euphoriant, and disinhibiting effects of these medications (with the possible exception of buspirone) and may abuse them to achieve the desired effects as tolerance develops. Psychological and physical dependence thus become potential hazards in long-term treatment.

Second, antianxiety agents may mask the symptom instead of treating the disease. Physicians who prescribe these medications as substitutes for time, concern, and support, do their patients a disservice.

How Do They Work?

The benzodiazepines alleviate anxiety through mechanisms that remain unclear, despite considerable research into this area of pharmacology. Investigators have demonstrated the existence of benzodiazepine receptors in the brain that are functionally linked with the receptors for gamma-aminobutyric acid (GABA) and with chloride ion channels. GABA is the major inhibitory neurotransmitter in the brain (see Chapter 8). Activation of the benzodiazepine receptor potentiates the actions of GABA, which, in turn, decrease neuronal activity. The mechanism by which buspirone exerts its anxiolytic effect is unclear.

Uses

The following are the major psychiatric disorders for which treatment with antianxiety agents is indicated.

Acute situational anxiety. Particularly when anxiety lies in the anticipation of some dreaded situation, these agents provide temporary relief. An important use is in relieving anxiety secondary to physical illness and prior to diagnostic, medical, or surgical procedures.

Generalized anxiety disorder. This more pervasive disorder is also effectively treated with antianxiety agents. They relieve both anxiety and somatic symptoms (e.g., gastrointestinal distress, palpitations). Psychotherapy of some variety is usually offered as well to help patients understand and manage situations that provoke anxiety. Medication is best used on a short-term basis as an adjunct to other forms of treatment.

Phobic disorders. Antianxiety agents do not treat the primary problem in the phobic disorders, but they do alleviate the concomitant anxiety and are useful in conjunction with other types of therapy, such as behavior modification (see Chapter 8).

Panic disorder. Panic attacks are effectively treated and prevented by certain high-potency benzodiazepines, particularly alprazolam, clonazepam, and lorazepam. Given that panic disorder may require prolonged pharmacological treatment, some clinicians prefer to use a tricyclic antidepressant (e.g., desipramine) to avoid the risk of dependence. However, a benzodiazepine often is used in conjunction with an antidepressant at the start of treatment, because the benzodiazepine can provide immediate relief from panic and anxiety while the patient waits for the antidepressant to take effect.

Insomnia. Benzodiazepines are useful in treating insomnia, but on a short-term or intermittent basis. The hypnotic effect of these medications typically wanes as patients become tolerant to them, so nightly use over long periods results in tolerance and the need for higher doses to achieve the desired effect. These medications are best used when insomnia is the result of a temporary situation (e.g., anxiety over upcoming surgery). They are a helpful adjunct to antidepressant therapy during the initial phases of treatment, when insomnia may be incapacitating and the antidepressant has not yet had time to exert its effect.

Drug withdrawal syndromes. The substitution of a long-acting benzodiazepine for the abused drug is an effective means of withdrawal from some agents, particularly alcohol, barbiturates, or nonbarbiturate sedatives, as well as for the treatment of delirium tremens.

Organic brain syndromes. Antianxiety agents can reduce dangerous hyperactivity and excitement, for example, in LSD hallucinosis and Alzheimer's disease, and in agitated elderly patients without Alzheimer's disease.

Extrapyramidal side effects. Antianxiety agents are somewhat useful in treating akathisia caused by antipsychotics.

Antianxiety agents are less useful in treating somatoform disorders, personality disorders, and severe depression. They are of little use in schizophrenia and other psychoses, but are sometimes used temporarily for sedation and to reduce doses of antipsychotics in patients with acute psychoses or mania.

Benzodiazepines

The benzodiazepines are the most commonly used antianxiety agents—so common, in fact, that Valium and Xanax have become household words. Benzodiazepines currently licensed for use in the United States for treatment of anxiety and insomnia are shown in Table 18-12.

All the benzodiazepines have similar effects, as follows.

Table 18-12. Characteristics of the benzodiazepines

Generic name	Trade name	Duration of action	Average daily dosage (mg)	Comments
Chlordiazepoxide	Librium and others	Long-acting	15–100	
Diazepam	Valium	Long-acting	6–30	Muscle-relaxant properties
Clorazepate	Tranxene, Azene	Long-acting	15–60	
Prazepam	Centrax, Verstran	Long-acting	20–60	
Flurazepam	Dalmane	Long-acting	15–30	Used primarily at bedtime for sleep
Halazepam	Paxipam	Long-acting	60–160	
Lorazepam	Ativan	Short-acting	2–6	Used to treat akathisia
Oxazepam	Serax	Short-acting	30–120	
Alprazolam	Xanax	Short-acting	0.75–1.5	Possible antidepressant effect and efficacy in panic disorders
Clonazepam	Klonopin	Long-acting	1.5–20	Prevention of petit mal, akinetic, and minor motor seizures
Temazepam	Restoril	Short-acting	30	
Triazolam	Halcion	Very short-acting	0.125–0.25	

Disinhibition. The benzodiazepines block conditioned fear and avoidance responses. This may be why the benzodiazepines cause increased hostility and aggressive behavior in some people.

Sedation. All the benzodiazepines are sedating. Although flurazepam (Dalmane) is highly touted for its usefulness as a hypnotic, studies have shown flurazepam to have no significant advantage over other benzodiazepines in producing sleep, and its very long duration of action often leads to a "hangover." People taking benzodiazepines must be cautioned about driving and about the use of alcohol. (The sedative effects of the benzodiazepines in combination with alcohol are greater than either alone.)

Anticonvulsant activity. Some benzodiazepines are used effectively in the treatment (diazepam) and prevention (clonazepam) of seizures.

Because their effects are similar, the major clinical difference among these medications is in their duration of action. Long-acting compounds (see Table 18-12) or their active metabolites are cleared from the body slowly and can build up to high levels in the bloodstream when taken over days or weeks. Because the antianxiety effects of long-acting agents last about as long as those of the short-acting compounds, the long-acting agents are given in frequent divided doses, despite their slow elimination from the body. Long-acting agents are metabolized and eliminated particularly slowly in people who have liver disease and in the elderly. Short-acting agents may have an advantage over long-acting ones in that, because they are more rapidly cleared from the body, they do not exert effects on the CNS much beyond the period of desired sedation and disinhibition. They may, however, be more addicting.

Side effects. *Sedation* is an effect that may or may not be desirable for patients on benzodiazepines. Patients must be warned that the medication may make them drowsy and impair their performance driving an automobile, operating machinery, or performing complex mental tasks. They must also be warned against taking other CNS depressants (particularly alcohol).

Memory impairment occurs with benzodiazepine use, particularly intravenous use during surgical procedures. However, oral benzodiazepine use may also cause memory impairment and dissociative reactions in the first several hours after each dose. (This problem has often been associated with triazolam.) Patients must be warned of this potential side effect.

Physical dependence is among the most worrisome of the untoward effects of the benzodiazepines. In rare instances, if these medications are precipitously discontinued after continuous use of high doses, a severe withdrawal syndrome can result, which includes hyperpyrexia, seizures, psychosis, and death. Whether such withdrawal can follow use of benzodiazepines at usual dosages is controversial. Some investigators have described a low-dose dependency that is followed by a mild withdrawal that includes muscle cramps, tachycardia, hypertension, panic, insomnia, anxiety, impaired memory and concentration, and perceptual disturbances. Withdrawal may begin within a day or up to a week after discontinuing the medication, and it may continue for weeks or months. Alprazolam and high doses of triazolam have been implicated in the occurrence of seizures following withdrawal of treatment, but it is not clear whether these two agents are more prone than other medications in this class to induce serious withdrawal symptoms.

To prevent withdrawal, it is best to taper benzodiazepines slowly over weeks to months, once they have been used for more than 2 or 3 months continuously. The dose can be reduced by 10% per week. Patients often find the last few doses difficult to discontinue and may require increased support from you as they do so.

Pregnancy and breast feeding are conditions that call for avoidance of benzodiazepine use when possible. The benzodiazepines may cause an increase in the incidence of congenital malformations, and they are passed on in breast milk.

Administration. Benzodiazepines may be given orally, intramuscularly (with the exception of diazepam), or intravenously. Most medication is given in oral form to outpatients. However, an agent such as lorazepam can be given intramuscularly for agitation when indicated. Intravenous administration is usually reserved for acute seizure activity, because one rare complication of this route of administration is respiratory depression or arrest.

Oral benzodiazepines are very safe in that it is virtually impossible to commit suicide by using one of these medications alone. However, they can be lethal when taken in combination with alcohol, other CNS depressants, or tricyclic antidepressants.

Buspirone

As noted above, buspirone is a new medication that is chemically unrelated to other anxiolytics. It is relatively nonsedating and does not interact with or show cross-tolerance to other sedating drugs (e.g., alcohol, barbiturates, benzodiazepines), so buspirone may be even less dangerous in overdose than the benzodiazepines. It does not impair motor performance and so can be used safely when operating potentially dangerous machinery. It does not appear to be prone to abuse. Because it does not exhibit cross-tolerance with other sedative-hypnotics, buspirone cannot be used to suppress withdrawal symptoms from drugs such as alcohol, or from the benzodiazepines themselves. (This latter fact is important to remember when switching a patient from a benzodiazepine to buspirone: withdrawal is a hazard unless benzodiazepines are tapered slowly.) Side effects of buspirone are few: primarily restlessness, nervousness, and occasional mild extrapyramidal symptoms.

The antianxiety effects of buspirone take approximately 2 weeks to appear once treatment is begun. Patients usually are maintained on 15 to 30 mg per day, typically starting at 5 mg tid, and the dosage may be increased by 5 mg every 2 or 3 days until a favorable response is seen. Maximum recommended daily dosage is 60 mg. Buspirone has proved both effective and safe in clinical trials, but wider experience with this medication over the next several years will provide more information about its clinical utility.

ELECTROCONVULSIVE THERAPY

Electroconvulsive therapy (ECT or "shock" therapy) may well be the most wrongly maligned treatment in medicine. Popular literature has depicted ECT as a repressive and cruel procedure. In one state, groups have even worked to outlaw it. Oddly enough, ECT is one of the most humane and most efficacious treatments available in mental health care. Its bad press stems largely from outdated information about how ECT is administered, and public concerns about the authoritarian aspects of the mental health system.

ECT involves the induction of a grand mal seizure by means of an electrical pulse through the brain. Each treatment consists of the induction of one seizure while the person is under anesthesia, and a course of ECT consists of several such treatments.

How Does Electroconvulsive Therapy Work?

As with other somatic therapies in psychiatry, we do not know the mechanism by which ECT exerts its therapeutic effects. ECT has been shown to affect a variety of neurotransmitters in the brain, including GABA, norepinephrine, serotonin, and dopamine. It also affects endogenous opiates. Also currently under investigation are the effects of ECT on regional cerebral blood flow.

Uses

Major depressive episodes. ECT is a uniquely advantageous treatment for severe major depressive episodes, because 1) it works more quickly than antidepressants to relieve symptoms (often within a few days); 2) it is safer for many frail, elderly people who have heart disease; and 3) it is probably more effective than TCAs in the treatment of depression, especially psychotic depression characterized by paranoid or somatic delusions. Major depressive episodes accompanied by severe vegetative melancholic disturbances respond remarkably well, with an improvement rate of 80% to 90%. ECT is effective for many severely depressed people who do not respond to medication. It is particularly useful when acute suicidal ideation and intent make rapid relief a priority; in pregnancy, when medication is less safely used; and in catatonia. However, ECT is not used in "neurotic" or "characterologic" depression (i.e., dysthymia).

Acute mania. ECT has been shown to be as effective in treating acute mania as in treating severe depression. Particularly for manic patients who are at risk of harming or exhausting themselves, ECT can give rapid relief.

Schizophrenia. Efficacy of ECT in schizophrenia has not been demonstrated, but some acutely ill schizophrenic patients with affective and catatonic symptoms may respond to ECT about as well as they do to antipsychotics. ECT is often used when other treatments have failed with schizophrenic patients.

Other disorders have not responded well to ECT, although the treatment has been tried in a wide variety of illnesses.

Administration

During the 1930s through 1950s, ECT was given to people who were awake and not premedicated. This made many patients fearful prior to the procedure and created an increased risk of fractures and bone dislocations because of violent movement during the seizure. Most ECT is now given with three types of medication prior to the treatment: 1) atropine, to reduce secretions; 2) general anesthesia with a very short-acting barbiturate (e.g., methohexital sodium), to reduce anxiety and discomfort; and 3) a depolarizing muscle relaxant (e.g., succinylcholine), to eliminate complications of the convulsion itself.

ECT is administered either *bilaterally* or *unilaterally*. That is, the two scalp electrodes that deliver the electrical stimulus are either placed over separate cerebral hemispheres or over the same (usually the nondominant) cerebral hemisphere. Although there is some evidence that unilateral ECT causes less memory loss than bilateral ECT, unilateral ECT may not be consistently as effective as bilateral ECT.

When the patient is fully anesthetized, the electrical stimulus is applied, usually 70 to 110 volts for 0.1 to 0.5 seconds at an amperage ranging from 200 to 1,600 milliamperes (mA). Sine-wave stimulation has traditionally been used, but newer ECT devices use brief square-wave pulse stimulation that can initiate a grand mal seizure with significantly less electrical energy and may therefore be more desirable. The tonic phase of the seizure begins immediately and lasts for about 10 seconds. Respiration returns to normal within a minute or two, and the person gradually recovers from the postconvulsive coma. The anesthetist administers oxygen to the patient during the procedure to prevent brain hypoxia.

The number of ECT treatments needed for each person is gauged individually according to the therapeutic response. Depressed people usually require an average of six to eight treatments. Treatments are commonly given three or four times a week (usually every other day).

When the patient has apparently achieved a maximal response— that is, when additional treatments yield no further beneficial effect—it is customary to give two or three additional treatments to help prevent relapse, although the efficacy of this practice remains to be proven. Following a course of ECT for depression, patients should be maintained on an antidepressant or lithium.

Preparations for Performing Electroconvulsive Therapy

Obtain informed consent. Explain the reasons for selecting this treatment, as well as the anticipated benefits and potential risks of ECT.

Medical history and physical examination. Pay particular attention to any history of cardiovascular disease, which may increase the risks involved in ECT. Severe high blood pressure may require increased medication to minimize the possibility of a stroke during ECT. People with musculoskeletal injuries may require additional muscle relaxants during the procedure. The only absolute contraindication to ECT is a space-occupying cerebral lesion that causes increased intracranial pressure, because ECT may cause a transient increase in intracranial pressure and might cause brain-stem herniation. A history of recent treatment with catecholamine-depleting medications (e.g., reserpine) is also a contraindication. ECT is particularly useful for elderly people, who frequently have cardiac and other major medical problems. The clinician must judge whether the risks of ECT are greater than the risks of allowing severe depression and agitation to go untreated. Often, ECT carries the lesser risk, and the person's response to treatment can be life-saving.

Laboratory workup. This workup includes routine blood chemistries (SMA-12), CBC, urinalysis, chest X-ray, spinal X-ray, EKG, and electroencephalogram (EEG).

Pretreatment regimen. If possible, all medications should be discontinued shortly before and during the course of ECT. If this is impossible, the dosages should be reduced as much as possible, particularly for medications that have cardiovascular effects or side effects. Lithium should not be used concurrently with ECT, because there is evidence of increased neurotoxicity with this combination. The patient should take nothing by mouth for 8 hours before treatment, to reduce the risk of vomiting and aspiration.

Side Effects

The most common side effects of ECT are shown in Table 18-13 and described below:

- Memory loss
- Headaches, which are responsive to acetaminophen or ibuprofen
- Muscle aches, which are transient

The acute brain syndrome (i.e., memory loss) that follows ECT is the most common and most widely publicized of its side effects. This syndrome consists of a confused state, variable intellectual impairment, and amnesia that may persist for several months following a course of treatment. The amnesia involves both memory for recent events (retrograde) and difficulty in retaining newly learned information (anterograde). The

Table 18-13. Common side effects of electroconvulsive therapy

Most common
  Memory loss
  Headaches
  Muscle aches
Less common
  Weight gain
  Amenorrhea
  Increase in permeability of the blood-brain barrier
  Systemic hypertension
  Apnea
  Cardiac arrhythmias

amnesia gradually lessens over the weeks following treatment and resolves completely in 6 to 9 months. People who have received unilateral
ECT tend to complain less of memory impairment than those who
received bilateral ECT. The question of whether memory impairment
persists beyond a few months is unresolved, but controlled studies have
failed to show permanent measurable memory loss or cognitive impairment in people who receive a course of ECT.

The less common side effects of ECT include the following:

- Weight gain, possibly due to treatment of anorexia
- Amenorrhea or other menstrual changes, lasting up to several
  months
- Transient increased permeability of the blood-brain barrier, which
  may alter the effects of certain medications
- Marked but transient systemic hypertension, which occurs rarely
  as a part of the generalized seizure
- Apnea following treatments (respiratory support should always
  be available)
- Cardiac arrhythmias—primarily premature ventricular contractions that occur during the brief period of slowed heartbeat that
  normally follows the seizure. This should be prevented by the use
  of atropine. However, cardiac arrests do very rarely occur during
  treatment, and resuscitation equipment must be on hand.

Risks Versus Benefits

Obviously, ECT is not an innocuous procedure, if only because of the
risks inherent in the use of general anesthesia. Although death due to
cardiac arrest occurs in fewer than 1 in 10,000 treatments, it nevertheless
constitutes an important risk. And memory impairment can be discon-
certing and even frightening.

Yet ECT is the most effective treatment available for serious melancholic depression, and its onset of action is more rapid than that of any of
the antidepressants or lithium. Large-scale studies have shown that the
risks of ECT are significantly lower than the risks of untreated severe
depression.

ECT is most clearly indicated under the following circumstances:

- In certain types of severe depression, e.g., depression accompanied
  by somatic delusions
- When other treatments for depression are likely to be more toxic
  to the patient, for example, in frail, elderly people who have severe
  heart disease

- When depression is life-threatening—as with actively suicidal people—and rapid remission is of the utmost importance

The risks of not using this relatively safe treatment must be weighed carefully. Unfortunately, the bad press that ECT has received has at times made patient acceptance of the procedure a problem. In such cases, other forms of treatment (e.g., TCAs) may be tried first, and ECT used as a last resort.

BIBLIOGRAPHY

Appleton WS: Practical Clinical Psychopharmacology, 3rd Edition. Baltimore, MD, Williams & Wilkins, 1988

Ayd FJ Jr (ed): International Drug Therapy Newsletter. Baltimore, MD, Ayd Medical Communications. (A monthly newsletter containing information on new research and use of psychotropic medications.)

Baldessarini RJ: Chemotherapy in Psychiatry: Principles and Practice. 2nd Edition. Cambridge, MA, Harvard University Press, 1985

Cade JFJ: Lithium salts in the treatment of psychotic excitement. Med J Aust 2:349–352, 1949

Cowdry RW, Gardner DL: Pharmacotherapy of borderline personality disorder: alprazolam, carbamazepine, trifluoperazine, and tranylcypromine. Arch Gen Psychiatry 45:111–119, 1988

Gilman AG, Goodman LS, Gilman A (eds): The Pharmacological Basis of Therapeutics, 7th Edition. New York, Macmillan, 1985

McElroy SL, Pope HG Jr (eds): Use of Anticonvulsants in Psychiatry: Recent Advances. Clifton, NJ, Oxford Health Care, 1988

Schatzberg AF, Cole JO: Manual of Clinical Psychopharmacology. Washington, DC, American Psychiatric Press, 1986

Silver JM, Yudofsky SC: Psychopharmacology and electroconvulsive therapy, in The American Psychiatric Press Textbook of Psychiatry. Edited by Talbott JA, Hales RE, Yudofsky SC. Washington, DC, American Psychiatric Press, 1988, pp 767–853

Squire LP, Chace PM: Memory function six to nine months after electroconvulsive therapy. Arch Gen Psychiatry 32:1557–1564, 1975

Weiner RD: The psychiatric use of electrically induced seizures. Am J Psychiatry 136:1507–1517, 1979

Appendix A

Sample Psychiatric Evaluation

The following is an example of an initial psychiatric evaluation summary of the kind described in Chapter 3. Each psychiatric facility has its own format for such write-ups, and you should follow the form used in the particular institution in which you work. The sample will give you a general idea of how these summaries are done. It is an outpatient evaluation; you may find that inpatient write-ups are more detailed.

HOSPITAL OUTPATIENT CLINIC EVALUATION SUMMARY AND TREATMENT PLAN

Patient: Doe, John

Evaluator: Mary Smith, Psychology Intern

Date: October 20, 1989

Identifying Data:

Mr. Doe is a 25-year-old single man who is a third-year law student at Eastern University. He lives by himself in an apartment in Boston and was referred to the Clinic by a friend who had been in treatment here 2 years ago.

Chief Complaint:

"I feel all screwed up. . . . I've got so many decisions to make in the next few months and all I'm doing is getting high."

History of Present Problem:

Mr. Doe dates his current difficulties as beginning 3 months ago, when he broke up with the woman with whom he had been living for the past year. The woman, Joan, moved out, and "had been dissatisfied with me because she said I wasn't giving her enough." In addition, in the last 8 weeks he has had increased distress from a duodenal ulcer (first diagnosed in 1977). He is being treated for this medical problem by Dr. Michael Jones, internist.

The patient is "worried and indecisive" about his future. He expects to graduate from law school this May but is pessimistic about finding a job. He is also indecisive about what legal area he would like to work in. He worries that he won't pass his bar exams this summer.

Mr. Doe reports awakening at 4:00 A.M. after 4 hours of sleep most every day for the past 2 months and is unable to get back to sleep. He feels more depressed in the early morning. He has been smoking two or three marijuana joints per day over the past 8 months, and states he feels more able to handle day-to-day responsibilities when he is high. Mr. Doe reports not feeling hungry in recent weeks, and he has lost 12 pounds in 2 months. At times he has had vague thoughts of suicide but has no plans to hurt himself and no history of self-destructive behavior. He reports frequent periods of weeping when he is alone and thinks of the loss of Joan. He notes a loss of interest in his schoolwork and in sports, and a general feeling of lethargy when he is not high. He is unable to reduce his use of marijuana, even though he states he wishes to do so. He denies any previous history of depressive symptoms and denies any history of euphoria, increased activity, or disordered thinking. He has had no previous psychiatric treatment.

Past History:

Mr. Doe is the only child born to parents of Scottish descent. Father, age 52, is a high school graduate and a machinist at a firm in Boston where he has been employed for the past 28 years. Mother, age 50, is employed as a part-time secretary and has been working on a part-time basis since the patient was 12 years old. Both mother and father are "hard workers." He continues to see parents at their home for dinner about once a month.

His earliest memory is at age 4, when he felt "very frightened and alone" during a hospitalization for a tonsillectomy. During preschool and latency years, patient and father often went on camping trips together, and he reports feeling closer to father. As a child, Mr. Doe received some instruction in the Presbyterian Church, but says religion was never that important in his life.

In elementary school and high school, Mr. Doe always received above-average grades. He paid great attention to detail in all his school assignments and at times was ridiculed by his peers for his overzealousness. In elementary school he was friendly with several boys, and was very active in Little League baseball and Boy Scouts. Mr. Doe began to date girls at age 16. He had several brief heterosexual relationships that ended as a result of his being "overbearing, demanding, and too controlling." He notes that he relates to women in this way when he finds himself getting "too close."

In college he remained very devoted to his studies, often preferring to study rather than to take part in social activities. He received his B.A. in English from Boston University in 1982 and hoped to gain admission to a prestigious law school. In college he received only average grades despite considerable effort, and was "disappointed" that he was unable to gain admission to a more prestigious law school. Both parents, especially father, always took great pride in Mr. Doe's academic achievements. Mr. Doe is the first college graduate in his extended family.

Family Psychiatric History:

Positive for depression: maternal grandfather suffered one episode of depression at age 65, which the patient believes resolved during a brief psychiatric hospitalization that included "shock treatments."

No other family history of affective illness, psychosis, or drug or alcohol abuse.

Medical History:

Negative except for duodenal ulcer (see above). Internist's report has been requested and will be forthcoming. Patient currently takes antacids infrequently, as needed for gastrointestinal discomfort, but no other prescribed or over-the-counter medications.

Drug and Alcohol History:

Marijuana use as noted above. Also drinks four or five beers per week.

No other current drug use. Experimented with LSD and "mushrooms" on several occasions in college.

Mental Status:

Mr. Doe presented as a neatly dressed man who looked his stated age of 25. He made little eye contact throughout the interview and appeared mildly anxious. Speech was clear, normal in rate, and somewhat monotonous in tone. He reported feeling "down in the dumps" and appeared sad, but affect varied little with thought content. He showed no evidence of a thought disorder, and no perceptual distortions. He reported vague suicidal ideation without any plan for harming himself, and denied any homicidal ideation. He was alert and oriented to time, place, and person. Concentration (digit span), memory, and judgment appeared to be within normal limits, as was his ability to interpret proverbs abstractly. He related to the interviewer in a formal and deferential manner.

Formulation:

Mr. Doe presents with a history of depression including anhedonia, lethargy, early morning awakening, and anorexia with weight loss over the past 2 months. He also reports continuous heavy marijuana use over the past 8 months. In recent weeks he has experienced difficulty doing his schoolwork and has lost interest in his usual social and recreational activities. All of this has occurred subsequent to losing his girlfriend and as he faces graduation from law school.

His clear depressive symptomatology over the past 2 months is complicated by marijuana abuse, and the extent to which cannabis has exacerbated his loss of motivation is unclear. A positive family history of affective disorder, as well as the presence of vegetative signs, suggests a significant biological component to this depressive episode and possible responsiveness to antidepressant medication.

His current symptoms occur in the context of more chronic emotional difficulties, particularly indecisiveness, difficulties with intimacy, and concerns about his own adequacy and self-worth. He is accustomed to being an achiever, and sees himself as falling short of his high standards for performance. The loss of his girlfriend and his fears about finding employment as graduation nears seem to have precipitated the present crisis. His usual obsessional defenses (intellectualization, isolation of affect), "self-medication" with cannabis, and his highly organized and somewhat rigid style of dealing with the world have not been successful in warding off his current depression.

Mr. Doe suffers from vegetative symptoms of depression, apparently precipitated by recent environmental stresses. He also reports long-standing emotional difficulties that impair his work and social life. Given this picture, a combination of psychotherapy and pharmaco-therapy may be an effective treatment plan. Career counseling might help to alleviate some of his anxiety about future employment. It will be important to keep Dr. Jones informed of the patient's treatment, in order to coordinate Mr. Doe's medical and psychiatric care.

Diagnosis:

Axis I	296.20	Major depression, Single Episode
	304.30	Cannabis dependence,continuous
Axis II		Obsessive-compulsive traits
Axis III		Duodenal ulcer
Axis IV		Psychosocial stressors

      a. Recent loss of girlfriend

      b. Increased academic pressures

      c. Fear of being unable to find employment as an attorney after graduation

      Severity: 4-Moderate

Axis V   Highest level of adaptive functioning past year: 3-Good

Treatment Plan:

1. Once-weekly individual psychotherapy to focus on patient's substance abuse, career and academic concerns, and difficulty in maintaining gratifying interpersonal relationships.
2. Referral for psychopharmacology consultation to assess suitability for treatment with antidepressant medication.
3. Referral to counselor at Careeer Planning Bureau at Eastern University to assist him in his job search.
4. Obtaining patient's written permission to speak with Michael Jones, M.D., regarding psychiatric and medical treatment.

_____

Mary Smith, Psychology Intern

_____

Frieda Mason, M.D., Supervisor

Appendix B

Table of Commonly Abused Drugs

Class	Trade name* (or source)	Street names
Opioids		
morphine	morphine sulfate	dope, M, Miss Emma, morpho, white stuff
heroin	none	H, hard stuff, horse, junk, skag, smack
hydromorphone	Dilaudid	DL's
oxymorphone	Numorphan	blues
meperidine	Demerol	
methadone hydrochloride	Dolophine	dollys, done
pentazocine	Talwin	
tincture of opium	paregoric	PG, licorice
cough preparations with codeine	Elixir terpin hydrate	schoolboy, blue velvet
	Robitussin A-C	Robby
hydrocodone	Hycodan	
oxycodone	Percodan	Percs

*Many of these drugs are sold under a variety of trade names; only one or two popular examples are used for each.

Source: *A Psychiatric Glossary*, 6th Edition. Edited by Stone EM. Washington, DC, American Psychiatric Association, 1980, pp. 58–62.

Class	Trade name* (or source)	Street names
Nonnarcotic analgesics		
propoxyphene	Darvon	
Barbiturates		barbs, candy, dolls, goofers, peanuts, sleeping pills
amobarbital	Amytal	blue angels, bluebirds, blue devils, blues, lily
pentobarbital	Nembutal	nebbies, yellow bullets, yellow dolls
secobarbital	Seconal	pink lady, red devils, reds, seccy, pinks
phenobarbital	Luminal	phennies, purple hearts
amobarbital/secobarbital	Tuinal	Christmas trees, double-trouble, rainbows, tooies
Other sedative-hypnotics		
glutethimide	Doriden	CIBA's, packs (with codeine)
methaqualone	Quaalude	sopors, ludes
methyprylon	Noludar	
Benzodiazepines		
alprazolam	Xanax	
chlordiazepoxide	Librium	
diazepam	Valium	
lorazepam	Ativan	
oxazepam	Serax	
Central nervous system stimulants		
d, di amphetamine	Biphetamine	black beauties
amphetamine sulfate	Benzedrine	A's, beans, bennies, cartwheels, crossroads, jelly beans, hearts, peaches, whites

---

*Many of these drugs are sold under a variety of trade names; only a single popular example is used for each.

Class	Trade name* (or source)	Street names
amphetamine sulfate/ amobarbital	Dexamyl	greenies
dextroamphetamine sulfate	Dexedrine	brownies, Christmas trees, dexies, hearts, wakeups
methamphetamine hydrochloride	Methedrine	bombit, crank, crystal, meth, speed
methylphenidate hydrochloride	Ritalin	
cocaine hydrochloride cocaine freebase	cocaine	coke, blow, toot, girl, crack, rock, base
chloral hydrate	Noctec	
ethchlorvynol	Placidyl	
paraldehyde	Paral	
scopolamine	Sominex	truth serum
meprobamate	Miltown	

Drugs with hallucinogenic properties

d lysergic acid diethylamide (LSD)	synthetic derivative (ergot fungus)	acid, pink wedges, sandos, sugar cubes, LSD
psilocin/psilocybin	mushroom (*Psilocybe mexicana*)	business man's acid, magic, mushroom
dimethyltryptamine (DMT)	synthetic	DMT, DET, DPT
morning glory seeds	bindweed (*Rivea corymbosa*)	flower power, heavenly blue, pearly gates
mescaline	peyote cactus	barf tea, big chief, buttons, cactus, mesc
methyldimethoxy- amphetamine (DOM)	synthetic (derivative)	STP
myristicin	nutmeg	MMDA
muscarine	mushroom (*Amanita muscaria*)	fly
phencyclidine		angel dust, dust, PCP

*Many of these drugs are sold under a variety of trade names; only a single popular example is used for each.

Class	Trade name* (or source)	Street names
Tetrahydrocannabinoids		
marijuana	*Cannabis sativa* (leaves, flowers)	grass, hay, joints, Mary Jane, pot, reefer, rope, smoke, weed
hashish	*Cannabis sativa*, resin	
Volatile solvents and gases		
benzine	gasoline	
toluol	glue vapor	
carbon tetrachloride	cleaning fluid	
naphtha	cleaning fluid	scrubwoman's kick
amyl nitrite	amyl nitrite	amys, pears, snappers, poppers
nitrous oxide	nitrous oxide	laughing gas, nitrous

*Many of these drugs are sold under a variety of trade names; only a single popular example is used for each.

Appendix C

Global Assessment of Functioning (GAF) Scale

Consider psychological, social, and occupational functioning on a hypothetical continuum of mental health–illness. Do not include impairment in functioning due to physical (or environmental) limitations.

Note: Use intermediate codes when appropriate, e.g., 45, 68, 72.

Code

90
        Absent or minimal symptoms (e.g., mild anxiety before an exam), **good functioning in all areas, interested and involved in a wide range of activities, socially effective, generally satisfied with life, no more than everyday problems or concerns**
81
        (e.g., an occasional argument with family members).

80
        If symptoms are present, they are transient and expectable reactions to psychosocial stressors (e.g., difficulty concentrating after family argument); **no more than slight impairment in social, occupational, or school functioning** (e.g., temporarily
71
        falling behind in school work).

70
        Some mild symptoms (e.g., depressed mood and mild insomnia) **OR some difficulty in social, occupational, or school functioning** (e.g., occasional truancy, or theft within the household), **but generally functioning pretty well, has some mean-**
61
        ingful interpersonal relationships.

60   **Moderate symptoms** (e.g., flat affect and circumstantial speech, occasional panic attacks) **OR moderate difficulty in social, occupational, or school functioning** (e.g., few friends, conflicts
51   with co-workers).

50   **Serious symptoms** (e.g., suicidal ideation, severe obsessional rituals, frequent shoplifting) **OR any serious impairment in social, occupational, or school functioning** (e.g., no friends,
41   unable to keep a job).

40   **Some impairment in reality testing or communication** (e.g., speech is at times illogical, obscure, or irrelevant) **OR major impairment in several areas, such as work or school, family relations, judgment, thinking, or mood** (e.g., depressed man avoids friends, neglects family, and is unable to work; child frequently beats up younger children, is defiant at home, and is
31   failing at school).

30   **Behavior is considerably influenced by delusions or hallucinations OR serious impairment in communication or judgment** (e.g., sometimes incoherent, acts grossly inappropriately, suicidal preoccupation) **OR inability to function in almost all
21   areas** (e.g., stays in bed all day; no job, home, or friends).

20   **Some danger of hurting self or others** (e.g., suicide attempts without clear expectation of death, frequently violent, manic excitement) **OR occasionally fails to maintain minimal personal hygiene** (e.g., smears feces) **OR gross impairment in
11   communication** (e.g., largely incoherent or mute).

10   **Persistent danger of severely hurting self or others** (e.g., recurrent violence) **OR persistent inability to maintain minimal personal hygiene OR serious suicidal act with clear expecta-
1   tion of death.**

0   **Inadequate information.**

Appendix D

Some Common
Psychotropic Medications
(classified by type)

Type of medication	Generic name	Trade name*
Antianxiety	alprazolam	Xanax
	chlordiazepoxide	Librium
	clonazepam	Klonopin
	clorazepate	Azene, Tranxène
	diazepam	Valium
	flurazepam	Dalmane
	halazepam	Paxipam
	lorazepam	Ativan
	meprobamate	Equanil, Miltown
	oxazepam	Serax
	prazepam	Centrax, Verstran
	tybamate	Solacen, Tybatran
Antidepressant	amitriptyline	Elavil
	amoxapine	Asendin
	bupropion	Wellbutrin
	doxepin	Adapin, Sinequan
	desipramine	Norpramin, Pertofrane
	fluoxetine	Prozac

*Many of these drugs are sold under a variety of trade names; only one or two popular examples are used for each.

Type of medication	Generic name	Trade name*
	imipramine	Tofranil
	isocarboxazid	Marplan
	maprotiline	Ludiomil
	nortriptyline	Aventyl
	phenelzine	Nardil
	protriptyline	Vivactil
	tranylcypromine	Parnate
	trazodone	Desyrel
Antimanic	lithium carbonate	Eskalith, Lithane
	lithium citrate	Cibalith-S
Antipsychotic	acetophenazine	Tindal
	chlorpromazine	Thorazine
	chlorprothixene	Taractan
	fluphenazine	Prolixin
	haloperidol	Haldol
	loxapine	Loxitane
	mesoridazine	Serentil
	molindone	Moban
	perphenazine	Trilafon
	piperacetazine	Quide
	reserpine	Serpasil
	thioridazine	Mellaril
	thiothixene	Navane
	trifluoperazine	Stelazine
Anticonvulsant	carbamazepine	Tegretol

*Many of these drugs are sold under a variety of trade names; only one or two popular examples are used for each.

Appendix E

Trade Names of
Psychotropic Medications

Trade name	Generic name	Type of medication
Adapin	doxepin	Antidepressant
Asendin	amoxapine	Antidepressant
Ativan	lorazepam	Antianxiety
Aventyl	nortriptyline	Antidepressant
Azene	clorazepate	Antianxiety
Centrax	prazepam	Antianxiety
Cibalith-S	lithium citrate	Antimanic
Dalmane	flurazepam	Antianxiety
Daxolin	loxapine	Antipsychotic
Desyrel	trazodone	Antidepressant
Elavil	amitriptyline	Antidepressant
Equanil	meprobamate	Antianxiety
Eskalith	lithium carbonate	Antimanic
Haldol	haloperidol	Antipsychotic
Klonopin	clonazepam	Antianxiety
Librium	chlordiazepoxide	Antianxiety
Lithane	lithium carbonate	Antimanic
Loxitane	loxapine	Antipsychotic
Ludiomil	maprotiline	Antidepressant

Trade name	Generic name	Type of medication
Marplan	isocarboxazid	Antidepressant
Mellaril	thioridazine	Antipsychotic
Miltown	meprobamate	Antianxiety
Moban	molindone	Antipsychotic
Nardil	phenelzine	Antidepressant
Navane	thiothixene	Antipsychotic
Norpramin	desipramine	Antidepressant
Parnate	tranylcypromine	Antidepressant
Paxipam	halazepam	Antianxiety
Pertofrane	desipramine	Antidepressant
Prolixin	fluphenazine	Antipsychotic
Quide	piperacetazine	Antipsychotic
Serax	oxazepam	Antianxiety
Serentil	mesoridazine	Antipsychotic
Serpasil	reserpine	Antipsychotic
Sinequan	doxepin	Antidepressant
Solacen	tybamate	Antianxiety
Stelazine	trifluoperazine	Antipsychotic
Taractan	chlorprothixene	Antipsychotic
Tegretol	carbamezepine	Anticonvulsant
Thorazine	chlorpromazine	Antipsychotic
Tindal	acetophenazine	Antipsychotic
Tofranil	imipramine	Antidepressant
Tranxene	clorazepate	Antianxiety
Trilafon	perphenazine	Antipsychotic
Tybatran	tybamate	Antianxiety
Valium	diazepam	Antianxiety
Verstran	prazepam	Antianxiety
Vivactyl	protriptyline	Antidepressant
Xanax	alprazolam	Antianxiety

Index

A

Abstraction, 72–73
A-L-Acetylmethadol (LAAM)
    opioid withdrawal, 427
Acquired immune deficiency
    syndrome (AIDS)
    and homosexuals, 411
    and intravenous drug use, 425, 428
Acrophobia, 66
Acting out, 31
Acute dystonia
    side effect of antipsychotic
        medications, 532
Adolescence, 29, 279, 284–286
    and depression, 317–318
    and psychiatric history, 46
    and suicide, 319
Adoption studies
    schizophrenia, 90
Adult children of alcoholics (ACOA),
    424
Affect, 61, 62
Affective disorders. *See* Mood
    disorders
Aging
    and dementia, 264

myths about, 233–235
processes, 235–237
and sex, 235, 389–390
See also Elderly
Agitated depression, 114, 543
Agoraphobia, 66, 202, 210
    differential diagnosis, 181
    with panic attacks, 202–203
    treatment, 204–205
Agranulocytosis
    side effect of antipsychotic
        medications, 534
Akathisia
    and mental status examination, 60
    side effect of antipsychotic
        medications, 533
    treatment with antianxiety
        medications, 565
Akinesia
    side effect of antipsychotic
        medications, 532–533
Al-Anon, 424
Alateen, 424
Alcohol amnestic disorder. *See*
    Korsakoff's syndrome
Alcoholic hallucinosis, 372, 421
Alcoholics Anonymous (AA), 423

Alcoholism and alcohol abuse
  abusers, 415
  and antisocial personality disorder,
    167, 169
  and borderline personality disorder,
    175
  causes, 415–417
  and depression, 114, 116
  diagnosis, 418–419
  diagnostic criteria of abuse,
    413–414
  and eating disorders, 439
  and generalized anxiety disorder,
    206
  and Korsakoff's syndrome, 372,
    422–423
  and passive-aggressive personality
    disorder, 188
  prevalence, 417–418
  and suicide, 418
  treatment, 420–425
  and violence, 470
  withdrawal, 420–422
Allergic hepatitis
  side effect of chlorpromazine, 535
Alpha-methyldopa
  and organic mood syndrome,
    depressed type, 374
Alprazolam
  panic disorder, 205
Altruism as a defense mechanism, 33
Alzheimer's disease, 254–256
  antianxiety medications, 565
  and violence, 471
Amitriptyline, 548
  sedating effects, 245
  suicidal ideation, 546
Amnesia, 71–72, 219–220, 372–374
Amnesic aphasia, 61
Amobarbital sodium
  psychogenic amnesia, 220
  psychogenic fugue, 220
  violent patients, 465
Amotivational syndrome and
    marijuana use, 435
Amoxapine, 548
Amphetamine psychosis, 430, 528
Amphetamines
  abuse, 430–431
  attention-deficit hyperactivity
    disorder, 299

and depression, 541
and violence, 470
Amytal interview
  psychogenic amnesia, 220
  psychogenic fugue, 220
Anafranil
  obsessive-compulsive disorder, 214
Anal character, 26–27
Androgen levels and violence, 471
Anergia, 107
Anhedonia, 106
Anomic aphasia, 61
Anorexia nervosa
  course and prognosis, 439
  and depression, 107, 122, 438–439
  differential diagnosis, 226
  etiology, 438
  morbidity and mortality, 439
  profile, 437–438
  treatment, 439–440
Antabuse, 424
Anterograde amnesia, 72, 219, 372
Antiandrogen agents
  sexual deviations, 407
  violence, 476
Antianxiety medications, 563–565
  depression, 124
  generalized anxiety disorder,
    208–209
  mechanisms of action, 517, 564
  multiple personality disorder, 223
  phobias, 211
  somatoform disorders, 229
  terminology, 517
  uses, 564–565
  See also Benzodiazepines
Anticipation as a defense mechanism,
  33
Anticonvulsant medications,
    561–563
  bipolar disorder, 137, 377
  depression as side effect, 243
  effects, 517
  sexual deviations, 407
Antidepressant medications
  agitated depression, 114
  anhedonia from cocaine
    withdrawal, 429
  attention-deficit hyperactivity
    disorder, 300
  bipolar disorder, 137, 138

classes, 541
clinical evaluation, 545–547
commonly used antidepressants
and their characteristics, 548
continuing therapy, 552–553
dementia, 264
dementia syndrome of depression,
260
depression, 105, 123
depression in children, 318
depression in the elderly, 244–246
dexamethasone suppression test,
120–121, 544–545
effects, 516–517
generalized anxiety disorder, 209
maintenance therapy, 553–554
medication interactions, 551
obsessive-compulsive disorder, 213,
214
panic disorder, 205
plasma levels and therapeutic
response, 551–552
posttraumatic stress disorder, 217
prescribing regimen, 551–552
psychotherapy versus medication,
541–544
responsiveness of symptoms to,
542–544
schizophrenia, 99
self-defeating personality disorder,
194
side effects, 245, 374, 550–551
sleep disturbance, 107
somatoform disorders, 229
suicidal ideation, 319, 546–547
tricyclic, 547–554
and violence, 470
Antihypertensive medications
and depression, 243
Antiparkinsonian medications
delusional disorder in the elderly,
241
treatment of extrapyramidal side
effects, 535–536
Antipsychotic medications
anxiety disorders in the elderly,
249
bipolar disorder, 136
and blunted affect, 62
borderline personality disorder,
176

choosing, 536–537
commonly used antipsychotics and
their characteristics, 537
delusional disorder in the elderly,
241
dementia in the elderly, 264
depression, 124
dosages, 529–531
effects, 516–517
indications for using, 527–529
maintenance therapy, 539–540
mania in the elderly, 247
mechanism of action, 527
medication interactions, 536
prescribing, 537–539
responsiveness of symptoms to,
529
schizophrenia, 89, 97–98
schizotypal personality disorder,
159
sexual deviations, 407
side effects, 531–536
types of, 529–531
Antisocial personality disorder
course and prognosis, 170
diagnosis, 167
differential diagnosis, 153, 165,
170–171, 191
epidemiology, 170
etiology, 167–169
and histrionic personality disorder,
160–161
profile, 166–167
treatment, 171–172
and violence, 469–470
Anxiety, 199–200
and depersonalization and
derealization, 66
and depression, 106, 116
illnesses accompanied by, 204
organic anxiety syndrome, 374
of physician in interviews, 15
Anxiety disorders
differential diagnosis, 106, 116,
208, 223
DSM-III-R classification system,
200
in the elderly, 248–250
profile, 199–200
See also specific anxiety disorders
Aphasia, 61

Appearance and mental status, 59–60
Arbitrary inference, 506
Arrhythmias
  side effect of antipsychotic
    medications, 535
Artane
  treatment of extrapyramidal side
    effects, 535–536
Asendin, 548
Assertiveness training for passive-
  aggressive personality disorder,
  188
Associations, 63–64
Atherosclerosis, 256–257
Attention-deficit hyperactivity
  disorder (ADHD)
  diagnosis, 298–299
  profile, 297–298
  treatment, 299–300
Attitude, 74
Atypical psychiatric disorders, 366
Auditory hallucinations, 67
  and alcohol abuse, 372
  and schizophrenia, 81
Autism, 308–309
Aventyl, 548
Aversive conditioning, 503–504
  alcoholism, 424
  paraphilias, 407
Avoidant personality disorder
  course and prognosis, 178
  diagnosis, 177
  differential diagnosis, 156, 178
  epidemiology, 178
  etiology, 177
  profile, 176–177
  treatment, 178–179

B

Barbiturates
  abuse, 431–433
  and depression, 107, 124, 243
  and organic mood syndrome,
    depressed type, 374
  and violence, 470
Bedwetting, 310–311
Behavioral medicine, 326
Behavior and mental status, 59–60
Behavior modification. *See* Behavior
  therapy

Behavior therapy
  agoraphobia, 205
  alcoholics, 424
  described, 486, 500–504
  functional encopresis, 311
  functional enuresis, 310
  obsessive-compulsive disorder, 186,
    214
  obsessive-compulsive personality
    disorder, 186
  sexual deviations, 407
  sexual dysfunction, 402
  types of, 501–504
La belle indifference, 227
Benadryl
  treatment of extrapyramidal side
    effects, 535
Benzamides, 541
Benzodiazepines, 563
  abuse, 431–433
  administration, 568
  anxiety disorders in the elderly,
    249
  avoidant personality disorder, 179
  dementia, 264
  and depression, 107, 124, 243
  effects, 563–564, 565–567
  generalized anxiety disorder,
    208–209
  insomnia in the elderly, 250
  mechanisms of action, 564
  panic disorder, 205
  phobias, 211
  side effects, 567–568
  treatment of akathisia, 533
  uses, 564–565
  and violence, 465, 470
Benztropine mesylate
  treatment of extrapyramidal side
    effects, 535, 536
Bereavement, 116, 121, 243
Beta-blocking agents
  intermittent explosive disorder,
    377
  panic attacks, 203
  performance anxiety, 211
  posttraumatic stress disorder, 217
Binge eating. *See* Bulimia
Biochemical theories of obsessive-
  compulsive disorder, 213
Biochemistry of the emotions, 326
Biopsychosocial medicine, 325

Bipolar disorder
  antidepressant medications, 543
  antipsychotic medications, 528
  clinical course, 132–133
  differential diagnosis, 116,
    130–132
  epidemiology, 133–134
  etiology, 134–135
  lithium, 556
  rapid cyclers, 133
  symptoms, 128–130
  treatment, 135–139
  valproate, 562
Bipolar II, 127
Bipolar mood disorders, 104, 127
  See also Bipolar disorder;
    Cyclothymia
Blocking, 63
Blunted affect, 62
Body dysmorphic disorder, 225–226
Borderline mental retardation, 307
Borderline personality disorder
  course and prognosis, 175
  and depersonalization and
    derealization, 66
  diagnosis, 173
  differential diagnosis, 152, 159,
    161–162, 165, 170–171, 175,
    223
  epidemiology, 174
  etiology, 173–174
  and labile affect, 62
  profile, 172–173
  treatment, 175–176
  and violence, 469
Bradykinesia
  side effect of antipsychotic
    medications, 532–533
Brain abnormalities. *See* Organic
    brain syndromes
Brain changes and aging, 235–236
Brain electrical activity mapping
    (BEAM), 352, 360–361
Brain trauma
  and amnesia, 72
  and dementia, 257–258
  and violence, 471
Brain tumors, 257
Brief reactive psychosis, 88
Briquet's syndrome, 226
Broca's aphasia, 61

Bulimarexia, 441
Bulimia, 436–437, 440–441
  antidepressant medications, 544
  and depression, 107
Buprenex
  opioid withdrawal, 427
Buprenorphine hydrochloride
  opioid withdrawal, 427
Bupropion, 550
Buspirone, 563, 568–569
  generalized anxiety disorder, 209
  panic disorder, 205

C

Cannabinoids
  and depression, 114
  substance abuse, 434–435
  and violence, 470
Carbamazepine
  depression, 561–562
  mania, 561
  mania in the elderly, 247
  side effects, 562
Castration anxiety, 28
Catatonia, 60
Catatonic type of schizophrenia, 85
Catecholamine hypothesis of
    depression, 119
Central nervous system depressants
    abuse, 431–433
Cerebral angiography, 352
Cerebrovascular dementia, 256–257
Character, 145–146
Chemical restraints, 94, 465
Child abuse, 319–322
  legal obligations, 191, 321–322
  and multiple personality disorder,
    222
  and posttraumatic stress disorder,
    215
Child development
  comparison of development stages
    of Freud and Erikson, 280
  Erikson's development stages,
    278–280
  factors influencing, 286–289
  Freud's psychosexual development
    stages, 24–30, 276–278
  importance of, 271–273

Mahler's separation-individuation concept, 273–276
motor and behavioral, 273
normal development, 280–286
Children
attention-deficit hyperactivity disorder, 297–300
autism, 308–309
conduct disorders, 300–302
depression in, 317–318
diagnostic evaluation, 289–291
factors influencing development, 286–289
functional encopresis, 311
functional enuresis, 310–311
gender identity disorder, 313–314
identity disorder, 314–315
interviewing, 293–296
interviewing parents, 291–293
and mental health professionals, 290–291
mental retardation, 305–308
psychiatric disorders, 296–297
and psychiatric history, 45–46, 291–293
psychological factors in physical illness, 315–317
school refusal, 312–313
separation anxiety disorder, 311–313
specific developmental disorders, 302–304
and suicide, 318–319
See also Child abuse; Child development
Chlordiazepoxide
alcohol withdrawal, 421
anxiety disorders in the elderly, 249
violent patients, 465
Chlorpromazine
bipolar disorder, 138
side effects, 534, 535
violent patients, 465
Circumstantiality, 63, 71
Clanging, 64, 129
Classical conditioning, 500–501
Claustrophobia, 66
Clomipramine
obsessive-compulsive disorder, 213, 214

panic disorder, 205
Clonazepam, 563
panic disorder, 205
Clonidine
opioid withdrawal, 427
Clozapine
schizophrenia, 541
side effects, 534
Cocaine Anonymous, 429
Cocaine use, 428–429
treatment, 429–430
and violence, 470
Codeine
substance abuse, 425
Cogentin
delusional disorder in the elderly, 241
treatment of extrapyramidal side effects, 535
Cognitive-behavior therapy, 505–508
anxiety disorders in the elderly, 249
borderline personality disorder, 176
depersonalization disorder, 224
depression, 126
generalized anxiety disorder, 208–209
obsessive-compulsive disorder, 214
obsessive-compulsive personality disorder, 186
phobias, 210
posttraumatic stress disorder, 217
Cognitive distortions, 506–508
Cognitive functioning and mental status, 68–74
Communication deviance and schizophrenia, 91
Compulsions, 182, 211–212
Computed tomography (CT) scanning, 352, 353
and Alzheimer's disease, 255
and schizophrenia research, 90
and subdural hematoma, 258
Computerized topographic brain mapping, 360–361
Concentration, 70–71
and depression, 108
Concrete thinking, 73
Condensation, 22
Conduct disorders, 300–302

Confabulation, 71
  and dementia, 252
  and Korsakoff's syndrome,
    422–423
Conflicts in psychodynamics,
  487–488
Congenital right-hemisphere
  syndrome, 375
Conscience, 23
Conscious, 20
Consciousness, 69
Consent
  electroconvulsive therapy, 571
  recording interviews, 6
Consultation-liaison psychiatry
  clinical approaches, 328–331
  history, 325–326
  illness-disease spectrum, 326–328
  interviewing, 335–339
  introducing yourself, 336
  medical-surgical patients, 340–343
  psychiatrist's role, 328
  reasons for, 332–335
  request for consultation, 331–332
  time, 336
  writing the consultation note,
    339–340
Control issues and sexual
  dysfunction, 394
Conversion as a defense mechanism,
  32
Conversion disorder, 227–228
Cooperative apartments, 97
Countertransference, 491–492
Couples therapy, 510–511
  sadistic personality disorder, 191
  self-defeating personality disorder,
    194
Covert sensitization
  paraphilias, 407
Crack. *See* Cocaine use
Criminality, 170
Cushing's syndrome, 374
Cyclothymia
  clinical course, 140
  diagnosis, 132, 139
  differential diagnosis, 140
  differentiated from bipolar
    disorder, 104, 127
  epidemiology, 139–140
  treatment, 141

D

Darvon
  substance abuse, 425
Day treatment programs, 97
Defense mechanisms, 30–33
Deficits in psychodynamics, 488–489
Deinstitutionalization, 93
Delirium
  causes, 265
  compared with dementia, 250–251
  diagnosis, 265
  differential diagnosis, 268
  managing the delirious patient,
    267–268
  and open-heart surgery, 265–266
  treatment, 266–267
  and violence, 471
Delirium tremens (DTs), 421
Delusional depression, 543
Delusional disorder, somatic subtype,
  226
Delusional (paranoid) disorder
  course and prognosis, 242
  diagnosis, 241
  differential diagnosis, 249
  in the elderly, 240–242
  etiology, 241
  onset, 240–241
  treatment, 241–242
Delusions, 65–66
  in the elderly, 243
  and mania, 130
  mood congruent, 108–109
  and schizophrenia, 81
Demence précoce, 79
Dementia
  and aging, 264
  antipsychotic medications, 528
  clinical picture, 252–254
  compared with delirium, 250–251
  and depression, 108, 115, 260–261
  diagnosis, 251–252
  differential diagnosis, 260–261
  diseases that may present with, 259
  interview and evaluation, 261
  irreversible causes, 254–257
  laboratory tests, 263
  mental status examination,
    262–263
  physical examination, 263

psychiatric history, 261–262
secondary to systemic illness,
    258–259
treatable causes, 257–261
treatment, 263–264
and violence, 471
Dementia syndrome of depression,
    242, 243, 260–261
Demerol
    substance abuse, 425
Denial, 31, 71
Depakene, 562
Depakote, 562
Dependent personality disorder
    course and prognosis, 180
    diagnosis, 179
    differential diagnosis, 181
    epidemiology, 180
    etiology, 179–180
    profile, 179
    treatment, 181
Depersonalization, 66
Depersonalization disorder, 223–224
Depo-Provera
    sexual deviations, 407
    violence, 476
Depression
    carbamazepine, 561–562
    in children and adolescents,
        317–319
    classification by systems other than
        DSM-III-R, 112–114
    clinical course, 116–117
    differential diagnosis, 86, 114–116,
        208, 213, 216, 223, 243
    DSM-III-R diagnostic categories,
        109–112
    in the elderly, 242–246, 250
    electroconvulsive therapy, 570
    epidemiology, 117–118, 244
    etiology, 118–122
    indications for hospitalization, 122
    medications that may cause, 114,
        243
    organic causes, 114–115
    in psychiatric history, 42
    psychodynamic factors, 121–122
    psychotherapy versus medication,
        541–544
    responsiveness to antidepressant
        medications, 542–544
    and schizophrenia, 99

and sexual dysfunction, 391–393
    symptoms, 105–109
    treatment, 122–127
    tricyclic antidepressants, 547–548
    valproate, 562
    and violence, 468–469
Depression with melancholia, 111
Depressive neurosis, 111–112
Derealization, 66
Dermatitis
    side effect of antipsychotic
        medications, 534
Desipramine, 548
    cocaine abuse, 429
    dementia, 264
    depression in the elderly, 245
    panic disorder, 205
Desyrel, 548
Developmental arithmetic disorder,
    303
Developmental articulation disorder,
    304
Developmental coordination
    disorder, 304
Developmental disorders, 302–304
Developmental expressive writing
    disorder, 304
Developmental language disorder,
    303
Developmental reading disorder, 303
Dexamethasone suppression test
    (DST), 120–121, 544–545
Dextropropoxyphene hydrochloride
    substance abuse, 425
*Diagnostic and Statistical Manual of
    Mental Disorders, Third
    Edition–Revised* (DSM-III-R)
    antisocial personality disorder, 169
    avoidant personality disorder, 177
    borderline personality disorder,
        173
    conduct disorders, 300
    cyclothymia, 139
    delirium, 265
    dementia, 252
    dependent personality disorder,
        179
    diagnosis organization, 50–51
    dissociative disorders, 218
    histrionic personality disorder, 160
    mania and hypomania, 128
    mood disorders, 109–112

narcissistic personality disorder,
    165
paranoid personality disorder, 151
passive-aggressive personality
    disorder, 187
personality disorders, 149
psychiatric disorders of children,
    290
psychoactive substance abuse, 413
psychoactive substance
    dependence, 413–414
removal of homosexuality, 410
schizoaffective disorder, 87
schizophrenia, 80
schizotypal personality disorder,
    157
Diazepam
    abuse, 431–433
    anxiety disorders in the elderly,
        249
    hallucinogen withdrawal, 434
    terminology, 517
    violent patients, 465
Dichotomous thinking, 507
Digitalis
    and depression, 243
Digit span, 71
Dilaudid
    substance abuse, 425
Dimethyltryptamine (DMT)
    substance abuse, 433–434
Diphenhydramine
    treatment of extrapyramidal side
        effects, 535
Disorganized type of schizophrenia,
    85
Displacement, 22, 32, 294
Dissociation as a defense mechanism,
    32
Dissociative disorders, 217–224
Dissociative episodes, 66, 218
Distractibility and mania, 129
Disulfiram
    alcoholism, 424
Diurnal variation in mood, 107, 111
Doctor-patient relationship
    countertransference, 491–492
    doctor's attitudes about sex, 385
    doctor's reactions to patient,
        15–16
    doctor's reactions to violence,
        477–478

duty to warn, 475
identification, 485
narcissistic patients, 166
paranoid patients, 153
patient attitude, 74
personality disorders patients, 195
psychotherapy, 483–486
resistance in, 492–493
schizoid patients, 154
suicidal patients, 443–444
transference, 484, 490–491
Dolophine
    substance abuse, 425
Dopamine
    and aging, 235
    and depression, 119
    and electroconvulsive therapy, 569
Dopamine hypothesis of
    schizophrenia, 89
Dorsolateral convexity lesions,
    367–369
Down's syndrome, 305
Doxepin, 548
    depression in the elderly, 245
Dream analysis, 493
Dreams, 21–22
Duty to warn, 475
Dyslexia, 303
Dysmorphophobia, 225–226
Dyspareunia, 396
Dysthymia
    antidepressant medications, 543
    clinical course, 117
    diagnosis, 111–112, 113
    differential diagnosis, 104, 109,
        110, 114–116, 216
    epidemiology, 117–118

E

Eating disorders, 436–441
Echolalia, 64
    and autism, 308
    and schizophrenia, 82
Education
    bipolar disorder, 138
    developmental disorders, 304
Ego, 23, 278
Ego ideal, 23
Ejaculatory incompetence, 398–399,
    401

Elation, 42, 127
Elavil, 548
Elderly
  anxiety disorder, 248–250
  assessing, 237–239
  delirium in, 264–268
  dementia in, 250, 251–264
  depression in, 242–246
  insomnia in, 249–250
  mania in, 246–247
  mood disorders in, 242–247
  psychosis in, 240–242
  special treatment considerations,
      239–240
  suicide risk, 243, 247–248
  See also Aging
Electroconvulsive therapy (ECT)
  administration, 570–571
  agitated depression, 114
  bipolar disorder, 137
  dementia syndrome of depression,
      260
  depression in the elderly, 246
  mechanism of action, 569
  mood disorders, 123, 124
  preparations, 571–572
  reactive depression, 113
  risks versus benefits, 573–574
  schizophrenia, 99
  side effects, 572–573
  uses, 570
Electroencephalograms (EEGs),
      354–355
  abnormalities, 357
  normal, 355
  ordering, 357
  technique, 355–357
Emotional disturbance and
      schizophrenia, 81–82
Emotions and mental status, 61–62
Endogenous depression, 112–113
Environmental factors
  and autism, 309
  and personality disorders, 147
  and schizophrenia, 91–92, 95–96
  and sexual deviations, 403
  and substance abuse, 416
  and violence, 473
Epidemiologic Catchment Area (ECA)
      Study
  depression in the elderly, 244

Epilepsy
  differential diagnosis, 222
  and electroencephalography, 357
  interictal behavior syndrome of
      temporolimbic epilepsy,
      370–372
Erikson, Erik, 278–280
Erogenous zone, 25
Event-related slow potentials (ERSPs),
      360
Evoked potentials (EPs), 352,
      358–360
Exhibitionism, 406
Experiential learning, 495–496
Exploratory psychotherapy, 497
Expressed emotion and
      schizophrenia, 95–96
Expressive language disorder, 303
Extinction, 503
Extrapyramidal diseases, 375–376
Extrapyramidal side effects
  of antipsychotic medications,
      532–534
  treatment, 535–536, 565
Eye contact and mental status, 60

F

Facial expression and mental status,
      60
Failure to thrive, 288, 320
Families
  and autism, 309
  and child development, 287–289
  interviewing parents, 291–293
  neuropsychiatric treatment, 378
  and personality disorders, 147
  psychiatric history, 43, 292–293,
      347
  and schizophrenia, 91–92, 95–96
  and sexual deviations, 403
  and substance abuse, 416
  and violence, 473
Family therapy, 511–512
  gender identity disorder, 314
  schizophrenia, 95–96
Fatigue and depression, 107
Fear, 199
Female sexual response, 388–389
Fetishism, 405

Financial resources and treatment plan, 52–53, 520
Flat affect, 62, 81
Flight of ideas, 64, 129
Flooding, 503
  obsessive-compulsive disorder, 214
  phobias, 211
  posttraumatic stress disorder, 217
Fluoxetine, 550
  obsessive-compulsive disorder, 214
Fluphenazine
  delusional disorder in the elderly, 242
  emergency dosage, 538
Fluphenazine decanoate
  schizophrenia treatment, 98
Flurazepam
  anxiety disorders in the elderly, 249
Fluvoxamine
  obsessive-compulsive disorder, 214
Free association, 493
Free-floating anxiety, 200
Freud, Anna, 272
Freud, Sigmund, 19, 20, 24, 34, 121, 207, 212, 276–278, 287–288, 486
Frigidity, 395
Frontal-lobe syndromes, 367–369
Functional encopresis, 311
Functional enuresis, 310–311
Fund of knowledge, 72

G

Gait apraxia, 258
Gender identity disorder, 313–314
Generalized anxiety disorder
  antianxiety medications, 564
  diagnosis, 206
  differential diagnosis, 208, 216
  in the elderly, 248–250
  etiology, 206–208
  symptoms, 205–206
  treatment, 208–209
Global Assessment of Functioning (GAF) Scale, 51, 585–586
Grief reactions, 116, 121, 243, 543
Grooming and mental status, 59–60
Group therapy, 508–510

avoidant personality disorder, 178–179
borderline personality disorder, 176
dependent personality disorder, 181
depression, 126
histrionic personality disorder, 162
narcissistic personality disorder, 166
obsessive-compulsive personality disorder, 187
schizoid personality disorder, 156
schizophrenia, 95
sexual dysfunction, 403
Gustatory hallucinations, 68

H

Haldol
  emergency dosage, 538
  schizophrenia, 98
  terminology, 517
  violent patients, 465
Halfway houses
  alcoholics, 424
  schizophrenics, 97
Hallucinations, 58, 67–68
  and alcohol abuse, 372
  and mania, 130
  and schizophrenia, 81
Hallucinogens
  abuse, 433–434
  and depression, 114
Haloperidol, 517
  delusional disorder in the elderly, 241
  dementia, 264
  emergency dosage, 538
  Tourette's syndrome, 528
  violent patients, 465
Haloperidol decanoate
  schizophrenia, 98
Hardening of the arteries, 256–257
Hartmann, Heinz, 29
Hashish, 434–435
  and violence, 470
Head injury, 369–370
Heroin abuse, 425
History. See Psychiatric history

Histrionic personality disorder
  course and prognosis, 161
  diagnosis, 160
  differential diagnosis, 161–162,
    165
  epidemiology, 161
  etiology, 160–161
  and hysteria, 259–260
  profile, 160
  and somatization disorder, 162
  treatment, 162
Homicide
  and bipolar disorder, 135
  determinants, 466
  and hospitalization, 474–475
  and mental status examination, 59,
    66–67
  and opioid addiction, 425
  and schizophrenia, 84–85
  See also Violence
Homosexuality
  aversive conditioning, 504
  causes, 409
  interviewing techniques, 411
  life-style, 409–410
  prevalence, 408–409
  psychopathology, 410
  treatment, 410–411
  and violence, 470
Hospitalization
  for cocaine abuse, 429
  for depression, 122
  for schizophrenia, 93–95
  violent patients, 474–475
  See also Consultation-liaison
    psychiatry
Humor
  as a defense mechanism, 33
  and interviewing, 13
  and patients with paranoid
    personality disorder, 153
Hydromorphone hydrochloride
  substance abuse, 425
Hyperactive child syndrome, 297
Hyperactivity
  and mania, 129
  See also Attention-deficit
    hyperactivity disorder (ADHD)
Hyperphagia and depression, 107
Hypersomnia, 107
Hypertensive crisis
  side effect of monoamine oxidase
    inhibitors, 555

Hyperthyroidism
  and anxiety, 374
  and organic mood syndrome,
    manic type, 374
Hypnagogic hallucinations, 68
Hypnosis, 504–505
  alcoholics, 424
  depersonalization disorder, 224
  psychogenic fugue, 220
  sexual dysfunction, 402
Hypnotic medications
  and depression, 107
Hypochondriasis, 228–229
  as a defense mechanism, 31
  in the elderly, 243
Hypomania, 127, 128
Hypothyroidism
  and organic mood syndrome,
    depressed type, 374
Hysteria, 159–160
Hysterical neurosis, conversion type,
  227–228

I

Id, 22–23
Ideas of reference, 66
Identification
  with parents, 28
  with patient, 15–16
  with therapist, 485
Identity disorder, 314–315
Idiot savants, 309
Illness-disease spectrum, 326–328
  See also Physical illness
Illusions, 67
Imipramine, 548
  cocaine abuse, 429
  and functional enuresis, 310–311
  panic disorder, 205
  phobias, 211
  posttraumatic stress disorder, 217
  suicidal ideation, 546
Immature defense mechanisms,
  31–33
Immediate memory, 71
Implosion, 503
Impotence, 396–397
  treatment, 401
Impulse disorders
  differential diagnosis, 153
Incest, 321

Incontinence, 258, 310–311
Infantile states, 26
Insight, 74
Insomnia
    antianxiety medications, 565
    and depression, 106–107, 124–125
    in the elderly, 249–250
Instinct theory, 24
Intellectualization, 32
Interictal behavior syndrome of
        temporolimbic epilepsy,
        370–372
Intermittent explosive disorder
    beta-blocking agents, 377
Interpersonal therapy (IPT)
    for depression, 125–126
The Interpretation of Dreams, 20
Interviews
    adolescents, 295–296
    children, 293–295
    closing, 16–17, 339
    consultation-liaison psychiatry,
        335–339
    defining goals, 7
    demented people, 261
    homosexuals, 411
    meeting the patient, 5–6, 336
    parents, 291–293
    patient's attitude toward
        interviewer, 74
    place, 5, 335
    process, 3–5
    purpose, 3
    reactions to patient, 15–16
    recording, 6
    sexual history questions, 385–386
    style, 8
    techniques, 8–12, 336–339
    time, 6–7, 336
    tips, 12–14
Involuntary commitment for violent
        patients, 475
Involutional melancholia, 111
Irritability, 41
Isolation of affect, 32–33

J

Judgment and psychiatric history, 73
Juvenile delinquency, 301

K

Kernberg, Otto, 166
Klonopin, 563
    panic disorder, 205
Klüver-Bucy syndrome, 371–372
Kohut, Heinz, 30, 165
Korsakoff's syndrome, 72, 372–374,
    422–423

L

Labile affect, 62
    and mania, 130
Language disorders
    and autism, 308
    See also Speech
Latency, 28–29, 283–284
Learned helplessness, 122
Learning theory
    of anxiety, 207–208
    of obsessive-compulsive disorder,
        213
Levodopa
    and depression, 243
    and violence, 470
Libido, 24
    effects of depression, 107
Librium, 517
    alcohol withdrawal, 421
    violent patients, 465
Light therapy, 125, 141
Lithium
    administration, 560
    bipolar disorder, 135, 136–138
    clinical evaluation, 559–560
    and depression, 123–124
    effects, 557
    maintenance, 561
    mania, 556, 557
    mania in the elderly, 247
    schizophrenia, 98–99, 541
    sexual deviations, 407
    side effects, 557–558
    toxicity, 558–559
    uses, 556–557
Locus coeruleus and panic attacks,
    203
Loose associations, 63
Lorazepam
    akathisia treatment, 533

Low birth weight and child abuse, 320
Ludiomil, 548
D-lysergic acid diethylamide (LSD), 433–434
and violence, 470

M

Magical thinking, 22
Magnetic resonance imaging (MRI), 352, 353–354
and schizophrenia research, 90
Magnification, 507
Mahler, Margaret, 273–276
Major depression, 104, 109–111
clinical course, 116–117
differential diagnosis, 114–116, 216
epidemiology, 117–118
etiology, 118–122
psychotherapy versus medication, 541–544
treatment, 122–127
Major depressive episode, 110–111, 113
electroconvulsive therapy, 570
psychotherapy, 543
Major tranquilizers, 517
depression, 124
Male sexual response, 389
Malingering, differential diagnosis, 216, 222–223
Mania, 127
carbamazepine, 561
clonazepam, 563
diagnosis, 130
diagnostic criteria, 128
differential diagnosis, 86, 171
in the elderly, 246–247
electroconvulsive therapy, 570
lithium, 556, 560
precipitation by monoamine oxidase inhibitors, 556
symptoms, 128–130
valproate, 562
and violence, 468
Manic-depressive illness. See Bipolar disorder
Mannerisms and mental status, 60
Maprotiline, 548

Marijuana, 434–435
and depression, 114
and violence, 470
Masked depressions in the elderly, 242
Masochism, 31, 191
sexual, 406, 407
Masters and Johnson's sex therapy techniques, 399–402
Mature defense mechanisms, 33
Mechanical restraints, 464–465
Medial frontal syndrome, 369
Medroxyprogesterone
sexual deviations, 407
violence, 476
Mellaril
and toxic retinopathy, 535
Memory, 71–72
and aging, 236
and depression, 108
Mental retardation
profile, 305
subtypes, 305–307
treatment, 307–308
Mental status examination (MSE)
dementia, 261, 262–263
determining the presence of psychosis, 57–59
elderly patients, 238–239
major areas of mental function, 348–349
outline, 55, 59–74
reporting, 74–76
using, 59
when to conduct, 56–57
Meperidine
substance abuse, 425
Mescaline
substance abuse, 433
Methadone
opioid maintenance, 427
opioid withdrawal, 427
substance abuse, 425
Methyldopa
and depression, 114
Methylphenidate
attention-deficit hyperactivity disorder, 299
and depression, 541
Milieu therapy, 94
Minimal brain dysfunction
and violence, 471

See also Attention-deficit
  hyperactivity disorder (ADHD)
Mini-Mental State Exam, 262–263
Minimization, 507
Minor tranquilizers, 517
  depression, 124
  violent patients, 465
Monoamine oxidase inhibitors
  (MAOIs), 554
  bipolar disorder, 124, 138
  borderline personality disorder,
    176
  depression, 123, 124
  depression in the elderly, 244–245
  dosages, 554
  drug interactions, 555–556
  lithium's potentiating effects, 123
  panic disorder, 205
  prescribing, 554–555
  psychotherapy versus medication,
    541–544
  side effects, 555
  suicidal ideation, 546
Mood and mental status, 61–62
Mood congruent delusions, 108–109
Mood disorders
  classification systems other than
    DSM-III-R, 112–114
  clinical course, 116–117
  diagnosis, 109–112
  differential diagnosis, 86, 114–116,
    175
  in the elderly, 242–247
  organic, 374–375
  profile, 103–104
Mood disturbance and mania, 128
Morality, 23–24
Morbid preoccupations, 66
Morel, Benedict-Augustin, 79
Morphine
  substance abuse, 425
Motor activity
  and mental status, 60
  psychomotility disorders, 375–376
  and schizophrenia, 82
Multiple personality disorder
  differential diagnosis, 222–223
  etiology, 222
  profile, 221
  treatment, 223
Mushroom
  substance abuse, 433

Mutism, 61
Mysophobia, 66

N

Naltrexone, 428
Narcissistic personality disorder
  and cocaine use, 429
  course and prognosis, 164
  diagnosis, 163
  differential diagnosis, 165
  epidemiology, 164
  etiology, 163
  and phallic stage of development,
    27
  profile, 162–163
  treatment, 165–166
Narcotics Anonymous, 428, 429,
    436
Nasopharyngeal (NP) leads, 357
Navane
  emergency dosage, 538
Negative reinforcement, 503
Neologisms, 64
  and schizophrenia, 82
Neuroendocrine systems and
  depression, 120–121
Neuroleptic malignant syndrome, 98,
    533
Neuroleptic medications
  bipolar disorder, 136
  and blunted affect, 62
  borderline personality disorder,
    176
  choosing, 536–537
  commonly used antipsychotics and
    their characteristics, 537
  delusional disorder in the elderly,
    241
  depression, 124
  dosages, 529–531
  indications for using, 527–529
  maintenance therapy, 539–540
  mania in the elderly, 247
  mechanism of action, 527
  medication interactions, 536
  prescribing, 537–539
  responsiveness of symptoms to,
    529
  schizophrenia, 89, 97–98
  side effects, 531–536

types of, 529–531
Neuropsychiatric disorders, 366–376
Neuropsychiatry
  common neuropsychiatric
    disorders, 366–376
  described, 345–346
  evaluation, 346–352
  examination, 348–349
  history, 363–364
  neurodiagnostic methods, 352–365
  neuropsychological testing,
    363–364
  treatment, 376–378
  written report, 349–352
Neuropsychological testing, 363–364
Neurotic, 28
Neurotic depression, 113
Neurotransmitters
  and aging, 235
  and depression, 119–120
  effects of electroconvulsive
    therapy, 569
  and generalized anxiety disorder,
    206–207
  receptors and depression, 120
  and schizophrenia, 89–90
  and violence, 471
Normal-pressure hydrocephalus
  (NPH), 258
Norpramin, 548
Nortriptyline, 548
  depression in the elderly, 245
Numorphan
  substance abuse, 425

O

Object constancy, 276, 282
Object-relations theory, 29–30
Obsessions, 182, 211
Obsessive-compulsive disorder (OCD)
  antidepressant medications, 544
  differential diagnosis, 204, 213
  differentiated from obsessive-
    compulsive personality
    disorder, 182, 184
  etiology, 212–213
  profile, 211–212
  treatment, 214
Obsessive-compulsive personality
  disorder

course and prognosis, 184
diagnosis, 184
differential diagnosis, 165,
  184–185
differentiated from obsessive-
  compulsive disorder, 182, 184
epidemiology, 184
etiology, 184
profile, 183–184
treatment, 185–186
and violence, 469
Obsessive-compulsive style, 182–183
Oedipus complex, 27–28
Olfactory hallucinations, 68
Open-heart surgery and delirium,
  265–266
Operant conditioning, 501
Opioids, 425
  overdose, 425–426
  treatment for abuse, 427–428
  and violence, 470
  withdrawal, 426
Oral contraceptives
  and depression, 114
Oral personalities, 26
Orbitofrontal cortex damage, 367
Organic amnestic syndromes, 72,
  372–374
Organic anxiety syndrome, 374
Organic brain syndromes, 250, 345
  antianxiety medications, 565
  common neuropsychiatric
    disorders, 366–377
  differential diagnosis, 87, 216
  in the elderly, 240, 242
  neurodevelopmental signs, 348
  treatment, 376–378
Organic delusional syndrome, 372
Organic mood disorders, 131,
  374–375
Organic personality syndromes
  diagnostic criteria, 367
  explosive type, 377
  frontal-lobe syndromes, 367–369
  head injury, 369–370
  interictal behavior syndrome of
    temporolimbic epilepsy,
    370–372
  treatment, 376–378
Organic psychotic syndromes, 240,
  372
Orgastic dysfunction, 395–396

Orientation, 70
Overdose
    central nervous system depressants,
        431–432
    opioids, 425–426
Overgeneralization, 506–507
Oxazepam
    panic disorder, 205
Oxycodone
    substance abuse, 425
Oxymorphone hydrochloride
    substance abuse, 425

P

Panic disorder
    antianxiety medications, 565
    antidepressant medications, 544
    clonazepam, 563
    differential diagnosis, 204, 208
    in the elderly, 248
    etiology, 203–204
    profile, 200–203
    treatment, 204–205
Paraldehyde
    violent patients, 465
Paranoid personality disorder
    course and prognosis, 152
    diagnosis, 151
    differential diagnosis, 88, 152–153,
        156
    epidemiology, 152
    etiology, 152
    profile, 149–151
    treatment, 153
    and violence, 469
Paranoid thinking
    and violence, 467–468
Paranoid type of schizophrenia, 85
Paraphilias
    behavior therapy, 407
Paraphrenia. See Delusional
    (paranoid) disorder
Parents. See Families
Parkinsonism
    side effect of antipsychotic
        medications, 532
    treatment, 535–536
Passive-aggressive personality
    disorder

course and prognosis, 188
diagnosis, 187
differential diagnosis, 188
epidemiology, 188
etiology, 187
profile, 186–187
treatment, 188–189
Patient attitude, 74
Pavlov, Ivan, 500
Pedophilia, 405–406
Peer relationships
    and child development, 29, 46,
        285, 286, 289
    and violence, 473
Pentazocine
    substance abuse, 425
Pentobarbital tolerance test, 432–433
Perception, 67–68
Percocet
    substance abuse, 425
Performance anxiety
    propranolol, 211
Permeable mind, 58
Perphenazine
    emergency dosage, 538
Perseveration, 63
Personality disorders
    antidepressant medications, 543
    antipsychotic medications, 528
    course and prognosis, 148
    and depression, 116
    diagnosis, 148–149
    differential diagnosis, 87–88, 175
    etiology, 147–148
    group therapy, 510
    profile, 146–147
    special treatment considerations,
        195
    and violence, 469–470
    See also specific personality
        disorders
Personality types, 340–342
Personalization, 507
Pervasive developmental disorder,
    308–309
Peyote cactus
    substance abuse, 433
Pharmacotherapy
    administration of psychotropic
        medications, 521–522
    advising patients, 522–523

attention-deficit hyperactivity
disorder, 299
borderline personality disorder,
176
choosing a medication, 519–520
combining medications, 524–525
dementia, 264
dosage determination, 520–521
failure of, 525
major groups of psychotropic
medications, 516–518
managing side effects, 523–524
obsessive-compulsive disorder, 214
phobias, 211
posttraumatic stress disorder, 217
prescribing principles, 518–527
risks of treatment, 519
schizophrenia, 97–99
table of common medications,
587–588
trade names of medications,
589–590
treatment team, 526–527
violence, 476
*See also specific drugs and classes
of drugs*
Phencyclidine (PCP)
and antipsychotic medications, 528
substance abuse, 434
and violence, 470
Phenelzine
depression in the elderly, 245
phobias, 211
posttraumatic stress disorder, 217
sexual dysfunction as side effect,
555
Phenobarbital
withdrawal from central nervous
system depressants, 433
Phenylketonuria (PKU), 305, 309
Pheochromocytoma
anxiety as side effect, 374
Phobias
antianxiety medications, 564
defined, 66, 209
differential diagnosis, 213–214
in the elderly, 248
major categories, 209–210
treatment, 210–211
Physical illness
accompanied by anxiety, 204

accompanied by dementia, 259
accompanied by mental symptoms,
332
and depression, 115
illness-disease spectrum, 326–328
and personality disorders, 148
psychological factors in children,
315–317
Physical restraints, 94, 135, 464–465
Pick's disease, 256
Pimozide
Tourette's syndrome, 528
Play therapy, 294–296
depression in children, 318
Pleasure principle, 23
Positive reinforcement, 503
Positron-emission tomography (PET),
352, 361–363
and Alzheimer's disease, 255
and schizophrenia research, 90
Postpartum depression
and violence, 469
Posttraumatic stress disorder (PTSD)
differential diagnosis, 216, 223
etiology, 216
profile, 215
treatment, 217
Postural hypotension
side effect of antipsychotic
medications, 534
Posture and mental status, 60
Preconscious, 20–21
Pregenital, 28
Premature birth and child abuse, 320
Premature ejaculation, 397–398
treatment, 401
Preoccupations, 66
Pre-oedipal, 28
Preschool child development, 283
Presenile dementia, 254–256
Primary gain
somatoform disorders, 227
Primary process thinking, 21–22
Projection, 31–32
Prolixin
emergency dosage, 538
and schizophrenia treatment, 98
Propranolol
akathisia, 533
depression, 114

organic mood syndrome, depressed type, 374
panic disorder, 203
phobias, 211
posttraumatic stress disorder, 217
Protriptyline, 548
Prozac, 550
obsessive-compulsive disorder, 214
Pseudodementia, 242, 260–261
Psilocybin
substance abuse, 433
Psychiatric evaluation sample, 575–579
Psychiatric history
case formulation, 48–50
chief complaint, 40
children, 291–293
demented patients, 261–262
diagnostic impression, 50–51
drug and alcohol history, 48
elderly patients, 237–238
family history of mental illness, 43, 47
history of current problem, 40–43
identifying data, 39–40
medical history, 47–48
mental status examination, 48
neuropsychiatric, 346–348
organization of, 37–38
outline, 38–39
past history, 43–47
referral source, 40
sample, 575–579
treatment plan, 51–53
Psychic numbing, 215
Psychoanalysis, 496–497
Psychodynamic psychotherapy
countertransference, 491–492
goals of, 500
misconceptions, 499–500
model of change, 486–493
process of change, 494–496
resistance in, 492–493
sources of data, 489–490
transference, 490–491
types of, 496–499
See also Psychotherapy
Psychodynamics, 19–33
in clinical practice, 33–34
See also Psychodynamic psychotherapy

Psychodynamic theory of obsessive-compulsive disorder, 212–213
Psychogenic amnesia
differential diagnosis, 219, 222
etiology, 219
profile, 219
treatment, 220
Psychogenic fugue, 220–221, 222
Psychomotility disorders, 375–376
Psychomotor agitation and depression, 107
Psychomotor retardation and depression, 107
Psychosexual development
perspective on, 29–30
stages, 24–29, 276–278
Psychosis, 58–59
and depression, 108–109
in the elderly, 240–242
Psychosomatic medicine, 325–326
Psychotherapy
alcoholics, 424
anxiety disorders in the elderly, 249
avoidant personality disorder, 178
bipolar disorder, 139
borderline personality disorder, 175–176
defined, 483
dependent personality disorder, 181
depersonalization disorder, 224
depression, 125
depression in children and adolescents, 318
depression in the elderly, 246
doctor-patient relationship, 483–486
exploratory, 497
gender identity disorder, 314
generalized anxiety disorder, 207, 208–209
goals of, 483–484
histrionic personality disorder, 162
identity disorder, 315
integrating the psychotherapies, 512–513
medical-surgical patients, 340–343
modalities of, 486, 508–513
multiple personality disorder, 223
narcissistic personality disorder, 166

obsessive-compulsive disorder, 214
obsessive-compulsive personality
    disorder, 186–187
opioid abuse, 428
panic disorder, 205
passive-aggressive personality
    disorder, 188
phobias, 211
posttraumatic stress disorder, 217
psychodynamic psychotherapy,
    486–500
psychogenic fugue, 220–221
resistance in, 492–493
sadistic personality disorder, 191
schizoid personality disorder, 156
schizophrenia, 95–96
schizotypal personality disorder,
    159
self-defeating personality disorder,
    194
sexual dysfunction, 402, 403
short-term, 498–499
somatoform disorders, 229
sources of data, 489–490
substance abuse, 436
supportive, 498
violence, 476
Psychotic depression, 113, 243
Psychotropic medications
    administration of, 521–522
    advising patients, 522–523
    choosing a medication, 519–520
    clinical evaluation, 518
    combining medications, 524–525
    commonly abused drugs, 414,
        581–584
    common medications, 587–588
    course of illness, 518–519
    dosage determination, 520–521
    failure of pharmacotherapy, 525
    major groups, 516–518
    managing side effects, 523–524
    obsessive-compulsive disorder, 214
    principles of prescribing, 518–527
    psychiatric use, 515–516
    risks of treatment, 519
    trade names, 589–590
    treatment team, 526–527
    See also specific drugs and classes
        of drugs
Puberty, 29, 279, 284–286

Punishment in behavior
    modification, 503
Punning, 64

R

Racing thoughts, 63
Reaction formation, 32
Reactive depression, 112–113, 543
Reality testing, 58
Recent memory, 71
Receptive language disorder, 303
Receptors and depression, 120
Regional cerebral blood flow (RCBF)
        studies
    and schizophrenia research, 90
Rehabilitation
    alcoholics, 424–425
    from brain injuries, 377–378
    cocaine addicts, 429
    and schizophrenia, 96
    and schizotypal personality
        disorder, 159
    substance abusers, 436
Relaxation techniques
    alcoholics, 424
    posttraumatic stress disorder, 217
Remote memory, 71
Repression
    as a defense mechanism, 31
    in hysterical people, 160
    and psychodynamic
        psychotherapy, 494
Reserpine
    depression as side effect, 114
    organic mood syndrome, depressed
        type as side effect, 374
Resistance in psychotherapy,
    492–493
Restraints, 94, 135, 464–465
Retarded depression, 114
Retarded ejaculation, 398–399, 401
Retarded thoughts, 63
Retroflexion, 31
Retrograde amnesia, 72, 219
Retrograde ejaculation
    and thioridazine, 535
Ritalin
    attention-deficit hyperactivity
        disorder, 299

Rules and rituals
  and autism, 308–309
  child development, 29

S

Sadistic personality disorder
  course and prognosis, 190
  diagnosis, 189
  differential diagnosis, 191
  epidemiology, 190
  etiology, 189
  legal issues, 191
  profile, 189
  treatment, 191
Satiation, 407–408
Schizoaffective disorder, 87,
    115–116, 131–132
  antidepressant medications, 543
  lithium, 557
  valproate, 562
Schizoid personality disorder
  course and prognosis, 156
  diagnosis, 154
  differential diagnosis, 156,
    158–159
  epidemiology, 155–156
  etiology, 155
  profile, 154
  treatment, 156
Schizophrenia
  active phase, 83
  aftercare, 97
  antidepressant medications, 99
  antipsychotic medications,
    527–528
  and brain dysfunction, 90
  clinical picture, 82–85
  and depression, 99, 115
  diagnosis, 80
  differential diagnosis, 86–88, 131,
    152, 156, 213, 222
  dopamine hypothesis, 89
  in the elderly, 240, 242, 249
  electroconvulsive therapy, 99, 570
  and environment, 91–92
  epidemiology, 88
  etiology, 88–89
  factors that affect outcomes, 84
  and genetics, 90–91

  hospitalization, 93–95
  lithium, 98, 541
  and neurotransmitter systems,
    89–90
  pharmacotherapy, 97–99
  prodromal phase, 82
  profile, 79–80
  psychotherapy, 95–96
  rehabilitation, 96
  residual phase, 83–84
  subtypes, 85–86
  symptoms, 80–82
  treatment, 92–100
  valproate, 562
  and violence, 468
Schizotypal personality disorder
  course and prognosis, 158
  diagnosis, 157
  differential diagnosis, 156,
    158–159
  epidemiology, 157
  etiology, 157
  profile, 157
  treatment, 159
School refusal, 312–313
Seasonal affective disorder, 141
Seasonal pattern depression, 111
Seclusion, 94, 135–136
Secondary gain
  posttraumatic stress disorder, 216
  somatoform disorders, 227, 228
Secondary process thinking, 21
Sedative-hypnotics, 517
Sedatives, 517
  depression, 124
Selective abstraction, 506
Self-defeating personality disorder
  course and prognosis, 193–194
  diagnosis, 192
  differential diagnosis, 194
  epidemiology, 193
  etiology, 192
  profile, 192
  term, 191
  treatment, 194
Self-esteem
  and antidepressant medications,
    542, 543
  and bulimia, 441
  and cocaine use, 429
  and conduct disorders, 300

and depression, 108, 121
and developmental disorders, 304
and mania, 129
and narcissistic personality
disorder, 163
and phallic stage of development,
27
and sexual dysfunction, 394
Senile dementia, 254–256
Separation anxiety disorder, 311–313
Separation-individuation concept of
child development, 273–276
Serotonin reuptake blockers
obsessive-compulsive disorder, 213,
214
Sex and aging, 235, 389–390
Sex chromosome abnormalities and
violence, 471
Sex therapy, 399–402, 512
Sexual abuse, 321–322
and multiple personality disorder,
222
and pedophilia, 406
Sexual deviations, 403–407
versus dysfunction, 390
treatment, 407–408
Sexual dysfunction
and antidepressant medications,
550
and depression, 107
deviation versus dysfunction, 390
female, 394–396
male, 394, 396–399
and monoamine oxidase inhibitors,
555
physical causes, 391
psychological causes, 391–394
treatment, 399–403
and violence, 470
Sexual history, 383–386
Sexual masochism, 406–407
Sexual response cycle, 386–390
Sexual sadism, 407
Short-term psychotherapy, 498–499
Sibling relationships, 43, 288–289
See also Families
Signal anxiety, 207
Silent assumptions, 507–508
Simple phobias, 210
differential diagnosis, 204
Sinequan, 548

Single-photon–emission computed
tomography (SPECT), 352, 363
Situational anxiety, 200
antianxiety medications, 564
Sleep
and aging, 235
and depression, 106–107
in the elderly, 249–250
and mania, 129
Sleep manipulation, 125
Slowed thoughts, 63
Social phobias, 210
differential diagnosis, 204
Sociopath, 166
Sodium amobarbital
psychogenic amnesia, 220
psychogenic fugue, 220
violent patients, 465
Sodium lactate, 203
Sodium valproate, 562
Somatic complaints
and masked depression in the
elderly, 242–243
Somatic delusions, 65
Somatic therapies. *See*
Electroconvulsive therapy (ECT);
Pharmacotherapy
Somatization disorder, 226–227
Somatoform disorders
categories, 225
primary gain, 227
profile, 224–225
secondary gain, 227, 228
treatment, 229
Somatoform pain disorder, 228
Speech
developmental articulation
disorder, 304
and mania, 129
and mental status, 60–61
and schizophrenia, 82
Speech impediments, 61
Speech therapy, 304
Sphenoidal leads, 357
Splitting, 32
Stelazine, 517
emergency dosage, 538
Steroids
depression, 114
side effects, 374

Stimulants, 517
  organic mood syndrome, manic
    type as side effect, 374
  substance abuse, 428–431
Stranger anxiety, 276
Structural family therapy, 511–512
Stuttering, 61
Subdural hematoma, 258
Sublimation, 33
Substance abuse
  abusers, 415
  amphetamines, 430–431
  antipsychotic medications, 528
  and anxiety, 374
  cannabinoids, 434–435
  causes, 415–417
  central nervous system depressants,
    431–433
  central nervous system stimulants,
    428–431
  cocaine, 428–430
  commonly abused drugs, 414,
    581–584
  and conduct disorders, 301, 302
  and cyclothymia, 140
  and delirium, 265
  diagnostic criteria, 412
  differential diagnosis, 171, 204
  and generalized anxiety disorder,
    206
  hallucinogens, 433–434
  and multiple personality disorder,
    221
  opioids, 425–428
  and panic disorder, 202
  and passive-aggressive personality
    disorder, 188
  phencyclidine (PCP), 434
  and posttraumatic stress disorder,
    215
  and somatization disorder, 226
  treatment of polydrug abuse,
    435–436
  and violence, 470
  See also Alcoholism and alcohol
    abuse
Substance dependence
  diagnostic criteria, 413–414
Suicide
  and alcohol, 418
  and antidepressant medications,
    546

and antisocial personality disorder,
    167
  assessing the suicidal patient,
    448–455
  biological factors, 447–448
  and bipolar disorder, 135
  and borderline personality disorder,
    175
  in children and adolescents,
    318–319
  and dementia syndrome of
    depression, 261
  and depression, 108, 117, 122
  in the elderly, 243, 247–248
  epidemiology, 445
  mental status examination, 59,
    66–67
  and multiple personality disorder,
    221
  myths, 444–445
  and opioid addiction, 425
  profile of suicidal patients,
    443–444
  restraints, 94
  risk factors, 445–447
  and schizophrenia, 84
  treating the suicidal patient,
    455–457
Superego, 23–24
Supportive psychotherapy, 498
Suppression, 33
Survivor guilt, 215
Symbiotic relationship and child
    development, 273–276
Symbolism, 22
Synthetic tetrahydrocannabinol
    and violence, 470
Systematic desensitization, 501–502
  alcoholics, 424
  generalized anxiety disorder, 208
  obsessive-compulsive disorder, 214
  phobias, 210–211
  posttraumatic stress disorder, 217
  sexual dysfunction, 402

T

Tactile hallucinations, 68
Talwin
  substance abuse, 425
Tangentiality, 64

Tape recording interviews, 6
Tardive dyskinesia, 60, 98, 533–534
Tegretol
  depression, 561–562
  mania, 561
  side effects, 562
Thiamine deficiency and Korsakoff's
    syndrome, 372, 422, 423
Thioridazine
  side effects, 535
Thiothixene
  emergency dosage, 538
Thorazine
  bipolar disorder, 136
  violent patients, 465
Thought broadcasting, 66
Thought content, 64–67
Thought disorder, 63
Thought process, 63–64
Thought-stopping
  posttraumatic stress disorder, 217
Toddler development, 282
Tofranil, 548
Toilet training, 26–27, 310, 311
Token economy, 503
Topographic model of the mind,
    20–22
Tourette's syndrome, 376
  treatment, 528
Toxic retinopathy
  side effect of thioridazine, 535
Tranquilizers
  dementia, 264
  depression, 124
  terminology, 517
Transference, 484, 490–491
Transsexualism, 404
  differential diagnosis, 226
Transvestitism, 404–405
Tranylcypromine
  depression in the elderly, 245
Trazodone, 548
  depression in the elderly, 244–245,
    245
Tricyclic antidepressant medications,
    547–554
  agitated depression, 114
  anhedonia from cocaine
    withdrawal, 429
  attention-deficit hyperactivity
    disorder, 300

commonly used antidepressants
    and their characteristics, 548
continuing therapy, 552–553
dementia, 264
depression, 114, 123
depression in children, 318
depression in the elderly, 245–246
generalized anxiety disorder, 209
maintenance therapy, 553–554
medication interactions, 551
obsessive-compulsive disorder, 213,
    214
panic disorder, 205
plasma levels and therapeutic
    response, 551–552
prescribing regimen, 551–552
psychotherapy versus medication,
    541–544
side effects, 245, 550–551
suicidal ideation, 319, 546–547
and violence, 470
Trifluoperazine, 517
  emergency dosage, 538
Trihexyphenidyl hydrochloride
  treatment of extrapyramidal side
    effects, 535, 536
Trilafon
  emergency dosage, 538
Tripartite model of the mind, 22–24
Twin studies
  antisocial personality disorder, 169
  bipolar disorder, 134
  depression, 118
  panic disorder, 203
  schizophrenia, 90–91

U

Unconscious, 20, 21–22
Unipolar disorders
  classification systems other than
    DSM-III-R, 112–114
  clinical course, 116–117
  differential diagnosis, 114–116
  DSM-III-R categories, 104,
    109–112
  epidemiology, 117–118
  etiology, 118–112
  factors that affect course, 117
  lithium, 556–557

symptoms, 105–109
treatment, 122–126

V

Vaginismus, 396
  treatment, 401
Valium, 517, 565
  abuse, 431–433
  violent patients, 465
Valproate, 562
Videotaping interviews, 6
Violence
  assessing the violent patient,
    471–474
  basic principles, 460–461
  and bipolar disorder, 135
  childhood correlates of violence in
    adults, 467
  clues to, 461–462
  doctor's reactions to, 477–478
  etiologies, 467–471
  managing the violent patient, 94,
    462–465
  and mental illness, 459–460
  profiles, 466–467
  and schizophrenia, 85, 94
  treatment, 474–476
Visual hallucinations, 67
Vivactil, 548
Volitional disturbance
  and schizophrenia, 82
Voyeurism, 406

W

Wellbutrin, 550
Wernicke's aphasia, 61
Wernicke's encephalopathy,
    372–374, 422–423
Wilson's disease, 376
Withdrawal
  alcohol, 420–422
  central nervous system depressants,
    432–433
  and depression, 114
  differential diagnosis, 204
  opioids, 426
  treatment with antianxiety
    medications, 565
Word salad, 64
Working through, 495

X

Xanax, 565
  panic disorder, 205
Xenophobia, 66

Z

Zoophilia, 405